Combined Nutrition and Exercise Interventions in Community Groups

Combined Nutrition and Exercise Interventions in Community Groups

Editor

Carlos Vasconcelos

MDPI • Basel • Beijing • Wuhan • Barcelona • Belgrade • Manchester • Tokyo • Cluj • Tianjin

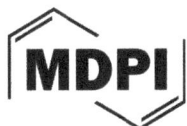

Editor
Carlos Vasconcelos
Sport Sciences and Motricity
Higher School of Education,
Polytechnic Institute of Viseu
Viseu
Portugal

Editorial Office
MDPI
St. Alban-Anlage 66
4052 Basel, Switzerland

This is a reprint of articles from the Special Issue published online in the open access journal *Nutrients* (ISSN 2072-6643) (available at: www.mdpi.com/journal/nutrients/special_issues/Combined_Nutrition_Exercise).

For citation purposes, cite each article independently as indicated on the article page online and as indicated below:

LastName, A.A.; LastName, B.B.; LastName, C.C. Article Title. *Journal Name* **Year**, *Volume Number*, Page Range.

ISBN 978-3-0365-6272-8 (Hbk)
ISBN 978-3-0365-6271-1 (PDF)

© 2023 by the authors. Articles in this book are Open Access and distributed under the Creative Commons Attribution (CC BY) license, which allows users to download, copy and build upon published articles, as long as the author and publisher are properly credited, which ensures maximum dissemination and a wider impact of our publications.

The book as a whole is distributed by MDPI under the terms and conditions of the Creative Commons license CC BY-NC-ND.

Contents

About the Editor vii

Preface to "Combined Nutrition and Exercise Interventions in Community Groups" ix

Erin Nitschke, Kimberly Gottesman, Peggy Hamlett, Lama Mattar, Justin Robinson and Ashley Tovar et al.
Impact of Nutrition and Physical Activity Interventions Provided by Nutrition and Exercise Practitioners for the Adult General Population: A Systematic Review and Meta-Analysis
Reprinted from: *Nutrients* **2022**, *14*, 1729, doi:10.3390/nu14091729 1

Daniela de Sousa, Adriana Fogel, José Azevedo and Patrícia Padrão
The Effectiveness of Web-Based Interventions to Promote Health Behaviour Change in Adolescents: A Systematic Review
Reprinted from: *Nutrients* **2022**, *14*, 1258, doi:10.3390/nu14061258 35

Mamaru Ayenew Awoke, Cheryce L. Harrison, Julie Martin, Marie L. Misso, Siew Lim and Lisa J. Moran
Behaviour Change Techniques in Weight Gain Prevention Interventions in Adults of Reproductive Age: Meta-Analysis and Meta-Regression
Reprinted from: *Nutrients* **2022**, *14*, 209, doi:10.3390/nu14010209 59

Li Zhang, Yuan Liu, Ying Sun and Xin Zhang
Combined Physical Exercise and Diet: Regulation of Gut Microbiota to Prevent and Treat of Metabolic Disease: A Review
Reprinted from: *Nutrients* **2022**, *14*, 4774, doi:10.3390/nu14224774 75

Phrashiah Githinji, John A. Dawson, Duke Appiah and Chad D. Rethorst
A Culturally Sensitive and Theory-Based Intervention on Prevention and Management of Diabetes: A Cluster Randomized Control Trial
Reprinted from: *Nutrients* **2022**, *14*, 5126, doi:10.3390/nu14235126 91

Aysegul Baltaci, Ghaffar Ali Hurtado Choque, Cynthia Davey, Alejandro Reyes Peralta, Silvia Alvarez de Davila and Youjie Zhang et al.
Padres Preparados, Jóvenes Saludables: A Randomized Controlled Trial to Test Effects of a Community-Based Intervention on Latino Father's Parenting Practices
Reprinted from: *Nutrients* **2022**, *14*, 4967, doi:10.3390/nu14234967 105

Patrice A. Hubert, Holly Fiorenti and Valerie B. Duffy
Feasibility of a Theory-Based, Online Tailored Message Program to Motivate Healthier Behaviors in College Women
Reprinted from: *Nutrients* **2022**, *14*, 4012, doi:10.3390/nu14194012 117

Daniel Wilson, Matthew Driller, Paul Winwood, Tracey Clissold, Ben Johnston and Nicholas Gill
The Effectiveness of a Combined Healthy Eating, Physical Activity, and Sleep Hygiene Lifestyle Intervention on Health and Fitness of Overweight Airline Pilots: A Controlled Trial
Reprinted from: *Nutrients* **2022**, *14*, 1988, doi:10.3390/nu14091988 139

Tanisha F. Aflague, Grazyna Badowski, Hyett Sanchez, Dwight Sablan, Catherine M. Schroeder and Eloise Sanchez et al.
Improving Willingness to Try Fruits and Vegetables and Gross Motor Skills in Preschool Children in Guam
Reprinted from: *Nutrients* **2021**, *14*, 93, doi:10.3390/nu14010093 155

Daniel Wilson, Matthew Driller, Paul Winwood, Ben Johnston and Nicholas Gill
The Effects of a Brief Lifestyle Intervention on the Health of Overweight Airline Pilots during COVID-19: A 12-Month Follow-Up Study
Reprinted from: *Nutrients* **2021**, *13*, 4288, doi:10.3390/nu13124288 167

Scott B. Maitland, Paula Brauer, David M. Mutch, Dawna Royall, Doug Klein and Angelo Tremblay et al.
Evaluation of Latent Models Assessing Physical Fitness and the Healthy Eating Index in Community Studies: Time-, Sex-, and Diabetes-Status Invariance
Reprinted from: *Nutrients* **2021**, *13*, 4258, doi:10.3390/nu13124258 183

Cally Jennings, Elsie Patterson, Rachel G. Curtis, Anna Mazzacano and Carol A. Maher
Effectiveness of a Lifestyle Modification Program Delivered under Real-World Conditions in a Rural Setting
Reprinted from: *Nutrients* **2021**, *13*, 4040, doi:10.3390/nu13114040 209

Inge Huybrechts, Nathalie Kliemann, Olivia Perol, Anne Cattey-Javouhey, Nicolas Benech and Aurelia Maire et al.
Feasibility Study to Assess the Impact of a Lifestyle Intervention during Colorectal Cancer Screening in France
Reprinted from: *Nutrients* **2021**, *13*, 3685, doi:10.3390/nu13113685 221

So Young Kim, Dae Myoung Yoo, Chanyang Min and Hyo Geun Choi
Changes in Dietary Habits and Exercise Pattern of Korean Adolescents from Prior to during the COVID-19 Pandemic
Reprinted from: *Nutrients* **2021**, *13*, 3314, doi:10.3390/nu13103314 233

Alejandro Martínez-Rodríguez, Bernardo J. Cuestas-Calero, María Martínez-Olcina and Pablo Jorge Marcos-Pardo
Benefits of Adding an Aquatic Resistance Interval Training to a Nutritional Education on Body Composition, Body Image Perception and Adherence to the Mediterranean Diet in Older Women
Reprinted from: *Nutrients* **2021**, *13*, 2712, doi:10.3390/nu13082712 243

Shannon M. Robson, Samantha M. Rex, Katie Greenawalt, P. Michael Peterson and Elizabeth Orsega-Smith
Utilizing Participatory Research to Engage Underserved Populations to Improve Health-Related Outcomes in Delaware
Reprinted from: *Nutrients* **2021**, *13*, 2353, doi:10.3390/nu13072353 255

Samira Amil, Isabelle Lemieux, Paul Poirier, Benoît Lamarche, Jean-Pierre Després and Natalie Alméras
Targeting Diet Quality at the Workplace: Influence on Cardiometabolic Risk
Reprinted from: *Nutrients* **2021**, *13*, 2283, doi:10.3390/nu13072283 265

Kelsey Fortin and Susan Harvey
Hunger and Health: Taking a Formative Approach to Build a Health Intervention Focused on Nutrition and Physical Activity Needs as Perceived by Stakeholders
Reprinted from: *Nutrients* **2021**, *13*, 1584, doi:10.3390/nu13051584 281

Jae Hyun Lee, Ae Wha Ha, Woo Kyoung Kim and Sun Hyo Kim
The Combined Effects of Milk Intake and Physical Activity on Bone Mineral Density in Korean Adolescents
Reprinted from: *Nutrients* **2021**, *13*, 731, doi:10.3390/nu13030731 295

About the Editor

Carlos Vasconcelos

Carlos Vasconcelos is a Professor in the Department of Sport Sciences and Motricity at High School of Education of Viseu, Polytechnic Institute of Viseu since 2007. His PhD focused on Lifestyle Interventions in patients with type 2 diabetes: exercise plus food education. Additionally, he is member of the Investigation Center CI&DEI and his investigation is focused on the relationship between lifestyle and health-related factors.

Preface to "Combined Nutrition and Exercise Interventions in Community Groups"

Diet and physical activity are two key modifiable lifestyle factors that influence health across the lifespan (prevention and management of chronic diseases and reduction of the risk of premature death through several biological mechanisms). Community-based interventions contribute to public health, as they have the potential to reach high population-level impact, through the focus on groups that share a common culture or identity in their natural living environment. While the health benefits of a balanced diet and regular physical activity are commonly studied separately, interventions that combine these two lifestyle factors have the potential to induce greater benefits in community groups rather than strategies focusing only on one or the other. Thus, this Special Issue entitled "Combined Nutrition and Exercise Interventions in Community Groups" is comprised of manuscripts that highlight this combined approach (balanced diet and regular physical activity) in community settings. The contributors to this Special Issue are well-recognized professionals in complementary fields such as education, public health, nutrition, and exercise. This Special Issue highlights the latest research regarding combined nutrition and exercise interventions among different community groups and includes research articles developed through five continents (Africa, Asia, America, Europe and Oceania), as well as reviews and systematic reviews.

Carlos Vasconcelos
Editor

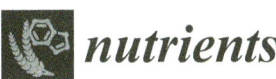

Systematic Review

Impact of Nutrition and Physical Activity Interventions Provided by Nutrition and Exercise Practitioners for the Adult General Population: A Systematic Review and Meta-Analysis

Erin Nitschke [1], Kimberly Gottesman [2], Peggy Hamlett [3], Lama Mattar [4], Justin Robinson [5], Ashley Tovar [6] and Mary Rozga [7,*]

1. Department of Exercise Science, Laramie County Community College, 1400 E College Drive, Cheyenne, WY 82007, USA; erinmd03@gmail.com
2. Department of Kinesiology, Nutrition and Food Science, California State University Los Angeles, 5151 South University Drive, Los Angeles, CA 90032, USA; kgottes@calstatela.edu
3. Department of Movement Sciences, University of Idaho, 875 Perimeter Drive, Moscow, ID 83844, USA; peghamlett@gmail.com
4. Department of Natural Sciences, School of Arts and Sciences, Lebanese American University, Beirut 10110, Lebanon; lama.mattar@lau.edu.lb
5. Kinesiology Department, Point Loma Nazarene University, 3900 Lomaland Dr, San Diego, CA 92106, USA; jrobins1@pointloma.edu
6. Gilead Sciences, 333 Lakeside Dr, Foster City, CA 94404, USA; ashleytovar@gmail.com
7. Evidence Analysis Center, Academy of Nutrition and Dietetics, 120 S Riverside Plaza, Suite 2190, Chicago, IL 60606, USA
* Correspondence: mrozga@eatright.org; Tel.: +1-(312)-899-1758

Abstract: Healthy dietary intake and physical activity reduce the risk of non-communicable diseases. This systematic review and meta-analysis aimed to examine the effect of interventions including both nutrition and physical activity provided by nutrition and exercise practitioners for adults in the general population (those without diagnosed disease). The MEDLINE, CINAHL, Cochrane Central, Cochrane Database of Systematic Reviews and SportDiscus databases were searched for randomized controlled trials (RCTs) published from 2010 until April 2021. Outcomes included physical activity, fruit and vegetable intake, waist circumference, percent weight loss, quality of life (QoL) and adverse events. Grading of Recommendations Assessment, Development and Evaluation (GRADE) methods were used to synthesize and grade evidence. Meta-analyses were stratified according to participant health status. The database search identified 11,205 articles, and 31 RCTs were included. Interventions increased physical activity amount [standardized mean difference (SMD) (95% CI): 0.25 (0.08, 0.43)] (low certainty evidence); increased vegetable intake [SMD (95% CI): 0.14 (0.05, 0.23)] (moderate certainty evidence); reduced waist circumference [MD (95% CI): −2.16 cm (−2.96, −1.36)] (high certainty evidence); and increased likelihood of achieving 5% weight loss for adults with overweight and obesity [relative risk (95% CI): 2.37 (1.76, 3.19)] (high certainty evidence). Very low and low certainty evidence described little-to-no effect on QoL or adverse events. Nutrition and exercise practitioners play key roles in facilitating positive lifestyle behaviors to reduce cardiometabolic disease risk in adults.

Keywords: primary prevention; nutrition; physical activity; nutritionists; counseling; systematic review; meta-analysis; randomized controlled trial

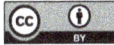

1. Introduction

Modifiable behaviors, such as unhealthy diet and sedentary lifestyle by physical inactivity, increase the risk of premature death from non-communicable diseases [1–3], which annually contribute to 71% of all deaths globally [2]. Nutrition recommendations for a healthy diet generally include individualizing intake to promote consumption of nutrient-dense foods such as vegetables and fruits, whole grains, lean proteins and healthy fats, and limit intake of added sugars, sodium, saturated fat and alcohol across the lifespan [4]. Physical activity recommendations for adults generally include performing 150 min to 300 min a week of moderate-intensity aerobic activity, or 75 min to 150 min a week of vigorous-intensity aerobic activity, or a combination of those activities. Additionally, resistance training activities focusing on all major muscle groups is recommended for adults at least two days a week [5]. Nutrition and physical activity significantly impact disease prevention; however, most adults fail to meet recommendations for the general population [1,4]. The World Health Organization (WHO) describes unhealthy diet and sedentary lifestyle by physical inactivity as leading global health risks [2].

A recent systematic review from the United States Preventive Services Task Force (USPSTF) demonstrated that behavioral interventions including both healthy diet and physical activity interventions collectively resulted in reduced risk of cardiovascular disease events and associated risk factors after 1–2 years in adults with cardiovascular disease risk [6] and can improve lifestyle behaviors and intermediate cardiometabolic outcomes in adults without cardiovascular disease risk factors [7]. Adults without diagnosed disease may have multiple risk factors such as overweight or obesity, impaired glucose tolerance, pre-hypertension, unhealthy diet, or sedentary lifestyle [8–12]. These adults may prefer to access allied healthcare practitioners who are available to the general population rather than seek medical care. With individualized, timely, and strategic interventions, allied healthcare practitioners can improve behaviors in adults who are healthy or have cardiometabolic risk factors to prevent disease development.

In the greater context of preventive medicine, specific allied healthcare practitioners such as registered dietitians or international equivalents (referred to as 'dietitians' in this manuscript), exercise practitioners, and health coaches receive unique training which positions them to enable meaningful lifestyle changes to improve health and well-being in clients. Though each of these professional groups has a distinct scope of practice [13–16], they share the common goal of facilitating lifestyle changes through nutrition and physical activity to prevent the development of cardiometabolic diseases [14,15,17]. Dietitians are credentialed nutrition practitioners who work in a variety of settings to provide quality nutrition services with an aim to improve health and well-being [13]. In contrast, exercise practitioners are certified professionals who develop safe, effective, goal-driven physical activity programs [14,15]. This two-pronged nutrition and physical activity approach to health and well-being is needed to address high population rates of unhealthy lifestyle behaviors and associated non-communicable diseases [2]. Thus, synthesized evidence is needed to determine the efficacy of nutrition and exercise practitioners in reducing cardiometabolic risk for adults prior to disease development.

The aim of this systematic review was to investigate the effects of nutrition and physical activity interventions provided by nutrition and exercise practitioners to healthy adults and those with cardiometabolic risk factors to deliver evidence-based information for practitioners and policy makers working to prevent incidence of cardiometabolic diseases. The objective of this systematic review was to examine the research question: In adults who are healthy or have cardiometabolic risk factors, what is the effect of nutrition and physical activity interventions provided by nutrition and exercise practitioners, compared to control conditions, on defined behavioral and anthropometric outcomes and quality of life?

2. Methods

This systematic review adhered to Grading of Recommendations, Assessment, Development and Evaluations (GRADE) methods described by the Cochrane Collaboration [18] as well as PRISMA guidelines [19] and was prospectively registered at PROSPERO (CRD42021247447) [20].

2.1. Eligibility Criteria

A full description of eligibility criteria can be found in Table 1. Studies were required to include adult participants (≥18 years of age) who were healthy or who had cardiometabolic risk factors, but no diagnosed disease. Cardiometabolic risk factors were overweight or obesity, and/or impaired glucose tolerance or diabetes risk or pre-hypertension, as defined by study authors. Interventions were required to include both nutrition and physical activity, last at least one month in duration, and be delivered by nutrition and/or exercise practitioners and/or health coaches. For this systematic review, nutrition practitioners were defined as registered dietitians or international equivalents [21]. Qualifying exercise practitioners were personal trainers, exercise physiologists, and those with other professional certifications recognized by the United States Registry of Exercise Professionals [22]. Health coaches were identified according to the authors' definition. The comparison group could not receive nutrition or physical activity counseling or coaching. Outcomes of interest included: physical activity (amount and intensity), fruit and vegetable intake (measured using a validated tool), waist circumference, percent weight loss (for adults with overweight or obesity), quality of life (QoL) and adverse events. Glucose homeostasis outcomes and anxiety/depression symptoms were also examined as outcomes of interest, but results are not published in this manuscript. Randomized controlled trials (RCTs) published from January 2010 until the search date were eligible. The publication cut-off date of 2010 was selected because a recent scoping review identified several relevant articles published since this period [23] and to reflect contemporary practice. Only peer reviewed articles published in the English language were included due to resource constraints.

Table 1. Eligibility criteria for systematic review examining the effect of nutrition and physical activity interventions provided by nutrition and exercise practitioners.

Category	Inclusion	Exclusion
Setting	Community, work, university, research and other "public" settings, primary care settings	In-patient
Population	Humans Adults ≥ 18 years of age Health Status: Healthy or with cardiometabolic risk factors (including overweight or obesity, pre-diabetes and pre-hypertension) but no diagnosed disease. Studies targeting women who are postpartum/lactating are included	Animal studies <18 years of age Professional or elite athletes Family is the target population Health Status: Any diagnosed disease or conditions limiting generalizability to individuals in the general population including but not limited to: Type 2 diabetes mellitus Cardiovascular disease Non-alcoholic fatty liver disease Chronic kidney disease Cancer Eating disorders Chronic obstructive pulmonary disorder Human immunodeficiency virus infection and acquired immune deficiency syndrome Heart failure, stroke Post-bariatric surgery Severe or persistent mental illness Hypertension Dyslipidemia Metabolic syndrome Frail elderly Osteoarthritis Pregnancy Diagnosed sleep apnea Cognitive impairment

Table 1. Cont.

Category	Inclusion	Exclusion
Intervention	Must include nutrition AND physical activity Multi-disciplinary beyond nutrition and physical activity are included (e.g., includes intervention from behavioral therapist, nurse, etc.)	Only includes nutrition OR physical activity
Intervention Provider	Interventions delivered by a dietitian or international equivalent, exercise practitioner (see below), or health coach Exercise practitioners as defined by United States Registry of Exercise Professionals http://usreps.org/Pages/credentials.aspx (accessed on 20 February 2022) [22] If the interventionist was defined as a "nutritionist", the authors checked the following website to determine if this was a dietitian equivalent in the country of interest or emailed the corresponding author: https://www.internationaldietetics.org/NDAs.aspx (accessed on 20 February 2022) [21] "Health Coaches" were identified according to the author's definition.	Interventions provided by professionals not specified in inclusion. Practitioner delivering the intervention is not specified. Interventions provided by lifestyle coaches Health coaches
Intervention Duration	≥ 1 month	<1 month
Control and Comparison Groups	Control group for the overarching question is no intervention, wait list, or other control that is not a nutrition or exercise intervention. Comparisons defined in sub-questions are investigated with sub-analyses (ex: efficacy of interventions delivered by telehealth (vs control) compared to efficacy of interventions delivered in-person (vs control)).	Comparison group receives the same level of nutrition and/or physical activity intervention compared to the intervention group.
Outcomes	Quality of life, anxiety/depression, physical activity (exercise duration (ex: min/week) or intensity measured as heart rate, rated perceived exertion or metabolic equivalents, fruit and vegetable intake (measured using a validated tool), waist circumference, percent weight loss (measured as a continuous variable for those with overweight/obesity or as proportion of participants achieving 5 percent weight loss)	Outcomes not defined in inclusion criteria.
Study Design	Randomized controlled trials Relevant systematic reviews and meta-analyses are searched for potentially included articles missed by the database search.	Non-randomized trials, non-controlled trials, observational studies, commentaries, narrative reviews.
Sample size	≥ 10 in each group	<10 in each group
Year	January 2010–2 April 2021	Prior to January 2010 or after the search date of 2 April 2021
Publication	Peer-reviewed publications.	Grey literature, conference abstracts
Language	Articles published in the English language.	Articles published in languages other than English.
Databases Searched	MEDLINE, CINAHL, SportsDiscus, Cochrane Database of Systematic Reviews, Cochrane Database of Controlled Trials	-

2.2. Information Sources

The full search strategy is described in Supplementary Table S1. Search strategies were written by an Information Specialist for the following databases via the Ebsco interface: Medline Complete; CINAHL Complete; Cochrane Database of Systematic Reviews;

Cochrane Central Register of Controlled Trials, and SportDiscus. Searches were conducted on 2 April 2021 for articles published since 1 January 2010. Two methodological filters were used, one for systematic reviews and meta-analyses; and another for randomized controlled trials. Results were limited to the English language. Results were managed and deduplicated in Endnote Software [24]. Relevant systematic reviews were hand-searched for potentially included articles that may have been missed by the database searches.

2.3. Selection Process

Titles and abstracts of articles identified in the databases searched were uploaded and screened using the online Rayyan screening tool, which allows each reviewer to independently review each title and abstract and then unblind results to compare judgements with other reviewers [25]. Two reviewers independently reviewed each abstract, and discrepancies were settled using consensus or a third review. The full texts of each included title/abstract were screened by two independent reviewers to determine eligibility. Discrepancies were settled by consensus or by a third review from a content expert.

2.4. Data Items and Extraction

Study and intervention characteristics were extracted by trained evidence analysts and were reviewed by a lead analyst and project manager. Quantitative data were extracted by the project manager and reviewed by content experts.

Data were extracted onto a standardized template and included bibliographic information, eligibility criteria, study location and funding source, sample sizes and dropout rates, and participant characteristics (age, sex, comorbidities). Analysts also extracted information on intervention details (practitioners providing nutrition and physical activity interventions, remote vs. in-person contacts, group vs. individual contacts, number of nutrition and physical activity contacts, study duration and follow up duration, prescribed diet and physical activity) and outcomes of interest.

For outcomes measured as continuous variables, quantitative data extracted included sample size, and mean change and variance (or pre/post study mean and variance) in the intervention and control groups with an aim to calculate mean difference (MD) and 95% confidence intervals for the outcome of interest between groups. When measurement methods or units were heterogeneous, standardized mean differences (SMD) were reported. For categorical variables, the sample size and number of events were extracted for each group to calculate the relative risk (RR) of events in the intervention groups compared to the control groups. If authors reported an outcome but did not include data required for the meta-analysis, corresponding authors were contacted to request additional data. If additional data were not shared, the result was included in the narrative synthesis only.

2.5. Risk of Bias Assessment for Each Study

Each study was assessed for risk of bias using the updated tool for assessing RCTs from the Cochrane Collaboration, the RoB 2 tool [26]. This tool assesses risk of bias due to the randomization process, deviations from intended interventions, missing outcome data, measurement of the outcome and selection of the reported result. Each study is assigned an overall rating of "High," "Some Concerns" or "Low" risk of bias. Risk of bias was assessed independently by two reviewers using the Cochrane Collaboration's online algorithm tool [27]. Discrepancies in ratings for specific domains and overall ratings were settled by a third review.

2.6. Synthesis Methods

All studies meeting eligibility criteria and reporting at least one outcome of interest (even if full data were not available), were included in the evidence synthesis and described in the study and intervention characteristics tables. All studies reporting a particular outcome of interest were pooled using a meta-analysis when data were available. Results of studies not included in the meta-analysis were described narratively only. An overview of results for each outcome was reported on a summary of findings table, adapted from the template developed by the Cochrane Collaboration [28]. Results from risk of bias assessments were presented based on the robvis tool [29].

Meta-analyses were conducted and forest plots were created using OpenMetaAnalyst [30] and RStudio [31] software. The methodologist utilized a random-effects model to accommodate the wide range of studies included. Sensitivity analyses were conducted using leave-one-out analysis and by examining effect size according to study quality. Publication bias was described using funnel plots and Egger's statistics. Heterogeneity was examined using the I^2 statistic. Sub-group analyses were conducted to examine efficacy of interventions on outcomes according to whether participants were healthy or had cardiometabolic risk factors.

2.7. Certainty Assessment

Certainty of evidence was assessed for each outcome using the GRADE method [18,28]. Grade for certainty of evidence considered study design, number of studies and participants, risk of bias in included studies, directness of findings, precision of findings, consistency among studies, publication bias and other factors. Certainty of evidence was graded as "High," "Moderate," "Low," or "Very Low" [32].

3. Results

3.1. Literature Search

The database search identified 11,205 unique articles; 472 full texts were reviewed, and 31 RCTs were included in this systematic review. Several studies reported results in more than one article, and, thus, forty-eight articles, describing results from the 31 RCTs, were included in this systematic review (Figure 1) [33–80].

3.2. Study Characteristics and Risk of Bias

Study and intervention characteristics are described in Tables 2 and 3. Fourteen RCTs were conducted in the United States [36,38,45,49–51,55,59,61,65,66,69,75,78] and 17 RCTs were conducted outside of the United States [35,42,43,46,47,54,56,57,60,62,63,67,70,71,73,76,77]. Sample sizes ranged from 23 [67] to 553 [71] participants; and study durations ranged from three [43,47,50] to 48 months [54,70].

Seven RCTs targeted adults without cardiometabolic risk factors [42,43,51,57,63,66,77], while the remaining 24 RCTs targeted adults with overweight or obesity [35,36,38,45–47,49,50,54–56,59,60,62,65,67,69,73,75,76,78], diabetes risk [54,59,61,67,70,73,78], or other cardiometabolic risk factors [71]. Practitioners providing nutrition and physical activity interventions were dietitians in 12 RCTs [35,36,38,43,47,51,59,61,63,66,71,78], dietitians and exercise practitioners were combined in ten RCTs [45,46,49,50,56,57,62,67,70,75], and health coaches in six RCTs [42,55,65,69,73,77]. Three additional RCTs described dietitians that provided both nutrition and physical activity interventions and were thus included, but in these studies, their interventions included an exercise practitioner that did not meet inclusion criteria [76], an exercise practitioner was available only if requested [60], or the practitioner description was inconsistent between articles [54,72]. Exercise practitioners in included studies were primarily exercise physiologists [36,42–45,48,49,52,57,59,66,74,78,79] and trainers [55,56,61,69].

The risk of bias of included RCTs is described in Figure 2. The most prevalent sources of bias were due to the randomization process, typically from lack of information regarding allocation concealment [36,43,49–51,54,73,76], and deviations from intended interventions and/or lack of information on intervention adherence [35,42,43,45,47,50,54,56,59–62,65,69–71,75–77]. Of the 31 included RCTs, six demonstrated Low risk of bias [38,46,55,57,63,66], 22 demonstrated Some Concerns [36,43,45,47,49–51,54,56,59,61,62,65,67,69–71,73,75–78] and three demonstrated High risk of bias [35,42,60].

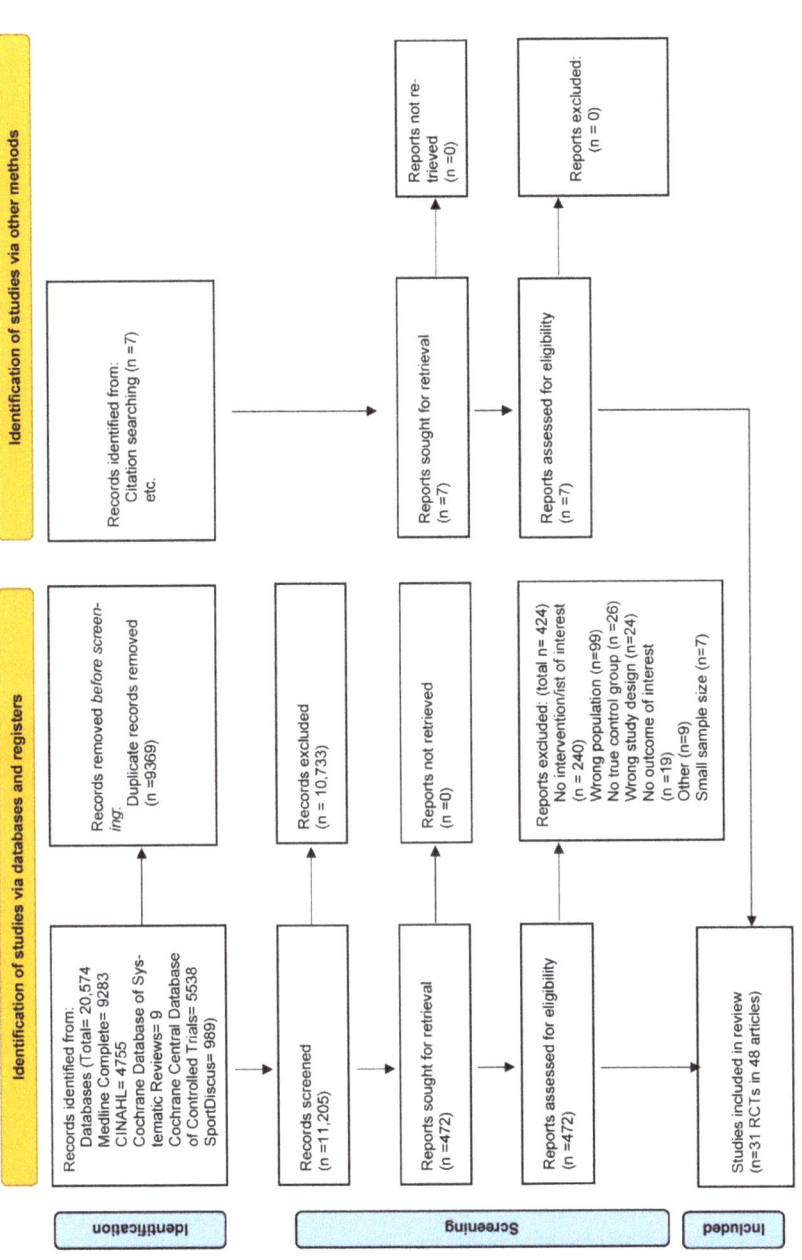

Figure 1. PRISMA 2020 flow diagram [19] for systematic review examining effect of nutrition and physical activity interventions provided by nutrition and exercise practitioners for the general population. *From:* Page, M.J.; McKenzie, J.E.; Bossuyt, P.M.; Boutron, I.; Hoffmann, T.C.; Mulrow, C.D.; et al. The PRISMA 2020 statement: an updated guideline for reporting systematic reviews. BMJ 2021;372:n71. doi: 10.1136/bmj.n71. For more information, visit: http://www.prisma-statement.org/ (accessed on 20 February 2022) [19].

Table 2. Study characteristics of randomized controlled trials included in the systematic review examining effect of nutrition and physical activity interventions provided by nutrition and exercise practitioners for the general population.

Trial Name (If Applicable), Author, Year	Country	Setting	Target Population	Mean Age (Years)	Sample Size (Final N)	Duration (Months)	Funding Source	Risk of Bias
40-Something Trial Hollis et al. 2015 [46] Williams et al. 2014 [79] Williams et al. 2019 [80]	Australia	Research/University	Female adults (44–50 years) with healthy weight or overweight (BMI = 18.5–29.9 kg/m^2)	Intervention: 47.6 Control: 46.9	40	12	University/Hospital	Low Risk
Beleigoli et al. 2020 [35]	Brazil	Research/University	Adults with overweight or obesity (BMI ≥ 25 kg/m^2)	Intervention (mean): 33.0 Control: 33.4	473	6	Government	High Risk
Colleran et al. 2012, [38,39]	United States	Community	Female adults with overweight or obesity (BMI 25–30 kg/m^2), postpartum	Intervention: 30.3 Control: 31.9	27	4	Government, University/Hospital	Low Risk
Finnish DPS Trial Lindstrom et al. 2013 [54] Ruusunen et al. 2012 [72]	Finland	Outpatient/Primary Care	Adults with type 2 diabetes risk, overweight or obesity (BMI ≥ 25 kg/m^2)	Intervention: 55 Control: 55	480	48	Government, University/Hospital, Not-for-profit	Some Concerns
Forsyth et al. 2015 [43]	Australia	Outpatient/Primary Care	Adults with anxiety/depression (Mean BMI 31.6 and 31.8 kg/m^2 for Intervention and Control)	NR	94	3	Government	Some Concerns
GHSH Trial Fjeldsoe et al. 2016 [42] Fjeldsoe et al. 2019 [41]	Australia	Community	Adults (Mean BMI 29.5 kg/m^2)	Intervention: 55.5 Control: 51.2	211	6	Government, University/Hospital	High Risk
Johnson et al. 2019 [50]	United States	Research/University	Adults with obesity (BMI ≥ 30 kg/m^2)	Intervention: 42.2 Control: 44.5	20	3	Government, Industry	Some Concerns
Kennedy et al. 2015 [51]	United States	Community	Adults identified as African American (BMI ≥ 23 kg/m^2)	Intervention: 54 Control: 54	37	12	Not-for-profit	Some Concerns

Table 2. Cont.

Trial Name (If Applicable), Author, Year	Country	Setting	Target Population	Mean Age (Years)	Sample Size (Final N)	Duration (Months)	Funding Source	Risk of Bias
LEVA in Real Life Trial Huseinovic et al. 2016 [47] Huseinovic et al. 2018 [48]	Sweden	Outpatient/Primary Care	Female adults with overweight or obesity (BMI ≥ 27 kg/m^2), postpartum	Intervention: 31.8 Control: 32.6	89	3	Government, Not-for-profit	Some Concerns
Maddison et al. 2019 [56]	New Zealand	Community	Male adults with overweight or obesity (BMI ≥ 25 kg/m^2)	Intervention: 40.6 Control: 44.7	80	4	NR	Some Concerns
Maruyama et al. 2010 [57]	Japan	Community	Adults (Mean BMI 25.7 and 25.8 for Intervention and Control)	Intervention: 43.1, 7.7 Control: 35.5, 8.1	87	4	Not-for-profit	Low Risk
MEDIM Trial Siddiqui et al. 2017 [73] Siddiqui et al. 2018 [74]	Sweden	Research/University	Adults with type 2 diabetes risk, overweight or obesity (BMI ≥ 28 kg/m^2)	Intervention: 47.9 Control: 48.9	67	4	Industry, University/Hospital	Some Concerns
Miller et al. 2015 [59]	United States	Research/University	Adults with type 2 diabetes risk (no information on BMI)	Intervention: 51.6 Control: 50.8	68	4	Government	Some Concerns
Neale et al. 2017 [60]	Australia	Community	Adults with overweight or obesity (BMI ≥ 25–40 kg/m^2)	Intervention: 43.79 Control: 42.10	189	12	Industry, Government, Not-for-profit	High Risk
NEW Trial Abbenhardt et al. 2013 [33] Campbell et al. 2012 [37] Duggan et al. 2016 [40] Foster-Schubert et al. 2012 [44] Imayama et al. 2011 [49] Mason et al. 2011 [58]	United States	Research/University	Female adults with overweight or obesity (BMI ≥ 25 kg/m^2)	Intervention: 58.0 Control: 57.4	188	12	Government	Some Concerns
Nicklas et al. 2014 [61]	United States	Community	Female adults with type 2 diabetes risk, postpartum (Mean BMI 31.2 and 31.6 kg/m^2 in the Intervention and Control groups)	Intervention: 33.6 Control: 33.3	71	12	Government	Some Concerns

Table 2. *Cont.*

Trial Name (If Applicable), Author, Year	Country	Setting	Target Population	Mean Age (Years)	Sample Size (Final N)	Duration (Months)	Funding Source	Risk of Bias
Pablos et al. 2017 [62]	Italy	Research/University	Adults with overweight or obesity (BMI ≥ 25 kg/m^2)	Intervention: 49.80 Control: 51.25	68	8	University/Hospital	Some Concerns
Perri et al. 2020 [65]	United States	Community	Adults with obesity (BMI 35–40 kg/m^2)	Intervention: 55.9 (individual counseling) and 55.4 (group counseling) Control: 54.8	260	6	Government	Some Concerns
RAINBOW Trial Ma et al. 2019 [55] Rosas et al. 2021 [68]	United States	Outpatient/Primary Care	Adults with overweight or obesity (BMI ≥ 30 kg/m^2 or ≥27 kg/m^2 if Asian)	Intervention: 50.9 Control: 51.0	371	12	Government	Low Risk
Rich-Edwards et al. 2019 [66]	United States	Community	Adults, postpartum (BMI ≥ 18.5–40 kg/m^2)	Intervention: 30.5 Control: 31.7	139	9	Government	Low Risk
Rollo et al. 2020 [67]	Australia	Community	Female adults with risk of type 2 diabetes, overweight or obesity (BMI ≥ 18.5–50 kg/m^2), postpartum	Intervention: 34.0 Control: 33.6	23	6	Not-for-profit	Some Concerns
Rosas et al. 2020 [69]	United States	Outpatient/Primary Care	Adults with overweight or obesity (BMI ≥ 24 kg/m^2)	Intervention: 50.3 Control: 50.1	183	12	Government	Some Concerns
Roumen et al. 2011 [70]	Netherlands	Research/University	Adults with type 2 diabetes risk (Mean BMI 29.9 kg/m^2 and 29.7 kg/m^2 for Intervention and Control groups)	Intervention: 55.0 Control: 58.8	109	48	Government, Not-for-profit	Some Concerns
Rubinstein et al. 2016 [71]	Argentina, Guatemala, Peru	Community	Adults with pre-hypertension (Mean BMI 30.2 kg/m^2 and 30.8 kg/m^2 for Intervention and Control groups)	Intervention: 48.6 Control: 43.2	553	12	Government, Industry	Some Concerns

Table 2. Cont.

Trial Name (If Applicable), Author, Year	Country	Setting	Target Population	Mean Age (Years)	Sample Size (Final N)	Duration (Months)	Funding Source	Risk of Bias
Shape Trial Bennett et al. 2013 [36] Krishnan et al. 2019 [52]	United States	Outpatient/Primary Care	Female adults with overweight or obesity (BMI 25–34.9 kg/m^2)	Intervention: 35.6 Control: 35.2	177	12	Government	Some Concerns
Thomas et al. 2019 [75]	United States	Research/University	Adults with overweight or obesity (BMI 25–45 kg/m^2)	NR	125	18	Government	Some Concerns
Toji et al. 2012 [76]	Japan	Community	Adults with overweight or obesity (BMI 24–28 kg/m^2)	Intervention: 61 Control: 62	32	6	Government	Some Concerns
TXT2BFiT Trial Allman-Farinelli et al. 2016 [34] Partridge et al. 2015 [63] Partridge et al. 2016 [64]	Australia	Telehealth	Adults at risk of weight gain (BMI 23–32 kg/m^2)	18–35	248	9	Government, Not-for-profit	Low Risk
Viester et al. 2018 [77]	Netherlands	Workplace	Male adults (Mean BMI 27.4 kg/m^2)	Intervention: 46.3 Control: 47.0	277	6	Foundation	Some Concerns
Weinhold et al. 2015 [78]	United States	Workplace, Research/University	Adults with type 2 diabetes risk, overweight or obesity (BMI 25–50 kg/m^2)	Intervention: 51.6 Control: 51.0	67	4	Government	Some Concerns
WOMAN Trial Gabriel et al. 2011 [45] Kuller et al. 2012 [53]	United States	Research/University	Female adults with overweight or obesity (BMI 25–39.9 kg/m^2)	Intervention: 56.9 Control: 57.1	400	36	Government	Some Concerns

BMI = body mass index; NR = not reported.

Table 3. Intervention characteristics of randomized controlled trials included in the systematic review examining effect of nutrition and physical activity interventions provided by nutrition and exercise practitioners for the general population.

Trial Name (If Applicable), Study, Author, Year	Nutrition Practitioner	PA Practitioner	Intervention Duration (Months)	Number of Contacts	In-Person, Remote, Blended	Group, Individual, Blended	Diet (Caloric Restriction, Macronutrient Change, Dietary Pattern, Unspecified, Individual)	PA Time (Minutes/Week) and Type (Aerobic, Resistance)	Outcomes Reported
40-Something Trial Hollis 2015 [46] Williams et al. 2014 [79] Williams et al. 2019 [80]	Dietitian or international equivalent	Exercise practitioner	12	5	Exclusively In-person	Exclusively Individual	Caloric Restriction, Individualized	150–250, NR	PA F&V Intake WC QoL
Beleigoli et al. 2020 [35]	Dietitian or international equivalent	Dietitian or international equivalent	6	Unclear	Exclusively Remote	Exclusively Individual	NR, Individualized	NR, NR	PA F&V % Weight Loss
Colleran et al. 2012, 2012b [38,39]	Dietitian or international equivalent	Dietitian or international equivalent	4	32	Blended	Exclusively Individual	Caloric Restriction, Dietary Pattern	NR, Both	F&V WC % Weight Loss
Finnish DPS Trial Lindstrom et al. 2013 [54] Ruusunen et al. 2012 [72]	Dietitian or international equivalent	Dietitian or international equivalent, Exercise practitioner (description varied between articles)	48	19	Blended	Blended	Caloric Restriction, Macronutrient change, Dietary Pattern, Individualized	240, Both	PA % Weight Loss
Forsyth et al. 2015 [43]	Dietitian or international equivalent	Dietitian or international equivalent	3	4	Exclusively In-person	Exclusively Individual	NR, Individualized	NR, NR	F&V
GHSH Trial Fjeldsoe et al. 2016 [42] Fjeldsoe et al. 2019 [41]	Health coach	Health coach	6	2	Exclusively Remote	Exclusively Individual	NR, Individualized	NR, NR	PA F&V WC
Johnson et al. 2019 [50]	Dietitian or international equivalent	Exercise practitioner	3	24	Exclusively In-person	Exclusively Individual	NR, Individualized	150, NR	% Weight Loss

Table 3. Cont.

Trial Name (If Applicable), Study, Author, Year	Nutrition Practitioner	PA Practitioner	Intervention Duration (Months)	Number of Contacts	In-Person, Remote, Blended	Group, Individual, Blended	Diet (Caloric Restriction, Macronutrient Change, Dietary Pattern, Unspecified, Individual)	PA Time (Minutes/Week) and Type (Aerobic, Resistance)	Outcomes Reported
Kennedy et al. 2015 [51]	Dietitian or international equivalent	Dietitian or international equivalent	12	12	Exclusively In-person	Exclusively Group	Unspecified	210, Aerobic	F&V QoL
LEVA in Real Life Trial Husenovic et al. 2016 [47] Husenovic et al. 2018 [48]	Dietitian or international equivalent	Dietitian or international equivalent	3	16	Blended	Exclusively Individual	Caloric Restriction, Macronutrient change, Dietary Pattern	NR, NR	WC % Weight Loss
Maddison et al. 2019 [56]	Dietitian or international equivalent	Exercise practitioner	4	12 to 24	Exclusively In-person	Exclusively group	NR	120–150, Both	PA WC
Maruyama et al. 2010 [57]	Dietitian or international equivalent	Exercise practitioner	4	4	Blended	Exclusively Individual	Dietary Pattern, Individualized	NR, NR	WC
MEDIM Trial Siddiqui et al. 2017 [73] Siddiqui et al. 2018 [74]	Health coach	Health coach	4	7	Exclusively In-Person	Exclusively group	Dietary Pattern	10,000 steps/day Aerobic	PA WC % Weight Loss
Miller et al. 2015 [59]	Dietitian or international equivalent	Dietitian or international equivalent	4	16	Exclusively In-person	Exclusively Group	Caloric Restriction, Macronutrient change	150, Aerobic	F&V % Weight Loss Adverse events
Neale et al. 2017 [60]	Dietitian or international equivalent	Dietitian or international equivalent OR Exercise practitioner if requested	12	NR	Nutrition: Blended PA: Blended	Nutrition: Exclusively Individual PA: Exclusively Individual	Dietary Pattern, Individualized	NR, NR	PA F&V QoL

Table 3. Cont.

Trial Name (If Applicable), Study, Author, Year	Nutrition Practitioner	PA Practitioner	Intervention Duration (Months)	Number of Contacts	In-Person, Remote, Blended	Group, Individual, Blended	Diet (Caloric Restriction, Macronutrient Change, Dietary Pattern, Unspecified, Individual)	PA Time (Minutes/Week) and Type (Aerobic, Resistance)	Outcomes Reported
NEW Trial Abbenhardt et al. 2013 [33] Campbell et al. 2012 [37] Duggan et al. 2016 [40] Foster-Schubert et al. 2012 [44] Imayama et al. 2011 [49] Mason et al. 2011 [58]	Dietitian or international equivalent	Exercise practitioner	12	62	Exclusively In-person	Exclusively Individual	Caloric Restriction, Macronutrient change	225, Aerobic	PA WC % Weight Loss QoL Adverse events
Nicklas et al. 2014 [61]	Dietitian or international equivalent	Dietitian or international equivalent	12	18	Exclusively Remote	Exclusively Individual	Macronutrient change	≤150, Both	PA
Pablos et al. 2017 [62]	Dietitian or international equivalent	Exercise practitioner	8	144	Exclusively In-person	Blended	Caloric Restriction, Macronutrient change, Individualized	140–180, Both	WC
Perri et al. 2020 [65]	Health coach	Health coach	6	18	Exclusively Remote	Individual or Group	Dietary Pattern	210, NR	% Weight Loss
RAINBOW Trial Ma et al. 2019 [55] Rosas et al. 2021 [68]	Health coach	Health coach	12	15	Blended	Exclusively Individual	Caloric Restriction	150, NR	PA F&V % Weight Loss
Rich-Edwards et al. 2019 [66]	Dietitian or international equivalent	Dietitian or international equivalent	9	Unclear	Exclusively Remote	Exclusively Individual	Dietary Pattern, Individualized	NR, NR	PA

Table 3. Cont.

Trial Name (If Applicable), Study, Author, Year	Nutrition Practitioner	PA Practitioner	Intervention Duration (Months)	Number of Contacts	In-Person, Remote, Blended	Group, Individual, Blended	Diet (Caloric Restriction, Macronutrient Change, Dietary Pattern, Unspecified, Individual)	PA Time (Minutes/Week) and Type (Aerobic, Resistance)	Outcomes Reported
Rollo et al. 2020 [67]	Dietitian or international equivalent	Exercise practitioner	6	6	Exclusively Remote	Exclusively Individual	NR	NR, Both	PA WC % Weight Loss QoL
Rosas et al. 2020 [69]	Health coach	Health coach	12	22	Exclusively In-person	Blended	Caloric Restriction, Macronutrient change, Dietary Pattern	150, NR	PA F&V WC % Weight Loss QoL
Roumen et al. 2011 [70]	Dietitian or international equivalent	Exercise practitioner	48	16	Exclusively In-person	Exclusively Individual	Caloric Restriction, Macronutrient change, Dietary Pattern, Individualized	150, Both	WC
Rubinstein et al. 2016 [71]	Dietitian or international equivalent	Dietitian or international equivalent	12	12	Exclusively Remote	Exclusively Individual	Macronutrient change, Dietary Pattern, Individualized	NR, NR	PA F&V WC
Shape Trial Bennett et al. 2013 [36] Krishnan et al. 2019 [52]	Dietitian or international equivalent	Dietitian or international equivalent	12	12	Exclusively Remote	Exclusively Individual	Caloric Restriction	NR, NR	WC QoL
Thomas et al. 2019 [75]	Dietitian or international equivalent	Exercise practitioner	18	42	Exclusively In-person	Exclusively Group	Caloric Restriction, Macronutrient change	200, NR	% Weight Loss

Table 3. Cont.

Trial Name (If Applicable), Study, Author, Year	Nutrition Practitioner	PA Practitioner	Intervention Duration (Months)	Number of Contacts	In-Person, Remote, Blended	Group, Individual, Blended	Diet (Caloric Restriction, Macronutrient Change, Dietary Pattern, Unspecified, Individual)	PA Time (Minutes/Week) and Type (Aerobic, Resistance)	Outcomes Reported
Toji et al. 2012 [76]	Dietitian or international equivalent	Dietitian or international equivalent, Health fitness programmer	6	7	Exclusively In-person	Blended	Caloric Restriction, Individualized	NR, Both	WC
TXT2BFiT Trial Allman-Farinelli et al. 2016 [34] Partridge et al. 2015 [63] Partridge et al. 2016 [64]	Dietitian or international equivalent	Dietitian or international equivalent	9	7	Exclusively Remote	Exclusively Individual	Dietary Pattern	NR, NR	PA F&V
Viester et al. 2018 [77]	Health coach	Health coach	6	2 to 4	Blended	Exclusively Individual	NR Individualized	NR, Resistance	PA F&V WC
Weinhold et al. 2015 [78]	Dietitian or international equivalent	Dietitian or international equivalent	4	12	Exclusively In-person	Blended	Caloric Restriction, Macronutrient change, Individualized	≤150, NR	PA WC % Weight Loss
WOMAN Trial Gabriel et al. 2011 [45] Kuller et al. 2012 [53]	Dietitian or international equivalent	Exercise practitioner	36	64	Exclusively In-person	Blended	Caloric Restriction, Dietary Pattern	NR, NR	PA WC % Weight Loss

F&V = fruit and vegetable, NR = not reported, PA = physical activity, QoL = quality of life, WC = waist circumference.

	Risk of Bias Domains (D)					
	D1[a]	D2[b]	D3[c]	D4[d]	D5[e]	Overall
40-Something Trial	+	+	+	+	+	+
Beleigoli et al 2020	-	-	+	×	+	×
Colleran et al 2012	+	+	+	+	+	+
Finnish DPS Trial	-	-	+	+	+	-
Fjeldsoe et al 2016, 2019	+	-	-	×	+	×
Forsyth et al 2015	-	-	+	+	+	-
Johnson et al 2019	-	-	+	+	+	-
Kennedy et al 2015	-	+	+	+	+	-
LEVA in Real Life	+	-	+	+	+	-
Maddison et al 2019	+	-	+	+	+	-

Figure 2. *Cont.*

Study						
Maruyama et al 2010	+	+	+	+	+	+
MEDIM Trial	-	+	+	+	+	-
Miller et al 2015	+	-	+	-	+	-
Neale et al 2017	+	-	x	+	+	x
NEW Trial	-	+	+	+	+	-
Nicklas et al 2015	+	-	+	+	-	-
Pablos et al 2017	+	-	+	+	+	-
Perri et al 2020	+	-	+	+	+	-
RAINBOW Trial	+	+	+	+	+	+
Rich-Edwards et al 2019	+	+	+	+	+	+
Rollo et al 2020	+	+	+	+	-	-
Rosas et al 2020	+	-	+	+	+	-

Figure 2. *Cont.*

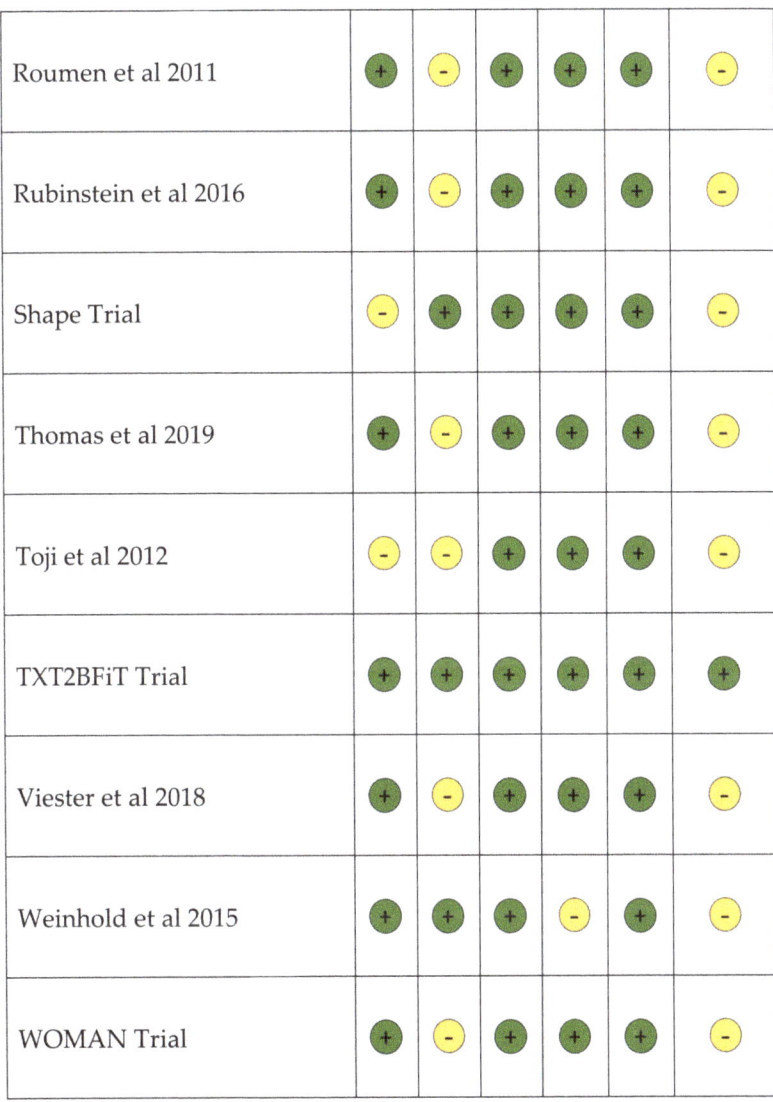

⊗ = High Risk of Bias, ⊖ = Some Concerns, ⊕ = Low Risk of Bias

Figure 2. Risk of bias in the systematic review examining effect of nutrition and physical activity interventions provided by nutrition and exercise practitioners for the general population [33–80]. [a] D1: Bias arising from the randomization process; [b] D2: Bias due to deviations from intended interventions; [c] D3: Bias due to missing outcome data; [d] D4: Bias in measurement of the outcome; [e] D5: Bias in selection of the reported result.

A summary of findings for all included outcomes can be found in Table 4. Publication bias is described in Supplementary Figure S1.

Table 4. Summary of findings describing effect of nutrition and physical activity interventions provided by nutrition and exercise practitioners for the general population.

Outcome Number of Participants (Studies)	Anticipated Absolute Effects (95% Confidence Interval (CI))	Risk of Bias	Inconsistency	Indirectness	Imprecision	Other	Evidence Certainty	What Happens
Physical activity amount Participants: 3339 (13 randomized controlled trials (RCTs))	Standardized Mean Difference (SMD) 0.25 SD higher (0.08 higher to 0.42 higher)	■[a]	■	☐[b]	☐	☐	⊕⊕◯◯ LOW	In adults who are healthy or have cardiometabolic risk factors, nutrition and physical activity interventions from nutrition and exercise practitioners may increase physical activity amount.
Fruit Participants: 1839 (9 RCTs)	SMD 0.38 SD higher (0.12 higher to 0.63 higher)	■	■	☐	☐	☐	⊕⊕◯◯ LOW	In adults who are healthy, nutrition and physical activity interventions from nutrition and exercise practitioners may increase fruit intake, but results are more heterogeneous for adults with cardiometabolic risk factors.
Vegetable intake Participants: 1839 (9 RCTs)	SMD 0.14 SD higher (0.05 higher to 0.23 higher)	■	☐	☐	☐	☐	⊕⊕⊕◯ MODERATE	In adults who are healthy, nutrition and physical activity interventions from nutrition and exercise practitioners likely increases vegetable intake slightly, but results were not significant for adults with cardiometabolic risk factors.
Waist circumference (cm) Participants: 2776 (18 RCTs)	Mean Difference (MD) 2.16 cm lower (2.96 lower to 1.36 lower)	■	☐	☐	☐	■[c]	⊕⊕⊕⊕ HIGH	In adults who have cardiometabolic risk factors, nutrition and physical activity interventions from nutrition and exercise practitioners reduce waist circumference compared to controls across a wide range of interventions, but results were not significant in studies targeting healthy adults.
Achieving 5% Weight Loss For participants with overweight or obesity Participants: 1112 (8 RCTs)	Relative Risk 2.37 (1.76 to 3.19)	■	☐	☐	☐	■[d]	⊕⊕⊕⊕ HIGH	In adults with overweight or obesity but no diagnosed disease, nutrition and physical activity interventions from nutrition and exercise practitioners improved likelihood of achieving 5% weight loss compared to controls.

Table 4. Cont.

Outcome Number of Participants (Studies)	Anticipated Absolute Effects (95% Confidence Interval (CI))	Risk of Bias	Inconsistency	Indirectness	Imprecision	Other	Evidence Certainty	What Happens
Percent weight loss (continuous) For participants with overweight or obesity Participants: 1030 (7 RCTs)	MD 2.37% lower (5.51 lower to 0.77 higher)	■	■	□	□	□	⊕⊕○○ LOW	In adults with overweight or obesity but no diagnosed disease, nutrition and physical activity interventions from nutrition and exercise practitioners, there was no significant reduction in percent weight loss as a continuous variable compared to controls and heterogeneity was high.
Quality of Life Participants: 295 (3 RCTs)	MD 3.91 higher (0.21 lower to 8.03 higher)	■	■	□	■	□	⊕○○○ VERY LOW	In adults who are healthy or have cardiometabolic risk factors, the evidence is very uncertain about the effect of nutrition and physical activity interventions provided by nutrition and exercise practitioners on physical and mental quality of life but suggests little-to-no effect.
Adverse events Participants: (3 RCTs)	not pooled	■	□	□	■	□	⊕⊕○○ LOW	Nutrition and physical activity interventions provided by nutrition and exercise practitioners may result in little to no difference in adverse events, though postmenopausal women receiving the intervention had reduced bone mineral density compared to the control group in one study.

[a] ■ Indicates certainty of evidence was marked down for risk of bias, inconsistency, indirectness and imprecision or marked up or down for other reasons. [b] □ indicates certainty of evidence was not marked up or down for the respective reason. [c] Dose-Response effect demonstrated [d] Large effect size.

3.3. Primary Outcomes

Physical Activity

Seventeen RCTs represented in 22 articles examined the effect of nutrition and physical activity interventions provided by nutrition and exercise practitioners on the outcome of physical activity [34,35,41,42,44–46,53,56,60,61,63,64,66–69,71,72,74,77,78]. Thirteen RCTs reported quantitative data that could be pooled in a meta-analysis [35,42,44,46,53,64,66–69,72,77,78]. In a meta-analysis of 13 RCTs, the intervention resulted in a small but significant effect on physical activity amount [SMD (95% CI): 0.25 (0.08, 0.43) (I^2 = 80.4%)] (Figure 3), and findings were significant for both participants with and without cardiometabolic risk factors. Maddison et al. reported heart rate as a measure of physical activity intensity and was not included in the meta-analysis, but the authors did report a significant reduction in resting heart rate in the intervention group compared to the control group [56]. Studies for which authors did not provide data that could be pooled in the meta-analysis reported no difference in physical activity amount between groups [60,61,71]. In adults who were healthy or had cardiometabolic risk factors, nutrition and physical activity interventions provided by nutrition and exercise practitioners may increase physical activity amount (Certainty of Evidence: Low).

Study, Year	Intervention			Comparison			SMD	Weight	SMD, 95% CI
	N	Mean	SD	N	Mean	SD			
Cardiometabolic Risk									
Beleigoli et al., 2020	408	23	144.28	470	2.4	2.21		9.96%	0.21 [0.08, 0.34]
Foster-Schubert et al., 2012	117	204.4	145.06	87	40	104.74		7.93%	1.27 [0.96, 1.57]
Hollis et al, 2015	27	-8.92	138.23	26	-54.96	147.9		5.11%	0.32 [-0.22, 0.86]
Kuller et al, 2012	210	1.9	12.5	223	-0.02	16.1		9.38%	0.13 [-0.06, 0.32]
Rollo et al, 2020	15	182	428.8	14	-42	433.35		3.53%	0.51 [-0.23, 1.24]
Rosas et al, 2021	205	-72.7	1283.7	204	9.6	1174.9		9.32%	-0.07 [-0.26, 0.13]
Rosas et al, 2020	85	35.8	226.3	98	-36.6	277.5		8.08%	0.28 [-0.01, 0.57]
Ruusunen et al, 2012	69	56.3	381.2	71	66.7	461.6		7.57%	-0.02 [-0.36, 0.31]
Weinhold et al, 2015	35	23.9	70.99	34	2.2	72.3		5.82%	0.30 [-0.18, 0.77]
Random Effects Model for Subgroup (Q = 57.92, df = 8, p = 0.00, I^2 = 86.2%)									0.31 [0.06, 0.55]
Healthy									
Fjeldsoe et al, 2016	104	7.41	67.75	114	-16.1	68.1		8.40%	0.34 [0.08, 0.61]
Partridge et al, 2016	123	784.85	2437.93	125	671.52	2512.1		8.65%	0.05 [-0.20, 0.29]
Rich-Edwards et al, 2018	69	3.1	25.74	70	-0.5	27.12		7.55%	0.14 [-0.20, 0.47]
Viester et al, 2018	127	62.9	570.07	129	-16.4	672.6		8.69%	0.13 [-0.12, 0.37]
Random Effects Model for Subgroup (Q = 2.73, df = 3, p = 0.43, I^2 = 0.0%)									0.16 [0.03, 0.29]
Random Effects Model for All Studies (Q = 61.28, df = 12, p = 0.00, I^2 = 80.4%)								100.00%	0.25 [0.08, 0.42]

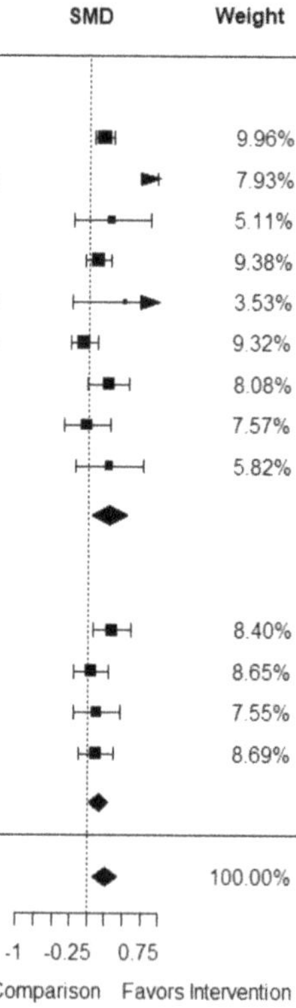

-1 -0.25 0.75
Favors Comparison Favors Intervention

Figure 3. Forest plot for physical activity amount in the systematic review examining effect of nutrition and physical activity interventions provided by nutrition and exercise practitioners for the general population [35,42,44,46,53,64,66–69,72,77,78].

3.4. Fruit and Vegetable Intake

Thirteen RCTs represented in 16 articles met inclusion criteria and reported the outcome of fruit and vegetable intake [34,35,39,41–43,46,51,59,60,63,64,68,69,71,77]. Ten RCTs reported fruit and vegetable intake separately [35,39,42,43,46,51,59,60,64,77], and three RCTs reported fruit and vegetable intake combined [68,69,71].

Nine of ten included RCTs reporting fruit and vegetable intake separately could be pooled in a meta-analysis [35,39,42,43,46,51,59,64,77]. In adults who were healthy, there was a small-to-moderate but significant effect of interventions on fruit intake with no heterogeneity [SMD (95% CI): 0.26 (0.13, 0.40) (I^2 = 0%)] [42,43,51,64,77], but effect size was more heterogeneous and not significant in participants with cardiometabolic risk factors [0.65 (−0.15, 1.44) (I^2 = 91.9%)] [35,39,46,59] (Figure 4A). Participants who were healthy experienced a small but significant increase in vegetable intake [SMD (95% CI): 0.15 (0.01, 0.28) (I^2 = 0%)] [42,43,51,64,77], as did participants with cardiometabolic risk factors [0.13 (0.01, 0.26) (I^2 = 0%)] [35,39,46,59] (Figure 4B). Neale et al. did not report data that could be included in a meta-analysis, but found no difference in fruit or vegetable intake between the intervention and control groups [60]. Three RCTs reported fruit and vegetable intake combined [68,69,71]. In the pooled analysis, there was no significant increase in fruit and vegetable intake in the intervention compared to control groups [SMD (95% CI): 0.10 (−0.03, 0.23) (I^2 = 20.5%)].

In adults who are healthy, nutrition and physical activity interventions provided by nutrition and exercise practitioners increased fruit and vegetable intake, but efficacy was more heterogeneous and less certain for adults with cardiometabolic risk factors (Certainty of Evidence: Moderate).

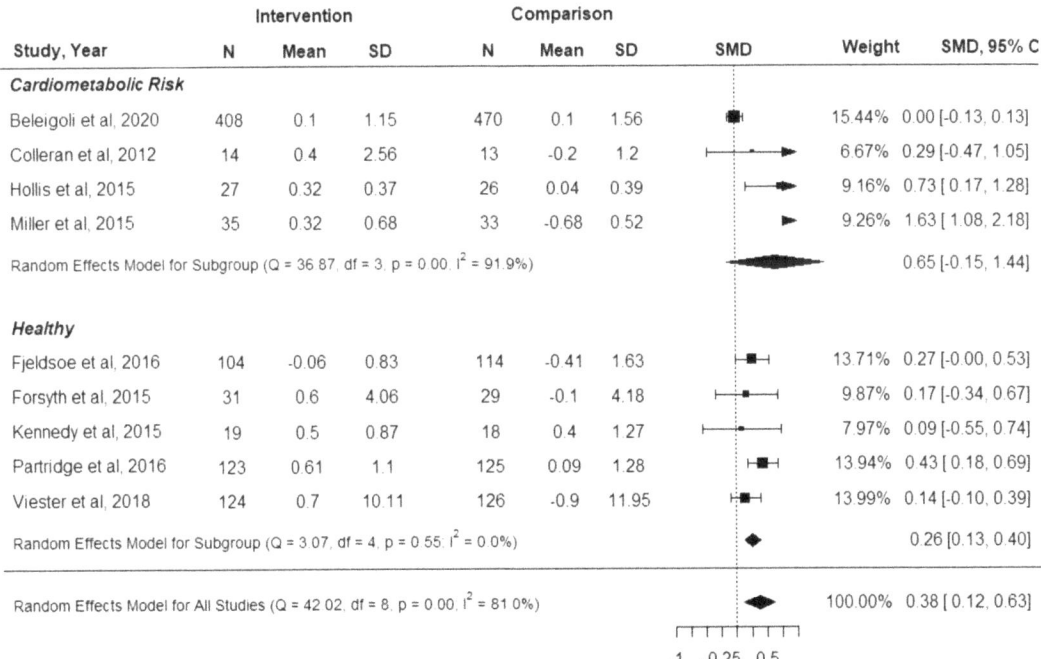

(A)

Figure 4. Cont.

| | Intervention | | | Comparison | | | | | |
Study, Year	N	Mean	SD	N	Mean	SD	SMD	Weight	SMD, 95% CI
Cardiometabolic Risk									
Beleigoli et al, 2020	408	0.2	1.46	470	0	1.56		47.70%	0.13 [-0.00, 0.26]
Colleran et al, 2012	14	0.7	3.84	13	-0.2	2.42		1.46%	0.27 [-0.49, 1.03]
Hollis et al, 2015	27	0.72	1.35	26	0.13	1.509		2.84%	0.41 [-0.14, 0.95]
Miller et al, 2015	35	-1.1	0.89	33	-1.01	0.91		3.71%	-0.10 [-0.57, 0.38]
Random Effects Model for Subgroup (Q = 2.01, df = 3, p = 0.57; I^2 = 0.0%)									0.13 [0.01, 0.26]
Healthy									
Fjeldsoe et al, 2016	104	-0.17	1.51	114	-0.41	1.63		11.87%	0.15 [-0.11, 0.42]
Forsyth et al, 2015	31	0.5	3.12	29	0.6	3.18		3.28%	-0.03 [-0.54, 0.48]
Kennedy et al, 2015	19	0.2	1.31	18	0.6	1.27		2.00%	-0.30 [-0.95, 0.35]
Partridge et al, 2016	123	0.85	1.73	125	0.35	1.663		13.42%	0.29 [0.04, 0.54]
Viester et al, 2018	125	-0.2	10.57	126	-1.3	10.198		13.71%	0.11 [-0.14, 0.35]
Random Effects Model for Subgroup (Q = 3.76, df = 4, p = 0.44; I^2 = 0.0%)									0.15 [0.01, 0.28]
Random Effects Model for All Studies (Q = 5.78, df = 8, p = 0.67; I^2 = 0.0%)								100.00%	0.14 [0.05, 0.23]

-1 -0.25 0.5
Favors Comparison   Favors Intervention

(**B**)

Figure 4. Forest plot for (**A**) fruit and (**B**) vegetable intake in the systematic review examining effect of nutrition and physical activity interventions provided by nutrition and exercise practitioners for the general population [35,39,42,43,46,51,59,64,77].

3.5. Waist Circumference

Twenty-one articles representing 18 RCTs reported the effect of interventions on waist circumference [36,38,41,42,44,45,48,53,56,57,62,67,69–71,73,76–80]. All studies provided results that could be included in a meta-analysis [36,38,42,44,48,53,56,57,62,67,69–71,73,76–78,80]. In adults with cardiometabolic risk factors, nutrition and physical activity interventions from nutrition and exercise practitioners reduced waist circumference compared to control conditions across a wide range of interventions [SMD (95% CI): −2.58 cm (−3.62, −1.53) (I^2 = 62.7%)] [36,38,44,48,53,56,62,67,69–71,73,76,78,80], but results were not significant in studies targeting healthy adults [−0.95 (−2.01, 0.12) (I^2 = 0%)] [42,57,77] (Figure 5) (Certainty of Evidence: High).

3.6. Percent Weight Loss

A priori, the expert panel specified that percent weight loss would be analyzed as an outcome for participants with overweight or obesity only. Studies were required to report the number of participants achieving 5% weight loss or percent weight loss as a continuous variable.

Eight RCTs reported the outcome of achieving 5% weight loss in adults with overweight or obesity [47,50,53,55,67,69,73,78]. In the meta-analysis, adults receiving nutrition and physical activity interventions had a RR (95% CI) of 2.37 (1.76, 3.19) ($p < 0.01$) of achieving 5% weight loss compared to control groups (I^2 = 28.6%) (Figure 6). Seven RCTs represented in nine articles reported the outcome percent weight loss as a continuous variable [33,39,40,50,54,58,59,75,78]. In a pooled analysis of three RCTs, there was no significant effect of interventions on percent weight loss [MD (95% CI): −2.37% (−5.51, 0.77) (I^2 = 79.9%)] [50,75,78]. In the remaining four studies, authors did not provide variance to the mean weight loss percentages reported, but all reported increased percent weight loss in participants who received the interventions compared to the controls [39,54,58,59].

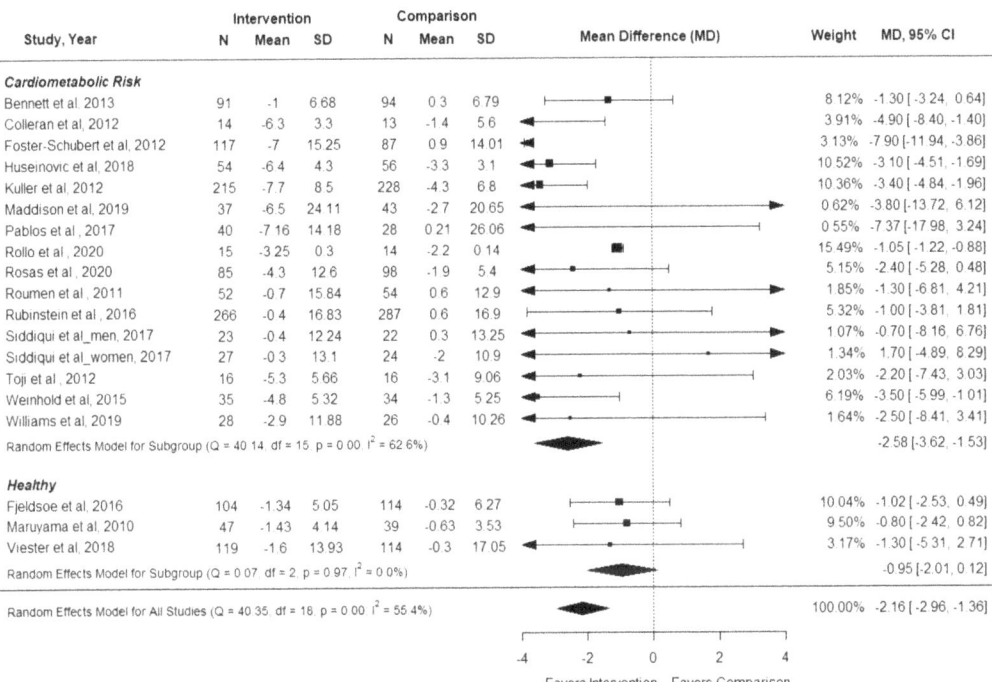

Figure 5. Forest plot for waist circumference in the systematic review examining effect of nutrition and physical activity interventions provided by nutrition and exercise practitioners for the general population [36,38,42,44,48,53,56,57,62,67,69–71,73,76–78,80].

Post-hoc, authors investigated if percent weight loss results varied according to if authors described caloric reduction as part of the intervention. Of the 13 RCTs that reported percent weight loss as an outcome for adults with overweight or obesity [39,47,50,53–55,58,59,67,69,73,75,78], authors of ten studies described that caloric reduction was advised and participants experienced significant percent weight loss or increased likelihood of reaching 5% weight loss in nine of these ten RCTs [39,47,53–55,58,59,69,78], but no effect in one RCT [75]. Three RCTs that did not describe prescribed caloric reduction did not result in significant percent weight loss [50,67,73].

In adults with overweight or obesity but no diagnosed disease, nutrition and physical activity interventions from nutrition and exercise practitioners improved likelihood of achieving 5% weight loss compared to controls, but there was no effect on percent weight loss as a continuous variable. Percent weight loss was generally only significant compared to controls when caloric reduction was prescribed (Certainty of Evidence: Moderate).

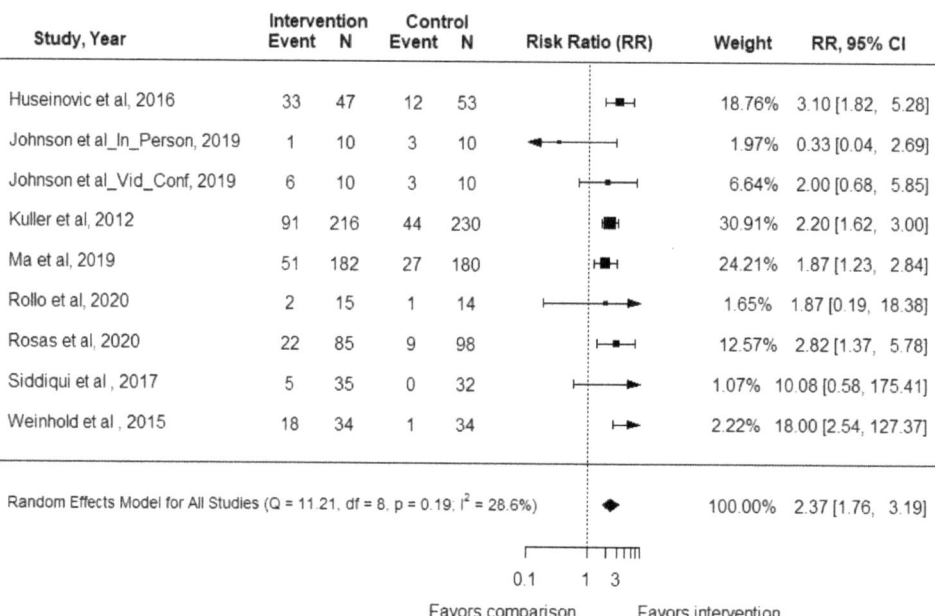

Figure 6. Forest plot for 5% weight loss in the systematic review examining effect of nutrition and physical activity interventions provided by nutrition and exercise practitioners for the general population [47,50,53,55,67,69,73,78].

3.7. Quality of Life

Seven included RCTs reported the outcome of QoL [49,51,52,60,67,69,80]. Study authors used a variety of tools to measure QoL. Because three RCTs utilized the Short Form-36 (SF-36), a common tool for determining QoL, these studies were included in the meta-analysis [49,51,80] and demonstrated no significant effect in the intervention groups compared to control groups on SF-36 Physical QoL [MD (95% CI): 3.91 (−0.21, 8.03) (I^2 = 57.3%)] or Mental QoL [0.19 (−4.04, 4.42) (I^2 = 33.1%)]. In Rosas et al., an Obesity-related Problems Scale was used to measure QoL, in which a lower number is a better outcome. There was no difference in outcomes between groups [69]. In a study by Krishnan et al., transformed weight was used as a proxy for QoL, and there was a greater increase in QoL in the intervention group, but there was no statistical comparison between groups [52]. When the Assessment of QoL 6-dimension tool was used in a small sample, QoL was improved in the intervention group compared to the control group [67]. In a study by Neale et al., the authors used the Short Form-12 to measure QoL and results were reported as medians (interquartile range). The authors reported no difference in QoL between groups [60].

In adults who are healthy or have cardiometabolic risk factors, the evidence is very uncertain about the effect of nutrition and physical activity interventions provided by nutrition and exercise practitioners on physical and mental quality of life but suggests little-to-no effect (Certainty of Evidence: Very Low).

3.8. Adverse Events

Three included RCTs reported adverse events [37,55,69]. In Ma et al. [55] and Rosas et al. [69], serious and nonserious adverse events were comparable between intervention and control groups. However, in a study targeting postmenopausal women, musculoskeletal injuries and hot flash number as well as severity were not significantly different between groups, but bone mineral density was decreased in the diet and exercise group compared to the control group (−1.7% compared with 0% change in the control group) [37]. In adults who were healthy or had cardiometabolic risk factors, nutrition and physical interventions provided by nutrition and exercise practitioners may result in little to no difference in adverse events, though postmenopausal women in an intervention group had reduced bone mineral density compared to the control group in one study (Certainty of Evidence: Low).

4. Discussion

The results of this systematic review demonstrate that combined nutrition and physical activity interventions provided by nutrition and exercise practitioners may increase physical activity amount (low certainty of evidence) and fruit and vegetable intake (low-to-moderate certainty of evidence), decrease waist circumference (high certainty of evidence), and improve the likelihood of achieving a 5% weight loss for adults with overweight or obesity (high certainty of evidence). Interventions may result in little to no difference in QoL (very low certainty of evidence), and adverse events (low certainty of evidence). The results demonstrated that interventions were more effective for fruit intake among healthy adults and were more effective for anthropometric outcomes among adults with cardiometabolic risk factors.

The evidence from this systematic review is consistent with findings from similar reviews. A 2020 systematic review conducted by the USPSTF demonstrated that medium- and high-contact multisession behavioral coaching nutrition and physical activity interventions were effective in reducing cardiovascular events, lowering blood pressure, and improving blood lipid levels in adults with cardiovascular risk factors [6]. A systematic review by Abbate et al. similarly demonstrated beneficial effects of diet and physical activity training in adults with cardiometabolic risk factors [81]. For adults without cardiovascular risk factors, findings from the current systematic review aligned with those from a 2022 systematic review by the USPSTF that nutrition and physical activity interventions improved dietary intake and physical activity amount [7]. Other systematic reviews have focused on the effectiveness of nutrition or physical activity interventions alone. For example, a 2021 systematic review by Jinnette et al. found that personalizing nutrition advice improved dietary intake compared to generalized nutrition advice [82], which supports the need for individualized client counseling. The current systematic review is unique because it specifically considers the effect of interventions including both nutrition and physical activity provided by nutrition and exercise health practitioners and targets participants who may be at risk for cardiometabolic disease due to poor lifestyle behaviors or cardiometabolic risk factors. This focus is important because clients can access such allied healthcare practitioners outside of traditional clinical and medical organizations. In addition, it provides policy makers with information on specific means (nutrition and exercise practitioners) to deliver effective interventions for disease prevention. The evidence from this and other current systematic reviews supports the importance and efficacy of early interventions to reduce cardiometabolic disease risk.

Interestingly, the results of this review revealed little to no effect on QoL. A 2021 systematic review by Jones et al. demonstrated that behavioral weight management interventions improved mental QoL and reduced depression [83], and a 2021 systematic review by the Academy of Nutrition and Dietetics found that overweight and obesity treatment interventions provided by a dietitian improved physical and mental QoL [84]. Conclusions related to the impact that lifestyle interventions have on psychosocial outcomes are, at this point, uncertain, and specific lifestyle interventions that improve QoL, particularly mental QoL, are unknown.

The efficacy of nutrition and physical activity interventions demonstrated in this review is encouraging. However, it is important to note and recognize the varying scopes of practice for each nutrition and exercise allied health practitioner, including when it may be appropriate for a practitioner to give general health recommendations outside of their area of expertise and when it is appropriate to refer to another allied health practitioner.

An allied health practitioner's nutritional scope of practice is determined by a combination of national certification and credentialing [85], state laws and regulations, and the professional's education, experience, and skillset. Thus, a high degree of variability among different practitioners exists regarding what advice and interventions they can ethically provide when dispensing nutrition and physical activity guidance and designing interventions. For example, dietitians have a wider and more sophisticated scope of practice as it relates to nutrition, medical nutrition therapy, nutrient analysis, and individualized meal planning compared to an exercise practitioner or health coach [13,16]. An exercise practitioner, such as a certified personal trainer and/or health coach, has a more limited scope with respect to nutrition, and would likely benefit from referring clients with metabolic risk factors, such as obesity, to dietitians. However, exercise professionals may discuss certain aspects of nutrition with clients. Exercise practitioners, including health coaches, who have earned an accredited certification [85] can and should educate clients and discuss the following: principles of healthy nutrition and food preparation, characteristics of a balanced diet, essential nutrients, actions of nutrients, effects of deficiencies and excess of nutrients, nutrient requirements throughout the lifespan, principles of pre and post-workout fueling, and information about nutrients in foods or supplements [15]. Certified health coaches, more specifically, can apply effective communication skills to assist clients in taking ownership of their behavior changes. Additionally, health coaches support and empower clients to develop measurable goals and the internal strength to achieve those goals [14].

Alternatively, it may be appropriate for dietitians or health coaches to provide generalized physical activity guidance to adults who are apparently healthy or who do not have physical activity limitations [13,16]. However, in more complex cases such as when clients have limited mobility due to obesity, limited experience with physical activity, or highly specific physical activity goals such as building muscle mass, referral to exercise practitioners may be warranted. Multidisciplinary collaboration allows allied health practitioners to share expertise, provides a trustworthy system for client referrals and increases access to interventions to empower adults to prevent disease.

5. Strengths and Limitations

Strengths of this systematic review and meta-analysis included rigorous methods that adhered to GRADE and PRISMA standards. In addition, included studies examined a wide range of nutrition and physical activity interventions provided by a variety of nutrition and exercise practitioners. This systematic review was conducted using a multidisciplinary team of researchers and practitioners in the fields of nutrition, physical activity, and behavior change. Finally, this meta-analysis examined multiple outcomes of interest that are commonly collected in practice and important to population health.

A limitation of this systematic review was that the limited number of studies for each outcome and the heterogeneous interventions and results prevented the team from drawing generalizable conclusions regarding the efficacy of specific types of interventions that include nutrition and physical activity, such as delivering intervention using telehealth or in a group setting. The GRADE method specifies that the number of outcomes selected for analysis are limited to seven outcomes, thus limiting examination of other important healthy dietary components such as intake of whole grains and added sugars. Further, this review relied on exclusively peer-reviewed literature, and there is the potential that unpublished, but applicable, literature relevant to the research question was not included. Finally, this review does not include an intentional analysis of specific sub-populations who are at higher risk for cardiometabolic disease, such as those with low socioeconomic status or who identify as members of racial or ethnic minority groups. Evidence for some outcomes was limited by the risk of bias of included studies or by the lack of studies reporting the outcome of interest, such as QoL.

6. Future Research

Future research should aim to investigate the effects of nutrition and physical activity interventions in underserved populations, such as those with low socioeconomic status or who identify as members of racial or ethnic minority groups, and others who are at higher risk for developing non-communicable diseases. Another goal of future research is to examine nutrition and physical activity interventions that specifically investigate a behavior change-based approach compared to education/information only based interventions. Investigations comparing process (behavior) goals versus product (outcome) goals would provide significant value. A third goal of future research is to examine the optimal number of sessions, types of interactions (e.g., one-on-one vs. group or in-person vs. remote), and/or number of contacts between a client and nutrition and/or exercise practitioners for effectively eliciting behavior change and positive habit development that promote sustainable and meaningful lifestyle changes.

7. Conclusions

Recent research demonstrates that allied health practitioners including dietitians, exercise practitioners and health coaches may facilitate improvement of lifestyle behaviors and anthropometric outcomes, and thus play a key role in improving population health by collaborating with clients who are healthy or who have cardiometabolic risk factors to reduce disease risk. However, more research is needed to determine consistent and effective delivery of interventions to a diversity of clients. Adults would benefit from improved access to allied health practitioners prior to disease development to establish healthy lifestyle behaviors through encouragement, education and skill development. Complementary practitioners can team up to provide multidisciplinary, comprehensive services to their clients while staying within their scopes of practice.

Supplementary Materials: The following supporting information can be downloaded at: https://www.mdpi.com/article/10.3390/nu14091729/s1. Figure S1. Publication Bias of Studies Included in the Systematic Review Examining the Effects of Nutrition and Physical Activity Interventions Provided by Qualified Practitioners; Table S1. Full search strategy for literature search of databases for the systematic review examining the effect of nutrition and physical activity interventions.

Author Contributions: Conceptualization, E.N., K.G., P.H., L.M., J.R., A.T. and M.R.; methodology, M.R.; formal analysis, M.R.; writing—original draft preparation, E.N. and M.R.; writing—review and editing, E.N., K.G., P.H., L.M., J.R., A.T. and M.R.; project administration, M.R. All authors have read and agreed to the published version of the manuscript.

Funding: This systematic review, including APC, was funded by the Academy of Nutrition and Dietetics and the American Council on Exercise (no grant number).

Institutional Review Board Statement: Not applicable.

Informed Consent Statement: Not applicable.

Data Availability Statement: No new data were created or analyzed in this study. Data sharing is not applicable to this article.

Acknowledgments: The authors would like to thank Kathy Keim, who worked as an analyst on this systematic review, as well as the information specialist who conducted the literature searches. In addition, the authors would like to thank the evidence analysts who extracted data and rated the risk of bias of the included articles.

Conflicts of Interest: Authors have no conflict of interest to disclose. Funders had no role in the design, execution, interpretation, or writing of the study.

References

1. World Health Organization. Physical Activity. Available online: https://www.who.int/news-room/fact-sheets/detail/physical-activity (accessed on 27 October 2021).
2. World Health Organization. Noncommunicable Diseases. Available online: https://www.who.int/news-room/fact-sheets/detail/noncommunicable-diseases (accessed on 27 October 2021).
3. Schwingshackl, L.; Bogensberger, B.; Hoffmann, G. Diet Quality as Assessed by the Healthy Eating Index, Alternate Healthy Eating Index, Dietary Approaches to Stop Hypertension Score, and Health Outcomes: An Updated Systematic Review and Meta-Analysis of Cohort Studies. *J. Acad. Nutr. Diet.* **2018**, *118*, 74–100.e111. [CrossRef] [PubMed]

4. U.S. Department of Agriculture and U.S. Department of Health and Human Services. *Dietary Guidelines for Americans, 2020–2025*, 9th ed.; U.S. Department of Agriculture and U.S. Department of Health and Human Services: Washington, DC, USA, 2020.
5. U.S. Department of Health and Human Services. *Physical Activity Guidelines for Americans*, 2nd ed.; U.S. Department of Health and Human Services: Washington, DC, USA, 2018.
6. O'Connor, E.A.; Evans, C.V.; Rushkin, M.C.; Redmond, N.; Lin, J.S. Behavioral Counseling to Promote a Healthy Diet and Physical Activity for Cardiovascular Disease Prevention in Adults With Cardiovascular Risk Factors: Updated Evidence Report and Systematic Review for the US Preventive Services Task Force. *JAMA* **2020**, *324*, 2076–2094. [CrossRef] [PubMed]
7. Patnode, R.N.; Iacocca, M.O.; Henninger, M. *Behavioral Counseling to Promote a Healthy Diet and Physical Activity for Cardiovascular Disease Prevention in Adults Without Known Cardiovascular Disease Risk Factors: Updated Systematic Review for the U.S. Preventive Services Task Force*; Agency for Healthcare Research and Quality, U.S. Department of Health and Human Services: Rockville, MD, USA, 2022.
8. Leite, N.N.; Cota, B.C.; Gotine, A.; Rocha, D.; Pereira, P.F.; Hermsdorff, H.H.M. Visceral adiposity index is positively associated with blood pressure: A systematic review. *Obes. Res. Clin. Pract.* **2021**, *15*, 546–556. [CrossRef] [PubMed]
9. Babaee, E.; Tehrani-Banihashem, A.; Eshrati, B.; Purabdollah, M.; Nojomi, M. How Much Hypertension is Attributed to Overweight, Obesity, and Hyperglycemia Using Adjusted Population Attributable Risk in Adults? *Int. J. Hypertens.* **2020**, *2020*, 4273456. [CrossRef]
10. Gupta, A.K.; Brashear, M.M.; Johnson, W.D. Coexisting prehypertension and prediabetes in healthy adults: A pathway for accelerated cardiovascular events. *Hypertens. Res.* **2011**, *34*, 456–461. [CrossRef]
11. Biddle, S.J.H.; García Bengoechea, E.; Pedisic, Z.; Bennie, J.; Vergeer, I.; Wiesner, G. Screen Time, Other Sedentary Behaviours, and Obesity Risk in Adults: A Review of Reviews. *Curr. Obes. Rep.* **2017**, *6*, 134–147. [CrossRef]
12. Mu, M.; Xu, L.-F.; Hu, D.; Wu, J.; Bai, M.-J. Dietary Patterns and Overweight/Obesity: A Review Article. *Iran. J. Public Health* **2017**, *46*, 869–876.
13. Academy of Nutrition and Dietetics: Revised 2017 Scope of Practice for the Registered Dietitian Nutritionist. *J. Acad. Nutr. Diet.* **2018**, *118*, 141–165. [CrossRef]
14. American Council on Exercise. *The Professional's Guide to Health and Wellness Coaching*; American Council on Exercise: San Diego, CA, USA, 2019; ISBN 9781890720711.
15. American Council on Exercise. *The Exercise Professional's Guide to Personal Training*; American Council on Exercise: San Diego, CA, USA, 2020; ISBN 78-1-890720-76-6.
16. Daigle, K.; Subach, R.; Valliant, M. Academy of Nutrition and Dietetics: Revised 2021 Standards of Practice and Standards of Professional Performance for Registered Dietitian Nutritionists (Competent, Proficient, and Expert) in Sports and Human Performance Nutrition. *J. Acad. Nutr. Diet.* **2021**, *121*, 1813–1830.e1855. [CrossRef]
17. Academy of Nutrition and Dietetics. Fitness. Available online: https://www.eatright.org/fitness (accessed on 27 October 2021).
18. The GRADE Working Group. GRADE Handbook for Grading Quality of Evidence and Strength of Recommendations. Available online: https://gdt.gradepro.org/app/handbook/handbook.html (accessed on 31 August 2021).
19. Page, M.J.; McKenzie, J.E.; Bossuyt, P.M.; Boutron, I.; Hoffmann, T.C.; Mulrow, C.D.; Shamseer, L.; Tetzlaff, J.M.; Akl, E.A.; Brennan, S.E.; et al. The PRISMA 2020 statement: An updated guideline for reporting systematic reviews. *BMJ* **2021**, *372*, n71. [CrossRef]
20. Rozga, M.Y.A.; Robinson, J.; Gottesmoan, K.; Hamlett, P.; Mattar, L.; Nitschke, E.; Tovar, A. Nutrition and Physical Activity Interventions Provided by Nutrition and Exercise Practitioners for the General Population: A Systematic Review PROSPERO 2021 CRD42021247447. Available online: https://www.crd.york.ac.uk/prospero/display_record.php?ID=CRD42021247447 (accessed on 31 August 2021).
21. International Confederation of Dietetic Associations. National Dietetic Associations (NDAs). Available online: https://www.internationaldietetics.org/NDAs.aspx (accessed on 31 August 2021).
22. US Registry of Exercise Professionals. Credentials. Available online: http://usreps.org/Pages/credentials.aspx (accessed on 31 August 2021).
23. Rozga, M.; Jones, K.; Robinson, J.; Yahiro, A. Nutrition and physical activity interventions for the general population with and without cardiometabolic risk: A scoping review. *Public. Health. Nutr.* **2021**, 1–19. [CrossRef] [PubMed]
24. The EndNote Team. *EndNote*; Clarivate: Philadelphia, PA, USA, 2013.
25. Ouzzani, M.; Hammady, H.; Fedorowicz, Z.; Elmagarmid, A. Rayyan-a web and mobile app for systematic reviews. *Syst. Rev.* **2016**, *5*, 210. [CrossRef] [PubMed]
26. Sterne, J.A.C.; Savović, J.; Page, M.J.; Elbers, R.G.; Blencowe, N.S.; Boutron, I.; Cates, C.J.; Cheng, H.Y.; Corbett, M.S.; Eldridge, S.M.; et al. RoB 2: A revised tool for assessing risk of bias in randomised trials. *BMJ* **2019**, *366*, l4898. [CrossRef] [PubMed]
27. Cochrane Collaboration. *Excel Tool to Implement RoB 2*; Cochrane Collaboration: London, UK, 2021.
28. McMaster University and Evidence Prime, Inc. GRADEpro GDT: GRADEpro Guideline Development Tool [Software]. 2020. Available online: https://www.gradepro.org/ (accessed on 25 February 2022).
29. McGuinness, L.A.; Higgins, J.P.T. Risk-of-bias VISualization (robvis): An R package and Shiny web app for visualizing risk-of-bias assessments. *Res. Synth. Methods* **2021**, *12*, 55–61. [CrossRef] [PubMed]
30. Wallace, B.C.; Dahabreh, I.J.; Trikalinos, T.A.; Lau, J.; Trow, P.; Schmid, C.H. Closing the gap between methodologists and end-users: R as a computational back-end. *J. Stat. Softw.* **2012**, *49*, 1–15. [CrossRef]

31. RStudio Team. *RStudio: Integrated Development for R*; RStudio, PBC: Boston, MA, USA, 2020.
32. Guyatt, G.; Oxman, A.D.; Sultan, S.; Brozek, J.; Glasziou, P.; Alonso-Coello, P.; Atkins, D.; Kunz, R.; Montori, V.; Jaeschke, R.; et al. GRADE guidelines: 11. Making an overall rating of confidence in effect estimates for a single outcome and for all outcomes. *J. Clin. Epidemiol.* **2013**, *66*, 151–157. [CrossRef]
33. Abbenhardt, C.; McTiernan, A.; Alfano, C.M.; Wener, M.H.; Campbell, K.L.; Duggan, C.; Foster-Schubert, K.E.; Kong, A.; Toriola, A.T.; Potter, J.D.; et al. Effects of individual and combined dietary weight loss and exercise interventions in postmenopausal women on adiponectin and leptin levels. *J. Intern. Med.* **2013**, *274*, 163–175. [CrossRef]
34. Allman-Farinelli, M.; Partridge, S.R.; McGeechan, K.; Balestracci, K.; Hebden, L.; Wong, A.; Phongsavan, P.; Denney-Wilson, E.; Harris, M.F.; Bauman, A. A Mobile Health Lifestyle Program for Prevention of Weight Gain in Young Adults (TXT2BFiT): Nine-Month Outcomes of a Randomized Controlled Trial. *JMIR Mhealth Uhealth* **2016**, *4*, e78. [CrossRef]
35. Beleigoli, A.; Andrade, A.Q.; Diniz, M.F.; Ribeiro, A.L. Personalized Web-Based Weight Loss Behavior Change Program With and Without Dietitian Online Coaching for Adults With Overweight and Obesity: Randomized Controlled Trial. *J. Med. Internet Res.* **2020**, *22*, e17494. [CrossRef]
36. Bennett, G.G.; Foley, P.; Levine, E.; Whiteley, J.; Askew, S.; Steinberg, D.M.; Batch, B.; Greaney, M.L.; Miranda, H.; Wroth, T.H.; et al. Behavioral treatment for weight gain prevention among black women in primary care practice: A randomized clinical trial. *JAMA Intern. Med.* **2013**, *173*, 1770–1777. [CrossRef]
37. Campbell, K.L.; Foster-Schubert, K.E.; Alfano, C.M.; Wang, C.C.; Wang, C.Y.; Duggan, C.R.; Mason, C.; Imayama, I.; Kong, A.; Xiao, L.; et al. Reduced-calorie dietary weight loss, exercise, and sex hormones in postmenopausal women: Randomized controlled trial. *J. Clin. Oncol.* **2012**, *30*, 2314–2326. [CrossRef] [PubMed]
38. Colleran, H.L.; Wideman, L.; Lovelady, C.A. Effects of energy restriction and exercise on bone mineral density during lactation. *Med. Sci. Sports Exerc.* **2012**, *44*, 1570–1579. [CrossRef] [PubMed]
39. Colleran, H.L.; Lovelady, C.A. Use of MyPyramid Menu Planner for Moms in a weight-loss intervention during lactation. *J. Acad. Nutr. Diet.* **2012**, *112*, 553–558. [CrossRef] [PubMed]
40. Duggan, C.; Tapsoba, J.D.; Wang, C.Y.; Campbell, K.L.; Foster-Schubert, K.; Gross, M.D.; McTiernan, A. Dietary Weight Loss, Exercise, and Oxidative Stress in Postmenopausal Women: A Randomized Controlled Trial. *Cancer Prev. Res.* **2016**, *9*, 835–843. [CrossRef]
41. Fjeldsoe, B.S.; Goode, A.D.; Phongsavan, P.; Bauman, A.; Maher, G.; Winkler, E.; Job, J.; Eakin, E.G. Get Healthy, Stay Healthy: Evaluation of the Maintenance of Lifestyle Changes Six Months After an Extended Contact Intervention. *JMIR Mhealth Uhealth* **2019**, *7*, e11070. [CrossRef]
42. Fjeldsoe, B.S.; Goode, A.D.; Phongsavan, P.; Bauman, A.; Maher, G.; Winkler, E.; Eakin, E.G. Evaluating the Maintenance of Lifestyle Changes in a Randomized Controlled Trial of the 'Get Healthy, Stay Healthy' Program. *JMIR Mhealth Uhealth* **2016**, *4*, e42. [CrossRef]
43. Forsyth, A.; Deane, F.P.; Williams, P. A lifestyle intervention for primary care patients with depression and anxiety: A randomised controlled trial. *Psychiatry Res.* **2015**, *230*, 537–544. [CrossRef]
44. Foster-Schubert, K.E.; Alfano, C.M.; Duggan, C.R.; Xiao, L.; Campbell, K.L.; Kong, A.; Bain, C.E.; Wang, C.Y.; Blackburn, G.L.; McTiernan, A. Effect of diet and exercise, alone or combined, on weight and body composition in overweight-to-obese postmenopausal women. *Obesity* **2012**, *20*, 1628–1638. [CrossRef]
45. Gabriel, K.K.; Conroy, M.B.; Schmid, K.K.; Storti, K.L.; High, R.R.; Underwood, D.A.; Kriska, A.M.; Kuller, L.H. The impact of weight and fat mass loss and increased physical activity on physical function in overweight, postmenopausal women: Results from the Women on the Move Through Activity and Nutrition study. *Menopause* **2011**, *18*, 759–765. [CrossRef]
46. Hollis, J.L.; Williams, L.T.; Morgan, P.J.; Collins, C.E. The 40-Something Randomised Controlled Trial improved fruit intake and nutrient density of the diet in mid-age women. *Nutr. Diet.* **2015**, *72*, 316–326. [CrossRef]
47. Huseinovic, E.; Bertz, F.; Leu Agelii, M.; Hellebö Johansson, E.; Winkvist, A.; Brekke, H.K. Effectiveness of a weight loss intervention in postpartum women: Results from a randomized controlled trial in primary health care. *Am. J. Clin. Nutr.* **2016**, *104*, 362–370. [CrossRef] [PubMed]
48. Huseinovic, E.; Bertz, F.; Brekke, H.K.; Winkvist, A. Two-year follow-up of a postpartum weight loss intervention: Results from a randomized controlled trial. *Matern. Child Nutr.* **2018**, *14*, e12539. [CrossRef] [PubMed]
49. Imayama, I.; Alfano, C.M.; Kong, A.; Foster-Schubert, K.E.; Bain, C.E.; Xiao, L.; Duggan, C.; Wang, C.Y.; Campbell, K.L.; Blackburn, G.L.; et al. Dietary weight loss and exercise interventions effects on quality of life in overweight/obese postmenopausal women: A randomized controlled trial. *Int. J. Behav. Nutr. Phys. Act.* **2011**, *8*, 118. [CrossRef] [PubMed]
50. Johnson, K.E.; Alencar, M.K.; Coakley, K.E.; Swift, D.L.; Cole, N.H.; Mermier, C.M.; Kravitz, L.; Amorim, F.T.; Gibson, A.L. Telemedicine-Based Health Coaching Is Effective for Inducing Weight Loss and Improving Metabolic Markers. *Telemed. J. e-Health* **2019**, *25*, 85–92. [CrossRef] [PubMed]
51. Kennedy, B.M.; Ryan, D.H.; Johnson, W.D.; Harsha, D.W.; Newton, R.L., Jr.; Champagne, C.M.; Allen, H.R.; Katzmarzyk, P.T. Baton Rouge Healthy Eating and Lifestyle Program (BR-HELP): A Pilot Health Promotion Program. *J. Prev. Interv. Community* **2015**, *43*, 95–108. [CrossRef]
52. Krishnan, A.; Finkelstein, E.A.; Levine, E.; Foley, P.; Askew, S.; Steinberg, D.; Bennett, G.G. A Digital Behavioral Weight Gain Prevention Intervention in Primary Care Practice: Cost and Cost-Effectiveness Analysis. *J. Med. Internet Res.* **2019**, *21*, e12201. [CrossRef]

53. Kuller, L.H.; Pettee Gabriel, K.K.; Kinzel, L.S.; Underwood, D.A.; Conroy, M.B.; Chang, Y.; Mackey, R.H.; Edmundowicz, D.; Tyrrell, K.S.; Buhari, A.M.; et al. The Women on the Move Through Activity and Nutrition (WOMAN) study: Final 48-month results. *Obesity* 2012, *20*, 636–643. [CrossRef]
54. Lindström, J.; Peltonen, M.; Eriksson, J.G.; Ilanne-Parikka, P.; Aunola, S.; Keinänen-Kiukaanniemi, S.; Uusitupa, M.; Tuomilehto, J. Improved lifestyle and decreased diabetes risk over 13 years: Long-term follow-up of the randomised Finnish Diabetes Prevention Study (DPS). *Diabetologia* 2013, *56*, 284–293. [CrossRef]
55. Ma, J.; Rosas, L.G.; Lv, N.; Xiao, L.; Snowden, M.B.; Venditti, E.M.; Lewis, M.A.; Goldhaber-Fiebert, J.D.; Lavori, P.W. Effect of Integrated Behavioral Weight Loss Treatment and Problem-Solving Therapy on Body Mass Index and Depressive Symptoms Among Patients With Obesity and Depression: The RAINBOW Randomized Clinical Trial. *JAMA* 2019, *321*, 869–879. [CrossRef]
56. Maddison, R.; Hargreaves, E.A.; Wyke, S.; Gray, C.M.; Hunt, K.; Heke, J.I.; Kara, S.; Ni Mhurchu, C.; Jull, A.; Jiang, Y.; et al. Rugby Fans in Training New Zealand (RUFIT-NZ): A pilot randomized controlled trial of a healthy lifestyle program for overweight men delivered through professional rugby clubs in New Zealand. *BMC Public Health* 2019, *19*, 166. [CrossRef]
57. Maruyama, C.; Kimura, M.; Okumura, H.; Hayashi, K.; Arao, T. Effect of a worksite-based intervention program on metabolic parameters in middle-aged male white-collar workers: A randomized controlled trial. *Prev. Med.* 2010, *51*, 11–17. [CrossRef] [PubMed]
58. Mason, C.; Foster-Schubert, K.E.; Imayama, I.; Kong, A.; Xiao, L.; Bain, C.; Campbell, K.L.; Wang, C.Y.; Duggan, C.R.; Ulrich, C.M.; et al. Dietary weight loss and exercise effects on insulin resistance in postmenopausal women. *Am. J. Prev. Med.* 2011, *41*, 366–375. [CrossRef] [PubMed]
59. Miller, C.K.; Weinhold, K.; Marrero, D.G.; Nagaraja, H.N.; Focht, B.C. A Translational Worksite Diabetes Prevention Trial Improves Psychosocial Status, Dietary Intake, and Step Counts among Employees with Prediabetes: A Randomized Controlled Trial. *Prev. Med. Rep.* 2015, *2*, 118–126. [CrossRef] [PubMed]
60. Neale, E.P.; Tapsell, L.C.; Martin, A.; Batterham, M.J.; Wibisono, C.; Probst, Y.C. Impact of providing walnut samples in a lifestyle intervention for weight loss: A secondary analysis of the HealthTrack trial. *Food Nutr. Res.* 2017, *61*, 1344522. [CrossRef] [PubMed]
61. Nicklas, J.M.; Zera, C.A.; England, L.J.; Rosner, B.A.; Horton, E.; Levkoff, S.E.; Seely, E.W. A web-based lifestyle intervention for women with recent gestational diabetes mellitus: A randomized controlled trial. *Obs. Gynecol.* 2014, *124*, 563–570. [CrossRef] [PubMed]
62. Pablos, A.P.; Drehmer, E.; Ceca, D.; Fargueta, M.; Pablos, C.; García-Esteve, A.; López-Hernández, L.; Romero, F.J. Effects of a lifestyle intervention program for treating obesity in lower socioeconomic status adults: A randomized controlled trial. *Gazz. Med. Ital. Arch. Sci. Med.* 2017, *176*, 467–477. [CrossRef]
63. Partridge, S.R.; McGeechan, K.; Hebden, L.; Balestracci, K.; Wong, A.T.; Denney-Wilson, E.; Harris, M.F.; Phongsavan, P.; Bauman, A.; Allman-Farinelli, M. Effectiveness of a mHealth Lifestyle Program With Telephone Support (TXT2BFiT) to Prevent Unhealthy Weight Gain in Young Adults: Randomized Controlled Trial. *JMIR Mhealth Uhealth* 2015, *3*, e66. [CrossRef]
64. Partridge, S.R.; McGeechan, K.; Bauman, A.; Phongsavan, P.; Allman-Farinelli, M. Improved eating behaviours mediate weight gain prevention of young adults: Moderation and mediation results of a randomised controlled trial of TXT2BFiT, mHealth program. *Int. J. Behav. Nutr. Phys. Act.* 2016, *13*, 44. [CrossRef]
65. Perri, M.G.; Shankar, M.N.; Daniels, M.J.; Durning, P.E.; Ross, K.M.; Limacher, M.C.; Janicke, D.M.; Martin, A.D.; Dhara, K.; Bobroff, L.B.; et al. Effect of Telehealth Extended Care for Maintenance of Weight Loss in Rural US Communities: A Randomized Clinical Trial. *JAMA Netw. Open* 2020, *3*, e206764. [CrossRef]
66. Rich-Edwards, J.W.; Stuart, J.J.; Skurnik, G.; Roche, A.T.; Tsigas, E.; Fitzmaurice, G.M.; Wilkins-Haug, L.E.; Levkoff, S.E.; Seely, E.W. Randomized Trial to Reduce Cardiovascular Risk in Women with Recent Preeclampsia. *J. Womens Health (Larchmt)* 2019, *28*, 1493–1504. [CrossRef]
67. Rollo, M.E.; Baldwin, J.N.; Hutchesson, M.; Aguiar, E.J.; Wynne, K.; Young, A.; Callister, R.; Haslam, R.; Collins, C.E. The Feasibility and Preliminary Efficacy of an eHealth Lifestyle Program in Women with Recent Gestational Diabetes Mellitus: A Pilot Study. *Int. J. Env. Res. Public Health* 2020, *17*, 7115. [CrossRef] [PubMed]
68. Rosas, L.G.; Xiao, L.; Lv, N.; Lavori, P.W.; Venditti, E.M.; Snowden, M.B.; Smyth, J.M.; Lewis, M.A.; Williams, L.M.; Suppes, T.; et al. Understanding mechanisms of integrated behavioral therapy for co-occurring obesity and depression in primary care: A mediation analysis in the RAINBOW trial. *Transl. Behav. Med.* 2021, *11*, 382–392. [CrossRef] [PubMed]
69. Rosas, L.G.; Lv, N.; Xiao, L.; Lewis, M.A.; Venditti, E.M.J.; Zavella, P.; Azar, K.; Ma, J. Effect of a Culturally Adapted Behavioral Intervention for Latino Adults on Weight Loss Over 2 Years: A Randomized Clinical Trial. *JAMA Netw. Open* 2020, *3*, e2027744. [CrossRef] [PubMed]
70. Roumen, C.; Feskens, E.J.; Corpeleijn, E.; Mensink, M.; Saris, W.H.; Blaak, E.E. Predictors of lifestyle intervention outcome and dropout: The SLIM study. *Eur. J. Clin. Nutr.* 2011, *65*, 1141–1147. [CrossRef] [PubMed]
71. Rubinstein, A.; Miranda, J.J.; Beratarrechea, A.; Diez-Canseco, F.; Kanter, R.; Gutierrez, L.; Bernabé-Ortiz, A.; Irazola, V.; Fernandez, A.; Letona, P.; et al. Effectiveness of an mHealth intervention to improve the cardiometabolic profile of people with prehypertension in low-resource urban settings in Latin America: A randomised controlled trial. *Lancet Diabet. Endocrinol.* 2016, *4*, 52–63. [CrossRef]
72. Ruusunen, A.; Voutilainen, S.; Karhunen, L.; Lehto, S.M.; Tolmunen, T.; Keinänen-Kiukaanniemi, S.; Eriksson, J.; Tuomilehto, J.; Uusitupa, M.; Lindström, J. How does lifestyle intervention affect depressive symptoms? Results from the Finnish Diabetes Prevention Study. *Diabet. Med.* 2012, *29*, e126–e132. [CrossRef]

73. Siddiqui, F.; Kurbasic, A.; Lindblad, U.; Nilsson, P.M.; Bennet, L. Effects of a culturally adapted lifestyle intervention on cardiometabolic outcomes: A randomized controlled trial in Iraqi immigrants to Sweden at high risk for Type 2 diabetes. *Metabolism* **2017**, *66*, 1–13. [CrossRef]
74. Siddiqui, F.; Koivula, R.W.; Kurbasic, A.; Lindblad, U.; Nilsson, P.M.; Bennet, L. Physical Activity in a Randomized Culturally Adapted Lifestyle Intervention. *Am. J. Prev. Med.* **2018**, *55*, 187–196. [CrossRef]
75. Thomas, J.G.; Bond, D.S.; Raynor, H.A.; Papandonatos, G.D.; Wing, R.R. Comparison of Smartphone-Based Behavioral Obesity Treatment With Gold Standard Group Treatment and Control: A Randomized Trial. *Obesity* **2019**, *27*, 572–580. [CrossRef]
76. Toji, C.; Okamoto, N.; Kobayashi, T.; Furukawa, Y.; Tanaka, S.; Ueji, K.; Fukui, M.; Date, C. Effectiveness of diet versus exercise intervention on weight reduction in local Japanese residents. *Env. Health Prev. Med.* **2012**, *17*, 332–340. [CrossRef]
77. Viester, L.; Verhagen, E.; Bongers, P.M.; van der Beek, A.J. Effectiveness of a Worksite Intervention for Male Construction Workers on Dietary and Physical Activity Behaviors, Body Mass Index, and Health Outcomes: Results of a Randomized Controlled Trial. *Am. J. Health Promot.* **2018**, *32*, 795–805. [CrossRef] [PubMed]
78. Weinhold, K.R.; Miller, C.K.; Marrero, D.G.; Nagaraja, H.N.; Focht, B.C.; Gascon, G.M. A Randomized Controlled Trial Translating the Diabetes Prevention Program to a University Worksite, Ohio, 2012–2014. *Prev. Chronic. Dis.* **2015**, *12*, E210. [CrossRef] [PubMed]
79. Williams, L.T.; Hollis, J.L.; Collins, C.E.; Morgan, P.J. Can a relatively low-intensity intervention by health professionals prevent weight gain in mid-age women? 12-Month outcomes of the 40-Something randomised controlled trial. *Nutr. Diabetes* **2014**, *4*, e116. [CrossRef] [PubMed]
80. Williams, L.T.; Collins, C.E.; Morgan, P.J.; Hollis, J.L. Maintaining the Outcomes of a Successful Weight Gain Prevention Intervention in Mid-Age Women: Two Year Results from the 40-Something Randomized Control Trial. *Nutrients* **2019**, *11*. [CrossRef] [PubMed]
81. Abbate, M.; Gallardo-Alfaro, L.; Bibiloni, M.D.M.; Tur, J.A. Efficacy of dietary intervention or in combination with exercise on primary prevention of cardiovascular disease: A systematic review. *Nutr. Metab. Cardiovasc. Dis.* **2020**, *30*, 1080–1093. [CrossRef] [PubMed]
82. Jinnette, R.; Narita, A.; Manning, B.; McNaughton, S.A.; Mathers, J.C.; Livingstone, K.M. Does Personalized Nutrition Advice Improve Dietary Intake in Healthy Adults? A Systematic Review of Randomized Controlled Trials. *Adv. Nutr.* **2021**, *12*, 657–669. [CrossRef] [PubMed]
83. Jones, R.A.; Lawlor, E.R.; Birch, J.M.; Patel, M.I.; Werneck, A.O.; Hoare, E.; Griffin, S.J.; van Sluijs, E.M.F.; Sharp, S.J.; Ahern, A.L. The impact of adult behavioural weight management interventions on mental health: A systematic review and meta-analysis. *Obes. Rev.* **2021**, *22*, e13150. [CrossRef]
84. Academy of Nutrition and Dietetics' Evidence Analysis Center. Nutrition and Physical Activity. Available online: https://andeal.org/npa (accessed on 2 November 2021).
85. Institute for Credentialing Excellence. NCAA Accreditation. Available online: https://www.credentialingexcellence.org/Accreditation/Earn-Accreditation/NCCA (accessed on 20 February 2022).

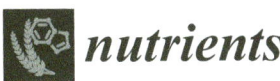

Systematic Review

The Effectiveness of Web-Based Interventions to Promote Health Behaviour Change in Adolescents: A Systematic Review

Daniela de Sousa [1,2], Adriana Fogel [1,2], José Azevedo [1,2,3] and Patrícia Padrão [1,2,4,*]

1. EPIUnit—Instituto de Saúde Pública, Universidade do Porto, 4050-600 Porto, Portugal; daniela.sousa@ispup.up.pt (D.d.S.); adriana.fogel@gmail.com (A.F.); azevedo@letras.up.pt (J.A.)
2. Laboratório para a Investigação Integrativa e Translacional em Saúde Populacional (ITR), 4050-600 Porto, Portugal
3. Faculdade de Letras, Universidade do Porto, 4150-564 Porto, Portugal
4. Faculdade de Ciências da Nutrição e Alimentação, Universidade do Porto, 4150-180 Porto, Portugal
* Correspondence: patriciapadrao@fcna.up.pt; Tel.: +351-22-5074320

Abstract: Although web-based interventions are attractive to researchers and users, the evidence about their effectiveness in the promotion of health behaviour change is still limited. Our aim was to review the effectiveness of web-based interventions used in health behavioural change in adolescents regarding physical activity, eating habits, tobacco and alcohol use, sexual behaviour, and quality of sleep. Studies published from 2016 till the search was run (May-to-June 2021) were included if they were experimental or quasi-experimental studies, pre-post-test studies, clinical trials, or randomized controlled trials evaluating the effectiveness of web-based intervention in promoting behaviour change in adolescents regarding those health behaviours. The risk of bias assessment was performed by using the Effective Public Health Practice Project (EPHPP)—Quality Assessment Tool for Quantitative Studies. Fourteen studies were included. Most were in a school setting, non-probabilistic and relatively small samples. All had a short length of follow-up and were theory driven. Thirteen showed significant positive findings to support web-based interventions' effectiveness in promoting health behaviour change among adolescents but were classified as low evidence quality. Although this review shows that web-based interventions may contribute to health behaviour change among adolescents, these findings rely on low-quality evidence, so it is urgent to test these interventions in larger controlled trials with long-term maintenance.

Keywords: systematic review; web-based intervention; health behaviour; behaviour change; adolescents

1. Introduction

A major concern to public health researchers is lifestyle behaviours. Risky behaviours, such as tobacco and alcohol use, unhealthy food habits, physical inactivity, risky sexual practices, and insufficient sleep duration, play a significant role in many of the leading causes of death worldwide [1]. According to data from 2015, 70% of all preventable deaths from non-communicable diseases in adults are related to lifestyle risk factors adopted during adolescence [2].

Adolescence is a critical period since many unhealthy habits and risky behaviours begin at this age. However, it is also a window of opportunity for the development of health-protective behaviours since health-related habits adopted at this age tend to persist into adulthood [3]. For this reason, it is suggested that public health interventions aimed to prevent or stop risky behaviours should target this life period [4], knowing that improving adolescents' health now is also ensuring a better future for the next generations [5,6].

A positive aspect for health promotion is that, since behaviours are modifiable health-related variables, the threat they represent is greatly preventable [7–9] and even minor changes in human behaviours can improve the overall population's health [1]. However, the drawback is that behaviour change is a very complex and iterative process, in which even individuals who are aware of better health practices still fall short in adjusting their behaviour [10].

Therefore, focusing on achieving and maintaining successful behavioural change in individuals and communities is a key question for health research [10]. Over the years, theories, models, and techniques have been suggested to understand and predict behaviour [11], contributing to the support of planners in handling challenges in the research concept, implementation, and evaluation to improve the effectiveness of behavioural interventions [12].

Until this moment, there has been no consensus on the key role that these behavioural interventions can play in population-level health. However, there is already agreement that understanding theories of behaviour change is an essential element of successful health-related interventions [13].

The relationship between the healthcare provider and the patient is now much more different than it was before, and at the end of the 20th century, researchers and health professionals began to realize how important shared decision-making is in healthcare service. Additionally, a growing interest in participatory approaches to health promotion has been observed, especially in interventions targeting children and adolescents. So, as the medical paradigm was changing, digital technologies able to raise patient empowerment were also becoming more readily available [14].

Thus, digital health promotion interventions, especially internet-based technologies, have been suggested as important tools to improve individuals' health and the quality of healthcare services and to reduce health inequalities due to their large-scale availability. Although there is a lack of robust evidence to support the effectiveness of web-based interventions, it seems to be a promising approach to support behavioural health change [15], which is becoming increasingly attractive to researchers [16].

The interest in using web-based interventions in the health field is still growing. The number of publications reveals this interest since this amount increased from 770 in 2016 to 1464 in 2020. In this same period, there was an increase of 683% in Pubmed/MEDLINE publication results for "health AND web-based intervention" (Figure 1).

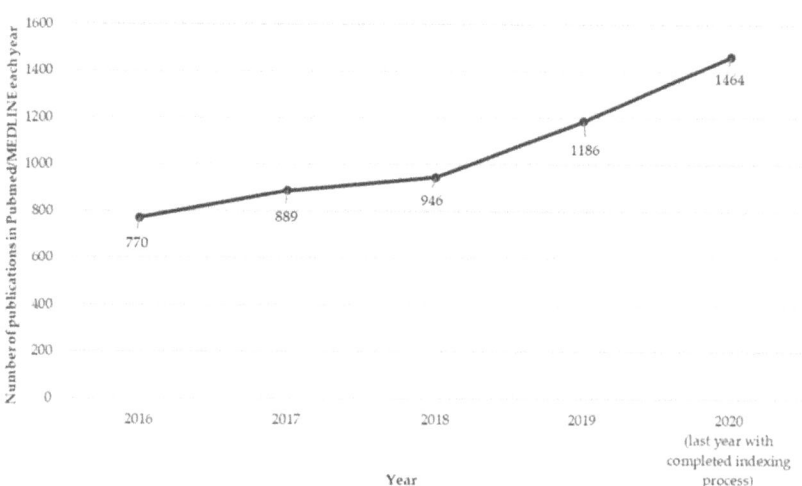

Figure 1. Self-elaborated graph of trends by year of publication for search terms "health AND web-based intervention" from PubMed/MEDLINE data on 26 August 2021.

Although web-based interventions may be attractive to both users and researchers, it is crucial to summarize evidence about their effectiveness. It is essential to identify which are the delivery modes and the behavioural change theories and techniques most frequently used to promote positive health behavioural change and its maintenance in the long term [13].

Since there is a wide range of digital technologies (e.g., social media, telemedicine, data analytics, artificial intelligence, personalized medicine, wearables, mobile apps, electronic medical records, web-resources for health education, among others) and each of them has unique capabilities and specificities [17], characterizing each one individually will help researchers construct more robust evidence to better explain their impact on different health outcomes.

So, it is valuable to summarize the recent findings concerning the effectiveness of web-based interventions in adolescents' health, especially those more critical to the 10–24-year-old age range, namely physical activity, eating, smoking, alcohol use, sexual behaviour, and quality of sleep. Additionally, it is important to evaluate how these interventions are modelled and used to support and maintain behavioural health change in this population. The main objective of this study is to respond to this need by systematically reviewing the literature published in the last 5 years.

2. Methods

2.1. Data Sources

This systematic review was prepared in accordance with the Preferred Reporting Items for Systematic Reviews and Meta-Analyses (PRISMA) statement [18]. The review protocol was registered on the International Prospective Register of Systematic Reviews (PROSPERO) (registration number CRD42021275508).

The electronic databases of PubMed/MEDLINE, Scopus, APA Journals, Web of Science and SAGE Journal were searched from May to June 2021. The search terms used were organized in three main sections: population, intervention, and health outcomes, each illustrated by keywords and synonyms. All the terms used in the search strategy were connected by the Boolean operator AND, between each main section, and OR, within each section, as detailed in Table S1. We set the alerts for each database to reach new added results. Additional articles were identified from the reference list of retrieved articles by applying a reverse snowballing search.

2.2. Inclusion and Exclusion Criteria

Studies were eligible for inclusion if their full text was published in scientific journals in English, Portuguese, or Spanish. Only studies published from 2016 till June of 2021 were included, considering the wide range of digital technologies [17], the raising of patient empowerment and their relationship with technology [14], as well as the exponential and rapid development of digital technology in this last five-year period [19].

Considering the PICO-S framework (population, intervention, comparison, outcomes, study design), we defined the other inclusion and exclusion criteria that we described below. Articles that cover all inclusion criteria were considered in this systematic review.

2.2.1. Participants/Population

Inclusion Criteria

The population included only adolescents according to the definition used by Sawyer et al., (2018), which corresponds to people between 10 and 24 years old [20] and who have participated in web-based health interventions.

Exclusion Criteria

Interventions targeted not directly to participants aged 10 to 24 years old but targeted their parents, educators, or healthcare professionals were excluded. Interventions targeting multiple ages were excluded if it was not possible to isolate the desired target age group.

Specific subgroups such as disabled people or people with irreversible clinical conditions or major chronic diseases were excluded since the review focused on general adolescents.

2.2.2. Intervention/Exposure

Inclusion Criteria

In our review, we considered the definition described by Barak et al., (2009), which mentions that a web-based intervention is "a primarily self-guided intervention programme that is executed using a prescriptive online programme operated through a website and used by consumers seeking health and mental-health related assistance. The intervention programme itself attempts to create positive change and or improve/enhance knowledge, awareness, and understanding via the provision of sound health-related material and use of interactive Web-based components" [21]. We considered web-based interventions developed for health promotion to improve and/or maintain positive health behaviours. To be included, the web-based intervention can be a stand-alone intervention or a multicomponent intervention where the use of web-based resources is one of the intervention's components.

Exclusion Criteria

We excluded articles if they do not report a web-based intervention, if the intervention does not aim to reduce lifestyle risk factors (non-health promotion interventions) or if the interventions aim to improve disease screening or to control major chronic diseases.

2.2.3. Comparator(s)/Control

Inclusion Criteria

Studies that compare the proposed intervention/exposure to another intervention or a non-intervention group, as well as studies with a pre-test and post-test design, were considered in this review.

Exclusion Criteria

Studies with no control group and only with a post-test design were excluded.

2.2.4. Outcome(s)

Inclusion Criteria

Regarding the main objective of this systematic review, we included studies if they analysed the effectiveness of the intervention to promote desired behavioural change using quantitative or mixed methods. This may include outcomes such as the extent and maintenance of behaviour changes, risk reduction, cognitions and attitudes, behavioural intention, subjective norm, self-efficacy, perceived behavioural control and pre-conditions for practising and maintaining the desired behaviours (regarding physical activity, eating habits and weight control, smoking, alcohol use, sexual behaviour, and quality of sleep).

Secondary outcomes such as adoption and adherence rates of the web-based intervention, patient-reported experience, feasibility and usability assessments, and coherence of the technology with behavioural change techniques will also be analysed when available.

Exclusion Criteria

Articles only evaluating the effectiveness of the intervention by qualitative methods were excluded, as well as those that did not have a measurement of the effectiveness. Additionally, studies not evaluating health outcomes related at least to one of these health behaviours were excluded: physical activity, eating habits and weight control, smoking, alcohol use, sexual behaviour, and quality of sleep.

2.2.5. Study Design
Inclusion Criteria

The final set of included studies was limited to quantitative or mixed methods studies as experimental studies, quasi-experimental studies, before-and-after studies/pre-post-test studies, clinical trials, and randomized control trials.

Exclusion Criteria

Other types of publications, such as case studies, systematic reviews, meta-analyses, case reports and series, ideas, editorials, opinions, study protocols and studies using only qualitative methods were not included.

2.3. Data Extraction

The main author (DS) performed a search of the electronic databases. The articles found by databases search, after applying the filters, were imported into Endnote TM20 software and the duplicate records were removed by automation tools and manual search. Early screening by titles and abstracts was performed by one author (DS) based on the aim of the study and the eligibility criteria. Those articles identified as being potentially eligible were fully examined by two researchers (DS and AF) separately to make sure they met the inclusion criteria. In case of discrepancies, the decision was discussed and deliberated by both reviewers. If the disagreement persisted, it was solved by two other authors (PP and JA).

The articles that met the specified inclusion criteria had their data extracted by the main reviewer (DS) and validated by a second reviewer (AF) using a table developed in Microsoft® Excel by the study team (Table S2).

Two researchers (DS and AF) independently performed the risk of bias assessment for all included studies using the Effective Public Health Practice Project—Quality Assessment Tool for Quantitative Studies (EPHPP), which has been validated for use in public health research [22]. Even though we considered several tools, we chose the Effective Public Health Practice Project (EPHPP) tool because it was a validated tool that could be used across multiple study designs and had been developed to be used in systematic reviews about effectiveness to questions related to public health programs [22,23].

The global rating for each article was assessed by evaluation as weak, moderate, or strong regarding six domain ratings: selection bias, study design, confounders, blinding, data collection methods, withdrawals, and drop-outs, according to a standardized guide and dictionary (Table 1). Those with no weak ratings and at least four strong ratings were considered strong. Those with less than four strong ratings and one weak rating were considered moderate. Finally, those with two or more weak ratings were considered weak. Two other domains were included in the assessment, but they were not included in the overall score (the integrity of the intervention and analysis) [23]. After classifying all dimensions, both reviewers (DS and AF) discussed and compared their assessments. When discrepancies occurred, the reason was identified as oversight, differences in interpretation of criteria or differences in interpretation of the study. After discussion, both researchers agreed on a final decision.

Table 1. Quality assessment components and ratings for EPHPP instruments reproduced from Thomas BH, Ciliska D, Dobbins M, Micucci S. A process for systematically reviewing the literature: providing the research evidence for public health nursing interventions. Worldviews Evid Based Nurs. 2004. [23], with permission from John Wiley and Sons, Copyright © 2004 (License number 5266150531479 obtained on 11 March 2022).

Components	Strong	Moderate	Weak
Selection bias	Very likely to be representative of the target population and greater than 80% participation rate	Somewhat likely to be representative of the target population and 60–79% participation rate	All other responses or not stated
Study design	RCT and CCT	Cohort analytic, case–control, cohort. Or an interrupted time series	All other designs or not stated
Confounders	Controlled for at least 80% of confounders	Controlled for 60–79% of confounders	Confounders not controlled for or not stated
Blinding	Blinding of outcome assessor and study participants to intervention status and/or research question	Blinding of either outcome assessor or study participants	Outcome assessor and study participants are aware of intervention status and/or research question
Data collection methods	Tools are valid and reliable	Tools are valid but reliability is not described	No evidence of validity or reliability
Withdrawals and drop-outs	Follow up rate >80% of participants	Follow-up rate of 60–79% of participants	Follow-up rate of <60% of participants or withdrawals and drop-outs not described

2.4. Data Synthesis

Considering the broad health behaviours included in our research question, substantial heterogeneity between studies was found regarding their aims, methods and reported outcomes. Thus, we decided to perform a qualitative synthesis to summarize the extracted data rather than perform a meta-analysis. By doing so, we intended to systematically review web-based interventions related to health behaviour change to interpret the results and draw conclusions about their effectiveness, feasibility, usability, and use of behaviour changing techniques. Furthermore, we also identified the limitations and proposed directions for future research.

3. Results

Table 2 encompasses the summary of narrative synthesis, and it includes authors, publication year, country/region, setting of the study, study design, health outcomes and main findings. More detailed information is available in Tables S3–S5.

3.1. Study Selection

As described in the PRISMA flowchart (Figure 2), 449 results were found through the search in the five electronic databases. Of those, 189 results were marked as ineligible by automated tools of the databases, the remaining articles were imported into Endnote TM20 software, and 77 results were found to be duplicate records. In total, 266 results were removed before the screening. One of the authors (DS) screened the title and abstracts of 183 studies and, based on the purpose of the study and the inclusion and exclusion criteria, DS identified 65 studies sought for retrieval. The full texts of those potentially eligible studies were independently assessed by two reviewers (DS and AF) using the inclusion and exclusion criteria. In cases of discrepancies, the decision was discussed and deliberated by both reviewers. If the disagreement persisted, it was solved by the two other authors (PP and JA).

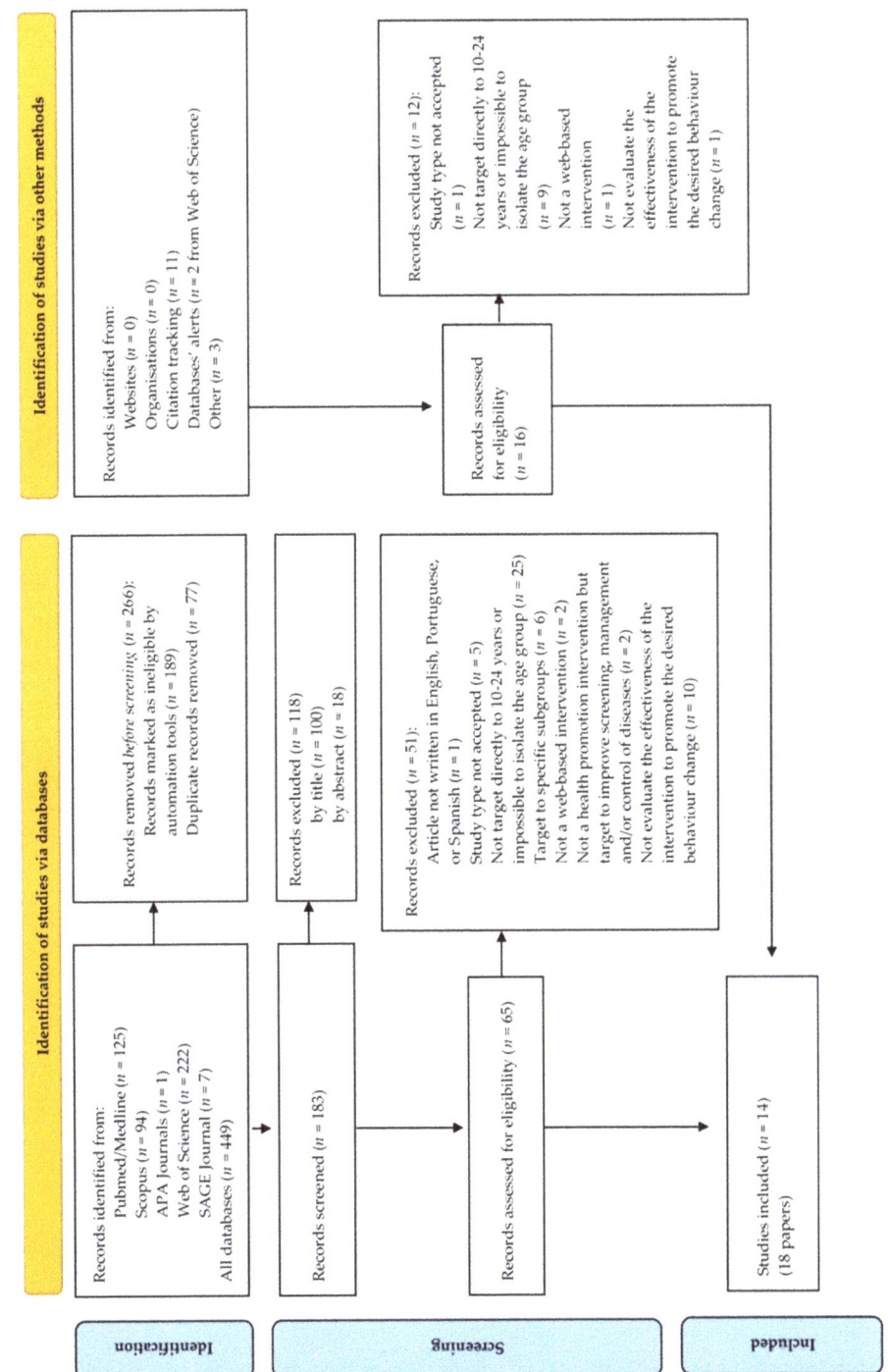

Figure 2. Study Flow Diagram adapted from: [18]. For more information, visit: http://www.prisma-statement.org/ (accessed on 29 January 2022).

The reference list of retrieved articles was searched, which resulted in 11 articles being added to be assessed for eligibility, two others were identified from databases' alerts and three more were found by searching the intervention names of the articles excluded because they did not evaluate the effectiveness of the intervention. In total, 16 records were identified via other methods, and their full texts were compared with our eligibility criteria; of those, 12 were excluded.

In total, 18 records met all the inclusion criteria, describing a total of 14 different interventions. We found five records with the same main author describing the same intervention (The eCHECKUP TO GO) [24–28], so prevent duplicate studies that might lead to biased results, we assessed the time of recruitment, the sample size, and the time of follow-up [29]. The decision was to include in the narrative synthesis the work of Doumas, D. M. et al., (2021) since it had the best combination of the longest time of follow-up (6 months) with the greatest sample size ($n = 311$) [28].

3.2. Description of the Studies

From among the 14 included studies, 6 were conducted in the United States of America (42.9%) [28,30–34], 3 in European countries (21.4%) [35–37], 3 in Asian countries (21.4%) [38–40] and 2 in Mexico (14.3%) [41,42]. Of those, 10 were implemented in an educational setting (71.4%) [28,30,32,33,37–42].

Concerning study design, seven studies were randomized controlled trials (50.0%) [28,32,33,35–37,40], four were quasi-experimental studies (28.6%) [38,39,41,42] and three had a pre and post-test design (21.4%) [30,31,34].

Regarding the desired behaviour change, four interventions intended to promote physical activity (28.6%) [30,31,38,39], one aimed to modify physical activity simultaneously with fruit and vegetable consumption (7.1%) [40], four were related to alcohol use (28.6%) [28,34,35,37], four tried to prevent risky sexual behaviours (28.6%) [33,36,41,42] and one proposed preventing tobacco use (7.1%) [32]. None of the sleep hygiene interventions records was found to meet the inclusion criteria.

Table 2. Summary of narrative synthesis of included studies.

Author, Year, Country	Setting	Study Design	Participants	Web-Based Intervention	Health Outcomes of Interest	Main Findings
Wilson, M. et al., (2017) [30] USA, North-western United States	School	One-group pre-/post-test design (pre-experimental)	N = 20 students (convenience sample) Mean age of 16.8 years.	Multicomponent Intervention: wearable digital tracking device using an Internet-based platform + group physical activities + nutrition group education/individual counselling session on healthy eating + weekly goal-setting sessions.	Measured at baseline and post-intervention: BMI calculation. Blood glucose level. Blood pressure and pulse measurements. Fitness and cardiovascular fitness. Cognitive and affective variables related to health behaviours. Adolescents' physical activity (PA) and healthy eating. Self-efficacy for PA and healthy eating. Self-determination. Screen time.	Participants showed improvements from pre-test to post-test in health and fitness markers (positive changes in weight, fitness, and cardiovascular measurements) and improved motivation toward PA and reduced screen time.
Larsen, B. et al., (2018) [31] USA (San Diego, CA)	Hispanic community	Pre/post-test design (Single-arm pilot trial)	N = 21 Latina adolescents Mean age of 14.7 years.	Website mobile phone friendly (tailored Internet-delivered activity manuals, computer-expert system tailored reports, activity tip sheets, and a guide of local activity resources)	Measured at baseline and follow-up (12 weeks): PA by 7-day physical activity recall (PAR) interview and ActiGraph GT3X+ accelerometers.	Results from the 7-day PAR showed that positive changes in PA at 12 weeks were seen not just in quantity but also in type. The usage of validated self-report measures showed to be better across accelerometers among this population since there are some activities in which the accelerometer may not be worn or that were not well measured by the accelerometer.
Huang, S.J. et al., (2019) [39] Taiwan, Taipei City	School	Quasi-experimental (Three-armed)	N initial = 617 students Mean age of 11.4 years.	Two experimental groups: One using a web-based exercise program applying a self-management strategy combined with geographical information system (GIS) mapping function with a narrative animated cartoon. The other was knowledge-only using only the animated story.	Measured at baseline, immediately post and 3-month follow-up: PA by the Chinese version of the Child/Adolescent Activity Log. Exercise-related self-efficacy using a 5-item Exercise-Related-Self-Efficacy Scale. Perceived benefit of PA using a self-developed 7-item Perceived-Benefit-of-Exercise Scale.	This intervention using self-management strategy + GIS mapping function was effective in producing small but significant increases in school children's self-efficacy and PA. The perceived benefit and self-efficacy of regular PA might have partly affected the participants' PA levels because the self-efficacy factor was always higher for both experimental groups than for the control at the post-test and follow-up; it was also higher for the self-management group than for the knowledge-only group. The intervention was more effective for male students than females.

Table 2. *Cont.*

Author, Year, Country	Setting	Study Design	Participants	Web-Based Intervention	Health Outcomes of Interest	Main Findings
Pirzadeh, A. et al., (2020) [38] Iran, Isfahan	University	Quasi-experimental	N = 278 high school students. Mean age is not described.	Two web-based intervention groups. One group received education through a website with tailored education strategies based on TTM. The second group only received general education by the same website but without tailored materials.	Measured before intervention and 6 months after: Stage of exercise behaviour change questionnaire. Processes of change questionnaire. Decision-making balance questionnaire. Exercise self-efficacy scale. International PA questionnaire short form.	Education on PA based on the website can be effective. The percentage of students with low, moderate, and severe levels of physical activity in the two intervention groups has increased significantly after the intervention. Participants showed significant progress during stages of change post-intervention and changes were greater in the group who was trained by the TTM.
Duan, Y. P. et al., (2017) [40] China, Central Region	University	Randomized controlled trial	N initial = 493 N post-intervention = 337 N 1-month follow-up = 142 Mean age of 19.2 years.	Web-based intervention modules target social–cognitive indicators for health behaviour change for Physical Activity and Fruit and Vegetable Intake (FVI) (information about risks and benefits, motivating intentions to change, identification of barriers, goal setting, development of action plans, coping plans and social support, providing tailored normative feedback).	PA by Chinese short version of the International Physical Activity Questionnaire (IPAQ-C). FVI in the past 7 days. Stages of behavioural change for PA and FVI. Social–cognitive indicators of behaviour change: positive and negative outcome expectancies for PA and FVI; self-efficacy for PA and FVI; action planning; coping planning; social support; intentions for PA and FVI; habit scale.	Students in the intervention group reported more FVI over time. Average FVI for the intervention group were all greater than the recommended amounts at the end of the 8-week intervention and the 1-month follow-up. In terms of PA behaviour, there was no significant interaction effect. Positive results on stage progression for the PA and FVI. All 6 tests revealed significant treatment effects on motivational, volitional, and distal indicators of PA and FVI over time.
Khalil, G. E. et al., (2017) [32] USA, Texas, Houston	School	Randomized controlled trial (2-arm single-blinded)	N = 101 adolescents Mean age of 13.4 years.	Two web-based intervention groups: One features interactivity and entertainment to engage adolescent users (text, animations, videos, task-oriented activities, two-dimensional environment to explore health information and make a virtual character). The second included the same health information but without any features of interactivity or entertainment.	Measured at baseline and follow-up: Intention to smoke using items adapted from the susceptibility to smoke scale.	The more participants considered intervention interactive and entertaining, the more they were probably going to show a reduction in their intention to smoke. Perceived interactivity had a more grounded relationship with the reduction in intention to smoke than perceived entertainment.

Table 2. Cont.

Author, Year, Country	Setting	Study Design	Participants	Web-Based Intervention	Health Outcomes of Interest	Main Findings
Castillo-Arcos L del, C. et al., (2016) [42] Mexico, Urban Mexico	School	Quasi-experimental (single-stage cluster sampling)	N = 193 participants Mean age of 15.8 years.	Multicomponent intervention: 6 online sessions + 2 face-to-face activities aimed at increasing levels of social competence and resilience about sexual behaviours.	Measured pre-and post-intervention: Self-reported risky sexual behaviours (defined as self-reporting unprotected sex, multiple concurrent sexual partners, and alcohol or drug use during sex). Resilience to risky sexual behaviour (defined as the ability to identify and practice strategies to avoid risky sexual behaviour).	The intervention was independently associated with improved self-reported resilience to risky sexual behaviours though not with a significant reduction in those behaviours in multivariate analyses. Participant age mediated the effect of the intervention on resilience, influencing the effectiveness of the intervention.
Doubova, S. V. et al., (2017) [41] Mexico, Mexico City	School	Quasi-experimental (field trial)	N = 833 adolescents Mean age is not described.	Multicomponent intervention: Educational sessions through a website displayed by two central characters + class discussions Main topics: dating, courtship, sexual relationships, misconceptions and myths about gender roles and sexual relationships, partner abuse, STIs, early pregnancy, self-esteem, safe sex, use of condoms and condom negotiation.	Measured at baseline, at the end of the four educational sessions (first month), and the end of the follow-up period (fourth month): Knowledge of STIs. Multidimensional Condom Attitudes Scale measuring attitudes regarding condom use. Self-efficacy toward consistent condom use.	The intervention had a positive effect on improving adolescents' knowledge of STIs, attitudes and self-efficacy toward consistent condom use. In the intervention group, the average knowledge of STIs increased by 30 points compared to the control group. An increase in positive attitudes and self-efficacy toward consistent condom use was also observed more often in the intervention group.
Brown, K. E. et al., (2018) [36] United Kingdom (UK), Midlands	Clinical (sexual health service)	Pilot randomized controlled trial (two-armed parallel-group)	N initial = 88 integrated sexual health service attendees N follow-up = 67 Mean age of 20.0 years.	Multicomponent intervention: brief tailored web-based programme + paper-based action planning card. Content about contraceptive pills and/or condoms use using characters with audio to take the user through the process of identifying environmental cues to key target behaviours and planning to perform those behaviours when the environmental cue is present.	Measured at baseline and 3-month follow-up: Self-reported contraceptive pill or condom "mishaps" in the past 3 months. Contraceptive pill or condom use intention. Attitude toward contraceptive pill or condom use. Perceived behavioural control over pill or condom use. Subjective norm relating to pill or condom use. Trait self-control.	The intervention supported pill and condom users to produce quality plans since potential improvements were identified. Bivariate correlations suggest that perceived behavioural control may have a role over method use within intervention content. Additionally, having greater levels of trait self-control may negatively affect plan quality. The study suggests early indications that the intervention could reduce the number of mishaps of intervention participants.

Table 2. *Cont.*

Author, Year, Country	Setting	Study Design	Participants	Web-Based Intervention	Health Outcomes of Interest	Main Findings
Widman, L. et al., (2018) [33] USA, South-eastern	School	Randomized Controlled Trial	N = 222 tenth-grade girls Mean age of 15.2 years.	Interactive, skills-focused web-based intervention. The intervention includes 5 modules about safer sex motivation, HIV and other STDs, sexual norms and attitudes, safer sex self-efficacy, sexual communication skills that can be completed on a computer, tablet, or smartphone device. Each module used audio and video clips, tips from other adolescents, interactive games and quizzes, infographics, and skill-building exercises with self-feedback given in real-time).	Measured at pre-test, post-test and 4-month follow-up: Behavioural assessment of sexual assertiveness skills (at refusing unwanted sexual activity and negotiating condom use). Self-reported sexual assertiveness by Multidimensional Sexual Self Concept Scale. Knowledge regarding HIV and other STDs. Intentions to use condoms and to communicate about sex with items from the AIDS Risk Behaviour Assessment. Sexual Self-Efficacy from self-efficacy for HIV prevention scale.	Immediately post-test, the intervention group showed better sexual assertiveness skills measured with a behavioural task, higher self-reported assertiveness, intentions to communicate about sexual health, knowledge regarding HIV and other STDs, safer sex norms and attitudes, and condom self-efficacy compared with the control condition. At a 4-month follow-up, group differences remained in knowledge regarding HIV and other STDs, condom attitudes, and condom self-efficacy.
Arnaud, N. et al., (2016) [35] European countries (Sweden, Germany, Belgium, and the Czech Republic)	Online	Randomized controlled trial (Two-armed multisite)	N initial = 1449 adolescents (Convenience sample) N follow-up = 211 Mean age of 16.8 years.	Interactive web-based system to generate individually tailored content. Generated information in small units using text and graphics and referred to previous participants' statements.	Measured at baseline and 3-month follow-up: Self-reported drinking index (drinking frequency, frequency of binge drinking, and typical quantity of drinks) using AUDIT-C screening tool.	Self-reported risky drinking as measured by a drinking index was significantly reduced for participants in the intervention group. Statistically significant mean differences at follow-up in favour of the intervention were found for drinking frequency and binge drinking frequency but not for quantity when missing follow-up data were not imputed. In contrast, analyses using an EM-imputed dataset revealed drinking quantity as the only significant secondary effect.

Table 2. *Cont.*

Author, Year, Country	Setting	Study Design	Participants	Web-Based Intervention	Health Outcomes of Interest	Main Findings
Norman, P. et al., (2018) [37] UK, large city	University	Randomized controlled trial (full-factorial design)	N initial = 2,951 students before starting university N post-intervention = 2681 Mean age of 18.8 years.	Brief online intervention combining self-affirmation x TPB-based messages x implementation intentions in a factorial design.	Measured at baseline, 1-week, 1-month and 6-month follow-up: Self-reported alcohol intake (total number of units consumed and number of binge drinking sessions/week). Hazardous and harmful patterns of alcohol use from 10-item AUDIT (only at 6-month follow-up). Cognitions about binge drinking (intention, affective attitude, cognitive attitude, subjective norms, descriptive norms, and perceived control) and extent of endorsement for the beliefs (Engaging in binge drinking at university would be fun; engaging in binge drinking at university would have a negative impact on my studies; my friends engaging in binge drinking would make my binge drinking at university more likely).	TPB-based messages had significant effects on reducing the quantity of alcohol consumed, frequency of binge drinking and harmful patterns of alcohol use over the first 6 months at university. Its effects did not diminish over time. The messages also had significant positive effects on intentions to binge drink, cognitive attitudes, subjective norms, descriptive norms, and self-efficacy, although some effects weakened over time. The effects on the quantity of alcohol and frequency of binge drinking were mediated by TPB variables with significant indirect effects through intention and self-efficacy. The effect sizes for the TPB-based messages on the quantity of alcohol consumed (d = 0.20) and the frequency of binge drinking (d = 0.17) were small. Messages were sufficiently relevant and persuasive to produce changes in behaviour without the need to form if-then plans. Non-significant effects were found for self-affirmation and forming implementation intentions.
Coughlin, L. N. et al., (2021) [34] USA, Michigan	Online	Pre/post-test design (Pilot study)	N = 39 participants Mean age of 20.7 years.	Mobile intervention with tailored messages and tips, inspirational images to reinforce content, web links to articles, or other web-based resources, based on users' responses to daily and weekly surveys. The intervention included gamification through a virtual aquarium environment.	Measured at baseline and 1-month follow-up: Concerning alcohol use (quantity and frequency of use, consequences of use, intention, importance confidence of change, perceived risk, reasons for use, and past month driving under influence of use).	Participants' substance use declined over time, and those reporting using the app more often reported less substance use (including fewer days drinking alcohol, binge drinking, fewer consequences of use and episodes of driving after drinking) at the 1-month follow-up than those who reported using the app less often.

Table 2. *Cont.*

Author, Year, Country	Setting	Study Design	Participants	Web-Based Intervention	Health Outcomes of Interest	Main Findings
Doumas, D. M. et al., (2021) [28] USA, Northwest region	School	Randomized controlled trial	$N = 311$ high school seniors. Mean age of 17.1 years old.	Online personalized normative feedback intervention via text, graphs, and video recordings. The program is intended to reduce risk factors for alcohol use and increase protective behaviours.	Measured at baseline, 30-day and 6-month follow-up: Weekly drinking quantity. Estimated peak blood alcohol concentration (eBAC). Self-reported peak alcohol volume. Classification of High-Risk vs. Low-Risk drinkers by participants' report on the frequency of binge drinking in the past month.	The intervention effects were moderated by risk status, such that high-risk students in the intervention condition reported a greater reduction in alcohol use relative to students in the control condition. For weekly drinking quantity, intervention effects were limited to the baseline to 30-day follow-up period. Among high-risk students was found a significant decrease in weekly drinking in the intervention condition. However, intervention effects from baseline to the 6-month follow-up were not significant since the control condition also reported significant decreases in weekly drinking. For eBAC, intervention effects were evident at the 30-day follow-up and were sustained at the 6-month follow-up. Specifically, among high-risk students, we found a significant decrease in eBAC relative at the 30-day and 6-month follow-up. It is unclear why sustained intervention effects were found for eBAC but not for weekly drinking. Non-significant intervention effects for low-risk drinkers.

3.3. Recruitment and Participants

Our review encompasses data from 7616 participants, with 10 included studies having relatively small size samples (≤150 subjects per study's condition or control) [28,30–34,36,38,39,42]. Sample sizes ranged from 20 subjects in the published work from Wilson, M. et al., (2017) [30] to almost 3000 participants in the study from Norman, P. et al., (2018) [37].

Data included in our review were collected from participants aged 10 to 24 years old, with an average mean age of 16.7, from all studies, except two of them who did not indicate the mean age of subjects [38,41]. The majority of the studies included older adolescents (aged > 14 years old) [28,30,33,35,37,38,41,42], only one was focused only on younger adolescents [39], two also encompassed younger adolescents (aged ≤ 14 years old) alongside older ones [31,32], and three also analysed emerging adults (aged < 25 years old) [34,36,40].

Concerning ethnic background, most interventions were tested in Caucasian participants [28,30,33–37], three focused on Asian participants [38–40], another three were implemented in Hispanic participants [31,41,42] and one mostly included both Hispanic (43.6%) and Afro-American participants (41.6%) [32].

There were more females than males in most studies [28,30,34,37,40–42], with two of the included studies only targeting girls [31,33], yet none were targeted only to male participants. In three studies, slightly more than half of the sample were men [32,35,39]. No information about sex representativity was available in Brown, K. E. et al., (2018) [36] and Pirzadeh, A. et al., (2020) [38].

In most of the studies, recruitment was achieved through educational institutions using institution-wide announcements, information sessions in lectures, classrooms, or after-school program meetings, and by sending emails and letters to participants and parents when applied [28,30,32,33,37–42]. Social media advertisements [34,35], announcements in health promotion sites, open access to the intervention's website landing page [35], printed promotion materials distributed in public areas (such as schools, cafes, bars, stores, youth meetings and health-focused community events) [31,35], referencing by other participants [31] and using a brief verbal introduction and printed material presented by the staff to clinical attendees [36] were other recruitment strategies identified in the included studies.

These recruitment strategies resulted in non-probabilistic samples in all these trials, so results may not be generalized to out-of-sample contexts.

In eight studies, financial rewards, gift cards, giveaway items and prize draws were used as incentives for retention [28,30,32–35,37,42].

Only three studies had 6 months of follow up [28,37,38]. The others had a shorter length of study follow-up (<6 months) [31,33–36,39–41] and three of them did not include follow-up measurements aside from the moment immediately post-intervention [30,32,42].

3.4. Web-Based Interventions

A variety of web-based interventions were evaluated in the included articles, from brief online interventions based on text messaging delivered through e-mail with multimedia content links [37] or wearable digital tracking devices to record data and provide feedback on progress using an internet-based platform [30], to websites using narrative and animation to deliver content and challenges into a real-life context combined with a geographical information system to record progress [39].

Nearly half of them were at least somewhat tailored [33–36,38,40] and the degree of customization was also variable, ranging from interactive systems designed to generate individually tailored content matching participants' response choices [35,36] to intervention elements that were consistent with the participants' level of motivation/readiness to change and personalized reports on the participants' progress [29] according to their questionnaire responses.

From among our 14 included articles, 10 interventions were exclusively internet-based and used the web to deliver all intervention components including the online data collection [26,29,32–34,36–39]. Most were delivered through a website and one of them was presented as a mobile application to create a gamification environment, a data collection field and shared affiliation links to other web-based resources [30]. However, in the other four studies, the web-based component was merely one element of a multicomponent intervention, such as using a wearable digital tracking device to record progress in an internet-based platform combined with workshops, lectures, and goal setting counselling face-to-face with professionals [31] or a brief tailored web-based programme with paper-based action planning cards [35], or to support online educational sessions with face-to-face sessions [41] or class discussions [40].

All our identified trials were health promotion interventions and included content to promote behavioural change on a range of topics, such as dietary patterns and healthy eating, physical activity, alcohol and tobacco use, and sexual behaviour.

3.5. Behaviour Change Theories and Techniques

All the included studies were theory-based interventions. Some of them were constructed based on only one theory or model, such as the Transtheoretical Model/Stages of Change [37], Operant Conditioning Theory [30], Information–Motivation–Behavioural Skills Model [40], Conceptual Framework of Adolescent Sexual Resilience [41], Theory of Motivational Interviewing [34], Health Action Process Approach [39], and the Self-efficacy Theory as a subset of the Social Cognitive Theory [31]. In contrast, other studies relied on more than one theoretical model, combining, namely: the Social Cognitive Theory with the Transtheoretical/Stages of Change Model [29], the Experiential Learning Theory and the Extended Elaboration Likelihood Model [32], the Theory of Planned Behaviour with the Health Action Process Approach [35] or with Self-affirmation and Implementation Intentions [36], the Social Cognitive Theory and the Health Belief Model [38], the Social Norming Theory with Motivational Enhancement models [26], as well as the Reasoned Action Model and Fuzzy Trace Theory with multiple others psychological and health behaviour change techniques [33].

3.6. Effectiveness of the Web-Based Interventions

Among the 14 included studies, three used differences between pre and post-test assessment [30,31,34] to document their effectiveness, while the remaining 11 based their findings on differences from intervention group to control groups, using active and non-active-control groups. Namely, six studies used a control group as assessment-only [28,35–38,40]; three studies used a non-web-based educational intervention as the control group, with one regarding the study outcome [41], while the other two were about generic health themes other than the one being studied [39,42]; the last two were web-based interventions, where one was about an unrelated health theme [33] and the other used a website with only written content and without interactivity or entertainment features [32].

Thirteen of the fourteen studied interventions revealed significant positive findings that support web-based intervention effectiveness in promoting health behaviour change, namely in improving motivation [30] and the practice of physical activity [31,38,39] as well as positive changes in weight, fitness and cardiovascular measurements [30]; in decreasing self-reported problematic alcohol use [28,34,35,37] and alcohol-related consequences [34]; in improving sex norms and attitudes, self-efficacy, self-reported sexual assertiveness skills, intentions to communicate about sexual health, knowledge concerning to sexually transmitted diseases and condom use [33,41] and to mitigate the numbers of mishaps in pill and condom use [36]; in reducing intention to smoke in non-smokers [32]; and in increasing fruit and vegetable intake [40].

Although the study from Castillo-Arcos Ldel, C. et al., (2016) had observed a crude reduction in risky sexual behaviours in the intervention group, they were not able to show a significant reduction in those behaviours using multivariate analyses since unexpected effects in pre and post-test scores occurred in the control group. It is important to note that the control group was subjected to the visualization of an educational video aimed to improve general health status, focusing on unhealthy food habits, mental health disorders, drug use, violence, and accidents [42].

3.7. Other Outcomes

The most frequent non-health-related outcome measured in the included studies was acceptability [30,31,34,36,39,41], but feasibility [30,31,36], engagement [32,34], adherence [30,31] and usability [30] were also evaluated in some studies.

The main aim of some of the studies was even to test feasibility and acceptability, being the evaluation of potential efficacy, a secondary objective given the pilot nature of those trials [30,31,34,36].

In these studies, the interventions overall proved to have reasonable levels of acceptability (ranging from moderate [31,36] to good [30,34,39,41]) and good feasibility [30,31,36,42]. As positive features, web-based interventions were classified by participants as easy to use [34], interactive and entertaining [32]. The time demanded to accomplish proposed activities [41], technical problems [34] and high drop-out rates [35,40] were negative aspects of some of these interventions.

3.8. Risk of Bias Assessment

The critical appraisal of individual studies performed using the Effective Public Health Practice Project—Quality Assessment Tool for Quantitative Studies (EPHPP) [23] for selection bias, study design, confounders, blinding, data collection methods, withdrawals and drop-outs are described in Table 3. Overall, the EPHPP tool showed the low quality of study methodology since 12 studies were classified as weak [28,30,31,33–40,42] and two as moderate [32,41].

Table 3. Risk of Bias Assessment—EPHPP Assessment Tool for Quantitative Studies.

Author, Year	Section Rating						Global Rating
	Selection Bias	Study Design	Confounders	Blinding	Data Collection Methods	Withdrawals and Drop-Outs	
Doumas, D. M. et al., (2021) [28]	WEAK	STRONG	STRONG	WEAK	STRONG	MODERATE	WEAK
Wilson, M. et al., (2017) [30]	WEAK	MODERATE	STRONG	WEAK	STRONG	MODERATE	WEAK
Larsen, B. et al., (2018) [31]	WEAK	MODERATE	STRONG	WEAK	STRONG	STRONG	WEAK
Khalil, G. E. et al., (2017) [32]	WEAK	STRONG	STRONG	WEAK	WEAK	NOT APPLICABLE	WEAK
Widman, L. et al., (2018) [33]	MODERATE	STRONG	STRONG	WEAK	WEAK	STRONG	WEAK
Coughlin, L. N. et al., (2021) [34]	WEAK	MODERATE	STRONG	WEAK	STRONG	STRONG	WEAK
Arnaud, N. et al., (2016) [35]	WEAK	STRONG	STRONG	WEAK	STRONG	WEAK	WEAK
Brown, K. E. et al., (2018) [36]	MODERATE	STRONG	STRONG	WEAK	STRONG	STRONG	MODERATE
Norman, P. et al., (2018) [37]	WEAK	STRONG	STRONG	WEAK	STRONG	WEAK	WEAK
Pirzadeh, A. et al., (2020) [38]	WEAK	STRONG	WEAK	WEAK	STRONG	STRONG	WEAK
Huang, S. J. et al., (2019) [39]	MODERATE	STRONG	STRONG	WEAK	MODERATE	WEAK	WEAK
Duan, Y. P. et al., (2017) [40]	MODERATE	STRONG	WEAK	WEAK	STRONG	WEAK	WEAK
Doubova, S. V. et al., (2017) [41]	WEAK	STRONG	STRONG	MODERATE	STRONG	STRONG	MODERATE
Castillo-Arcos Ldel, C. et al., (2016) [42]	WEAK	STRONG	STRONG	WEAK	WEAK	MODERATE	WEAK

4. Discussion
4.1. Summary of Findings

Most previous systematic reviews about digital health interventions are limited to the self-management of clinical conditions or symptoms instead of focusing on health promotion [43–47] or try to understand only one major health outcome change such as nutrition-related behaviours [48–51], sedentary behaviours [52] and physical activity [53], depression and mental health [54], alcohol-related problems [55] and their target population is other than adolescents such as adults [56] and older adults [57].

Although one previous review and meta-analysis performed by Wantland, D. J. et al., (2004) had found substantial evidence that the use of web-based interventions could improve knowledge and/or behavioural change outcomes when compared with non-web-based interventions, that one focused on the general population [58].

Since we hypothesized that its effectiveness could be more relevant in a very digital-skilled population, such as young people, our review intended to evaluate the effectiveness of web-based interventions in health behaviour change in adolescents. Moreover, due to the rapid growth of the technological field, an update focused on the most recent literature was justified.

As well as the work from Wantland, D. J. et al., (2004) [58], our systematic review also showed positive effects of internet-based interventions to achieve health behaviour change, including increased motivation [30] and physical activity level [30,31,38,39], decreased harmful alcohol use and its consequences [28,34,35,37], improved attitudes, self-efficacy, assertiveness skills, intentions to communicate and knowledge concerning to sexual behaviours [33,36,41], decreased intention to smoke [32], and increased fruit and vegetable consumption [40].

However, these findings relied mostly on small sample sizes [28,30–34,36,38,39,42], non-probabilistic samples, and studies with a lower length of follow-up, very context-specific [28,30–42], which limits the generalizability of the results, as already described in the literature [59].

In addition, although all studies analysed presented statistically significant differences between groups (control vs. intervention or pre-test vs. post-test), not all evaluated the intervention effect size [31,36] and when they do, different analytic estimators were used, compromising the quantitative summary and interpretation of the dimension of the differences.

In addition to the widely used statistical significance, the use of effect size for each outcome should also be promoted, as it would allow for more detailed reading and interpretation of results [60].

Although our review suggests that web-based interventions are a promising approach to achieve health behaviour change, robust evidence from larger randomized controlled trials, from the population's representative samples, with proven relevant effects, is still needed.

A wide range of web-based interventions was found. It is worth noticing that the more interactive and entertaining the intervention was, the higher was the participants' retention in the study. It also increases the intervention's acceptability and feasibility [32]. Overall, web-based interventions seem to have moderate to good acceptability and feasibility [30,31,34,36,39,41,42].

In contrast to the previous literature [61], we found that researchers are largely developing interventions based on theoretical frameworks and models, which has been shown to improve an intervention's effectiveness [62]. Critical points to the quality of evidence seem to be mainly related to sampling issues, representativeness of populations and absence of blinding. We identified that some important information, which is required by risk assessment tools, is sometimes non-available or unclear. The previous literature also underlines that researchers should include more detailed descriptions of their web-based interventions to achieve improved research designs [63]. Therefore, examining in advance all the domains evaluated in these tools may help researchers to conduct more robust methodological studies with a higher quality of evidence.

Even though web-based interventions seem to be a promising approach in health behaviour change with positive acceptability among adolescents, robust evidence is still lacking. We keep making the same errors as in the past since we still lack results from larger randomized controlled trials from high-quality papers (lower risk of bias), with representative samples and testing the long-term maintenance of these health behaviour changes (time of follow-up > 6 months). These limitations are known by most of the authors, who refer to them in their papers [28,30–35,39–41]. Nonetheless, it is crucial to identify why they keep being reported repeatedly and, moreover, try to overcome them. It was also frequent that studies were being classified as pilot projects, highlighting the need to study the effectiveness of the intervention in other studies, but never publishing those randomized controlled trials with the sample size needed for the effect size wanted. This may partially be explained by the lack of financial resources as well as time availability. Planning, developing, ensuring internal testing and usability testing is very time-demanding and costly research since the development of a web-based intervention is often a back and forward process [15]. With limited funding and restricted time to accomplish the intervention, most researchers will fail in providing robust evidence. We suggest that more than developing new web-based interventions, researchers should unify their strengths and resources to largely test the existing intervention in different cultural contexts within different populations.

4.2. Limitations of This Review

The present review is intended to summarize the most relevant evidence available to assess the effectiveness of web-based interventions to promote health behaviour change in adolescents. We acknowledge that our selection of 2016 as the oldest reference comports the risk of excluding previous robust evidence. However, the recent global increment of the importance of the web in our daily life and the emergence of other digital innovative technologies justify our focus.

It is also a fact that in the last two years, the resources and efforts of the worldwide scientific community have focused on the issue of COVID-19, mitigating the investment in health-promotion interventions for children and adolescents, since the educational context where these interventions were often implemented has undergone critical adaptations. This may partially justify the reduced number of included papers despite the growing trend observed during the last years. Nevertheless, the mandatory lockdown reinforced the need to invest in technological health promotion strategies that may be implemented at a distance, large scale and with almost the same financial and human resources.

We are aware that, due to time restrictions, we left out other databases relevant to this topic, such as EMBASE, ERIC, B-on, and Emerald, among others. It has been suggested that piloting a sample of records through every review's step, such as producing a "mini" review, could be used to effectively change the criteria in the data extraction table to ensure that the full review would include the most useful and relevant information, removing the need to re-visit the papers at a later phase [58]. Thus, we can consider this work as a "mini" systematic review since an update should be performed by running the search query in other relevant databases. In addition, searching in grey literature, which was not included in this review, could expand the number of eligible publications. Even though publication bias has been largely documented in the literature, it seems that this bias is increasing. It could be explained by the higher competition between researchers that tend to publish positive results rather than negative ones [59]. For this reason, searching the grey literature would give us a more realistic summary of evidence.

The main limitations of the present review include the combination of results from well-designed and less rigorously designed studies, their heterogeneity of studies in terms of setting, interventions, methods and outcome measures, and the lack of included records on sleep hygiene. Additionally, the absence of analysis by subgroups of health outcomes and active components of the behaviour change intervention may be considered a limitation.

However, the low number of studies that used each health area and each behaviour change technique did not allow this analysis to be performed.

In addition to these limitations, to our knowledge, this is the first systematic review summarizing the effectiveness of web-based interventions in promoting a wide range of health behaviour changes focused specifically on adolescents. Important findings were highlighted to help researchers to reach high-quality evidence in the development and evaluation of web-based interventions. Authors should discuss the results and how they can be interpreted from the perspective of previous studies and of the working hypotheses. The findings and their implications should be discussed in the broadest context possible. Future research directions may also be highlighted.

5. Conclusions

Our findings support that web-based interventions significantly contribute to achieving health behaviour change among adolescents, regarding physical activity, eating habits, tobacco and alcohol use and sexual behaviour, with reasonable levels of acceptability and feasibility. Additionally, more evidence is needed to prove their effectiveness in long-term maintenance, since there are few studies with follow-up assessments longer than 6 months. As shown by the critical assessment of the risk of bias, these findings are of low-quality evidence, so it is urgent to test these web-based interventions in larger randomized controlled trials, within probabilistic samples, ideally in single or double-blinded design and testing the long-term maintenance of these health behaviour changes (time of follow-up > 6 months).

Supplementary Materials: The following are available online at https://www.mdpi.com/article/10.3390/nu14061258/s1, Table S1: Search terms. Table S2: Excel spreadsheet with extracted data from included studies. Table S3: Data extracted about Recruitment and Participants. Table S4: Data extracted about web-based intervention and behaviour change theories. Table S5: Data extracted about secondary outcomes.

Author Contributions: D.d.S. was responsible for the first draft of this manuscript and this systematic review's protocol. D.d.S. and A.F. performed the full-text screening against eligibility criteria, risk of bias (quality) assessment and data extraction. P.P. and J.A. contributed to this study protocol conception and design. All the authors critically revised the manuscript and gave their final approval. All authors have read and agreed to the published version of the manuscript.

Funding: This review was funded by national funds through the FCT—Foundation for Science and Technology, I.P., under the project UIDB/04750/2020. Additionally, an individual PhD grant attributed to AF (2021.08877.BD) was funded by FCT—Fundação para a Ciência e a Tecnologia and the European Social Fund (ESF).

Institutional Review Board Statement: Not applicable.

Informed Consent Statement: Not applicable.

Conflicts of Interest: The authors declare no conflict of interest. The funders had no role in the design, analysis or writing of this paper.

References

1. Davis, R.; Campbell, R.; Hildon, Z.; Hobbs, L.; Michie, S. Theories of behaviour and behaviour change across the social and behavioural sciences: A scoping review. *Health Psychol. Rev.* **2015**, *9*, 323–344. [CrossRef]
2. Every Woman Every Child. *The Global Strategy for Women's, Children's and Adolescents' Health (2016–2030)*; United Nations: New York, NY, USA, 2015.
3. National Research Council (US) and Institute of Medicine (US) Committee on Adolescent Health Care Services and Models of Care for Treatment Prevention, and Healthy Development. Adolescents Health Status. In *Adolescent Health Services-Missing Opportunities*; Robert, S., Lawrence, J.A.G., Leslie, J.S., Eds.; National Academies Press: Washington, DC, USA, 2009; pp. 52–133.
4. Kathryn, L.; Santoro, C.S.; Schoenman, J.; Myers, C.; Chockley, N. *The Case for Investing in Youth Health Literacy: One Step on the Path to Achieving Health Equity for Adolescents*; National Institute for Health Care Management Research and Educational Foundation: Washington, DC, USA, 2011.

5. World Health Organization. *Global Accelerated Action for the Health of Adolescents (AA-HA!): Guidance to Support Country Implementation*; Licence: CC BY-NC-SA 3.0 IGO.; World Health Organization: Geneva, Switzerland, 2017.
6. Lehtimaki, S.S.N.; Solis, L. *Adolescent Health: The Missing Population in Universal Health Coverage*; World Health Organization: Geneva, Switzerland, 2019.
7. Steinberg, L. How to Improve the Health of American Adolescents. *Perspect Psychol. Sci.* **2015**, *10*, 711–715. [CrossRef] [PubMed]
8. Kann, L.; McManus, T.; Harris, W.A.; Shanklin, S.L.; Flint, K.H.; Queen, B.; Lowry, R.; Chyen, D.; Whittle, L.; Thornton, J.; et al. Youth Risk Behaviour Surveillance-United States, 2017. *MMWR Surveill. Summ.* **2018**, *67*, 1–114. [CrossRef] [PubMed]
9. Tylee, A.; Haller, D.M.; Graham, T.; Churchill, R.; Sanci, L.A. Youth-friendly primary-care services: How are we doing and what more needs to be done? *Lancet* **2007**, *369*, 1565–1573. [CrossRef]
10. Petrescu, D.G.; Tribus, L.C.; Raducu, R.; Purcarea, V.L. Social marketing and behavioural change. *Rom. J. Ophthalmol.* **2021**, *65*, 101–103. [CrossRef]
11. Chichirez, C.M.; Purcărea, V.L. Health marketing and behavioural change: A review of the literature. *J. Med. Life* **2018**, *11*, 15–19.
12. Michie, S.; Richardson, M.; Johnston, M.; Abraham, C.; Francis, J.; Hardeman, W.; Eccles, M.P.; Cane, J.; Wood, C.E. The behaviour change technique taxonomy (v1) of 93 hierarchically clustered techniques: Building an international consensus for the reporting of behaviour change interventions. *Ann. Behav. Med.* **2013**, *46*, 81–95. [CrossRef]
13. Milne-Ives, M.; Lam, C.; De Cock, C.; Van Velthoven, M.H.; Meinert, E. Mobile Apps for Health Behaviour Change in Physical Activity, Diet, Drug and Alcohol Use, and Mental Health: Systematic Review. *JMIR Mhealth Uhealth* **2020**, *8*, e17046. [CrossRef]
14. Meskó, B.; Drobni, Z.; Bényei, É.; Gergely, B.; Gyorffy, Z. Digital health is a cultural transformation of traditional healthcare. *mHealth* **2017**, *3*, 38. [CrossRef]
15. Horvath, K.J.; Ecklund, A.M.; Hunt, S.L.; Nelson, T.F.; Toomey, T.L. Developing Internet-based health interventions: A guide for public health researchers and practitioners. *J. Med. Internet Res.* **2015**, *17*, e28. [CrossRef]
16. Teixeira, P.J.; Marques, M.M. Health Behaviour Change for Obesity Management. *Obes. Facts* **2017**, *10*, 666–673. [CrossRef]
17. Ronquillo, Y.; Meyers, A.; Korvek, S.J. Digital Health. In *StatPearls*; StatPearls Publishing LLC.: Treasure Island, FL, USA, 2021.
18. Page, M.J.; McKenzie, J.E.; Bossuyt, P.M.; Boutron, I.; Hoffmann, T.C.; Mulrow, C.D.; Shamseer, L.; Tetzlaff, J.M.; Akl, E.A.; Brennan, S.E.; et al. The PRISMA 2020 statement: An updated guideline for reporting systematic reviews. *BMJ* **2021**, *372*, n71. [CrossRef]
19. Schwab, K. *The Fourth Industrial Revolution: What It Means, How to Respond*; World Economic Forum (Cologny, Geneva): Geneva, Switzerland, 2016. Available online: https://www.weforum.org/agenda/2016/01/the-fourth-industrial-revolution-what-it-means-and-how-to-respond/ (accessed on 27 June 2021).
20. Sawyer, S.M.; Azzopardi, P.S.; Wickremarathne, D.; Patton, G.C. The age of adolescence. *Lancet Child. Adolesc. Health* **2018**, *2*, 223–228. [CrossRef]
21. Barak, A.; Klein, B.; Proudfoot, J.G. Defining Internet-Supported Therapeutic Interventions. *Ann. Behav. Med.* **2009**, *38*, 4–17. [CrossRef]
22. Armijo-Olivo, S.; Stiles, C.R.; Hagen, N.A.; Biondo, P.D.; Cummings, G.G. Assessment of study quality for systematic reviews: A comparison of the Cochrane Collaboration Risk of Bias Tool and the Effective Public Health Practice Project Quality Assessment Tool: Methodological research. *J. Eval. Clin. Pract.* **2012**, *18*, 12–18. [CrossRef]
23. Thomas, B.H.; Ciliska, D.; Dobbins, M.; Micucci, S. A process for systematically reviewing the literature: Providing the research evidence for public health nursing interventions. *Worldviews Evid. Based Nurs.* **2004**, *1*, 176–184. [CrossRef]
24. Doumas, D.M.; Esp, S. Reducing Alcohol-Related Consequences Among High School Seniors: Efficacy of a Brief, Web-Based Intervention. *J. Couns. Dev.* **2019**, *97*, 53–61. [CrossRef]
25. Doumas, D.M.; Esp, S.; Flay, B.; Bond, L. A Randomized Controlled Trial Testing the Efficacy of a Brief Online Alcohol Intervention for High School Seniors. *J. Stud. Alcohol Drugs* **2017**, *78*, 706–715. [CrossRef]
26. Doumas, D.M.; Esp, S.; Johnson, J.; Trull, R.; Shearer, K. The eCHECKUP TO GO for High School: Impact on risk factors and protective behavioural strategies for alcohol use. *Addict. Behav.* **2017**, *64*, 93–100. [CrossRef]
27. Doumas, D.M.; Hausheer, R.; Esp, S. Age of Drinking Initiation as a Moderator of the Efficacy of a Brief, Web-Based Personalized Feedback Alcohol Intervention. *J. Child Adolesc. Subst. Abus.* **2016**, *25*, 591–597. [CrossRef]
28. Doumas, D.M.; Esp, S.; Turrisi, R.; Bond, L. A Randomized Controlled Trial of the eCHECKUP to GO for High School Seniors across the Academic Year. *Subst. Use Misuse* **2021**, *56*, 1932. [CrossRef]
29. Donato, H.; Donato, M. Stages for Undertaking a Systematic Review. *Acta Med. Port.* **2019**, *32*, 227–235. [CrossRef]
30. Wilson, M.; Ramsay, S.; Young, K.J. Engaging Overweight Adolescents in a Health and Fitness Program Using Wearable Activity Trackers. *J. Pediatr. Health Care* **2017**, *31*, e25–e34. [CrossRef]
31. Larsen, B.; Benitez, T.; Cano, M.; Dunsiger, S.S.; Marcus, B.H.; Mendoza-Vasconez, A.; Sallis, J.F.; Zive, M. Web-Based Physical Activity Intervention for Latina Adolescents: Feasibility, Accept-ability, and Potential Efficacy of the Niñas Saludables Study. *J. Med. Internet Res.* **2018**, *20*, e170. [CrossRef]
32. Khalil, G.E.; Wang, H.; Calabro, K.S.; Mitra, N.; Shegog, R.; Prokhorov, A.V. From the Experience of Interactivity and Entertainment to Lower Intention to Smoke: A Randomized Controlled Trial and Path Analysis of a Web-Based Smoking Prevention Program for Adolescents. *J. Med. Internet Res.* **2017**, *19*, e44. [CrossRef]
33. Widman, L.; Golin, C.E.; Kamke, K.; Burnette, J.L.; Prinstein, M.J. Sexual Assertiveness Skills and Sexual Decision-Making in Adolescent Girls: Randomized Controlled Trial of an Online Program. *Am. J. Public Health* **2018**, *108*, 96–102. [CrossRef]

34. Coughlin, L.N.; Nahum-Shani, I.; Philyaw-Kotov, M.L.; Bonar, E.E.; Rabbi, M.; Klasnja, P.; Murphy, S.; Walton, M.A. Developing an Adaptive Mobile Intervention to Address Risky Substance Use Among Adolescents and Emerging Adults: Usability Study. *JMIR Mhealth Uhealth* **2021**, *9*, e24424. [CrossRef] [PubMed]
35. Arnaud, N.; Baldus, C.; Elgán, T.H.; De Paepe, N.; Tønnesen, H.; Csémy, L.; Thomasius, R.; Blankers, M.; Haug, S. Effectiveness of a Web-Based Screening and Fully Automated Brief Motivational Intervention for Adolescent Substance Use: A Randomized Controlled Trial. *J. Med. Internet Res.* **2016**, *18*, e103. [CrossRef]
36. Brown, K.E.; Beasley, K.; Das, S. Self-Control, Plan Quality, and Digital Delivery of Action Planning for Condom and Contraceptive Pill Use of 14–24-Year-Olds: Findings from a Clinic-Based Online Pilot Randomised Controlled Trial. *Appl. Psychol. Health Well Being* **2018**, *10*, 391–413. [CrossRef]
37. Norman, P.; Cameron, D.; Epton, T.; Webb, T.L.; Harris, P.R.; Millings, A.; Sheeran, P. A randomized controlled trial of a brief online intervention to reduce alcohol consumption in new university students: Combining self-affirmation, theory of planned behaviour messages, and im-plementation intentions. *Br. J. Health Psychol.* **2018**, *23*, 108–127. [CrossRef]
38. Pirzadeh, A.; Zamani, F.; Khoshali, M.; Kelishadi, R. Web-based intervention on the promotion of physical activity among Iranian youth using the transtheoretical model. *J. Educ. Health Promot.* **2020**, *9*, 118. [CrossRef] [PubMed]
39. Huang, S.J.; Hung, W.C.; Shyu, M.L.; Chang, K.C.; Chen, C.K. Web-based intervention to promote physical activity in Taiwanese children. *J. Pediatr. Nurs.* **2019**, *45*, e35–e43. [CrossRef] [PubMed]
40. Duan, Y.P.; Wienert, J.; Hu, C.; Si, G.Y.; Lippke, S. Web-Based Intervention for Physical Activity and Fruit and Vegetable Intake among Chinese University Students: A Randomized Controlled Trial. *J. Med. Internet Res.* **2017**, *19*, e106. [CrossRef] [PubMed]
41. Doubova, S.V.; Martinez-Vega, I.P.; Infante-Castañeda, C.; Pérez-Cuevas, R. Effects of an internet-based educational inter-vention to prevent high-risk sexual behaviour in Mexican adolescents. *Health Educ. Res.* **2017**, *32*, 487–498. [CrossRef]
42. Castillo-Arcos, L.C.; Benavides-Torres, R.A.; López-Rosales, F.; Onofre-Rodríguez, D.J.; Valdez-Montero, C.; Maas-Góngora, L. The effect of an Internet-based intervention designed to reduce HIV/AIDS sexual risk among Mexican adolescents. *AIDS Care* **2016**, *28*, 191–196. [CrossRef]
43. Nicholl, B.I.; Sandal, L.F.; Stochkendahl, M.J.; McCallum, M.; Suresh, N.; Vasseljen, O.; Hartvigsen, J.; Mork, P.J.; Kjaer, P.; Søgaard, K.; et al. Digital Support Interventions for the Self-Management of Low Back Pain: A Systematic Review. *J. Med. Internet Res.* **2017**, *19*, e179. [CrossRef]
44. Sin, J.; Galeazzi, G.; McGregor, E.; Collom, J.; Taylor, A.; Barrett, B.; Lawrence, V.; Henderson, C. Digital Interventions for Screening and Treating Common Mental Disorders or Symptoms of Common Mental Illness in Adults: Systematic Review and Meta-analysis. *J. Med. Internet Res.* **2020**, *22*, e20581. [CrossRef]
45. Brigden, A.; Anderson, E.; Linney, C.; Morris, R.; Parslow, R.; Serafimova, T.; Smith, L.; Briggs, E.; Loades, M.; Crawley, E. Digital Behaviour Change Interventions for Younger Children with Chronic Health Conditions: Systematic Review. *J. Med. Internet Res.* **2020**, *22*, e16924. [CrossRef]
46. Manby, L.; Aicken, C.; Delgrange, M.; Bailey, J.V. Effectiveness of eHealth Interventions for HIV Prevention and Management in Sub-Saharan Africa: Systematic Review and Meta-analyses. *AIDS Behav.* **2021**, *26*, 457–469. [CrossRef]
47. Pfaeffli Dale, L.; Dobson, R.; Whittaker, R.; Maddison, R. The effectiveness of mobile-health behaviour change interventions for cardiovascular disease self-management: A systematic review. *Eur. J. Prev. Cardiol.* **2016**, *23*, 801–817. [CrossRef]
48. Brown, V.; Tran, H.; Downing, K.L.; Hesketh, K.D.; Moodie, M. A systematic review of economic evaluations of web-based or telephone-delivered interventions for preventing overweight and obesity and/or improving obesity-related behaviours. *Obes. Rev.* **2021**, *22*, e13227. [CrossRef]
49. Ryan, K.; Dockray, S.; Linehan, C. A systematic review of tailored eHealth interventions for weight loss. *Digit. Health* **2019**, *5*, 1–29. [CrossRef]
50. Chen, Y.; Perez-Cueto, F.J.A.; Giboreau, A.; Mavridis, I.; Hartwell, H. The Promotion of Eating Behaviour Change through Digital Interventions. *Int. J. Environ. Res. Public Health* **2020**, *17*, 7488. [CrossRef]
51. Villinger, K.; Wahl, D.R.; Boeing, H.; Schupp, H.T.; Renner, B. The effectiveness of app-based mobile interventions on nutrition behaviours and nutrition-related health outcomes: A systematic review and meta-analysis. *Obes. Rev.* **2019**, *20*, 1465–1484. [CrossRef]
52. Stephenson, A.; McDonough, S.M.; Murphy, M.H.; Nugent, C.D.; Mair, J.L. Using computer, mobile and wearable technolo-gy-enhanced interventions to reduce sedentary behaviour: A systematic review and meta-analysis. *Int. J. Behav. Nutr. Phys. Act.* **2017**, *14*, 105. [CrossRef]
53. Wibowo, R.A.; Kelly, P.; Baker, G. The effect of smartphone application interventions on physical activity level among university/college students: A systematic review protocol. *Phys. Ther. Rev.* **2020**, *25*, 135–142. [CrossRef]
54. Young, C.L.; Trapani, K.; Dawson, S.; O'Neil, A.; Kay-Lambkin, F.; Berk, M.; Jacka, F.N. Efficacy of online lifestyle interventions targeting lifestyle behaviour change in depressed populations: A systematic review. *Aust. N. Z. J. Psychiatry* **2018**, *52*, 834–846. [CrossRef]
55. Kaner, E.F.; Beyer, F.R.; Garnett, C.; Crane, D.; Brown, J.; Muirhead, C.; Redmore, J.; O'Donnell, A.; Newham, J.J.; de Vocht, F.; et al. Personalised digital interventions for reducing hazardous and harmful alcohol consumption in community-dwelling populations. *Cochrane Database Syst. Rev.* **2017**, *9*, Cd011479. [CrossRef]

56. Newby, K.; Teah, G.; Cooke, R.; Li, X.; Brown, K.; Salisbury-Finch, B.; Kwah, K.; Bartle, N.; Curtis, K.; Fulton, E.; et al. Do automated digital health behaviour change interventions have a positive effect on self-efficacy? A systematic review and meta-analysis. *Health Psychol. Rev.* **2021**, *15*, 140–158. [CrossRef] [PubMed]
57. Sanyal, C.; Stolee, P.; Juzwishin, D.; Husereau, D. Economic evaluations of eHealth technologies: A systematic review. *PLoS ONE* **2018**, *13*, e0198112. [CrossRef]
58. Wantland, D.J.; Portillo, C.J.; Holzemer, W.L.; Slaughter, R.; McGhee, E.M. The effectiveness of Web-based vs. non-Web-based interventions: A meta-analysis of behavioural change outcomes. *J. Med. Internet Res.* **2004**, *6*, e40. [CrossRef] [PubMed]
59. Enam, A.; Torres-Bonilla, J.; Eriksson, H. Evidence-Based Evaluation of eHealth Interventions: Systematic Literature Review. *J. Med. Internet Res.* **2018**, *20*, e10971. [CrossRef] [PubMed]
60. Aarts, S.; Akker, M.V.D.; Winkens, B. The importance of effect sizes. *Eur. J. Gen. Pract.* **2014**, *20*, 61–64. [CrossRef] [PubMed]
61. Chang, S.J.; Choi, S.; Kim, S.-A.; Song, M. Intervention Strategies Based on Information-Motivation-Behavioural Skills Model for Health Behaviour Change: A Systematic Review. *Asian Nurs. Res.* **2014**, *8*, 172–181. [CrossRef]
62. Michie, S.; Johnston, M. Behaviour Change Techniques. In *Encyclopedia of Behavioural Medicine*; Gellman, M.D., Turner, J.R., Eds.; Springer: New York, NY, USA, 2013; pp. 182–187.
63. Murray, E. Web-Based Interventions for Behavior Change and Self-Management: Potential, Pitfalls, and Progress. *Medicina* **2012**, *1*, e3. [CrossRef]

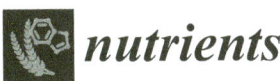

Review

Behaviour Change Techniques in Weight Gain Prevention Interventions in Adults of Reproductive Age: Meta-Analysis and Meta-Regression

Mamaru Ayenew Awoke, Cheryce L. Harrison, Julie Martin, Marie L. Misso, Siew Lim [†] and Lisa J. Moran *,[†]

Monash Centre for Health Research and Implementation (MCHRI), School of Public Health and Preventive Medicine, Monash University, Clayton, VIC 3168, Australia; mamaru.awoke@monash.edu (M.A.A.); cheryce.harrison@monash.edu (C.L.H.); juliechristine34@yahoo.com (J.M.); Marie.Misso@monash.edu (M.L.M.); siew.lim1@monash.edu (S.L.)
* Correspondence: lisa.moran@monash.edu; Tel.: +613-8572-2664
† These authors contributed equally to this work.

Abstract: Weight gain prevention interventions are likely to be more effective with the inclusion of behaviour change techniques. However, evidence on which behaviour change techniques (BCT) are most effective for preventing weight gain and improving lifestyle (diet and physical activity) is limited, especially in reproductive-aged adults. This meta-analysis and meta-regression aimed to identify BCT associated with changes in weight, energy intake and physical activity in reproductive-aged adults. BCT were identified using the BCT Taxonomy (v1) from each intervention. Meta-regression analyses were used to identify BCT associated with change in weight, energy intake and physical activity. Thirty-four articles were included with twenty-nine articles for the meta-analysis. Forty-three of the ninety-three possible BCT listed in the taxonomy were identified in the included studies. *Feedback on behaviour* and *Graded tasks* were significantly associated with less weight gain, and *Review behaviour goals* was significantly associated with lower energy intake. No individual BCT were significantly associated with physical activity. Our analysis provides further evidence for which BCT are most effective in weight gain prevention interventions. The findings support that the use of key BCT within interventions can contribute to successful weight gain prevention in adults of reproductive age.

Keywords: behaviour change techniques; weight gain prevention; reproductive age; meta-analysis; meta-regression

Citation: Awoke, M.A.; Harrison, C.L.; Martin, J.; Misso, M.L.; Lim, S.; Moran, L.J. Behaviour Change Techniques in Weight Gain Prevention Interventions in Adults of Reproductive Age: Meta-Analysis and Meta-Regression. *Nutrients* **2022**, *14*, 209. https://doi.org/10.3390/nu14010209

Academic Editor: Carlos Vasconcelos

Received: 30 November 2021
Accepted: 30 December 2021
Published: 3 January 2022

Publisher's Note: MDPI stays neutral with regard to jurisdictional claims in published maps and institutional affiliations.

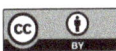

Copyright: © 2022 by the authors. Licensee MDPI, Basel, Switzerland. This article is an open access article distributed under the terms and conditions of the Creative Commons Attribution (CC BY) license (https://creativecommons.org/licenses/by/4.0/).

1. Introduction

Obesity is a pressing global health challenge. The prevalence of overweight and obesity affect one-third of the world's population and are escalating globally [1]. Both men and women of reproductive age are at increasing risk of longitudinal weight gain and development of obesity [2,3] with longitudinal data reporting they gained 0.5–0.8 kg per year [4,5]. Furthermore, women of reproductive age are at a particularly higher risk of weight gain and obesity exacerbated by excess gestational weight gain and postpartum weight retention. For example, reproductive age women in Australia had an average weight gain of 6.3 kg over 10 years [6] with this rate of weight gain greater in women 18–50 years (0.4–0.7 kg/year) compared to women above 50 years (0.2–0.5 kg/year) [7]. In addition to increasing the risk of obesity, weight gain in adults is associated with increased risk of various chronic diseases including type 2 diabetes, hypertension, cardiovascular diseases and cancer [8,9] and an overall increased risk of mortality [10].

Prevention of weight gain is considered less expensive, more feasible and effective than obesity treatment [11]. Once established, obesity treatment is more intensive, costly and largely unsustainable [12,13]. In response to this challenge, there is a need to consider a greater emphasis on weight gain prevention to curb the rising prevalence of overweight and obesity [14,15]. A recent meta-analysis of 29 studies by our group assessed the efficacy of lifestyle interventions for the prevention of weight gain in 37, 407 adults [16]. Overall, lifestyle interventions were effective in preventing weight gain in adults aged 18–50 years (MD −1.15 kg; 95% CI −1.50, −0.80) compared to control [16]. Interventions were effective for both women and men. The impact of the interventions was also more pronounced in non-obese adults and for prescriptive compared to non-prescriptive interventions. However, behaviour change strategies associated with the intervention effectiveness remain to be identified.

Lifestyle interventions are often complex and involve multiple components also known as active ingredients designed to change behaviour [17]. A behaviour change technique (BCT) has been previously defined as an "observable, replicable, and irreducible component of an intervention designed to alter or redirect causal processes that regulate behaviour; that is, a BCT is proposed to be an 'active ingredient'" [18]. A taxonomy of behaviour change technique (BCTTv1) has been developed for better understanding of complex interventions and identification of active ingredients of interventions that contribute to positive behaviour change. This taxonomy by Michie et al. [18] provides a standardized list of 93 BCT labels and detailed definitions. For example, some key BCTs are: *Goal setting behaviour* (e.g., eat 2 serves of fruit and 5 serves of vegetables each day, aim 8000–10,000 steps per day), *Problem solving* (e.g., identify barriers or facilitator for change, relapse prevention), *Self-monitoring of behaviour* (e.g., regular self-weighing, using pedometer or diary), *Review behavioural goals* (email or written feedback on energy intake and physical activity), *Social support* (unspecified, (encouraged to walk with friends or join compatible local group programs), *Graded tasks* (encourage a gradual increase in physical activity levels-working towards 150–300 min per week) and *Behavioural practice/rehearsal* (e.g., exercise classes with role play). Several previous meta-regression analyses have investigated BCTs associated with change in diet, physical activity and weight [19–23]. Several reviews have also identified effective BCTS within lifestyle interventions to improve outcomes in diet [24] and weight [25,26] using percentage effectiveness ratios and have reported that interventions are likely to be more effective with the inclusion of BCTs such as self-monitoring, goal setting and social support. These studies, however, have focused on specific population groups including younger adults [24,25], pregnant women [23], postpartum women [20] and participants with chronic conditions [19] which limits the generalizability of these findings to the broader population of adults of reproductive age who experience greater longitudinal weight gain. To date, no previous studies have evaluated BCTs associated with interventions specifically targeting weight gain prevention in adults of reproductive age (18–50 years); therefore, a greater understanding of specific BCTs or combination of BCTs associated with weight gain prevention and improvements in lifestyle outcomes is required to guide future intervention development. This study aims to identify the BCTs associated with change in weight, energy intake and physical activity in adults of reproductive age.

2. Methods

2.1. Protocol and Registration

This meta-analysis was reported according to the Preferred Reporting Items for Systematic Reviews and Meta-Analyses statement [27]. The review protocol was registered with PROSPERO (registration number CRD42018114156). This work is part of our recent published systematic review and meta-analysis of lifestyle intervention of randomized controlled trials (RCTs) for preventing weight gain in adults aged 18–50 years [16]. Here, we present a secondary analysis to identify the BCTs associated with change in weight, energy intake and physical activity.

2.2. Data Sources and Searches

Complete search strategies used in electronic databases, study selection, eligibility criteria, data extraction process and risk of bias assessments are reported in detail in the previous systematic review [16]. A systematic literature search was conducted with no time limit, inclusive to May 2020. Briefly, we included RCTs published in English that recruited men and women aged between 18 to 50 years, that exclusively aimed to prevent weight gain with lifestyle intervention (incorporating diet, physical activity and/or behaviour change strategies) of any duration compared with no/minimal intervention (waiting list, materials or information only interventions) and reported a weight or BMI (weight (kg)/height (m^2)) following intervention as either a change score or endpoint value. Adults aged 18–50 were defined as reproductive age as although females under 18 and males over 50 can reproduce, it is recognized that fertility is suboptimal in older males [28] and that there are biological and social ramifications of pregnancies in women under 18 [29]. We used study level data for the outcome of weight, diet and physical activity from our previous systematic review and meta-analysis of randomized controlled lifestyle interventions to prevent weight gain [16]. Overall, 29 studies across 34 publications were included. Results including detailed description of included studies, intervention effectiveness for weight, physical activity and energy intake outcomes as well as risk of bias are reported in detail in our previous systematic review [16]. In brief, lifestyle interventions resulted in significant reductions in weight (MD -1.15 kg, 95% CI -1.48, -0.81, 29 studies, 11874 participants, $I^2 = 35.83\%$, $p < 0.001$), energy intake (MD -111.21 kcal/day, 95% CI -115.44, -106.97, 13 studies, 4207 participants, $I^2 = 87\%$, $p < 0.001$) and significant increases in physical activity levels (MD 71.75 MET-min/week, 95%CI 22.72, 120.77, 6 studies, 1329 participants, $I^2 = 0\%$, $p = 0.004$) [16]. The majority ($n = 15$) of studies were classified as moderate risk of bias [16].

2.3. BCTs Coding

We used the BCTTv1 [18] to identify BCTs utilized within the lifestyle interventions. Intervention descriptions of each study were reviewed and coded as presence or absence of the 93 BCTs in the taxonomy. We also referred to intervention protocols and Supplementary Materials associated with the studies and coded these for BCTs. As stated in previous systematic reviews and meta-regressions of behaviour strategies [20,22], both the intervention and control groups were coded and only BCTs that were present in the intervention group and absent in the control group were included in the analyses. BCTs were coded independently by three reviewers who have completed the BCTTv1 online training course (http://www.bct-taxonomy.com/, accessed on 23 January, 2020). Each study was independently coded by two reviewers, in which one reviewer (M.A.A) independently coded all intervention descriptions in studies and the other two reviewers (L.M. and S.L. who are dietitians with experience in lifestyle intervention development) independently coded 50% of all studies. Discrepancies were resolved by consensus in discussion with all reviewers.

2.4. Data Synthesis and Analysis

Data analysis methods are previously reported in the original systematic review [16]. Briefly, outcomes were pooled using the inverse variance weighted random-effects meta-analysis with the restricted maximum-likelihood estimator and expressed as mean differences (MDs) for weight (kg) and energy intake (kilocalories) with 95% confidence intervals. While we report physical outcome only for six studies reported on similar scales (MET-min/week) in our previous paper [16], here, we analyzed studies reported on different scales which can be combined as standardized mean differences (SMDs) (calculated using Hedges' (g)) with 95% confidence interval. This was to maximize the sample size to provide sufficient power to perform meta-regression of BCTs where at least 10 studies are required. Chi-square tests were used to examine heterogeneity between studies with $p < 0.1$ considered statistically significant. The degree of inconsistency between studies was assessed using I^2 with values $\geq 25\%$, $\geq 50\%$, and $\geq 75\%$ indicating moderate, substantial and high heterogeneity, respectively [30]. Publication bias was assessed with the funnel plot and Egger's test for meta-analyses.

2.5. Analysis of BCTs: Meta-Regression and Percentage Effectiveness Ratio

The total number of BCTs used per study were calculated as the sum of BCTs that were present in the intervention but not in the control group. For meta-regression and percentage effectiveness ratio, BCTs were included in the analysis if they were present in three or more studies to minimize the impact of single studies or avoid inflation of results (i.e., to reduce type−1 error) [19,31]. Here, we used two approaches to analyse BCTs and results from both methods of analyses were triangulated to increase robustness of the findings. Percentage effectiveness ratio is descriptive in nature and has the advantage of being able to identify most BCTs that have the potential to be effective. However, it may have low specificity due to its binary nature of categorization (effective/non effective), potentially including large numbers of BCTs that may only have small contributions to effectiveness but are frequently included in intervention components [32]. Meta-regressions, on the other hand, are able to detect effects that are too small to be picked up in individual studies, but they require a large number of studies and a substantial heterogeneity between studies to detect associations.

Random effect meta-regression analyses with restricted maximum likelihood estimation were conducted to explore the associations between BCTs and changes in weight, energy intake and physical activity. Adjusted R^2 was used as a measure of variance accounted for by the covariates. A series of univariable meta-regression analyses were performed to explore the effect of individual BCTs, the total number of BCTs and number of BCTs congruent with control theory (i.e., all BCTs under *Goals and planning* and *Feedback and monitoring* group) [20] on intervention effect. The group of BCTs congruent with control theory were considered here as it has been found to be associated with greater effect sizes in weight loss with lifestyle interventions in previous meta-regressions [19,20].

Additionally, a descriptive analysis of BCTs was conducted using 'percentage effectiveness ratio' as described in previous reviews [24,25]. Firstly, studies were categorized as effective (a significant difference in outcomes between intervention and control groups) or non-effective (no significant differences in outcomes between groups). BCTs utilized in effective and non-effective interventions were identified. The percentage effectiveness ratio was calculated as the ratio of the number of times each BCT was identified in an effective study divided by the number of times it was a component of all studies, including in non-effective trials. BCTs with percentage effectiveness ratio >50% were considered a component of effective interventions [25]. All statistical analyses were performed with STATA statistical software version 16.1 (StataCorp, College Station, TX, USA).

3. Results

3.1. Study Selection and Intervention Efficacy Overview

Study selection and screening process are shown in Figure S1 and the intervention and comparator characteristics of included studies are shown in Table S1. As reported previously, 29 studies across 34 publications were included for weight, 13 studies for energy intake and 17 studies for physical activity. Most studies involved both male and female ($n = 17$) participants, were conducted in a community settings ($n = 18$) and utilized a mixed diet and physical activity intervention ($n = 14$ studies) or behaviour change approach ($n = 17$ studies) [16]. Intervention delivery was predominantly face-to-face group sessions ($n = 12$) with median intervention duration of 9 months. Here, combining studies that reported physical activity on different scales, the intervention effect remained significant on physical activity levels (SMD 0.13, 95% CI −0.05, 0.31, 17 studies, 4496 participants, $I^2 = 80.77\%$, $p < 0.001$) (Figure S2).

3.2. BCT Analysis

BCTs identified within intervention descriptions of each study have been published before [16]. Of 93 possible BCTs in the taxonomy, a total 43 BCTs unique to the intervention group were coded in the interventions (Figure 1). The number of BCTs per study ranged from 2 to 20, with an average of eight BCTs per study. The five most frequently coded BCTs were *Goal setting behaviour* (in 24 studies), *Self-monitoring of behaviour* (in 19 studies), *Action planning* (in 16 studies), *Social support (unspecified)* (16 studies) and *Instruction on how to perform the behaviour* (16 studies).

The associations between BCTs and changes in weight, energy intake and physical activity are shown in Table 1. *Feedback on behaviour* and *Graded tasks* were significantly associated with reduced weight gain (Table 1). *Review behaviour goals* was significantly associated with a greater decrease in energy intake (Table 1). No individual BCT was significantly associated with physical activity outcomes (Table 1). Both the total number of behaviour strategies and BCTs congruent with control theory were not significantly associated with weight, energy intake or physical activity (Table 1).

A summary of BCTs identified in effective and non-effective interventions for changes in weight, energy intake and physical activity are shown in Table 2. There were 23 BCTs identified in at least three studies for weight with 18 BCTs having a percentage effectiveness ratio >50% (Table 2). For energy intake, 16 BCTs were identified in at least three studies with 9 BCTS having a percentage effectiveness ratio >50% (Table 2). For physical activity, 19 BCTs were identified in at least three studies and no BCTs showed an effectiveness ratio >50% (Table 2).

Figure 1. *Cont.*

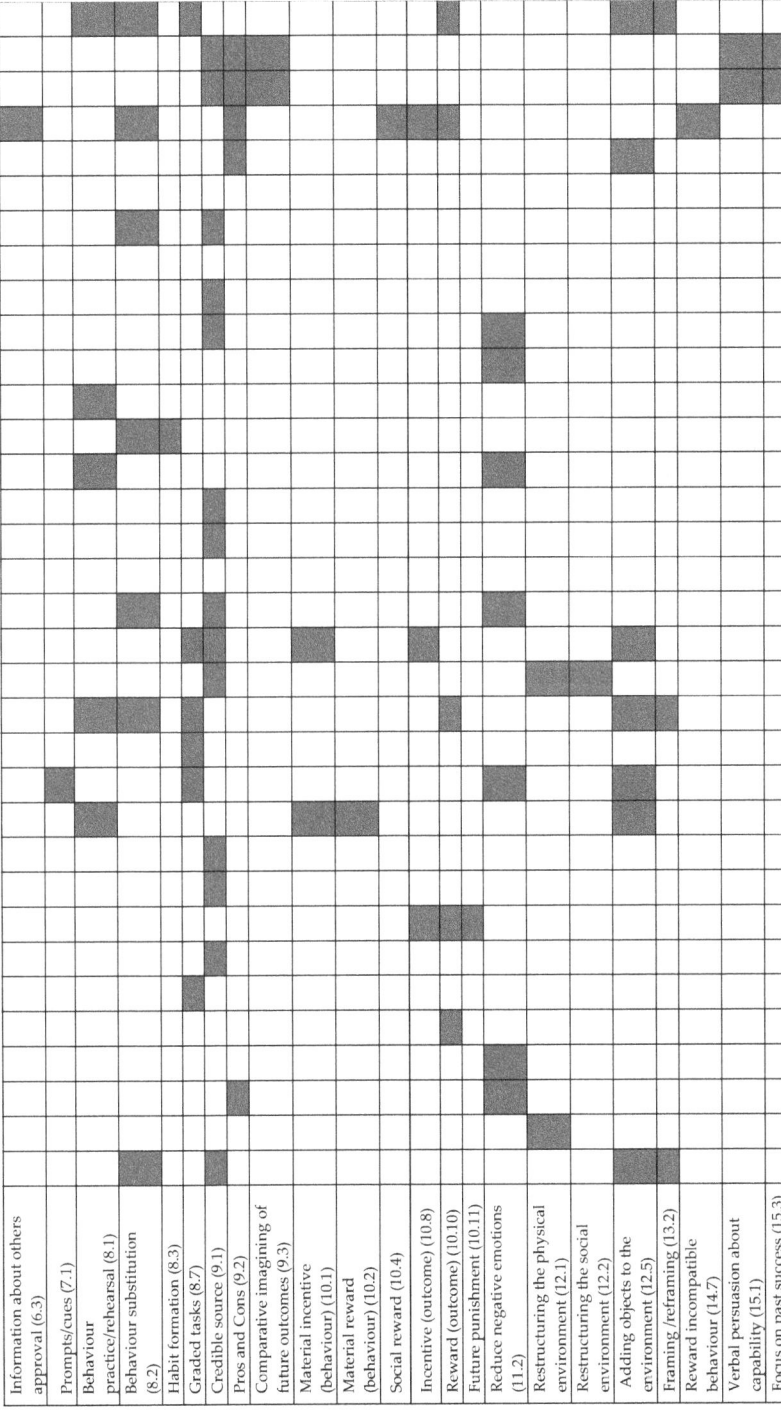

Figure 1. Identified behaviour change strategies in lifestyle interventions from the included studies ($n = 34$).

Table 1. Univariable meta-regression results for weight and energy intake by behaviour change techniques.

Behaviour Change Strategies	Weight (n = 29)			Energy Intake (n = 13)			Physical Activity (n = 17)		
	β (95%CI)	p Value	Adj. R^2 (%)	β (95%CI)	p Value	Adj. R^2 (%)	β (95%CI)	p Value	Adj. R^2 (%)
Total BCT	−0.03 (−0.10, 0.05)	0.475	0	−3.99 (−10.5, 2.48)	0.202	21.6	−0.04 (−0.08, 0.01)	0.107	30.12
Behaviour strategies consistent with control theory	0.46 (−0.48, 1.40)	0.323	0	−20.4 (−230.5, 189.8)	0.835	0	−0.26 (−0.90, 0.39)	0.413	0
Goal setting (behaviour) (1.1)	−0.06 (−0.78, 0.66)	0.867	0	−20.4 (−230.5, 189.8)	0.835	0	−0.26 (−0.90, 0.39)	0.413	0
Problem solving (1.2)	−0.18 (−0.91, 0.54)	0.604	0	−62.2 (−163.9, 39.0)	0.203	24.2	−0.04 (−0.41, 0.33)	0.817	0
Goal setting (outcome) (1.3)	−0.29 (−0.96, 0.38)	0.383	10.6	−24.2 (−124.5, 76.0)	0.605	0.11	−0.11 (−0.48, 0.26)	0.647	0
Action planning (1.4)	−0.09 (−0.78, 0.60)	0.795	0	−18.9 (−132.1, 94.2)	0.720	0	−0.06 (−0.47, 0.35)	0.763	0
Review behaviour goals (1.5)	−0.65 (−1.34, 0.08)	0.079	27.5	−90.6 (−164.6, −16.7)	0.021	52.6	−0.15 (−0.52, 0.22)	0.405	0
Discrepancy between current behaviour and goal (1.6)	−0.68 (−1.69, 0.33)	0.179	15.4	−60.4 (−135.2, 14.4)	0.103	43.4	NA	NA	NA
Review outcomes goals (1.7)	−0.38 (−1.43, 0.67)	0.462	5.33	−24.3 (−119.6, 71.1)	0.587	0	NA	NA	NA
Feedback on behaviour (2.2)	−0.73 (−1.43, −0.03)	0.042	40.1	−61.7 (−136.6, 13.1)	0.097	43.9	−0.05 (−0.47, 0.37)	0.798	0
Self-monitoring of behaviour (2.3)	−0.54 (−1.19, 0.11)	0.103	20.6	−20.9 (−117.6, 75.6)	0.642	0	0.22 (−0.11, 0.57)	0.174	21.12
Self-monitoring of outcomes of behaviour (2.4)	0.76 (0.16, 1.14)	0.015	29.7	6.3 (−91.4, 103.9)	0.890	0	0.09 (−0.32, 0.51)	0.644	0
Feedback on outcomes of behaviour (2.7)	0.61 (−0.18, 0.14)	0.123	25.6	NA	NA	NA	−0.36 (−0.74, 0.01)	0.053	34.2
Social support (unspecified) (3.1)	−0.32 (−1.02, 0.38)	0.350	8.2	26.2 (−61.7, 114.1)	0.525	0	0.17 (−0.21, 0.56)	0.358	0
Social support (emotional) (3.3)	−0.65 (−1.55, 0.26)	0.156	21.1	NA	NA	NA	−0.15 (−0.62, 0.32)	0.503	0
Instruction on how to perform the behaviour (4.1)	0.08 (−0.61, 0.78)	0.813	0	−33.9 (−119.5, 51.8)	0.403	0	0.04 (−0.35, 0.44)	0.811	0
Information about health consequences (5.1)	0.15 (−0.67, 0.98)	0.709	0	−21.9 (−114.2, 70.5)	0.623	0	−0.31 (−0.70, 0.09)	0.117	20.4
Information about social and environmental consequences (5.3)	0.71 (0.05, 1.37)	0.037	23.9	NA	NA	NA	−0.04 (−0.56, 0.44)	0.865	0
Demonstration of the behaviour (6.1)	0.00 (−0.87, 0.87)	0.998	0	−59.7 (−140.3, 20.9)	0.131	43.3	−0.07 (−0.52, 0.38)	0.750	0
Behaviour practice/rehearsal (8.1)	0.13 (−0.74, 1.01)	0.758	0	−0.81 (−102.2, 100.6)	0.986	0	−0.01 (−0.69, 0.68)	0.982	0
Behaviour substitution (8.2)	−0.54 (−1.33, 0.25)	0.171	22.0	NA	NA	NA	NA	NA	NA

Table 1. Cont.

Behaviour Change Strategies	Weight (n = 29)			Energy Intake (n = 13)			Physical Activity (n = 17)		
	β (95%CI)	p Value	Adj. R^2 (%)	β (95%CI)	p Value	Adj. R^2 (%)	β (95%CI)	p Value	Adj. R^2 (%)
Graded tasks (8.7)	−0.82 (−1.46, −0.17)	0.015	50.3	NA	NA	NA	0.45 (−0.04, 0.94)	0.070	32.72
Credible source (9.1)	−0.24 (−0.96, 0.49)	0.510	0	52.7 (−50.5, 155.9)	0.285	14.2	0.09 (−0.28, 0.46)	0.611	0
Reward (outcome) (10.10)	NA	NA	NA	−60.3 (−135.2, 14.6)	0.104	43.4	NA	NA	NA
Reduce negative emotions (11.2)	0.35 (−0.53, 1.23)	0.421	0	NA	NA	NA	0.03 (−0.47, 0.53)	0.894	0
Adding objects to the environment (12.5)	−0.46 (−1.15, 0.23)	0.185	15.4	NA	NA	NA	0.05 (−0.38, 0.48)	0.754	0

β = beta coefficient; CI = confidence interval; n = number of studies; NA = not applicable because a BCT is not present in at least three studies; Adj. R^2 = adjusted R^2 which measures percentage of variation. BCTs in bold text denote significant association.

Table 2. Percentage of behaviour change techniques used in effective and non-effective interventions for weight, energy intake and physical activity.

Behaviour Change Strategies	Weight (n = 29)			Energy Intake (n = 13)			Physical Activity (n = 17)		
	Effective	Non-Effective	Percentage of Effectiveness	Effective	Non-Effective	Percentage of Effectiveness	Effective	Non-Effective	Percentage of Effectiveness
Goal setting (behaviour) (1.1)	11	8	57.9	4	6	40.0	3	12	20.0
Problem solving (1.2)	6	4	60.0	4	3	57.1	2	6	25.0
Goal setting (outcome) (1.3)	8	3	72.7	3	2	60.0	1	5	16.7
Action planning (1.4)	8	4	66.7	3	4	42.9	2	9	18.2
Review behaviour goals (1.5)	4	3	57.1	4	2	66.7	2	4	33.3
Discrepancy between current behaviour and goal (1.6)	3	0	100	2	1	66.7	NA	NA	NA
Review outcomes goals (1.7)	NA	NA	NA	2	1	66.7	NA	NA	NA
Feedback on behaviour (2.2)	4	1	80.0	3	1	75.0	1	3	25.0
Self-monitoring of behaviour (2.3)	12	5	70.6	2	3	40.0	2	7	22.2
Self-monitoring of outcomes of behaviour (2.4)	7	5	58.3	1	2	33.3	1	3	25.0
Feedback on outcomes of behaviour (2.7)	1	2	33.3	NA	NA	NA	0	3	0

Table 2. Cont.

Behaviour Change Strategies	Weight (n = 29)			Energy Intake (n = 13)			Physical Activity (n = 17)		
	Effective	Non-Effective	Percentage of Effectiveness	Effective	Non-Effective	Percentage of Effectiveness	Effective	Non-Effective	Percentage of Effectiveness
Social support (unspecified) (3.1)	11	2	84.6	1	3	25.0	2	4	33.3
Social support (emotional) (3.3)	3	1	75.0	NA	NA	NA	1	3	25.0
Instruction on how to perform the behaviour (4.1)	8	6	57.1	4	6	40.0	3	9	25.0
Information about health consequences (5.1)	6	1	85.7	2	1	66.7	0	3	0
Information about social and environmental consequences (5.3)	2	3	40.0	NA	NA	NA	0	3	0
Demonstration of the behaviour (6.1)	3	1	75.0	2	2	50.0	1	2	33.3
Behaviour practice/rehearsal (8.1)	2	2	50.0	2	1	66.7	NA	NA	NA
Behaviour substitution (8.2)	4	1	80.0	NA	NA	NA	NA	NA	NA
Graded tasks (8.7)	5	0	100	NA	NA	NA	1	2	33.3
Credible source (9.1)	8	4	66.7	0	5	0	3	5	37.5
Reward (outcome) (10.10)	NA	NA	NA	3	0	100	NA	NA	NA
Reduce negative emotions (11.2)	2	5	28.6	NA	NA	NA	0	4	0
Adding objects to the environment (12.5)	4	2	66.7	NA	NA	NA	0	4	0

BCT is considered effective if identified in a significant effect size of outcomes (weight, energy intake and physical activity); NA = not applicable because a BCT is not present in at least three studies. BCTs in bold text denote that had a percentage effectiveness ratio >50%.

4. Discussion

This meta-analysis and meta-regression assessed for the first time BCTs within lifestyle intervention targeting weight gain prevention in healthy reproductive-age adult populations. As previously reported, weight gain prevention interventions prevented weight gain (1.15 kg), reduced energy intake (−111.21 kcal/day) and improved physical activity (71.75 MET-min/week) compared with controls [16]. We extended this work to report the effective BCTs associated with change in weight, diet and physical activity. While analysis from percentage effectiveness ratios suggest a number of BCTs are effective intervention components for reducing weight and energy intake, only *Feedback on behaviour* and *Graded tasks* were associated with weight and *Review behaviour goal(s)* associated with energy intake in meta-regression. No individual BCT was significantly associated with physical activity outcomes as a percentage effectiveness ratio or in meta-regression. The total number of BCTs and strategies congruent with Control Theory were not associated with any of outcomes.

A number of BCTs had a percentage effectiveness ratio >50% for weight and energy intake, but not for physical activity, with most of these related to self-regulation strategies (e.g., *Goal setting outcome*, *Review behaviour goals*, *Self-monitoring outcome(s) of behaviour*, *Feedback on behaviour*). This is consistent with a previous systematic review of electronic health interventions in young adults reporting self-regulation skills such as *Goal setting*, *Self-monitoring* and *Social support* were key strategies for weight gain prevention [33]. Self-regulation related BCTs were also previously associated with effective interventions for reducing energy intake in adults with obesity and chronic conditions [19,21,22]. Furthermore, interventions including *Self-monitoring* were associated with greater weight reduction in postpartum women [34], in children [35] and in adults with obesity and chronic conditions [19], although this is not consistently reported [36]. These inconsistent findings may be related to variations in methodology including BCT taxonomy used (e.g., 26-item CALO-RE taxonomy [37], redefined 40-item CALO-RE taxonomy [38], BCTT v1), population studied (young adults, postpartum women, adults with obesity and chronic conditions) and method of BCT analysis (e.g., meta-regression, percentage effectiveness ratio, Meta-CART analysis).

On meta-regression, *Feedback on behaviour* and *Graded tasks* were significantly associated with reduced weight gain. Studies evaluating specific BCTs or combination of BCTs within lifestyle interventions aimed at preventing weight gain, instead of weight management in general, in adults of reproductive age are limited. A recent review by Ashton et al. [25] identified *Goal-setting (outcome)* as an effective component for weight gain prevention interventions in young adults using percentage effectiveness ratios. We extend these findings by broadening the population studied to adults aged 18–50 years and by including a meta-regression analysis, which investigates the association between BCTs and effect sizes of intervention outcomes [21]. While the past finding on *Goal-setting (outcome)* was confirmed from our percentage effectiveness ratio analyses [25], this was not supported by the meta-regression in the current study.

In contrast to these results and previous findings on BCTs for weight gain prevention, meta regression analysis targeting weight loss interventions in adults with obesity (aged 40 years and above) reported that BCTs including *Provision of instructions*, *Self-monitoring of behaviour* and *Relapse prevention* were associated with greater weight loss [19]. None of these BCTs were associated with effect sizes of change in weight in current study. Most common BCTs associated with weight loss or weight management in previous reviews were within the BCT group of *Goals and planning* (e.g., *Goal setting*, *Problem solving*, *Action planning*) or *Feedback and monitoring* (e.g., *Self-monitoring*, *Personalized feedback*) [19,39]. In the current review only *Feedback on behaviour* within the *Feedback and Monitoring* BCT group was associated with weight change. These differences may be related to the fact that interventions targeting weight loss tend to be more prescriptive and intensive [40] than weight gain prevention interventions and, therefore, involve unique or distinct BCTs. Further research is needed to confirm this.

We report that *Review behaviour goal(s)* was significantly associated with a greater reduction in energy intake which is consistent with previous meta-regression analysis targeting healthy eating behaviour in adults [21]. A prior meta-regression in weight loss interventions in postpartum women reported several BCTs under *Goals and planning* BCT group (e.g., *Goal-setting of outcome, Problem-solving, Reviewing outcome goal*) and *Feedback and monitoring* BCT group (e.g., *Feedback on behaviour, Self-monitoring of behaviour*) were associated with greater decreases in energy intake [20]. However, only *Review behaviour goals* from the *Goals and planning* BCT group was associated with energy intake in the current study targeting weight gain prevention interventions. This indicates that *Review behaviour goal(s)* can be one of the active ingredients in interventions aiming at reducing energy intake with potential benefits for weight gain prevention. Fewer BCTs identified for weight gain prevention may again reflect the fact that prevention of weight gain requires a smaller change in energy intake [41] than weight loss (cumulative energy deficit of 3500 kcal per 0.5 kg weight loss) [42] and lifestyle interventions to prevent weight gain may, therefore, include less or distinct BCTs.

We did not find any individual BCTs significantly associated with physical activity. This is consistent with prior research in postpartum women [20] and in adults with obesity and obesity-related comorbidities [19] using meta-regression. In contrast, another review reported several BCTs including action planning, providing instruction and reinforcing effort towards behaviour were associated with physical activity in older adults [43]. However, this study used a different method of BCT identification instead of meta-regression and older version of BCT taxonomy that limits the comparison of findings. *Providing feedback, review of feedback* and *relapse prevention* have been previously suggested in a meta-review as effective BCTs in changing physical activity levels albeit with inconsistent findings [36]. However, specific BCTs or components of intervention to guide changes in physical activity and subsequently weight remain unclear in weight gain prevention trials. As weight gain prevention can be achieved by optimizing both diet and physical activity [44] and there are independent health benefits in engaging in a healthy diet and regular physical activity [45,46], there is a need for further research on identifying BCTs associated with physical activity in healthy adult populations of reproductive age.

Here, we also report that the total number of BCTs used in lifestyle interventions was not associated with weight, energy intake or physical activity consistent with prior research by Dombrowski et al. among adults in weight loss intervention using older version of the BCT taxonomy [19]. Similarly, another meta-regression found no significant association between number of BCTs and vegetable and fruit intake in adults of retirement age [47]. In contrast, a meta-regression in weight loss interventions in postpartum women found significant association between increased number of BCTs and decreases in energy but not weight and physical activity [20,22]. The exact reason for these inconsistent findings is not clear, although this may be related to the population studied. Using more BCTs may lead better outcomes for energy intake or eating behaviour in postpartum women [48] as they have additional barriers for healthy eating relating to their specific life stage. However, using a greater number of BCTS in interventions may increase the complexity of interventions [49], which may contribute to challenges in broader implementation [49]. Future research should determine the benefits of using effective types of numbers of BCTs or parsimonious set of BCTs for both efficacy and successful implementation [21].

The strength of this review were: (1) use of the most recent validated BCT taxonomy (BCTTv1) for BCTs coding; (2) coding of BCTs by trained three independent reviewers who also had experience in developing lifestyle interventions; use of rigorous method of BCT analysis using both percentage effectiveness ratio as explorative analysis and meta-regression to identify BCTs associated with intervention effectiveness effect size following previous recommendations [19,21]; focusing on weight gain prevention interventions in adults of reproductive age distinguishing it from previous reviews [22,24,25] through BCT taxonomy used, target outcomes and population studied.

However, the current study has several limitations. Firstly, our search was restricted to studies published in English language only. Secondly, most of the included studies provided insufficient studies in assessing the risk of bias. Thirdly, BCTs coding (presence or absence) depend on the description of interventions details reported in RCTs with an insufficiently detailed methodology precluding accurate analysis. This limitation was minimized through reviewing and coding methodology protocols and Supplementary Files or supporting documents for included studies. Fourth, we were unable to assess the relative effectiveness of different BCTs between men and women due to insufficient numbers of studies that present data sex differences. Fifth, the analysis was limited to the effect of individual BCTs and, therefore, does not show the effect of combination of BCTs. While this can be done using a meta-classification and regression trees (Meta-CART) analysis [50,51], we were unable to perform this due to insufficient number of studies. Lastly, this study was limited by the small number of studies which may reduce the chance of detecting the true effect with meta-regression. The lack of a significant effect of BCTs observed here may not indicate that these specific techniques are not important components of lifestyle interventions for weight gain prevention.

5. Conclusions

This meta-regression analysis showed that *Feedback on behaviour* and *Graded tasks* were associated with effect sizes in weight and *Review behaviour goal(s)* was associated with reduced energy intake. Further studies are required to confirm key BCTs associated with physical activity and to evaluate the interactive and synergetic effect of BCTs for intervention effectiveness.

Supplementary Materials: The following are available online at https://www.mdpi.com/article/10.3390/nu14010209/s1, Figure S1: Preferred Reporting Items for Systematic Reviews and Meta-analysis flow diagram of included studies., Table S1: Intervention and comparator characteristics of included studies, Figure S2: Forest plot for physical activity.

Author Contributions: Conceptualization, L.J.M., M.A.A. and C.L.H.; search strategy development, screening papers for eligibility, data extraction, quality appraisal, M.A.A. and J.M.; BCT identification and coding, M.A.A., S.L. and L.J.M.; data analysis and sole responsibility for initial draft of the manuscript., M.A.A.; manuscript review, interpretation of results and edits, M.L.M., S.L., C.L.H. and L.J.M.; supervision, L.J.M. All authors have read and agreed to the published version of the manuscript.

Funding: M.A.A. is funded by the Monash International Tuition Scholarship and Monash Graduate Scholarship; C.L.H. is funded by a Senior Postdoctoral Fellowship from the NHMRC Centre for Research Excellence for Health in Preconception and Pregnancy (CRE-HiPP; APP1171142); J.M is supported by the Australian Government Research Training Program (RTP) Stipend; L.J.M. is funded by the National Heart Foundation Future Leader Fellowship; and S.L. is funded by the National Medical Health and Research Council Fellowship.

Conflicts of Interest: The authors declare no conflict of interest.

References

1. Ng, M.; Fleming, T.; Robinson, M.; Thomson, B.; Graetz, N.; Margono, C.; Mullany, E. Global, regional, and national prevalence of overweight and obesity in children and adults during 1980–2013: A systematic analysis for the Global Burden of Disease Study 2013. *Lancet* **2014**, *384*, 766–781. [CrossRef]
2. Kimokoti, R.W.; Newby, P.; Gona, P.; Zhu, L.; McKeon-O'Malley, C.; Guzman, J.P.; D'Agostino, R.B.; Millen, B.E. Patterns of weight change and progression to overweight and obesity differ in men and women: Implications for research and interventions. *Public Health Nutr.* **2013**, *16*, 1463–1475. [CrossRef]
3. Mozaffarian, D.; Hao, T.; Rimm, E.B.; Willett, W.C.; Hu, F.B. Changes in diet and lifestyle and long-term weight gain in women and men. *N. Engl. J. Med.* **2011**, *364*, 2392–2404. [CrossRef] [PubMed]
4. Lewis, C.E.; Jacobs, D.R., Jr.; McCreath, H.; Kiefe, C.I.; Schreiner, P.J.; Smith, D.E.; Williams, O.D. Weight gain continues in the 1990s: 10-year trends in weight and overweight from the CARDIA study. *Am. J. Epidemiol.* **2000**, *151*, 1172–1181. [CrossRef]
5. Brown, W.J.; Kabir, E.; Clark, B.K.; Gomersall, S.R. Maintaining a healthy BMI: Data from a 16-year study of young Australian women. *Am. J. Prev. Med.* **2016**, *51*, e165–e178. [CrossRef]

6. Adamson, L.; Brown, W.; Byles, J.; Chojenta, C.; Dobson, A.; Fitzgerald, D.; Hockey, R.; Loxton, D.; Powers, J.; Spallek, M. *Women's Weight: Findings from the Australian Longitudinal Study on Women's Health: Report Prepared for the Australian Government Department of Health and Ageing*; Australian Government Department of Health and Ageing: Canberra, Australia, 2007.
7. Gomersall, S.; Dobson, A.; Brown, W. Weight gain, overweight, and obesity: Determinants and health outcomes from the Australian Longitudinal Study on Women's Health. *Curr. Obes. Rep.* **2014**, *3*, 46–53. [CrossRef] [PubMed]
8. Truesdale, K.P.; Stevens, J.; Lewis, C.E.; Schreiner, P.J.; Loria, C.M.; Cai, J. Changes in risk factors for cardiovascular disease by baseline weight status in young adults who maintain or gain weight over 15 years: The CARDIA study. *Int. J. Obes.* **2006**, *30*, 1397–1407. [CrossRef]
9. Zheng, Y.; Manson, J.E.; Yuan, C.; Liang, M.H.; Grodstein, F.; Stampfer, M.J.; Willett, W.C.; Hu, F.B. Associations of weight gain from early to middle adulthood with major health outcomes later in life. *JAMA* **2017**, *318*, 255–269. [CrossRef]
10. Chen, C.; Ye, Y.; Zhang, Y.; Pan, X.-F.; Pan, A. Weight change across adulthood in relation to all cause and cause specific mortality: Prospective cohort study. *BMJ* **2019**, *367*, l5584. [CrossRef]
11. Hall, K.D.; Kahan, S. Maintenance of lost weight and long-term management of obesity. *Med. Clin.* **2018**, *102*, 183–197. [CrossRef]
12. Nordmo, M.; Danielsen, Y.S.; Nordmo, M. The challenge of keeping it off, a descriptive systematic review of high-quality, follow-up studies of obesity treatments. *Obes. Rev.* **2020**, *21*, e12949. [CrossRef]
13. Proietto, J. Why is treating obesity so difficult? Justification for the role of bariatric surgery. *Med. J. Aust.* **2011**, *195*, 144–146. [CrossRef] [PubMed]
14. World Health Organization. *Global Action Plan for the Prevention and Control of Noncommunicable Diseases 2013–2020*; World Health Organization: Geneva, Switzerland, 2013.
15. World Health Organization. *Obesity: Preventing and Managing the Global Epidemic*; World Health Organization: Geneva, Switzerland, 2000.
16. Martin, J.C.; Awoke, M.A.; Misso, M.L.; Moran, L.J.; Harrison, C.L. Preventing weight gain in adults: A systematic review and meta-analysis of randomized controlled trials. *Obes. Rev.* **2021**, *22*, e13280. [CrossRef] [PubMed]
17. Davidson, K.W.; Goldstein, M.; Kaplan, R.M.; Kaufmann, P.G.; Knatterud, G.L.; Orleans, C.T.; Spring, B.; Trudeau, K.J.; Whitlock, E.P. Evidence-based behavioral medicine: What is it and how do we achieve it? *Ann. Behav. Med.* **2003**, *26*, 161–171. [CrossRef] [PubMed]
18. Michie, S.; Richardson, M.; Johnston, M.; Abraham, C.; Francis, J.; Hardeman, W.; Eccles, M.P.; Cane, J.; Wood, C.E. The behavior change technique taxonomy (v1) of 93 hierarchically clustered techniques: Building an international consensus for the reporting of behavior change interventions. *Ann. Behav. Med.* **2013**, *46*, 81–95. [CrossRef]
19. Dombrowski, S.U.; Sniehotta, F.F.; Avenell, A.; Johnston, M.; MacLennan, G.; Araújo-Soares, V. Identifying active ingredients in complex behavioural interventions for obese adults with obesity-related co-morbidities or additional risk factors for co-morbidities: A systematic review. *Health Psychol. Rev.* **2012**, *6*, 7–32. [CrossRef]
20. Lim, S.; Hill, B.; Pirotta, S.; O'Reilly, S.; Moran, L. What Are the Most Effective Behavioural Strategies in Changing Postpartum Women's Physical Activity and Healthy Eating Behaviours? A Systematic Review and Meta-Analysis. *J. Clin. Med.* **2020**, *9*, 237. [CrossRef]
21. Michie, S.; Abraham, C.; Whittington, C.; McAteer, J.; Gupta, S. Effective techniques in healthy eating and physical activity interventions: A meta-regression. *Health Psychol.* **2009**, *28*, 690. [CrossRef]
22. Samdal, G.B.; Eide, G.E.; Barth, T.; Williams, G.; Meland, E. Effective behaviour change techniques for physical activity and healthy eating in overweight and obese adults; systematic review and meta-regression analyses. *Int. J. Behav. Nutr. Phys. Act.* **2017**, *14*, 42. [CrossRef]
23. Hill, B.; Skouteris, H.; Fuller-Tyszkiewicz, M. Interventions designed to limit gestational weight gain: A systematic review of theory and meta-analysis of intervention components. *Obes. Rev.* **2013**, *14*, 435–450. [CrossRef]
24. Ashton, L.M.; Sharkey, T.; Whatnall, M.C.; Williams, R.L.; Bezzina, A.; Aguiar, E.J.; Collins, C.E.; Hutchesson, M.J. Effectiveness of interventions and behaviour change techniques for improving dietary intake in young adults: A systematic review and meta-analysis of RCTs. *Nutrients* **2019**, *11*, 825. [CrossRef]
25. Ashton, L.M.; Sharkey, T.; Whatnall, M.C.; Haslam, R.L.; Bezzina, A.; Aguiar, E.J.; Collins, C.E.; Hutchesson, M.J. Which behaviour change techniques within interventions to prevent weight gain and/or initiate weight loss improve adiposity outcomes in young adults? A systematic review and meta-analysis of randomized controlled trials. *Obes. Rev.* **2020**, *21*, e13009. [CrossRef]
26. Martin, J.; Chater, A.; Lorencatto, F. Effective behaviour change techniques in the prevention and management of childhood obesity. *Int. J. Obes.* **2013**, *37*, 1287–1294. [CrossRef]
27. Moher, D.; Liberati, A.; Tetzlaff, J.; Altman, D.G.; PRISMA Group. Preferred reporting items for systematic reviews and meta-analyses: The PRISMA statement. *PLoS Med.* **2009**, *6*, e1000097. [CrossRef]
28. Brandt, J.S.; Cruz Ithier, M.A.; Rosen, T.; Ashkinadze, E. Advanced paternal age, infertility, and reproductive risks: A review of the literature. *Prenat. Diagn.* **2019**, *39*, 81–87. [CrossRef]
29. Mann, L.; Bateson, D.; Black, K.I. Teenage pregnancy. *Aust. J. Gen. Pract.* **2020**, *49*, 310–316. [CrossRef]
30. Higgins, J.P.; Thompson, S.G.; Deeks, J.J.; Altman, D.G. Measuring inconsistency in meta-analyses. *BMJ* **2003**, *327*, 557–560. [CrossRef]

31. Bull, E.R.; McCleary, N.; Li, X.; Dombrowski, S.U.; Dusseldorp, E.; Johnston, M. Interventions to promote healthy eating, physical activity and smoking in low-income groups: A systematic review with meta-analysis of behavior change techniques and delivery/context. *Int. J. Behav. Med.* **2018**, *25*, 605–616. [CrossRef]
32. Michie, S.; West, R.; Sheals, K.; Godinho, C.A. Evaluating the effectiveness of behavior change techniques in health-related behavior: A scoping review of methods used. *Transl. Behav. Med.* **2018**, *8*, 212–224. [CrossRef]
33. Willmott, T.J.; Pang, B.; Rundle-Thiele, S.; Badejo, A. Weight management in young adults: Systematic review of electronic health intervention components and outcomes. *J. Med. Internet Res.* **2019**, *21*, e10265. [CrossRef]
34. Lim, S.; O'Reilly, S.; Behrens, H.; Skinner, T.; Ellis, I.; Dunbar, J.A. Effective strategies for weight loss in post-partum women: A systematic review and meta-analysis. *Obes. Rev.* **2015**, *16*, 972–987. [CrossRef]
35. Darling, K.E.; Sato, A.F. Systematic review and meta-analysis examining the effectiveness of mobile health technologies in using self-monitoring for pediatric weight management. *Child. Obes.* **2017**, *13*, 347–355. [CrossRef]
36. Spring, B.; Champion, K.E.; Acabchuk, R.; Hennessy, E.A. Self-regulatory behaviour change techniques in interventions to promote healthy eating, physical activity, or weight loss: A meta-review. *Health Psychol. Rev.* **2020**, 1–32. [CrossRef] [PubMed]
37. Abraham, C.; Michie, S. A taxonomy of behavior change techniques used in interventions. *Health Psychol.* **2008**, *27*, 379. [CrossRef]
38. Michie, S.; Ashford, S.; Sniehotta, F.F.; Dombrowski, S.U.; Bishop, A.; French, D.P. A refined taxonomy of behaviour change techniques to help people change their physical activity and healthy eating behaviours: The CALO-RE taxonomy. *Psychol. Health* **2011**, *26*, 1479–1498. [CrossRef] [PubMed]
39. Hutchesson, M.J.; Rollo, M.E.; Krukowski, R.; Ells, L.; Harvey, J.; Morgan, P.J.; Callister, R.; Plotnikoff, R.; Collins, C.E. eHealth interventions for the prevention and treatment of overweight and obesity in adults: A systematic review with meta-analysis. *Obes. Rev.* **2015**, *16*, 376–392. [CrossRef] [PubMed]
40. Singh, N.; Stewart, R.A.H.; Benatar, J.R. Intensity and duration of lifestyle interventions for long-term weight loss and association with mortality: A meta-analysis of randomised trials. *BMJ Open* **2019**, *9*, e029966. [CrossRef]
41. Hills, A.P.; Byrne, N.M.; Lindstrom, R.; Hill, J.O. 'Small Changes' to Diet and Physical Activity Behaviors for Weight Management. *Obes. Facts* **2013**, *6*, 228–238. [CrossRef]
42. Hall, K.D. What is the required energy deficit per unit weight loss? *Int. J. Obes.* **2008**, *32*, 573–576. [CrossRef]
43. Williams, S.L.; French, D.P. What are the most effective intervention techniques for changing physical activity self-efficacy and physical activity behaviour—And are they the same? *Health Educ. Res.* **2011**, *26*, 308–322. [CrossRef]
44. Lombard, C.; Harrison, C.; Kozica, S.; Zoungas, S.; Ranasinha, S.; Teede, H. Preventing weight gain in women in rural communities: A cluster randomised controlled trial. *PLoS Med.* **2016**, *13*, e1001941. [CrossRef]
45. Foster-Schubert, K.E.; Alfano, C.M.; Duggan, C.R.; Xiao, L.; Campbell, K.L.; Kong, A.; Bain, C.E.; Wang, C.Y.; Blackburn, G.L.; McTiernan, A. Effect of diet and exercise, alone or combined, on weight and body composition in overweight-to-obese postmenopausal women. *Obesity* **2012**, *20*, 1628–1638. [CrossRef]
46. Warburton, D.E.; Bredin, S.S. Health benefits of physical activity: A systematic review of current systematic reviews. *Curr. Opin. Cardiol.* **2017**, *32*, 541–556. [CrossRef]
47. Lara, J.; Evans, E.H.; O'Brien, N.; Moynihan, P.J.; Meyer, T.D.; Adamson, A.J.; Errington, L.; Sniehotta, F.F.; White, M.; Mathers, J.C. Association of behaviour change techniques with effectiveness of dietary interventions among adults of retirement age: A systematic review and meta-analysis of randomised controlled trials. *BMC Med.* **2014**, *12*, 177. [CrossRef]
48. Smith, D.M.; Taylor, W.; Lavender, T. Behaviour change techniques to change the postnatal eating and physical activity behaviours of women who are obese: A qualitative study. *BJOG Int. J. Obstet. Gynaecol.* **2016**, *123*, 279–284. [CrossRef]
49. Tate, D.F.; Lytle, L.; Polzien, K.; Diamond, M.; Leonard, K.R.; Jakicic, J.M.; Johnson, K.C.; Olson, C.M.; Patrick, K.; Svetkey, L.P. Deconstructing weight management interventions for young adults: Looking inside the black box of the EARLY consortium trials. *Obesity* **2019**, *27*, 1085–1098. [CrossRef]
50. Dusseldorp, E.; Van Genugten, L.; van Buuren, S.; Verheijden, M.W.; van Empelen, P. Combinations of techniques that effectively change health behavior: Evidence from Meta-CART analysis. *Health Psychol.* **2014**, *33*, 1530. [CrossRef] [PubMed]
51. Li, X.; Dusseldorp, E.; Meulman, J.J. Meta-CART: A tool to identify interactions between moderators in meta-analysis. *Br. J. Math. Stat. Psychol.* **2017**, *70*, 118–136. [CrossRef]

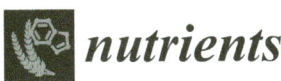

Review

Combined Physical Exercise and Diet: Regulation of Gut Microbiota to Prevent and Treat of Metabolic Disease: A Review

Li Zhang [1], Yuan Liu [1], Ying Sun [2] and Xin Zhang [2,*]

[1] Department of Physical Education, China University of Mining and Technology, Beijing 100083, China
[2] Department of Food Science and Engineering, Ningbo University, Ningbo 315211, China
* Correspondence: zhangxin@nbu.edu.cn

Abstract: Background: Unhealthy diet and sedentary lifestyle have contributed to the rising incidence of metabolic diseases, which is also accompanied by the shifts of gut microbiota architecture. The gut microbiota is a complicated and volatile ecosystem and can be regulated by diet and physical exercise. Extensive research suggests that diet alongside physical exercise interventions exert beneficial effects on metabolic diseases by regulating gut microbiota, involving in the changes of the energy metabolism, immune regulation, and the microbial-derived metabolites. Objective: In this review, we present the latest evidence in the modulating role of diet and physical exercise in the gut microbiota and its relevance to metabolic diseases. We also summarize the research from animal and human studies on improving metabolic diseases through diet-plus-exercise interventions, and new targeted therapies that might provide a better understanding of the potential mechanisms. Methods: A systematic and comprehensive literature search was performed in PubMed/Medline and Web of Science in October 2022. The key terms used in the searches included "combined physical exercise and diet", "physical exercise, diet and gut microbiota", "physical exercise, diet and metabolic diseases" and "physical exercise, diet, gut microbiota and metabolic diseases". Conclusions: Combined physical exercise and diet offer a more efficient approach for preventing metabolic diseases via the modification of gut microbiota, abating the burden related to longevity.

Keywords: metabolic diseases; gut microbiota; diet; physical exercise

1. Introduction

Sedentary lifestyle has progressively become a habitual way of life in modern societies, and so contributes to the rising incidence of metabolic diseases such as Type 2 diabetes (T2D), obesity, cardiovascular diseases (CVD) and non-alcoholic fatty liver disease (NAFLD) [1]. Metabolic risks (namely high body mass index (BMI), high blood sugar, high blood pressure, and high cholesterol) accounted for nearly 20 % of total health loss worldwide in 2019, according to the World Health Organization (WHO) database. The Lancet published that high blood pressure contributed to one in five deaths (almost 11 million) in 2019, followed by high blood sugar (6.5 million deaths), high BMI (5 million), and high cholesterol (4.4 million). The costs associated with these diseases are enormous, but it has been estimated that these diseases are preventable by regular and adequate levels of physical exercise. Practically, evidence showing the benefits of regular physical exercise for health, regardless of age, has grown in recent years. Habitual exercise contributes to decreasing blood pressure and serum triglyceride levels, as well as improving high-density lipoprotein cholesterol levels, insulin sensitivity and glucose homeostasis [2]. The health-promoting mechanisms of physical exercise are complex and multifaceted, including better regulate immune–inflammatory responses, reductions in oxidative stress and adiposity, acceleration of the elimination of damaged mitochondria, and so on [3]. Intriguingly, a new factor by which exercise may affect metabolic diseases has emerged: the interplay with gut microbiota (GM) [4].

GM is engaged in various interplays affecting the health during the host's entire life span. It acts as an endocrine organ, and the shifts of microbiota architecture and status promoted by exercise play an instrumental role in promoting the production of beneficial metabolites, stimulating/modulating the immune system, protecting the host from colonization of pathogens, and controlling lipid accumulation and insulin signaling [5]. In fact, positive effects have been reported, mainly in order to shape the diversity of microbiota, promote the formation of short-chain fatty acids (SCFAs), impact the integrity of the gut mucus layer, and maintain balance between beneficial and pathogenic bacterial communities [6]. Clinical research has revealed that α-diversity and SCFAs were increased and bacterial endotoxin lipopolysaccharide (LPS) was decreased in professional players than in non-athlete healthy subjects [7]. Meanwhile, regular exercise is a hormetic stressor to the gut that propels beneficial responses and improves the integrity of the intestinal barrier [8].

Diet is important in sculpting the microbial communities or metabolites in a manner that may affect disease [9]. The microbiota is exposed to healthy dietary components, such as dietary carbohydrates, proteins, vitamins, minerals and polyphenols, which can produce beneficial metabolites, in particular, SCFAs and tryptophan metabolites. These metabolites participate in the maintenance of intestinal mucosa integrity and also mediating host immune and homeostatic responses [6]. Conversely, an unhealthy diet, such as a high-fat diet (HFD), augments the production of pro-inflammatory cytokines, thereby leading to systemic chronic inflammation and LPS translocation, which increase the risk of metabolic diseases [4]. The effect of exercise on gut microbial composition or function is inextricably linked with dietary adjustments. The variety in the GM that seems to be associated with exercise may therefore be due to the combination with dietary intake, rather than exercise itself. According to the data from the WHO and The Centers for Disease Control and Prevention, regular physical exercise and dietary interventions can reduce the prevalence of gestational diabetes by 30% and the risk of death by 20% to 30% [1]. In this article, we review the research progress of the GM and its relationship with metabolic diseases, mainly including obesity, T2D, CVD, and NAFLD. We also focus on the effect of physical exercise, dietary components and dietary patterns on the GM. Importantly, this review presents some research and related mechanisms of preventing metabolic diseases by combining physical exercise and diet, which might provide a burgeoning avenue for the prevent of metabolic diseases.

2. Effect of Physical Exercise on Gut Microbiota

Physical exercise is defined as a subset of physical activity that is planned, structured and repetitive and aims to either improve or maintain physical fitness [10]. Research demonstrates that regular exercise is performing physical exercise of moderate intensity for a minimum of 30 min, 5 days a week, or of high intensity for a minimum of 20 min, 3 days a week [10]. Habitual exercise suppresses the expression of basal pro-inflammatory cytokines, but excessive exercise triggers the production of multiple pro-inflammatory mediators. Reasonable and moderate physical exercise protects against all-cause mortality, and only in extreme cases can these adaptations contribute to an increased risk of physical exercise-associated complications [11]. In fact, regular exercise training independently effects gut function and microbiome characteristics, and then has a beneficial role in preventing metabolic diseases (Figure 1).

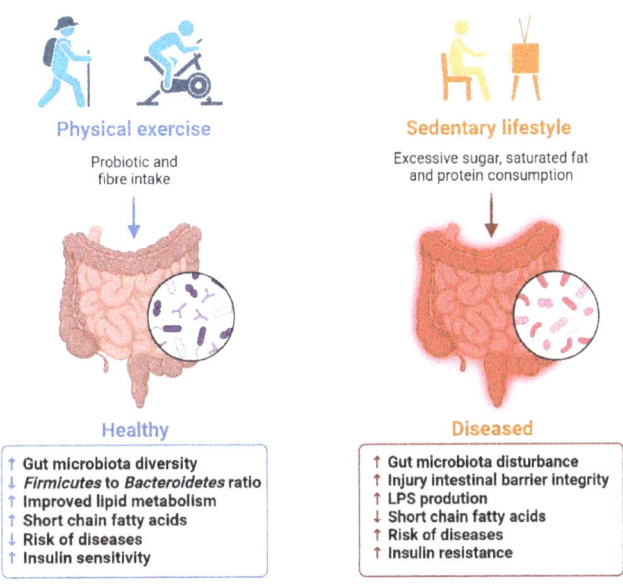

Figure 1. Effect of physical exercise on gut microbiota and host health.

The role of physical exercise in shaping the diversity of the GM and modulating its distribution has been demonstrated. The changes in the GM, under exercise conditions, can affect the absorption of nutrients, and then affect host metabolism. Data from the American Gut Project indicated that adopting moderate exercise (from never to daily) reshaped the alterations in microbial composition and function, and promoted a healthier gut environment of elderly individuals, especially overweight elderly individuals [12]. The GM of professional rugby players exhibited greater α-diversity and a decrease in the *Firmicutes* to *Bacteroidetes* ratio [13]. Women performing the regular dose of exercise displayed a higher abundance of health-promoting taxa, such as *Faecalibacterium prausnitzii*, *Roseburia hominis* and *Akkermansia muciniphila*, compared to sedentary counterparts [14]. Research revealed that these microbes are known butyrate producers, having a beneficial effect on promoting intestinal barrier integrity, regulating the host immune system and lipid metabolism [15–17]. Similar results have been yielded in animals. Mice that performed physical exercise typically showed an increase in commensal taxa such as *Bifidobacterium*, *Lactobacilli* and *Akkermansia* [8,18]. Moderate exercise also alleviated chronic stress-induced intestinal barrier impairment in mice, reducing bacterial translocations and maintaining intestinal permeability [19]. Furthermore, significant quantities of lactate are released during exercise and then secreted into the gut lumen, which can alter intestinal pH [6].

Conversely, high-intensity exercise may be having a deleterious influence on intestinal function. A total of 70% of athletes might experience abdominal pain, nausea, and diarrhea after strenuous exercises [20]. Prolonged exercise also results in less microbial diversity, increases the abundance of *Helicobacter*, as well as induces an increased intestinal permeability, promoting bacterial and their toxic products to enter into the bloodstream and activate systemic inflammation [21]. Exhaustive and acute endurance exercise, as observed in animal studies, has been indicated to induce altered permeability [22].

3. Effect of Diet on Gut Microbiota

3.1. Nutrients

3.1.1. Dietary Carbohydrates

A diet rich in different types and numbers of fruits, vegetables, and wholegrain cereals is the main sources of dietary carbohydrates (CHOs). In the human genome, less than 20 glycosidases have been identified as enzymes involved in digestion of dietary CHOs. Salivary α-amylase firstly breaks down complex CHOs into simple sugars in the mouth cavity, and digestible CHOs can be degraded and digested through pancreatic α-amylase, sucrase, maltase, galactose and lactase [23]. Complex non-digestible dietary CHOs drive our gut microbial to evolve an arsenal of carbohydrate-active enzymes in order to efficiently compete for nutrition [24].

The distal gut of the host is constantly inundated with a dynamic array of CHOs. It has been noted that simple CHOs (e.g., sucrose, fructose) cause rapid microbiota remodeling and hence metabolic disturbance in the host [25]. Complex CHOs, specifically, certain microbiota-accessible polysaccharides and dietary fiber, feed the dense consortium of microbes that compete in this habitat, having a major effect on gut microbial ecology and health [26]. A diet high in polysaccharides is related to up-regulated GM community diversity and promotes the growth of beneficial microbes, such as *Akkermansia*, *Bifidobacterium* and *Lactobacillus*. Meanwhile, GM can use intermediate oligosaccharides to generate host-beneficial SCFAs [27]. Pharmacological studies suggested *Dendrobium officinale* polysaccharides (DOPs) were indigestible and non-absorbing but promoted GM to produce more butyrate, mainly generated by *Parabacteroides*_sp_HGS0025, which mediated the improvement of intestinal health and immune function [28]. DOPs intervention also could reinforce the intestinal barrier function via promoting mucin synthesis, by acting on *Akkermansia muciniphila* [29]. Other polysaccharides from *Schisandra chinensis* also reversed the GM dysbiosis and upregulated the production of butyric acid and propionic acid, which is possibly involved in the anti-inflammation protective mechanism [30]. For dietary fiber, research indicated that an insulin-enriched diet reduced fasting blood glucose levels, as well as alleviated glucose intolerance and blood lipid panels in diabetic rats [31]. Remarkably, dietary fiber restriction not only contributes to a decrease in microbial diversity and the production of SCFAs, but also alters the metabolism of GM toward the utilization of less favorable substrates, which may be detrimental to the host [32].

3.1.2. Dietary Proteins

Dietary protein is another key macronutrient, which also modulates microbial composition and metabolite production. The relationship between protein intake and health follows a U-shaped curve, in which a lower protein intake is associated with undernutrition states, while intake above the tolerable limit is associated with overnutrition illnesses [24]. WHO recommends a daily protein intake of 0.83 g/kg for adults [33]. The products of dietary protein digestion are amino acids. Metabolites of amino acids by GM degradation include SCFAs, branched chain fatty acids, indoles, phenols, thiols, sulfides, ammonia and amines [24]. On the one hand, protein degradation provides essential free amino acids as an alternative energy source for colonocytes [9]. On the other hand, this process also releases toxic metabolic by-products such as ammonia, sulfides and phenols, which are detrimental for the local intestinal environment [9]. Research showed that moderate dietary protein restriction could shape the harmonious balance of the microbiota composition and diversity, and improve gut barrier function in adult pigs [34]. Higher protein diets show a reduction in the abundance of CHO utilizers belonging to *Lachnospiraceae*, *Ruminococcaceae* and *Akkermansia* [35]. In addition, proteins, especially from red meat and processed meat, are a source of L-carnitine and choline, which can be metabolized by GM and produce trimethylamine (TMA) [36], subsequently oxidized to trimethylamine N-oxide (TMAO) [37]. High TMAO concentrations are correlated with an increased risk of CVD or death [38]. It is important to note that athletes may have a higher protein requirement to support bone metabolism, keep adequate protein synthesis and energy metabolism, as well as sufficient immune function and intestinal integrity in the intensive/prolonged exercise routines [39]. Research recommends that the protein intake of endurance- and strength-trained athletes was 1.2–1.7 g/kg/day [40]. Lack of protein, for instance, could lead to menstrual disorders in female athletes [41].

3.1.3. Dietary Fats

Dietary fats from plants and animals are a reserve source of energy for the human growth and development. Fat is first digested by lingual and gastric lipases in the mouth. Dietary fat is hydrolyzed into free fatty acids (FFA) by pancreatic lipase; most of the FFA is absorbed in the small intestine, and a minority will pass through the gastrointestinal tract and directly alter GM composition [42]. A palm oil-based diet could induce body mass gains, negatively affect the microbiota diversity, and increase the ratio of *Firmicutes* to *Bacteroidetes*, compared to olive or safflower oil [43]. Regarding genera, saturated fatty acids decrease the abundance of *Bacteroides*, *Prevotella*, *Lactobacillus* spp. and *Bifidobacterium* spp. [44]. Consumption of HFD significantly also reduced the release of SCFAs compared with a low-fat diet [45]. The variation of the GM composition induced by dietary fats can also regulate the production of microbial-derived secondary bile acids (BAs). An HFD trigger enhanced BAs' discharge, resulting in increased colonic concentrations of primary BAs. However, 5% to 10% of BAs are not reabsorbed but are converted to secondary BAs by microbes in the large intestine, which are harmful and promote colon carcinogenesis [46]. Moreover, the microbiota dysbiosis observed in HFD mice favored the passage of LPS from the intestinal lumen to systemic circulation, which activated the host pro-inflammatory signaling pathway and then triggered a low-grade systemic inflammation [9,47].

3.1.4. Other Dietary Components

A stable gut microbial community is affected by several essential components, such as vitamins, minerals and polyphenols. Vitamins are required cofactors in small amounts for maintaining normal physiological function. Humans are incapable of synthesizing most vitamins to meet our daily needs, and they consequently have to be obtained exogenously. Remarkably, the GM has the capacity to regulate both the synthesis and metabolic output of various vitamins [24]. Subsequently, vitamins also can dramatically alter the abundance and diversity of the GM. Vitamin A, for example, can up-regulate the health-beneficial microbiota, including *Bifidobacterium*, *Lactobacillus* and *Akkermansia* genera [48]. Like vitamins, minerals are micronutrients that play an instrumental role for host metabolism and performing active interaction with the GM. It has been demonstrated that magnesium (Mg) deficiency is associated with an increased incidence of chronic disease [49] and reduces the *Bifidobacterial* content in Mg-deficient mice for four days [50]. While, with prolonged Mg deficiency (21 d), there is an increase in the abundance of *Bifidobacteria* and *Lactobacilli* [50]. Clinical trials are still necessary to identify the effects of magnesium deficiency and magnesium supplementation for avoiding adverse effects. In addition, polyphenols are a large and diverse family of compounds found widely in plant foods, several of which have been related to the gut health. Tea polyphenols could inhibit the growth of detrimental bacteria such as *Helicobacter pylori* and *Staphylococcus aureus*, and stimulate the growth or favor the growth of beneficial species of the GM, such as *Bifidobacterium* and *Akkermansia muciniphila* [51].

3.2. Dietary Patterns

It has been reported that dietary patterns may have a pronounced effect on the metabolic activity of the GM than individual nutrients. A single-nutrient dietary intervention has several limitations. Dietary habits worldwide are manifold, including the Western diet (WD), Mediterranean diet (MD), ketogenic diet (KD), intermittent fasting (IF) and so on (Table 1) [52]. In a WD, a large proportion of energy is provided by acellular nutrients, which are more easily digested by microbial and human cells [53]. Increased amounts of readily accessible acellular nutrients affect the regulation and maintenance of GM homeostasis by contributing to variations in pH, the GM composition and metabolism. On the other hand, the consumption of HFD also augmented the production of pro-inflammations cytokines, thereby leading to systemic chronic inflammation and LPS translocation [54]. As opposed to the WD, the MD is considered one of the most worldwide healthy dietary patterns. Greater adherence to the MD has been linked with a significant reduction in total mortality and reduces risk of immune system dysregulation, CVD, cognitive decline and cancer [55]. In addition, the MD changes the composition of the microbiota in favor of beneficial bacteria, such as *Parabacteroides distasonis*, *Bacteroides thetaiotaomicron*, and *Bifidobacterium adolescentis*, and counteracts the growth of pathogens, restoring potentially beneficial microbes [56]. The KD is a high-fat, adequate-protein, and low-CHOs diet. The body burns fats rather than CHOs to obtain calories by restricting the availability of CHOs. Research showed that the KD affected the GM with mixed results. On the one hand, the KD is at a greater risk of being nutritionally inadequate and may not maintain a healthy microbiota by lacking in fiber, necessary vitamins, minerals, and iron. On the other hand, research revealed that the KD conferred microbiota benefits and relieved colitis in a DSS-induced recipient, following the dramatic increase of the abundance of *Akkermansia* and butyric acid-producing *Roseburia*; additionally, the decrease of the abundance of *Escherichia/Shigella* was found in mice fed with a KD [57]. The IF is a dietary intervention similar to caloric restriction, encompassing various programs that manipulate meal time to improve body composition and overall health [58]. Overwhelming studies support the robust disease-modifying efficacy of the IF in animal models on a wide range of chronic disorders, including T2D, CVD, and brain function, in addition to weight loss [59]. The IF appears to have positive impacts on the GM. Preclinical studies consistently demonstrated the IF contributed to increasing the richness of gut microbes, enriching of the *Akkermansia muciniphila* and Lactobacillus, reducing putatively pro-inflammatory taxa *Desulfovibrio* and *Turicibacter*, and enhancing antioxidative microbial metabolic pathways [60].

Table 1. The effect of dietary patterns on health mediated by gut microbiota.

Dietary Pattern	Characteristic	Changes of Gut Microbiota	Effect	Reference
WD	High consumption of saturated and trans fatty acids, refined grains, sugar, salt, alcohol and other harmful elements; Low content of complex dietary fiber.	Firmicutes/Bacteroidetes ratio↑ *Alistipes*↑ *Bilophila*↑ *Bifidobacteria*↓	Systemic chronic inflammation and LPS translocation; Increase the risk of disease.	[61]
MD	High intake of whole grains and vegetables; Use olive oil as the lipid supply; A regular but moderate consumption of fish and other meat, dairy products and red wine.	*Bifidobacteria*↑ *Lactobacillus*↑ *Clostridium*↑ *Faecalibacterium*↑ *Oscillospira*↑ *Ruminococcus*↓ *Coprococcus*↓	Improve the gut barrier integrity; Protect against oxidative stress and inflammation; Reduce the total mortality and the risk of cardiovascular, metabolic and gastrointestinal diseases.	[56]
KD	High-fat, adequate-protein, and low-carbohydrate.	*Akkermansia*↑ *Parabacteroides*↑ *Escherichia*↓ *Shigella*↓	Nutritionally inadequate in fiber, necessary vitamins, minerals, and iron.	[57]

Table 1. Cont.

Dietary Pattern	Characteristic	Changes of Gut Microbiota	Effect	Reference
IF	Manipulate meal time to improve body composition and overall health, including of time-restricted feeding, alternate day fasting, and religious fasting.	*Akkermansia*↑ *Lactobacillus*↑ *Desulfovibrio*↓ *Turicibacter*↓	Improve gut epithelial integrity, the leaking LPS and blunted systemic inflammation; Improve metabolic profiles and reduce the risk of obesity, obesity-related conditions.	[62]
VD	Reduce or restrict of animal-derived foods; High intake of plant-source foods.	*Bacteroides* / *Prevotella* ratio↑ *Clostridium*↑ *Faecalibacterium*↑ *Bifidobacteria*↓	Reduce of caloric intake but nutritional deficiency of fatty acids, proteins, vitamins, and minerals; Prevent and better control of chronic diseases.	[63]
GD	The exclusion of gluten-containing cereals like wheat, rye, barley and hybrids.	*Bifidobacterium* ↓ *Lactobacillus*↓ *Enterobacteriaceae*↑ *Escherichia coli*↑	Appropriate for treatment of celiac disease, dermatitis herpetiformis and gluten ataxia.	[64]

WD = Western diet, MD = Mediterranean diet, KD = ketogenic diet, IF = intermittent fasting, VD = vegetarian diet, GD = gluten-free diet, ↑ = up-regulate, ↓ = down-regulate.

4. Gut Microbial Dysbiosis Linked to Metabolic Diseases

Traditionally, genetic variants have been thought to be the major drivers of metabolic diseases, but the heritability of these variants is fairly modest. The GM is recently suspected to be a contributor for driving metabolic diseases. Compared with healthy individuals, most populations with obesity, T2D, CVD and NAFLD show reduced gut microbial diversity. The GM's composition, if modified by external factors, leads to a dramatic change of the symbiotic relationship between GM and the host, which are essential for the development of metabolic diseases.

Alteration of the GM by behavioral changes, such as HFD and use of antibiotics, could be the robust drivers of the obesity pandemic. The researches concerning the role of the GM in mediating obesity pathogenesis, were based on findings from animal models firstly. The obese microbiota results in a significantly greater increase in harvesting energy from the diet. It has been observed that introduction of the microbiota from obese donors into germ-free (GF) mice results in an increased energy gain capacity, compared to those receiving the microbiota of lean donors [65]. Similarly, a transferrable obesity-associated microbiota contributes to the accumulation of total body fat than colonization with a 'lean microbiota' [66,67]. Following these phenomena, subsequent epidemiological studies have shown that GM composition differs between obese and lean individuals. [67]. Human studies observed that the microbiota of overweight individuals was characterized by a lower abundance of *Bacteroidetes* and a higher *Firmicutes* when compared with non-overweight individuals [68,69]. At the genus level, a metagenome-wide association study revealed the under-representation of *Bacteroides thetaiotaomicron* in obese individuals. Interestingly, gavage with *B. thetaiotaomicron* could alleviate diet-induced body weight gain and adiposity in mice, implying that probiotic or microbial compounds might be potential future modalities for anti-obesity [70].

T2D has also been considered to be under the influence of the dysregulated GM composition and functionality. Clinical reports have indicated the relative abundance of *Bifidobacterium*, *Lactobacillus* and butyrate-producing bacteria (*Akkermansia muciniphila*) were negatively associated with T2D, while the genera of *Clostridium* spp., *Ruminococcus*, *Fusobacterium* and *Blautia* were positively associated with T2D [71,72]. The dysregulation of the GM may impair intestinal barriers through damaging tight junction proteins (TJPs), subsequently causing a leaky mucosa and metabolic endotoxemia, which is one of the leading factors in insulin resistance and the development of T2D [73]. In addition, indirect evidence that the GM might be involved in glucose regulation comes from large-scale epidemiological studies, which revealed that patients with total colectomy had an increased risk of T2D compared with those without colectomy [74].

There are many pathological processes and risk factors of CVDs involved in obesity, T2D, dyslipidemia, hypertension, and an unhealthy lifestyle, such as partaking in smoking, lack of exercise and poor dietary habits [75]. Noteworthy, most of those factors are associated with the GM, and genome sequencing and metagenomic analyses also revealed the association between CVD phenotypes and changes of specific microbial taxa, or the GM richness and diversity. Early study demonstrated that bacterial DNA (mainly of *Chryseomonas*) was detected in atherosclerotic plaques with signatures that match taxa associated with disease states [76]. Moreover, a metagenomic analysis showed that the gut microbiome of CVD patients differed from those of healthy individuals, which was mainly manifested in elevated abundances of *Streptococcus* spp. and *Enterobacteriaceae* spp., and in the decreased abundances of *Bacteroides* spp., *Prevotella copri*, and *Alistipes shahii* [77,78]. At the mechanistic level, the effect of the GM on CVDs has been linked to modulation of inflammation, intestinal barrier function and metabolites. Dysbiosis-associated changes in the GM impair intestinal barriers, leading to an elevation in circulating LPS levels, and LPS can activate inflammatory signals through the toll-like receptor (TLR)-MyD88 signaling pathway, resulting in the release of pro-inflammatory cytokines that orchestrate an inflammatory state in the host [79]. Previous studies showed patients with heart failure displayed impaired intestinal integrity, and that elevated levels of pro-inflammatory cytokines in the blood are associated with symptom severity and poorer outcomes [80]. In metabolism-dependent pathways, GM cleaves some TMA-containing compounds to produce TMA, which can be further oxidized to TMAO by flavin monooxygenase. TMAO activates MAPK, NF-κB signaling pathways, contributing to inflammatory gene expression, which affects lipid metabolism and increases triglycerides, and decreases high-density lipoproteins in CVD patients [81].

NAFLD is a disorder associated with obesity, generally regarded as the hepatic manifestation of the metabolic syndrome. Multiple preclinical and clinical studies have highlighted a role of the GM in NAFLD pathogenesis, although we are still far from finding a causal link. In brief, individuals with NAFLDs harbor lower GM diversity than healthy subjects, having an increased abundance of species assigned to *Anaerobacter*, *Streptococcus*, *Escherichia* and *Lactobacillus*, and a lesser abundance of *Prevotella*, *Oscillibacter* and *Alistipes* spp [82–84]. The mechanism by which GM is proposed to affect NAFLD is in terms of the gut–liver axis. Aside from dysregulation of the GM, NAFLD is also related to the enterohepatic circulation of bile acids, GM-mediated inflammation of the intestinal mucosa and the related impairment in mucosal immune function [52].

5. Combined Physical Exercise and Diet for Preventing Metabolic Diseases by Modulating Gut Microbiota

Consumption of a calorie-rich diet and sedentary lifestyle have contributed to the rising incidence of obesity in the modern lifestyle, which is caused by energy intake exceeding energy expenditure to a large extent. Substantial epidemiologic evidence suggests obesity is a risk factor for inducing other metabolic diseases, including T2D, CVD and NAFLD. Identifying effective interventions is an important way for improving metabolic diseases. In fact, the majority of research concluded that when a program includes diet alongside physical exercise, there were more effective changes, compared with exercise or diet alone [85]. The diversity and function of GM are also affected by diet and physical exercise. Here, we will summarize the research from animal and human and potential mechanisms on improving metabolic diseases through diet-plus-exercise interventions.

5.1. Evidence from Animal Studies

The effects of exercise and diet on GM are more extensively focused on in HFD animal models. Repeated exercise increased the α-diversity and metabolic capacity of the mouse distal GM during diet-induced obesity [86]. Moderate exercise and a low-fat diet have beneficial effects on body weight loss and macrophage immunocompetence in HFD-induced obese mice [4]. Exercise plus curcumin in combination exhibited better effective in weight loss and improved glucose homeostasis and lipid profiles of diabetic rats, compared with exercise or diet alone interventions groups [87]. Besides, the combined treatment of isoflavones and exercise has a stronger impact on enhancing GM diversity and preventing HFD-induced inflammation [88].

5.2. Evidence from Human Studies

Although diet-plus-exercise interventions are classically accepted, few human studies deeply reveal the effect of the combination of physical exercise and diet on GM and metabolic diseases, which often focus on meta-analysis studies. A meta-analysis from Johns et al. identified that there was no difference in weight loss in the short-term for diet-only/exercise-only interventions than for combined physical exercise and diet, but in both the short and long term, weight had a greater reduction in the diet-plus-exercise interventions groups [36]. Wu et al. conducted a meta-analysis of weight loss studies published from 1997 to 2008. Results indicated that the weighted mean difference for the 1–2 year time point between combined physical exercise groups and diet-only controls was -2.29 vs. -0.67 kg/m^2 for BMI, respectively, implying that diet-plus-exercise interventions yielded a more long-term weight loss effect than diet-only interventions [89]. The diet-plus-exercise interventions was also found to be superior in improving the body weight and adiposity of overweight/obese postmenopausal women, compared with diet-only interventions [90]. Moreover, a 6 month randomized intervention program suggested that aerobic exercise and a low-CHO diet offer a more efficient approach for reducing liver fat and preventing diabetes via modification of GM composition [91]. A randomized controlled trial for overweight/obese Chinese females (BMI 25.1 ± 3.1 kg/m^2) revealed that a combined low-carbohydrate diet with exercise training increased the SCFAs-producing *Blautia* genus and reduced T2D-related genus *Alistipes*, caused significant weight loss, as well as improved blood pressure, insulin sensitivity and cardiorespiratory fitness, suggesting that a low-CHO diet and exercise interventions might play a role in cardiometabolic health by regulating the GM [92,93]. A recent randomized controlled trial demonstrated that diet-plus-exercise interventions could significantly reduce hepatic fat content and increase the diversity and stabilize of keystone microbes than exercise or diet alone interventions, which offered a more efficient avenue for developing diet-plus-exercise intervention strategies for preventing NAFLD [94].

5.3. Underlying Mechanisms

The key is to understand the potential mechanism that a combined diet and exercise strategy may prevent metabolic diseases (Figure 2). Several studies have elucidated that exercise in the fasted state generated advantageous metabolic adaptations, accompanying by stable blood glucose concentrations and elevated blood FFA concentrations, which may be more effective in improving insulin sensitivity and controlling glycemic in insulin-resistant individuals [95,96]. From the GM perspective, combining physical exercise and diet tempers intestinal barrier dysfunction, reserving mucous thickness and intestinal permeability. The intestinal barrier is a selective physical and immunological barrier that facilitates nutrient, water, and electrolyte absorption into circulation while deterring the translocation of harmful pathogens and noxious luminal substances [97]. As previously mentioned, one of the pathophysiological statuses by which metabolic diseases could be perpetuated and aggravated was intestinal homeostasis dysbiosis to release endotoxins, creating a leaky gut, which induces a chronic low-grade inflammatory state in the host [98]. Diet and exercise can modulate the expression of TJPs involved in the maintenance of epithelial membrane integrity, which improves intestinal permeability and reduces the risk for chronic disease [99].

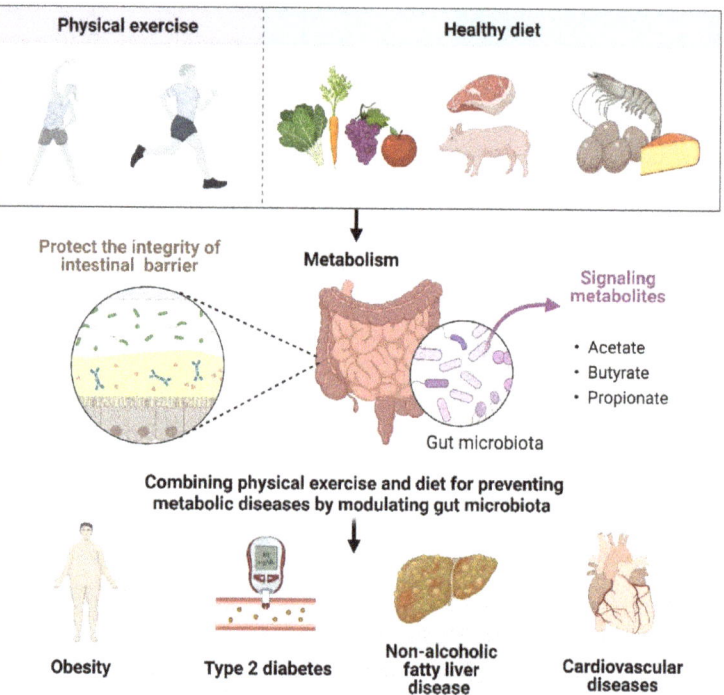

Figure 2. Combining physical exercise and diet for preventing metabolic diseases by modulating gut microbiota.

The combination of diet and exercise also can influence how the GM utilizes and synthesizes metabolites. The GM and the corresponding metabolites act in concert with the host in different ways, affecting intestinal homoeostasis and providing protective intervention for metabolic diseases. Specifically, SCFAs are one of the major end products of microbial fermentation or the transformation of dietary polysaccharides in the gut. Exercise is a potent modulator of SCFAs, exerting a particular influence on butyrate concentrations [16]. SCFAs are the primary energy source for the intestinal epithelial cells, participating in the maintenance of intestinal mucosa integrity, which also improves glucose and lipid metabolism, controls energy expenditure as well as regulates the immune system and inflammatory responses [100]. In animal models, the supplementation with SCFAs has been shown to improve the metabolic phenotype by increasing energy expenditure and glucose tolerance, and might help delay or attenuate diabetes and lead to weight reduction [101].

6. Conclusions and Future Perspectives

Regular and adequate levels of physical exercise and diet interventions abate the burden related to longevity and expand life expectancy of present days. Regular exercise is a hormetic stressor to the gut that propels beneficial responses, particularly in shaping the diversity of the GM and modulating its distribution. Healthy dietary components and patterns combined with physical exercise propels the production of beneficial metabolites and tempers intestinal barrier dysfunction, which protects the host against invading microorganisms, contributing to maintaining homeostasis and preventing metabolic diseases. However, additional challenges and limitations in the area of research are numerous. Although both interventions are traditionally accepted and implemented, few in-depth studies focus on the mechanism of microbiota-based strategies coupled with physical exercise programs to delay metabolic disease onset. More research is needed to determine whether the GM could be an important predictor of metabolic diseases in response to dietary and exercise interventions. Exercise intensity is a controversial issue; we must be take into consideration the various forms of exercise, and the exercise duration. Meanwhile, we should formulate different intervention plans according to different populations; the challenge is how to motivate the sedentary people to escape from unhealthy lifestyles.

Author Contributions: Conceptualization, writing—original draft, supervision, L.Z.; writing—conceptualization; investigation; writing—review & editing, Y.L.; writing—review and editing, Y.S.; supervision, writing—review and editing, X.Z. All authors have read and agreed to the published version of the manuscript.

Funding: This work was funded by the Ningbo Natural Science Foundation [2021J107].

Institutional Review Board Statement: Not applicable.

Informed Consent Statement: Not applicable.

Conflicts of Interest: The authors declare no conflict of interest.

References

1. Kramer, A. An overview of the beneficial effects of exercise on health and performance. *Adv. Exp. Med. Biol.* **2020**, *1228*, 3–22. [PubMed]
2. Wu, N.N.; Tian, H.; Chen, P.; Wang, D.; Ren, J.; Zhang, Y. Physical exercise and selective autophagy: Benefit and risk on cardiovascular health. *Cells* **2019**, *8*, 1436. [CrossRef]
3. Peeri, M.; Amiri, S. Protective effects of exercise in metabolic disorders are mediated by inhibition of mitochondrial-derived sterile inflammation. *Med. Hypotheses* **2015**, *85*, 707–709. [CrossRef] [PubMed]
4. Jeong, J.; Park, H.; Kwon, S.; Jang, H.; Jun, J.; Kim, M.-W.; Lee, S.K.; Lee, K.; Lee, W.L. Effect of moderate exercise training and low-fat diet on peritoneal macrophage immunocompetence in high-fat diet-induced obese mice model. *Phys. Act. Nutr.* **2012**, *16*, 133–142. [CrossRef]
5. Ejtahed, H.S.; Soroush, A.R.; Angoorani, P.; Larijani, B.; Hasani-Ranjbar, S. Gut microbiota as a target in the pathogenesis of metabolic disorders: A new approach to novel therapeutic agents. *Horm. Metab. Res.* **2016**, *48*, 349–358. [CrossRef]
6. Mailing, L.J.; Allen, J.M.; Buford, T.W.; Fields, C.J.; Woods, J.A. Exercise and the gut microbiome: A review of the evidence, potential mechanisms, and implications for human health. *Exerc. Sport Sci. Rev.* **2019**, *47*, 75–85. [CrossRef]
7. Chen, J.; Guo, Y.; Gui, Y.; Xu, D. Physical exercise, gut, gut microbiota, and atherosclerotic cardiovascular diseases. *Lipids Health Dis.* **2018**, *17*, 17. [CrossRef]
8. Hughes, R.L. A review of the role of the gut microbiome in personalized sports nutrition. *Front. Nutr.* **2019**, *6*, 191. [CrossRef]
9. Wolter, M.; Grant, E.T.; Boudaud, M.; Steimle, A.; Pereira, G.V.; Martens, E.C.; Desai, M.S. Leveraging diet to engineer the gut microbiome. *Nat. Rev. Gastroenterol. Hepatol.* **2021**, *18*, 885–902. [CrossRef]
10. Cordero, A.; Masia, M.D.; Galve, E. Physical exercise and health. *Rev. Esp. Cardiol.* **2014**, *67*, 748–753. [CrossRef]
11. Codella, R.; Luzi, L.; Terruzzi, I. Exercise has the guts: How physical activity may positively modulate gut microbiota in chronic and immune-based diseases. *Dig. Liver Dis.* **2018**, *50*, 331–341. [CrossRef] [PubMed]
12. Zhu, Q.; Jiang, S.; Du, G. Effects of exercise frequency on the gut microbiota in elderly individuals. *Microbiologyopen* **2020**, *9*, e1053. [CrossRef] [PubMed]
13. Clarke, S.F.; Murphy, E.F.; O'Sullivan, O.; Lucey, A.J.; Humphreys, M.; Hogan, A.; Hayes, P.; O'Reilly, M.; Jeffery, I.B.; Wood-Martin, R.; et al. Exercise and associated dietary extremes impact on gut microbial diversity. *Gut* **2014**, *63*, 1913–1920. [CrossRef] [PubMed]
14. Bressa, C.; Bailen-Andrino, M.; Perez-Santiago, J.; Gonzalez-Soltero, R.; Perez, M.; Montalvo-Lominchar, M.G.; Mate-Munoz, J.L.; Dominguez, R.; Moreno, D.; Larrosa, M. Differences in gut microbiota profile between women with active lifestyle and sedentary women. *PLoS ONE* **2017**, *12*, e0171352. [CrossRef]
15. Peng, L.; Li, Z.R.; Green, R.S.; Holzman, I.R.; Lin, J. Butyrate enhances the intestinal barrier by facilitating tight junction assembly via activation of AMP-activated protein kinase in Caco-2 cell monolayers. *J. Nutr.* **2009**, *139*, 1619–1625. [CrossRef]
16. Matsumoto, M.; Inoue, R.; Tsukahara, T.; Ushida, K.; Chiji, H.; Matsubara, N.; Hara, H. Voluntary running exercise alters microbiota composition and increases n-butyrate concentration in the rat cecum. *Biosci. Biotechnol. Biochem.* **2008**, *72*, 572–576. [CrossRef]
17. Canani, R.B.; Costanzo, M.D.; Leone, L.; Pedata, M.; Meli, R.; Calignano, A. Potential beneficial effects of butyrate in intestinal and extraintestinal diseases. *World J. Gastroenterol.* **2011**, *17*, 1519–1528. [CrossRef]
18. Liu, T.W.; Park, Y.M.; Holscher, H.D.; Padilla, J.; Scroggins, R.J.; Welly, R.; Britton, S.L.; Koch, L.G.; Vieira-Potter, V.J.; Swanson, K.S. Physical activity differentially affects the cecal microbiota of ovariectomized female rats selectively bred for high and low aerobic capacity. *PLoS ONE* **2015**, *10*, e0136150. [CrossRef]

19. Luo, B.; Xiang, D.; Nieman, D.C.; Chen, P. The effects of moderate exercise on chronic stress-induced intestinal barrier dysfunction and antimicrobial defense. *Brain Behav. Immun.* **2014**, *39*, 99–106. [CrossRef]
20. de Oliveira, E.P.; Burini, R.C. The impact of physical exercise on the gastrointestinal tract. *Curr. Opin. Clin. Nutr. Metab. Care* **2009**, *12*, 533–538. [CrossRef]
21. Karl, J.P.; Margolis, L.M.; Madslien, E.H.; Murphy, N.E.; Castellani, J.W.; Gundersen, Y.; Hoke, A.V.; Levangie, M.W.; Kumar, R.; Chakraborty, N.; et al. Changes in intestinal microbiota composition and metabolism coincide with increased intestinal permeability in young adults under prolonged physiological stress. *Am. J. Physiol. Gastrointest. Liver Physiol.* **2017**, *312*, G559–G571. [CrossRef]
22. Gutekunst, K.; Kruger, K.; August, C.; Diener, M.; Mooren, F.C. Acute exercises induce disorders of the gastrointestinal integrity in a murine model. *Eur. J. Appl. Physiol.* **2014**, *114*, 609–617. [CrossRef] [PubMed]
23. Kumar, J.; Rani, K.; Datt, C. Molecular link between dietary fibre, gut microbiota and health. *Mol. Biol. Rep.* **2020**, *47*, 6229–6237. [CrossRef] [PubMed]
24. Gentile, C.L.; Weir, T.L. The gut microbiota at the intersection of diet and human health. *Science* **2018**, *362*, 776–780. [CrossRef] [PubMed]
25. Sonnenburg, E.D.; Smits, S.A.; Tikhonov, M.; Higginbottom, S.K.; Wingreen, N.S.; Sonnenburg, J.L. Diet-induced extinctions in the gut microbiota compound over generations. *Nature* **2016**, *529*, 212–215. [CrossRef]
26. Moszak, M.; Szulinska, M.; Bogdanski, P. You are what you eat-the relationship between diet, microbiota, and metabolic disorders-a review. *Nutrients* **2020**, *12*, 1096. [CrossRef]
27. Sun, Y.; Zhang, Z.; Cheng, L.; Zhang, X.; Liu, Y.; Zhang, R.; Weng, P.; Wu, Z. Polysaccharides confer benefits in immune regulation and multiple sclerosis by interacting with gut microbiota. *Food Res. Int.* **2021**, *149*, 110675. [CrossRef] [PubMed]
28. Li, M.; Yue, H.; Wang, Y.; Guo, C.; Du, Z.; Jin, C.; Ding, K. Intestinal microbes derived butyrate is related to the immunomodulatory activities of *Dendrobium officinale* polysaccharide. *Int. J. Biol. Macromol.* **2020**, *149*, 717–723. [CrossRef] [PubMed]
29. Wang, Y.J.; Li, Q.M.; Zha, X.Q.; Luo, J.P. *Dendrobium fimbriatum* Hook polysaccharide ameliorates dextran-sodium-sulfate-induced colitis in mice via improving intestinal barrier function, modulating intestinal microbiota, and reducing oxidative stress and inflammatory responses. *Food Funct.* **2022**, *13*, 143–160. [CrossRef]
30. Yan, T.; Wang, N.; Liu, B.; Wu, B.; Xiao, F.; He, B.; Jia, Y. *Schisandra chinensis* ameliorates depressive-like behaviors by regulating microbiota-gut-brain axis via its anti-inflammation activity. *Phytother. Res.* **2021**, *35*, 289–296. [CrossRef]
31. Zhang, Q.; Yu, H.; Xiao, X.; Hu, L.; Xin, F.; Yu, X. Inulin-type fructan improves diabetic phenotype and gut microbiota profiles in rats. *PeerJ* **2018**, *6*, e4446. [CrossRef] [PubMed]
32. Makki, K.; Deehan, E.C.; Walter, J.; Backhed, F. The impact of dietary fiber on gut microbiota in host health and disease. *Cell Host Microbe* **2018**, *23*, 705–715. [CrossRef] [PubMed]
33. World Health Organization. *Protein and Amino Acid Requirements in Human Nutrition*; World Health Organization: Geneva, Switzerland, 2007; pp. 1–265.
34. Chen, X.; Song, P.; Fan, P.; He, T.; Jacobs, D.; Levesque, C.L.; Johnston, L.J.; Ji, L.; Ma, N.; Chen, Y.; et al. Moderate dietary protein restriction optimized gut microbiota and mucosal barrier in growing pig model. *Front. Cell Infect. Microbiol.* **2018**, *8*, 246. [CrossRef] [PubMed]
35. Mu, C.; Yang, Y.; Luo, Z.; Guan, L.; Zhu, W. The colonic microbiome and epithelial transcriptome are altered in rats fed a high-protein diet compared with a normal-protein diet. *J. Nutr.* **2016**, *146*, 474–483. [CrossRef]
36. Johns, D.J.; Hartmann-Boyce, J.; Jebb, S.A.; Aveyard, P. Behavioural weight management review. Diet or exercise interventions vs combined behavioral weight management programs: A systematic review and meta-analysis of direct comparisons. *J. Acad. Nutr. Diet* **2014**, *114*, 1557–1568. [CrossRef] [PubMed]
37. Koeth, R.A.; Wang, Z.; Levison, B.S.; Buffa, J.A.; Org, E.; Sheehy, B.T.; Britt, E.B.; Fu, X.; Wu, Y.; Li, L.; et al. Intestinal microbiota metabolism of L-carnitine, a nutrient in red meat, promotes atherosclerosis. *Nat. Med.* **2013**, *19*, 576–585. [CrossRef] [PubMed]
38. Tang, W.H.; Hazen, S.L. The contributory role of gut microbiota in cardiovascular disease. *J. Clin. Investig.* **2014**, *124*, 4204–4211. [CrossRef]
39. Karlund, A.; Gomez-Gallego, C.; Turpeinen, A.M.; Palo-Oja, O.M.; El-Nezami, H.; Kolehmainen, M. Protein supplements and their relation with nutrition, microbiota composition and health: Is more protein always better for sportspeople? *Nutrients* **2019**, *11*, 829. [CrossRef]
40. Rodriguez, N.R.; DiMarco, N.M.; Langley, S.; American Dietetic Association; Dietitians of Canada; American College of Sports Medicine: Nutrition; Performance, A. Position of the American dietetic association, dietitians of Canada, and the American College of Sports Medicine: Nutrition and athletic performance. *J. Am. Diet Assoc.* **2009**, *109*, 509–527.
41. Lagowska, K.; Kapczuk, K.; Friebe, Z.; Bajerska, J. Effects of dietary intervention in young female athletes with menstrual disorders. *J. Int. Soc. Sports Nutr.* **2014**, *11*, 21. [CrossRef]
42. Coelho, O.G.L.; Candido, F.G.; Alfenas, R.C.G. Dietary fat and gut microbiota: Mechanisms involved in obesity control. *Crit. Rev. Food Sci. Nutr.* **2019**, *59*, 3045–3053. [CrossRef] [PubMed]
43. de Wit, N.; Derrien, M.; Bosch-Vermeulen, H.; Oosterink, E.; Keshtkar, S.; Duval, C.; de Vogel-van den Bosch, J.; Kleerebezem, M.; Muller, M.; van der Meer, R. Saturated fat stimulates obesity and hepatic steatosis and affects gut microbiota composition by an enhanced overflow of dietary fat to the distal intestine. *Am. J. Physiol. Gastrointest. Liver Physiol.* **2012**, *303*, G589–G599. [CrossRef] [PubMed]

44. Zhang, H.; Cui, Y.; Zhu, S.; Feng, F.; Zheng, X. Characterization and antimicrobial activity of a pharmaceutical microemulsion. *Int. J. Pharm.* **2010**, *395*, 154–160. [CrossRef]
45. Parolini, C.; Bjorndal, B.; Busnelli, M.; Manzini, S.; Ganzetti, G.S.; Dellera, F.; Ramsvik, M.; Bruheim, I.; Berge, R.K.; Chiesa, G. Effect of dietary components from antarctic krill on atherosclerosis in apoE-deficient mice. *Mol. Nutr. Food Res.* **2017**, *61*, 10. [CrossRef]
46. Usuda, H.; Okamoto, T.; Wada, K. Leaky gut: Effect of dietary fiber and fats on microbiome and intestinal barrier. *Int. J. Mol. Sci.* **2021**, *22*, 7613. [CrossRef] [PubMed]
47. Boroni Moreira, A.P.; de Cassia Goncalves Alfenas, R. The influence of endotoxemia on the molecular mechanisms of insulin resistance. *Nutr. Hosp.* **2012**, *27*, 382–390. [PubMed]
48. Yang, Q.; Liang, Q.; Balakrishnan, B.; Belobrajdic, D.P.; Feng, Q.J.; Zhang, W. Role of dietary nutrients in the modulation of gut microbiota: A narrative review. *Nutrients* **2020**, *12*, 381. [CrossRef]
49. Grober, U.; Schmidt, J.; Kisters, K. Magnesium in prevention and therapy. *Nutrients* **2015**, *7*, 8199–8226. [CrossRef]
50. Pachikian, B.D.; Neyrinck, A.M.; Deldicque, L.; De Backer, F.C.; Catry, E.; Dewulf, E.M.; Sohet, F.M.; Bindels, L.B.; Everard, A.; Francaux, M.; et al. Changes in intestinal *bifidobacteria* levels are associated with the inflammatory response in magnesium-deficient mice. *J. Nutr.* **2010**, *140*, 509–514. [CrossRef]
51. Tomas-Barberan, F.A.; Selma, M.V.; Espin, J.C. Interactions of gut microbiota with dietary polyphenols and consequences to human health. *Curr. Opin. Clin. Nutr. Metab. Care* **2016**, *19*, 471–476. [CrossRef]
52. Aron-Wisnewsky, J.; Warmbrunn, M.V.; Nieuwdorp, M.; Clement, K. Nonalcoholic fatty liver disease: Modulating gut microbiota to improve severity? *Gastroenterology* **2020**, *158*, 1881–1898. [CrossRef] [PubMed]
53. Zinocker, M.K.; Lindseth, I.A. The Western diet-microbiome-host interaction and its role in metabolic disease. *Nutrients* **2018**, *10*, 365. [CrossRef] [PubMed]
54. Garcia-Montero, C.; Fraile-Martinez, O.; Gomez-Lahoz, A.M.; Pekarek, L.; Castellanos, A.J.; Noguerales-Fraguas, F.; Coca, S.; Guijarro, L.G.; Garcia-Honduvilla, N.; Asunsolo, A.; et al. Nutritional components in Western diet versus Mediterranean diet at the gut microbiota-immune system interplay. Implications for health and disease. *Nutrients* **2021**, *13*, 699. [CrossRef] [PubMed]
55. Martinez-Gonzalez, M.A.; Salas-Salvado, J.; Estruch, R.; Corella, D.; Fito, M.; Ros, E.; Predimed, I. Benefits of the Mediterranean diet: Insights from the PREDIMED study. *Prog. Cardiovasc. Dis.* **2015**, *58*, 50–60. [CrossRef]
56. Haro, C.; Garcia-Carpintero, S.; Alcala-Diaz, J.F.; Gomez-Delgado, F.; Delgado-Lista, J.; Perez-Martinez, P.; Rangel Zuniga, O.A.; Quintana-Navarro, G.M.; Landa, B.B.; Clemente, J.C.; et al. The gut microbial community in metabolic syndrome patients is modified by diet. *J. Nutr. Biochem.* **2016**, *27*, 27–31. [CrossRef]
57. Kong, C.; Yan, X.; Liu, Y.; Huang, L.; Zhu, Y.; He, J.; Gao, R.; Kalady, M.F.; Goel, A.; Qin, H.; et al. Ketogenic diet alleviates colitis by reduction of colonic group 3 innate lymphoid cells through altering gut microbiome. *Signal Transduct. Target Ther.* **2021**, *6*, 154. [CrossRef]
58. Nowosad, K.; Sujka, M. Effect of various types of intermittent fasting (IF) on weight loss and improvement of diabetic parameters in human. *Curr. Nutr. Rep.* **2021**, *10*, 146–154. [CrossRef]
59. Zhang, M.; Zhao, D.; Zhou, G.; Li, C. Dietary pattern, gut microbiota, and Alzheimer's disease. *J. Agric. Food. Chem.* **2020**, *68*, 12800–12809. [CrossRef]
60. Cignarella, F.; Cantoni, C.; Ghezzi, L.; Salter, A.; Dorsett, Y.; Chen, L.; Phillips, D.; Weinstock, G.M.; Fontana, L.; Cross, A.H.; et al. Intermittent fasting confers protection in CNS autoimmunity by altering the gut microbiota. *Cell Metab.* **2018**, *27*, 1222–1235.e6. [CrossRef]
61. Christ, A.; Lauterbach, M.; Latz, E. Western diet and the immune system: An inflammatory connection. *Immunity* **2019**, *51*, 794–811. [CrossRef]
62. Hatori, M.; Vollmers, C.; Zarrinpar, A.; DiTacchio, L.; Bushong, E.A.; Gill, S.; Leblanc, M.; Chaix, A.; Joens, M.; Fitzpatrick, J.A.; et al. Time-restricted feeding without reducing caloric intake prevents metabolic diseases in mice fed a high-fat diet. *Cell Metab.* **2012**, *15*, 848–860. [CrossRef] [PubMed]
63. Hargreaves, S.M.; Raposo, A.; Saraiva, A.; Zandonadi, R.P. Vegetarian diet: An overview through the perspective of quality of life domains. *Int. J. Environ. Res. Public Health* **2021**, *18*, 4067. [CrossRef] [PubMed]
64. Rinninella, E.; Cintoni, M.; Raoul, P.; Lopetuso, L.R.; Scaldaferri, F.; Pulcini, G.; Miggiano, G.A.D.; Gasbarrini, A.; Mele, M.C. Food components and dietary habits: Keys for a healthy gut microbiota composition. *Nutrients* **2019**, *11*, 2393. [CrossRef] [PubMed]
65. Backhed, F.; Ding, H.; Wang, T.; Hooper, L.V.; Koh, G.Y.; Nagy, A.; Semenkovich, C.F.; Gordon, J.I. The gut microbiota as an environmental factor that regulates fat storage. *Proc. Natl. Acad. Sci. USA* **2004**, *101*, 15718–15723. [CrossRef] [PubMed]
66. Turnbaugh, P.J.; Ley, R.E.; Mahowald, M.A.; Magrini, V.; Mardis, E.R.; Gordon, J.I. An obesity-associated gut microbiome with increased capacity for energy harvest. *Nature* **2006**, *444*, 1027–1031. [CrossRef]
67. Turnbaugh, P.J.; Baeckhed, F.; Fulton, L.; Gordon, J.I. Diet-induced obesity is linked to marked but reversible alterations in the mouse distal gut microbiome. *Cell Host Microbe* **2008**, *3*, 213–223. [CrossRef]
68. Kasai, C.; Sugimoto, K.; Moritani, I.; Tanaka, J.; Oya, Y.; Inoue, H.; Tameda, M.; Shiraki, K.; Ito, M.; Takei, Y.; et al. Comparison of the gut microbiota composition between obese and non-obese individuals in a Japanese population, as analyzed by terminal restriction fragment length polymorphism and next-generation sequencing. *BMC Gastroenterol.* **2015**, *15*, 100. [CrossRef]

69. Bervoets, L.; Van Hoorenbeeck, K.; Kortleven, I.; Van Noten, C.; Hens, N.; Vael, C.; Goossens, H.; Desager, K.N.; Vankerckhoven, V. Differences in gut microbiota composition between obese and lean children: A cross-sectional study. *Gut Pathog.* **2013**, *5*, 10. [CrossRef]
70. Liu, R.; Hong, J.; Xu, X.; Feng, Q.; Zhang, D.; Gu, Y.; Shi, J.; Zhao, S.; Liu, W.; Wang, X.; et al. Gut microbiome and serum metabolome alterations in obesity and after weight-loss intervention. *Nat. Med.* **2017**, *23*, 859–868. [CrossRef]
71. Wang, X.K.; Xu, X.Q.; Xia, Y. Further analysis reveals new gut microbiome markers of type 2 diabetes mellitus. *Anton. Leeuw. Int. J. G.* **2017**, *110*, 445–453. [CrossRef]
72. Larsen, N.; Vogensen, F.K.; van den Berg, F.W.J.; Nielsen, D.S.; Andreasen, A.S.; Pedersen, B.K.; Abu Al-Soud, W.; Sorensen, S.J.; Hansen, L.H.; Jakobsen, M. Gut microbiota in Hhuman adults with type 2 diabetes differs from non-diabetic adults. *PLoS ONE* **2010**, *5*, e9085. [CrossRef] [PubMed]
73. Thaiss, C.A.; Levy, M.; Grosheva, I.; Zheng, D.P.; Soffer, E.; Blacher, E.; Braverman, S.; Tengeler, A.C.; Barak, O.; Elazar, M.; et al. Hyperglycemia drives intestinal barrier dysfunction and risk for enteric infection. *Science* **2018**, *359*, 1376–1383. [CrossRef] [PubMed]
74. Jensen, A.B.; Sorensen, T.I.A.; Pedersen, O.; Jess, T.; Brunak, S.; Allin, K.H. Increase in clinically recorded type 2 diabetes after colectomy. *Elife* **2018**, *7*, e37420. [CrossRef] [PubMed]
75. Xu, H.; Wang, X.; Feng, W.; Liu, Q.; Zhou, S.; Liu, Q.; Cai, L. The gut microbiota and its interactions with cardiovascular disease. *Microb. Biotechnol.* **2020**, *13*, 637–656. [CrossRef] [PubMed]
76. Koren, O.; Spor, A.; Felin, J.; Fak, F.; Stombaugh, J.; Tremaroli, V.; Behre, C.J.; Knight, R.; Fagerberg, B.; Ley, R.E.; et al. Human oral, gut, and plaque microbiota in patients with atherosclerosis. *Proc. Natl. Acad. Sci. USA* **2011**, *108* (Suppl. 1), 4592–4598. [CrossRef] [PubMed]
77. Jie, Z.Y.; Xia, H.H.; Zhong, S.L.; Feng, Q.; Li, S.H.; Liang, S.S.; Zhong, H.Z.; Liu, Z.P.; Gao, Y.; Zhao, H.; et al. The gut microbiome in atherosclerotic cardiovascular disease. *Nat. Commun.* **2017**, *8*, 845. [CrossRef] [PubMed]
78. Emoto, T.; Yamashita, T.; Kobayashi, T.; Sasaki, N.; Hirota, Y.; Hayashi, T.; So, A.; Kasahara, K.; Yodoi, K.; Matsumoto, T.; et al. Characterization of gut microbiota profiles in coronary artery disease patients using data mining analysis of terminal restriction fragment length polymorphism: Gut microbiota could be a diagnostic marker of coronary artery disease. *Heart Vessels* **2017**, *32*, 39–46. [CrossRef]
79. Witkowski, M.; Weeks, T.L.; Hazen, S.L. Gut microbiota and cardiovascular disease. *Circ. Res.* **2020**, *127*, 553–570. [CrossRef]
80. Rauchhaus, M.; Doehner, W.; Francis, D.P.; Davos, C.; Kemp, M.; Liebenthal, C.; Niebauer, J.; Hooper, J.; Volk, H.D.; Coats, A.J.; et al. Plasma cytokine parameters and mortality in patients with chronic heart failure. *Circulation* **2000**, *102*, 3060–3067. [CrossRef]
81. Yang, G.; Wei, J.; Liu, P.; Zhang, Q.; Tian, Y.; Hou, G.; Meng, L.; Xin, Y.; Jiang, X. Role of the gut microbiota in type 2 diabetes and related diseases. *Metabolism* **2021**, *117*, 154712. [CrossRef]
82. Jiang, W.; Wu, N.; Wang, X.; Chi, Y.; Zhang, Y.; Qiu, X.; Hu, Y.; Li, J.; Liu, Y. Dysbiosis gut microbiota associated with inflammation and impaired mucosal immune function in intestine of humans with non-alcoholic fatty liver disease. *Sci. Rep.* **2015**, *5*, 8096. [CrossRef] [PubMed]
83. Raman, M.; Ahmed, I.; Gillevet, P.M.; Probert, C.S.; Ratcliffe, N.M.; Smith, S.; Greenwood, R.; Sikaroodi, M.; Lam, V.; Crotty, P.; et al. Fecal microbiome and volatile organic compound metabolome in obese humans with nonalcoholic fatty liver disease. *Clin. Gastroenterol. Hepatol.* **2013**, *11*, 868–875.e1–3. [CrossRef] [PubMed]
84. Del Chierico, F.; Nobili, V.; Vernocchi, P.; Russo, A.; De Stefanis, C.; Gnani, D.; Furlanello, C.; Zandona, A.; Paci, P.; Capuani, G.; et al. Gut microbiota profiling of pediatric nonalcoholic fatty liver disease and obese patients unveiled by an integrated meta-omics-based approach. *Hepatology* **2017**, *65*, 451–464. [CrossRef] [PubMed]
85. Sohail, M.U.; Yassine, H.M.; Sohail, A.; Thani, A.A.A. Impact of physical exercise on gut microbiome, inflammation, and the pathobiology of metabolic disorders. *Rev. Diabet. Stud.* **2019**, *15*, 35–48. [CrossRef]
86. Denou, E.; Marcinko, K.; Surette, M.G.; Steinberg, G.R.; Schertzer, J.D. High-intensity exercise training increases the diversity and metabolic capacity of the mouse distal gut microbiota during diet-induced obesity. *Am. J. Physiol. Endocrinol. Metab.* **2016**, *310*, E982–E993. [CrossRef]
87. Cho, J.A.; Park, S.H.; Cho, J.; Kim, J.O.; Yoon, J.H.; Park, E. Exercise and curcumin in combination improves cognitive function and attenuates ER stress in diabetic rats. *Nutrients* **2020**, *12*, 1309. [CrossRef]
88. Ortega-Santos, C.P.; Al-Nakkash, L.; Whisner, C.M. Exercise and/or genistein treatment impact gut microbiota and inflammation after 12 weeks on a high-fat, high-sugar diet in C57BL/6 mice. *Nutrients* **2020**, *12*, 3410. [CrossRef]
89. Wu, T.; Gao, X.; Chen, M.; van Dam, R.M. Long-term effectiveness of diet-plus-exercise interventions vs. diet-only interventions for weight loss: A meta-analysis. *Obes. Rev.* **2009**, *10*, 313–323. [CrossRef]
90. Foster-Schubert, K.E.; Alfano, C.M.; Duggan, C.R.; Xiao, L.; Campbell, K.L.; Kong, A.; Bain, C.E.; Wang, C.Y.; Blackburn, G.L.; McTiernan, A. Effect of diet and exercise, alone or combined, on weight and body composition in overweight-to-obese postmenopausal women. *Obesity* **2012**, *20*, 1628–1638. [CrossRef]
91. Liu, W.Y.; Lu, D.J.; Du, X.M.; Sun, J.Q.; Ge, J.; Wang, R.W.; Wang, R.; Zou, J.; Xu, C.; Ren, J.; et al. Effect of aerobic exercise and low carbohydrate diet on pre-diabetic non-alcoholic fatty liver disease in postmenopausal women and middle aged men–the role of gut microbiota composition: Study protocol for the AELC randomized controlled trial. *BMC Public Health* **2014**, *14*, 48. [CrossRef]
92. Sun, S.; Kong, Z.; Shi, Q.; Zhang, H.; Lei, O.K.; Nie, J. Carbohydrate restriction with or without exercise training improves blood pressure and insulin sensitivity in overweight women. *Healthcare* **2021**, *9*, 637. [CrossRef] [PubMed]

93. Sun, S.; Lei, O.K.; Nie, J.; Shi, Q.; Xu, Y.; Kong, Z. Effects of low-carbohydrate diet and exercise training on gut microbiota. *Front. Nutr.* **2022**, *9*, 884550. [CrossRef] [PubMed]
94. Cheng, R.; Wang, L.; Le, S.; Yang, Y.; Zhao, C.; Zhang, X.; Yang, X.; Xu, T.; Xu, L.; Wiklund, P.; et al. A randomized controlled trial for response of microbiome network to exercise and diet intervention in patients with nonalcoholic fatty liver disease. *Nat. Commun.* **2022**, *13*, 2555. [CrossRef] [PubMed]
95. Wilson, R.L.; Kang, D.W.; Christopher, C.N.; Crane, T.E.; Dieli-Conwright, C.M. Fasting and exercise in oncology: Potential synergism of combined interventions. *Nutrients* **2021**, *13*, 3421. [CrossRef]
96. Hansen, D.; De Strijcker, D.; Calders, P. Impact of endurance exercise training in the fasted state on muscle biochemistry and metabolism in healthy subjects: Can these effects be of particular clinical benefit to type 2 diabetes mellitus and insulin-resistant patients? *Sports Med.* **2017**, *47*, 415–428. [CrossRef]
97. Julio-Pieper, M.; Bravo, J.A.; Aliaga, E.; Gotteland, M. Review article: Intestinal barrier dysfunction and central nervous system disorders–a controversial association. *Aliment. Pharmacol. Ther.* **2014**, *40*, 1187–1201. [CrossRef]
98. Campbell, S.C.; Wisniewski, P.J., 2nd. Exercise is a novel promoter of intestinal health and microbial diversity. *Exerc. Sport Sci. Rev.* **2017**, *45*, 41–47. [CrossRef]
99. Campbell, S.C.; Wisniewski, P.J.; Noji, M.; McGuinness, L.R.; Haggblom, M.M.; Lightfoot, S.A.; Joseph, L.B.; Kerkhof, L.J. The effect of diet and exercise on intestinal integrity and microbial diversity in mice. *PLoS ONE* **2016**, *11*, e0150502. [CrossRef]
100. Agus, A.; Clement, K.; Sokol, H. Gut microbiota-derived metabolites as central regulators in metabolic disorders. *Gut* **2021**, *70*, 1174–1182. [CrossRef]
101. Lai, Z.L.; Tseng, C.H.; Ho, H.J.; Cheung, C.K.Y.; Lin, J.Y.; Chen, Y.J.; Cheng, F.C.; Hsu, Y.C.; Lin, J.T.; El-Omar, E.M.; et al. Fecal microbiota transplantation confers beneficial metabolic effects of diet and exercise on diet-induced obese mice. *Sci. Rep.* **2018**, *8*, 15625. [CrossRef]

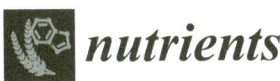

Article

A Culturally Sensitive and Theory-Based Intervention on Prevention and Management of Diabetes: A Cluster Randomized Control Trial

Phrashiah Githinji [1,2,*], John A. Dawson [1,3], Duke Appiah [4] and Chad D. Rethorst [2]

1. Department of Nutritional Science, Texas Tech University, 1301 Akron Ave., Lubbock, TX 79409, USA
2. Institute of Advancing Health through Agriculture, Texas A&M AgriLife Research, 17360 Coit Rd., 17360, Dallas, TX 77843, USA
3. Department of Economics, Applied Statistics, and International Business, New Mexico State University, 127, Las Cruces, NM 88003, USA
4. Department of Public Health, School of Population and Public Health, Texas Tech University Health Sciences Center, 3601 4th Street, Lubbock, TX 79410, USA
* Correspondence: phrashiah.githinji@ag.tamu.edu

Abstract: Type 2 diabetes is an emerging concern in Kenya. This clustered-randomized trial of peri-urban communities included a theory-based and culturally sensitive intervention to improve diabetes knowledge, health beliefs, dietary intake, physical activity, and weight status among Kenyan adults. Those in the intervention group (IG) received a culturally sensitive diabetes education intervention which applied the Health Belief Model in changing knowledge, health beliefs and behavior. Participants attended daily education sessions for 5 days, each lasting 3 h and received mobile phone messages for an additional 4 weeks. The control group (CG) received standard education on COVID-19. Data was collected at baseline, post-intervention (1 week), and follow-up assessment (5 weeks). Linear mixed effect analysis was performed to assess within and across group differences. Compared to the control, IG significantly increased diabetes knowledge ($p < 0.001$), health beliefs including perceived susceptibility ($p = 0.05$), perceived benefits ($p = 0.04$) and self-efficacy ($p = 0.02$). IG decreased consumption of oils ($p = 0.03$), refined grains ($p = 0.01$), and increased intake of fruits ($p = 0.01$). Perceived barriers, physical activity, and weight status were not significantly different between both groups. The findings demonstrate the potential of diabetes education in improving diabetes knowledge, health beliefs, and in changing dietary intake of among adults in Kenya.

Keywords: diabetes intervention; health belief model; culturally sensitive; diabetes prevention; health promotion; health behaviors; diet; physical activity; low and middle income and countries; community intervention

1. Introduction

Non-communicable diseases (NCDs) are responsible for 41 million annual deaths globally [1]. Approximately 77% of NCD deaths are in low-and middle-income countries (LMICs) in South East Asia and Africa [1]. In LMICs like Kenya, NCDs are responsible for over 50% of all reported adult hospital admissions and 55% of adult mortality [2]. In these regions, the burden of morbidity and mortality due to NCDs is often overshadowed by the infectious diseases [3]. For instance, NCDs resulted in 67% of disability-adjusted life years (DALYs) and accounted for 74% of deaths globally [1,4]. However, In LMICs, NCDs receive 2% of global funds allocated from governments, the private sector, or donors in comparison to the response given to the treatments of infectious diseases such as HIV/AIDS that accounts for 3% of DALYs yet receives 30% of global funds [5–8].

About three quarters of the global burden of type 2 diabetes (T2D) occur in LMICs [9]. In Kenya, the prevalence of diabetes is 12.2% in urban areas, higher than the global prevalence of 9.3% [10]. Kenya, like other LMICs, is undergoing a nutritional and epidemiological transition as the population increases the consumption of ultra-processed, high-caloric diets and adopts a sedentary lifestyle due to social-economic development and urbanization [11]. Dietary preferences are shifting from indigenous healthier food options, rich in micronutrients, high fiber and diverse, including a variety of fruits, vegetables, nuts, legumes, and root tubers to western-style diets that are energy-dense and ultra-processed, high in saturated fats, added sugar and sodium [9,10]. Additionally, countries in Sub-Saharan Africa, including Kenya, now have the highest smoking and alcohol consumption rates globally [11,12].

Besides the dietary shift, changes have also occurred in physical activity patterns. For instance, there is a shift away from the high-energy expenditure activities such as farming, mining, and forestry towards the service sector and white-collar jobs, with reduced energy expenditures [13]. Similarly, economic growth, urbanization, and technological changes have also influenced and simplified how people move, with more individuals now owning cars or using train systems to conveniently get from one place to another, rather than walking [14], and this has contributed to a reduction in overall energy expenditure. In addition, unlike in the recent past, where leisure time would be spent outdoors, it is now more common that leisure time will include sedentary activities such as watching TV or smart devices [14]. Diet and physical activity transitions have influenced the demographic characteristics of those affected with T2D. For example, T2D was often associated with older age (65 years or older), but research now shows that globally, the greatest number of people with diabetes are between 40–59 years of age, with increasingly more younger people diagnosed with pre-diabetes [15].

Another reason for the increase of T2D in Kenya is a lack of knowledge about diabetes and poor health attitudes [11]. Some studies report that low awareness of risk and preventive factors for T2D significantly contribute to the increasing cases of T2D in Kenya [10,16]. People are vulnerable to misinformation, unhealthy behavior, and poor health outcomes without proper health information [17]. Furthermore, the few existing T2D programs are primarily led by the government of Kenya through the Ministry of Health (MOH) [18]. However, according to the Ministry of Health, they face several challenges that prevent successful implementation of these programs, including a lack of capacity of the health workforce in terms of numbers, equipment, and skills and poor availability and affordability of quality, safe and efficient technologies and medications for screening, diagnosis and treatment [19]. As such, many of the available documented programs on T2D education are outdated and are not supported by behavior theories that offer a framework for understanding and predicting human behavior [18,19]. Additionally, many of the existing programs lack cultural tailoring, which is proven to be important in enhancing receptivity of health programs by adapting intervention materials to fit the needs, preferences, and norms of the population more appropriately [20].

Due to the increasing prevalence of T2D enabled by the above-mentioned factors, there is a need to provide culturally sensitive diabetes education, guided by theory-based behavioral oriented methods that are effective in motivation and behavior change [21]. Consequently, this study aimed to examine the effectiveness of a theory-based and culturally sensitive educational intervention on diabetes prevention knowledge, health beliefs, dietary intake, physical activity, and weight status among adults in peri-urban communities in Nairobi, Kenya.

2. Materials and Methods

2.1. Study Design

A cluster randomized control trial (cRCT) design was used in this study. Peri-urban communities were purposively selected as study locations as they are areas where towns and the countryside meet that are nutritional zones with observable changes in diet and lifestyle and increasing growth of overweight and obesity [22]. The specific locations were peri-urban communities in Embakasi constituency, which borders the city of Nairobi and was the area that where administrative access to do the study was granted. Sample size was calculated for a cRCT with fixed number of clusters ($n = 6$) and in consideration of a power of 90%, a 5% level of significance, an expected drop-out rate of 10%, an intra-cluster correlation coefficient of 0.01, to detect a difference of 2.5 points (or a standardized effect size d of 0.8) based on a similar intervention focusing on changing diabetes knowledge and attitudes [23–25]. In line with these calculations, 226 participants were enrolled in the study.

Six peri-urban communities in Nairobi County were randomized so that 3 were assigned to the intervention group (IG) and 3 were assigned to the control group (this 3&3 balance was enforced by the randomization scheme). An impartial statistician with no active role in the study conducted the random assignment.

Data was collected at baseline assessment, post-intervention assessment (1 week), and at a follow-up assessment (5 weeks after baseline). Adults 18 years and older, living within peri-urban communities in Embakasi constituency were recruited through flyers distributed at the chief's camp, religious centers, social media, and local community groups ('Nyumba Kumi'). Those excluded were pregnant women, and those with chronic diseases, as these conditions can affect dietary intake, metabolism, and physical activity [26].

2.2. Diabetes Education Intervention

The diabetes education intervention was designed based on established components associated with effective health interventions for adult populations, including having clear and focused objectives and using behavioral theory to guide the intervention. The intervention focused on the desired behavior and used an interactive teaching method, such as hands-on activities and group discussions. The intervention was delivered by Community health workers (CHW) that attended a 2-day training on the delivery of the intervention. The intervention was driven by the Health Belief Model (HBM) constructs (perceived susceptibility, perceived seriousness, perceived benefits, perceived barriers, self-efficacy), and it was informed by materials from scientific sources, including the American Diabetes Association [23], the Vanderbilt Medical University Diabetes Pride Study [26] and USDA's SNAP Education Program [27]. The intervention addressed diabetes knowledge, prevention, and management as directed by five modules: (i) understanding diabetes, (ii) preventing and managing diabetes through nutrition, (iii) physical activity, (iv) reducing tobacco and alcohol consumption, and (v) management of diabetes (Table 1). Each module was culturally tailored and designed to suit the population. For instance, the use of culturally relevant examples and use of cultural beliefs and behaviors to provide context to the content. The use of plain language, visual aids, large fonts, demonstrations were used as low health literacy strategies for teaching. Teach-back techniques were also employed to improve the understanding of diabetes concepts.

Table 1. Demographic characteristics of participants ($n = 226$).

	Total Participants	Intervention Group	Control Group	p-Value
	Mean ± SD			
Age (years)	37.5 ± 12.7	39.4 ± 12.6	35.5 ± 12.7	0.02
Weight (pounds)	169.9 ± 38.8	164.2 ± 31.1	175.9 ± 44.8	0.02
Height (inches)	65.0 ± 6.4	63.7 ± 8.5	66.0 ± 3.4	0.01
	Body Mass Index			
Underweight	4 (1.8)	3 (2.6)	1 (0.9)	
Normal weight	84 (37.2)	40 (34.8)	44 (40.0)	0.001
Overweight	51 (22.6)	22 (19.1)	29 (26.4)	
Obese	72 (31.9)	36 (31.3)	36 (32.7)	
	Gender			
Male	64 (28.3)	38 (32.8)	26 (23.6)	0.08
Female	158 (69.9)	74 (63.8)	84 (76.4)	

Table 1. Cont.

	Total Participants	Intervention Group	Control Group	p-Value
Education				
Primary School	9 (4.0)	5 (4.3)	4 (3.6)	
Secondary School	77 (34.1)	28 (24.1)	49 (44.5)	
College (2-year degree)	77 (34.1)	45 (38.8)	32 (29.1)	0.06
University Degree (4-year degree)	50 (22.1)	29 (25.0)	21 (19.1)	
Post-graduate Degree	12 (5.3)	8 (6.9)	4 (3.6)	
Occupation				
Government employed	87 (38.5)	49 (42.2)	38 (34.5)	
NGO employed	27 (11.9)	14 (12.1)	13 (11.8)	
Self employed	43 (19.0)	21 (18.1)	22 (20.0)	
Homemaker	9 (4.0)	3 (2.6)	6 (5.5)	0.81
Retired	7 (3.1)	4 (3.4)	3 (2.7)	
Not employed	50 (22.1)	23 (19.8)	27 (24.5)	
Unable to work	2 (0.9)	1 (0.9)	1 (0.9)	
Household Income				
100 USD or less	49 (21.7)	24 (20.7)	25 (22.7)	
100–299 USD	75 (33.2)	38 (32.8)	37 (33.6)	
300–499 USD	41 (18.1)	21 (18.1)	20 (18.2)	0.97
500–999 USD	35 (15.5)	19 (16.4)	16 (14.5)	
1000 USD and above	9 (4.0)	5 (4.3)	4 (3.6)	
Diabetes Diagnosis				
Yes	20 (8.8)	9 (45.0)	11 (55.0)	0.71
No	206 (91.2)	107 (51.9)	99 (48.1)	
Family history of diabetes				
Yes	75 (33.2)	36 (48.0)	39 (52.0)	0.67
No	151 (66.8%)	71 (47.0)	80 (53.0)	
Type of family member with diabetes				
dia	32 (42.6%)	14 (43.8)	18 (56.2)	
Extended	28 (37.33%)	17 (60.7)	11 (39.30)	0.63
Both	15 (20.0%)	6 (40)	9 (60)	

Guided by the participants' preferred availability, those in the IG attended 5 days of concurrent face-to-face sessions, each lasting 3 h and where each of the five modules was covered. Following the completion of the face-to-face sessions, participants received three mobile-phone and WhatsApp messages each week to reinforce the materials learned, such as MyPlate, portion control and physical activity reminders. The CG received the standard education by the World Health Organization on hygiene practices related to COVID-19 [28]. The topics included hand washing and sanitization, social and physical distancing, face masks and facial coverings, cleaning protocols, assessment of symptoms and quarantine measures. To avoid contamination between the IG and CG, participants from each group met at different sites.

2.3. Data Collection

The lead author and 16 CHWs did all the data collection. The CHWs attended 4 h of data collection training sessions by the lead author. The training session included the purpose of the study, the role of the CHWs, the questionnaires involved and maintaining data integrity. Participant's consent was obtained before data were collected. Participants' anthropometrics were measured, and a set of questionnaires was administered to collect data on diabetes knowledge, health beliefs, and dietary intake and physical activity at baseline (T1), post-intervention (1 week; T2), and follow-up (5 weeks; T3).

2.3.1. Knowledge Assessment

Diabetes knowledge was assessed using a questionnaire based on diabetes education objectives that reflected participants' culture and health literacy levels. The questionnaire consisted of thirty-nine questions informed by previously validated scales [29] that sought to measure knowledge on risk factors, symptoms, the role of nutrition and physical activity, alcohol and tobacco and other self-management skills. The questionnaire underwent face and content validation by experts and was pilot tested to identify potential problem areas and deficiencies in the instrument to improve accuracy, comprehension, appropriateness, and consistency. Out of 39 possible points, participants' knowledge was categorized as poor for scoring 13 points or less, acceptable for scoring between 14 and 26 points, and good knowledge for scoring 27 or more points.

2.3.2. Health Beliefs

Health beliefs related to diabetes were assessed using a validated HBM scale from a study of the relationship between health beliefs and prevention behaviors of T2D [30]. The questionnaire had 23 items which were grouped in categories related to the constructs of the HBM. These are perceived susceptibility, perceived seriousness, perceived benefits, and perceived barriers. All questions were evaluated on a 5-point Likert scale ranging from strongly disagree (coded as 1) to strongly agree (coded as 5).

2.3.3. Self-Efficacy

Self-efficacy was assessed using the validated scale from the Risk and Health Behavior Scales research [31]. The questionnaire consists of four sections with five items assessing self-efficacy related to nutrition, six items related to physical activity, five items related to alcohol and four related to smoking. The scale was based on a Likert scale of 4, where respondents are asked to rate their confidence in their ability to change their health behavior. The question responses ranged from strongly disagree (coded as 1), disagree (coded as 2), agree (coded as 3) to strongly agree (coded as 4).

2.3.4. Dietary Intake

Dietary intake was assessed using a validated and culturally sensitive semi-quantitative 30-day food frequency questionnaire (FFQ) designed for adults in urban populations in Nairobi, Kenya [32]. The FFQ consists of 123 food items contributing to the total energy. The portion size was estimated by asking participants to translate their usual consumption amount based on commonly locally used utensils that were provided for demonstration. The sizes used were small (250 mL), medium (360 mL) and large (750 mL) portions. The Kenyan food composition tables were used to convert and analyze nutrient estimates for each food item [33]. The period between baseline assessment and post-intervention assessment was one week, and therefore, the dietary intake of the participants was only assessed at two-time points, at baseline and four weeks after intervention at follow-up assessment.

2.3.5. Physical Activity

Physical activity was assessed using the International Physical Activity Questionnaire (IPAQ) [34]. The questionnaire consists of 27 items focusing on physical activity in household activities, activity during transportation and time spent on leisure activities. The Metabolic Equivalent of Task (METs) scores were assigned to the various activities. Physical activity was categorized as high if the participants achieved 3000 MET minutes per week with a combination of walking, moderate and vigorous activity, or three days or more of a combination of walking, moderate and vigorous activity with more than 1500 MET per week. Moderate activity consists of 600 MET per week or five or more days of any combination, including walking or moderate activity for at least 30 min per day. Participants were classified as having low activity levels if they had less than 600 MET per week and not less than 10 min of physical activity per day. Any activity less than 10 min was not considered. After that, physical activity was coded on a 3-point scale, with 1 being high, 2 moderate physical activity and 3-low physical activity.

2.3.6. Anthropometric Measures

The body weight of each participant was measured using a properly calibrated digital scale, and their information was recorded in kilograms in their individually labeled questionnaires. Weight was later converted to pounds. Height was measured in centimeters using a wall-mounted stadiometer and later converted to inches.

2.4. Data Analysis

Data were analyzed using SPSS system (Version 28, SPSS Inc, Chicago, IL, USA). Descriptive statistics were used to describe differences in demographic characteristics, knowledge, health beliefs, household food insecurity, physical activity, and dietary intake among groups. One-way Analysis of Variance (ANOVA) and chi-square (χ^2) tests were used to assess for equivalency between the demographic variables (age, income, marital status, education level, BMI) between the IG and CG. Linear mixed effect models with random effects for clusters and subjects were fit to assess within and between group differences in the outcomes from baseline to post-intervention and from to follow-up assessment. The change scores in diabetes knowledge, dietary intake, health beliefs, physical activity and weight status was compared between the IG (Δ_{IG}: change score in the IG) and CG (Δ_{CG}: change score in the CG). The linear mixed effect analysis adjusted for age and BMI. An alpha level of 0.05 was used as the threshold for statistical significance.

3. Results

A total of 226 adults completed the baseline assessment (116 adults in the IG; 110 in the CG). Ten participants (6 in the IG and 4 in the CG) dropped out of the study for personal reasons. A total of 216 adults attended the study and completed the post-test assessment (T2). An additional 28 adults (13 in the IG; 15 in the CG) dropped out from the study before the follow-up assessment. A total of 188 adults (83.2%) completed the study in its entirety (Figure 1).

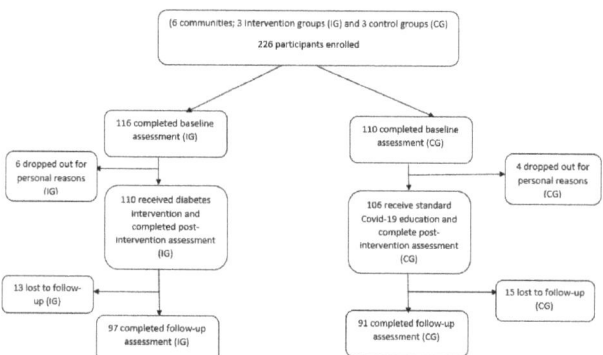

Figure 1. Flow diagram of recruitment and study participation.

A summary of the characteristics of the participants can be found in Table 1. Most participants were females (71.7%), with a mean age of 37.5 years with majority (54.5%) having overweight or obesity (54.5%). Statistical comparisons showed significant differences in age and BMI between the two groups ($p = 0.02$; $p < 0.001$) that were adjusted for in analysis. No other differences between the groups were significant (Table 1).

3.1. Effect of Intervention on Diabeteknowledge, Health beliefs, Physical Activity, Dietary Intake and Weight Status

3.1.1. Diabetes Knowledge

The mean diabetes knowledge score of participants in the IG at baseline was 1.43. After the intervention, this significantly increased to 2.80 at post-intervention and to 2.87 at follow-up. Compared to the CG, this increase in knowledge in the IG was significant over time from T1 to T3 ($p < 0.001$) (Table 2) and across the other assessment time points (Tables S1 and S2).

Table 2. Changes in diabetes knowledge and health beliefs from baseline (T1) to post-intervention (T2) and follow-up (T3) assessments.

Variables	Baseline Assessment (T1) Mean Change ± SD		Post-Intervention Assessment (T2) (1 Week after Baseline) Mean Change ± SD		Follow-Up Assessment (T3) (5 Weeks after Baseline) Mean Change ± SD		Δ_{T3-T1} (m ± sd)		p-Value [†] between Groups over Time
	IG	CG	IG	CG	IG	CG	IG	CG	
Diabetes Knowledge	1.43 ± 0.68	1.36 ± 0.61	2.80 ± 0.55	1.31 ± 0.59	2.87 ± 0.43	1.40 ± 0.69	1.44 ± 0.56	0.04 ± 0.65	0.001
Perceived Susceptibility	2.37 ± 1.06	2.21 ± 1.02	3.03 ± 0.53	2.27 ± 0.95	3.22 ± 1.11	2.34 ± 0.90	0.85 ± 1.09	0.13 ± 0.96	0.05
Perceived Seriousness	2.91 ± 0.83	3.13 ± 0.72	2.53 ± 0.39	3.03 ± 0.79	2.51 ± 0.97	2.99 ± 0.78	−0.4 ± 0.90	−0.14 ± 0.75	0.06
Perceived Benefits	3.63 ± 0.94	3.48 ± 0.95	4.30 ± 0.91	3.41 ± 0.89	3.64 ± 0.89	3.43 ± 0.85	0.01 ± 0.92	−0.05 ± 0.90	0.04
Perceived Barriers	2.58 ± 0.92	2.67 ± 0.92	2.54 ± 0.32	2.64 ± 0.81	2.45 ± 0.94	2.68 ± 0.75	−0.13 ± 0.93	0.01 ± 0.84	0.09
Self-efficacy-Nutrition	3.12 ± 0.74	3.09 ± 0.76	3.82 ± 0.62	3.08 ± 0.68	3.86 ± 0.72	3.06 ± 0.68	0.74 ± 0.73	−0.03 ± 0.72	0.02
Self-efficacy-Physical activity	2.98 ± 0.82	2.92 ± 0.83	3.03 ± 0.82	2.89 ± 0.79	3.05 ± 0.81	2.87 ± 0.77	0.07 ± 0.82	−0.05 ± 0.80	0.98
Self-efficacy-Alcohol (n = 76)	3.08 ± 0.81	3.04 ± 0.87	3.49 ± 0.29	2.99 ± 0.82	3.48 ± 0.81	2.86 ± 0.83	0.40 ± 0.81	−0.18 ± 0.85	0.02
Self-efficacy-Smoking (n = 30)	2.71 ± 1.02	2.33 ± 0.88	2.85 ± 0.32	2.89 ± 1.01	2.71 ± 1.02	2.89 ± 1.02	0.00 ± 1.02	0.56 ± 0.95	0.12

Note: Δ_{T3-T1}: change score from T1 to T3 assessment, calculated by subtracting score at T1 from score at T3; IG: intervention group; CG: control group. [†] Adjusted for cluster differences in age, and BMI.

3.1.2. Health Beliefs

Perceived Susceptibility

On a scale of 5, the perceived susceptibility to T2D in the IG significantly increased from 2.37 to 3.03 to 3.22 points (Table 2). Comparing the IG and the CG over the three assessment periods, there was a significant increase in the perceived susceptibility of participants in the IG versus the CG from T1 to T3 ($p = 0.05$; Table 2) and across the other assessment time points (Tables S1 and S2).

Perceived Seriousness

There was no significant change in the perceived seriousness of diabetes in both groups. At baseline, the mean score for the IG was 2.91 points, which changed to 2.53 at the post-test and 2.51 at the follow-up assessment. When comparing the two groups, the change in perceived seriousness was not significant for participants in the IG versus the CG at any of the three time points (Tables 2, S1 and S2).

Perceived Benefits

Perceived benefits of adopting healthier behaviors among the intervention group significantly increased in this study. For example, at baseline, IG participants scored an average of 3.63, 4.30 points at post intervention and 3.64 points at follow up assessment. This was a significant increase in perceived benefits of participants compared to the CG from T1 to T3 ($p = 0.04$; Table 2) and across the other assessment time points (Tables S1 and S2).

Perceived Barriers

The participant's perceived barriers to achieving a healthy lifestyle did not significantly change within and across groups (Table 2). The mean score for the IG was 2.58, 2.54, and 2.45 at the three respective time points, and this was not statistically different at any time. (Tables 2, S1 and S2).

Self-Efficacy

Self-efficacy related to nutrition and healthy eating significantly increased in the IG over the three assessment points from 3.12 to 3.82 to 3.86 points, respectively. When comparing the two groups over the three assessment periods, there was a significant increase in the self-efficacy (nutrition) of participants in the IG versus the CG (Tables 2, S1 and S2). The mean self-efficacy at baseline for those in the IG who consumed alcohol was 3.08 points at baseline, 3.49 at post-test and 3.48 at follow-up assessment. Self-efficacy for the CG was 3.04 at baseline, 2.99 at post-test and 2.86 at follow-up assessment. In comparison, there was a significant difference in self-efficacy relating to alcohol use by participants in the IG versus the CG from T1 to T3 ($p = 0.02$) and across the other assessment (Tables S1 and S2). Self-efficacy related to smoking and physical activity did not significantly increase for participants within and across both groups from T1 to T2 to T3 (Table 2).

3.1.3. Dietary Intake

As shown in Table 3, the intake of refined grains in the IG significantly decreased from a mean intake of 6.03 cups at baseline assessment to 5.43 cups at follow-up assessment $p = 0.004$). The CG refined grain intake was 6.01 cups at baseline and 6.13 at follow-up ($p = 0.363$). The IG had a significantly reduced intake of refined grains versus the CG ($p = 0.009$). The mean daily intake of oils in the IG significantly decreased from 42.53 g at baseline to 38.7 g at follow-up assessment ($p < 0.001$). While the CG intake of oils did not significantly change from 43.54 g at baseline and 44.72 g at follow-up assessment. Overall, the IG had a significantly reduced intake of oils versus the CG ($p = 0.030$). Additionally, mean daily fruit intake significantly increased for participants in the IG from 3.68 to 4.66 cups ($p = 0.002$) but did not significantly increase for the CG ($p = 0.663$). The dairy intake was 5.14 at baseline, and 4.41 cups at follow-up assessment ($p = 0.03$), and this was different compared to CG over time ($p = 0.05$) (Table 3).

Table 3. Changes in food groups consumption from baseline (T1) to follow-up assessment (T3).

Food Groups	Baseline Assessment Mean (SD)		Follow-Up Assessment Mean (SD)		Δ_{T3-T1} (m ± sd)		p-Value between Groups Over Time
	IG	CG	IG	CG	IG	CG	
Whole Grain [††]	2.40 (2.26)	2.28 (2.23)	2.09 (2.51)	2.30 (2.31)	−0.31 ± 2.385	0.02 ± 2.27	0.77
Refined Grains [††]	6.03 (1.89)	6.01 (1.92)	5.43 (1.29)	6.13 (1.03)	−0.6 ± 1.59	0.12 ± 1.48	0.01
Meat/poultry/eggs [φ]	1.48 (1.68)	1.52 (1.68)	2.38 (1.39)	1.72 (1.36)	0.9 ± 1.54	0.20 ± 1.52	0.34
Fish/seafood [φ]	3.36 (1.67)	3.01 (1.67)	3.22 (1.29)	3.38 (1.23)	−0.14 ± 1.48	0.37 ± 1.45	0.69
Dark green vegetable [Φ]	4.93 (2.21)	4.95 (2.22)	4.84 (1.49)	4.56 (1.81)	−0.09 ± 1.85	−0.39 ± 2.02	0.17
Red & orange vegetables [Φ]	6.15 (1.87)	6.14 (1.89)	6.23 (0.91)	6.22 (0.83)	0.08 ± 1.39	0.08 ± 1.36	0.56
Other vegetables [Φ]	3.98 (2.62)	3.99 (2.62)	3.86 (2.17)	3.87 (1.99)	−0.12 ± 2.39	−0.12 ± 2.31	0.51
Oils [¥]	42.53 (1.42)	43.54 (1.02)	38.7 (0.83)	44.72 (0.86)	−3.83 ± 1.13	1.18 ± 0.94	0.03
Starchy vegetables [Φ]	2.21 (0.31)	2.28 (0.31)	3.62 (0.57)	2.26 (3.09)	1.41 ± 0.44	−0.02 ± 1.70	0.001
Beans/peas/lentils [Φ]	2.19 (2.64)	2.17 (2.65)	2.47 (2.17)	2.37 (1.95)	0.28 ± 2.41	0.20 ± 2.30	0.29
Fruits [††]	3.68 (2.88)	3.66 (2.93)	4.66 (1.88)	3.81 (2.00)	0.98 ± 2.38	0.15 ± 2.47	0.01
Dairy [††]	5.14 (3.02)	5.02 (3.08)	4.41 (2.00)	4.92 (2.20)	−0.73 ± 2.50	−0.10 ± 2.64	0.05
Nuts/seeds/soy [φ]	0.75 (1.20)	0.82 (1.33)	0.78 (0.89)	0.75 (0.85)	0.03 ± 1.05	−0.07 ± 1.09	0.87

Note: Δ_{T3-T1}: change score from T1 to T3 assessment, calculated by subtracting score at T1 from score at T3; IG: intervention group; CG: control group. [φ] demotes dietary intake reported in ounce equivalents per day. [¥] demotes dietary intake reported in grams per day. [Φ] denotes dietary intake reported in cup equivalents per week. [††] denotes dietary intake reported in cup equivalents per day. Food group intake based on participant's mean caloric intake of 2200–2600.

3.1.4. Physical Activity and Weight Status

Physical activity measured in METs was categorized on a 3-point scale, with 1 being high, 2 moderate and 3-low physical activity. The mean scores on physical activity among participants in the IG were 1.92 at baseline, 1.96 at post-test and 1.89 at follow-up assessment ($p = 0.96$). The mean score for the CG was 1.90 at baseline, 1.94 at post-test, and 1.91 at follow-up assessment ($p = 0.99$). The mean weight for the IG was 164.16 at baseline, 162.26 at post-test and 166.96 pounds at follow-up assessment. The mean weight for the CG was 174.34, 175.45, and 179.45 pounds within the three respective time points. There were no significant differences in changes in weight status within and across groups from baseline to post-intervention and follow-up assessment ($p = 0.96$).

4. Discussion

Findings from this study showed that a theory-based intervention was effective in increasing diabetes knowledge and improving health beliefs (perceived susceptibility to diabetes, perceived benefits, and self-efficacy) in adopting a healthier lifestyle. The intervention also improved dietary intake with reduced intake of refined grains and oils and increased intake of fruits. However, the intervention did not result in a significant improvement in the other food groups, perceived seriousness, perceived barriers, physical activity and weight status.

The findings of this study showed an improvement in knowledge of diabetes risk factors, symptoms, role of nutrition and physical activity, alcohol and tobacco and other self-management skills. These findings are similar to other studies conducted in LMICs, including by Muchiri and colleagues, where participants in the treatment group who received a diabetes education intervention had higher knowledge scores than the control group [23]. Similarly, Chawla and colleagues found that participants that received education showed a significant increase in knowledge from baseline to endpoint compared to the control group [35]. Diabetes education interventions can lead to an increase in knowledge, as demonstrated by a systematic review that looked at over 19 heterogeneous trials and found that education interventions led to a significant increase in knowledge of T2D [35].

Perceived susceptibility to diabetes, perceived benefits and self-efficacy improved in this study. However, perceived seriousness and barriers did not improve. Like these findings, several studies have found that while perceived susceptibility, benefits, and self-efficacy improve, there may be an inverse relationship with perceived seriousness. For instance, in a similar study where participants received an education intervention on calcium intake, the perceived seriousness of osteoporosis declined with increased knowledge, improved benefits and self-efficacy [36]. Likewise, Suratman and colleagues, in an educational intervention to improve perceptions for reducing exposure to pesticides in farmers, found a decrease in perceived seriousness with improved perceived susceptibility [37]. It is possible that as participants increase their knowledge and perceived benefits of adopting healthier behaviors and improve their self-efficacy, these improvements contribute to a decrease in the perceived seriousness of disease as participants feel empowered by the knowledge and skills to change their behavior to a healthier lifestyle.

This study looked at barriers at the inter-personal level in the socio-ecological context, such as taste, time management, cost of food, social influences from family and friends, motivation, and stress [38,39]. These perceived barriers did not significantly improve. A possible reason for the lack of change is that the study was conducted during the COVID-19 pandemic and effects of the lockdowns could have exacerbated health barriers. Furthermore, barriers addressed were at the individual level, and yet there may be others at the macro level, such as lack of employment opportunities, gender inequalities, inhibitive policies, poverty, and insecurity [40]. Therefore, future studies can incorporate a broader scope while addressing perceived barriers to diabetes health.

The intake of whole grains was low at 2.4 cups compared to the recommended 2.5–4.5 cup equivalents per day. Refined grain intake was high, with average intake of 6.03 cups compared to the recommended intake of 3.5–4.5 cup eq/day. These findings are consistent with other studies investigating dietary patterns that have found that the average diet in Nairobi, Kenya is heavily reliant on carbohydrates as a source of energy intake with primary staples being maize products, wheat, rice and cooking bananas [41]. A time series study assessing staple food consumption patterns in households in Nairobi, and its environs, found that there was a significant increase in consumption of milled and refined grains overtime at the expense of whole grains [41]. This could explain the high intake of refined carbohydrates versus whole grains in this study. The intake of refined grains significantly reduced after the diabetes intervention, and this was ultimately a positive effect as there's higher risks of obesity and associated chronic diseases, with increased intake of refined grains [42]. However, while refined grains reduced, the intake of starchy vegetables increased. This may signify a dietary compensation mechanism that has been observed in some studies, and that needs further investigation, where in response to adjustments in energy intake, individuals compensate by increasing intake of certain foods to maintain satiety and regardless of portion control there's constant energy intake [43]. The high mean intake of dark green vegetables (4.95 vs. 2.0–2.5 cups/week), red and orange vegetables (6.15 vs. 6.0 cups/week), and fruits (3.68 vs. 2.0 cups/day) at baseline could explain the lack of significant change in intake after the intervention [44]. Nyanchoka and colleagues had similar findings in a study in Kenya where 78% of the respondents met fruits, vegetables and beans/peas/lentils recommendations [45]. Regarding the lack of change in physical activity, participants in this study already had a high physical activity of 3000 MET minutes per week with a combination of walking and moderate and vigorous activity at baseline assessment. It is possible that this contributed to the lack of observable change in the amount of physical activity at post-test and follow-up assessment. Weight status did not change significantly after the intervention. Notably, there was a significant portion of the sample in the underweight and normal weight categories, and this could have statistically affected the ability to observe significant change in weight. Additionally, weight loss is extremely challenging due to interactions between our biology, behavior, and obesogenic environments [46]. Change in body weight also requires consistent behavior change and long-term observation, which could explain the lack of significant change in this study [47]. It is recommended that future interventions that hope to observe a significant change in weight status have a longer post-intervention period, preferably longer than the four weeks applied in this study.

Implications and Recommendations

The findings of this study have several implications and recommendations for policy and future research. The increase in diabetes knowledge, perceived susceptibility, benefits, and self-efficacy after the intervention, amplifies the importance of educating people to prevent and manage T2D. Education interventions should target improving awareness of T2D and increasing perceived threats to diabetes, and the benefits of adopting healthier behavior while addressing barriers and building self-efficacy.

The CHWs were instrumental in implementing the intervention, since they are well known to the community, they can be tapped into to educate the community on T2D as a sustainable measure and can facilitate the scaling up of existing or future T2D programs. Lastly, the cultural and theory-based aspects of the intervention were a crucial part of ensuring that there was increased knowledge, perceived susceptibility, perceived benefits, self-efficacy and improving dietary intake. These have important implications for the designing of future community-based health interventions focusing on T2D prevention and management. It is recommended that similar health education interventions be culturally tailored, theory-driven and should also apply low health literacy strategies. They should also extend their duration to measure sustained behavioral changes.

This study had some limitations. For instance, some data were self-reported and may be subject to bias resulting from recall or social desirability, especially in reporting dietary intake data and health beliefs. Additionally, while the diabetes knowledge questionnaire was pilot tested and underwent face and content validation by experts, it may benefit from further confirmatory analyses to establish reliability before use in other settings. Again, the study was not powered to detect non-primary outcomes, which may have affected our ability to observe changes in physical activity and body weight. Lastly, the short study period may have limited the ability to detect body weight changes and hindered the evaluation of the long-term effects of the intervention effects.

5. Conclusions

The findings of this study demonstrate that the culturally sensitive and theory-based diabetes intervention was effective in increasing diabetes knowledge and improving health beliefs, including perceived seriousness, perceived benefits, and self-efficacy. It also effectively improved the dietary intake of refined grains, oils, fruits, and dairy among adults in peri-urban communities in Nairobi, Kenya.

Supplementary Materials: The following supporting information can be downloaded at: https://www.mdpi.com/article/10.3390/nu14235126/s1, Table S1: Changes in diabetes knowledge and health beliefs from baseline (T1) to post-intervention assessment (T2); Table S2: Changes in diabetes knowledge and health beliefs from post-intervention (T2) to follow-up assessment (T3).

Author Contributions: Conceptualized the study, P.G.; developed the methodology of the study, P.G., J.A.D. and D.A.; oversaw recruitment of participants, implementing the intervention and all project administration, P.G.; performed data analysis with guidance and feedback from P.G. and J.A.D. All the authors played a role in discussing the results and interpreting the data findings. validated the study, C.D.R.; wrote the manuscript while all authors reviewed and gave substantive feedback, P.G. and C.D.R. All authors have read and agreed to the published version of the manuscript.

Funding: This research was partially supported by the Graduate School and the Nutritional Sciences department at Texas Tech University.

Institutional Review Board Statement: The study was conducted in accordance with the Declaration of Helsinki and approved by the Institutional Review Board of Texas Tech University (IRB 2020-497) and the Kenya National Commission for Science, Technology, and Innovation granted a permit.

Informed Consent Statement: Informed consent was obtained from all subjects involved in the study.

Acknowledgments: The authors would like to thank the Community Health Workers for their assistance with the study recruitment and intervention. We would also like to thank all the individuals and community groups through the Nyumba Kumi program, that participated in the study. We would also like to especially thank the Community and International Nutrition Research Laboratory at the Nutrition Sciences department at Texas Tech University which provided support during the dissertation process.

Conflicts of Interest: The authors declare no conflict of interest.

References

1. WHO, (World Health Organization). Non-Communicable Diseases. Available online: https://www.who.int/news-room/fact-sheets/detail/noncommunicable-diseases (accessed on 9 September 2021).
2. Phaswana-Mafuya, N.; Peltzer, K.; Chirinda, W.; Musekiwa, A.; Kose, Z.; Hoosain, E.; Davids, A.; Ramlagan, S. Self-Reported Prevalence of Chronic Non-Communicable Diseases and Associated Factors among Older Adults in South Africa. *Glob. Health Action* **2017**, *6*, 20936. [CrossRef] [PubMed]
3. Melaku, Y.A.; Gill, T.K.; Taylor, A.W.; Appleton, S.L.; Gonzalez-Chica, D.; Adams, R.; Achoki, T.; Shi, Z.; Renzaho, A. Trends of Mortality Attributable to Child and Maternal Undernutrition, Overweight/Obesity and Dietary Risk Factors of Non-Communicable Diseases in Sub-Saharan Africa, 1990–2015: Findings from the Global Burden of Disease Study 2015. *Public Health Nutr.* **2019**, *22*, 827–840. [CrossRef]
4. Gouda, H.N.; Charlson, F.; Sorsdahl, K.; Ahmadzada, S.; Ferrari, A.J.; Erskine, H.; Leung, J.; Santamauro, D.; Lund, C.; Aminde, L.N.; et al. Burden of Non-Communicable Diseases in Sub-Saharan Africa, 1990–2017: Results from the Global Burden of Disease Study 2017. *Lancet Glob. Health* **2019**, *7*, e1375–e1387. [CrossRef]
5. Remais, J.V.; Zeng, G.; Li, G.; Tian, L.; Engelgau, M.M. Convergence of Non-Communicable and Infectious Diseases in Low- and Middle-Income Countries. *Int. J. Epidemiol.* **2013**, *42*, 221–227. [CrossRef]
6. Jailobaeva, K.; Falconer, J.; Loffreda, G.; Arakelyan, S.; Witter, S.; Ager, A. An Analysis of Policy and Funding Priorities of Global Actors Regarding Noncommunicable Disease in Low- and Middle-Income Countries. *Glob. Health* **2021**, *17*, 68. [CrossRef]

7. Roser, M.; Ritchie, H. Burden of Disease. Available online: https://ourworldindata.org/burden-of-disease (accessed on 29 August 2022).
8. Allen, L. Non-Communicable Disease Funding. *Lancet Diabetes Endocrinol.* **2017**, *5*, 92. [CrossRef] [PubMed]
9. Manne-Goehler, J.; Geldsetzer, P.; Agoudavi, K.; Andall-Brereton, G.; Aryal, K.K.; Bicaba, B.W.; Bovet, P.; Brian, G.; Dorobantu, M.; Gathecha, G.; et al. Health System Performance for People with Diabetes in 28 Low- and Middle-Income Countries: A Cross-Sectional Study of Nationally Representative Surveys. *PLoS Med.* **2019**, *16*, e1002751. [CrossRef] [PubMed]
10. Kiberenge, M.W.; Ndegwa, Z.M.; Njenga, E.W.; Muchemi, E.W. Knowledge, Attitude and Practices Related to Diabetes among Community Members in Four Provinces in Kenya: A Cross-Sectional Study. *Pan. Afr. Med. J.* **2017**, *7*, 2.
11. Popkin, B.M.; Adair, L.S.; Ng, S.W. Global Nutrition Transition and the Pandemic of Obesity in Developing Countries. *Nutr. Rev.* **2012**, *70*, 3–21. [CrossRef]
12. Popkin, B.M. The Nutrition Transition: An Overview of World Patterns of Change. *Nutr. Rev.* **2004**, *62*, S140–S143. [CrossRef]
13. McCloskey, M.L.; Tarazona-Meza, C.E.; Jones-Smith, J.C.; Miele, C.H.; Gilman, R.H.; Bernabe-Ortiz, A.; Miranda, J.J.; Checkley, W. Disparities in Dietary Intake and Physical Activity Patterns across the Urbanization Divide in the Peruvian Andes. *Int. J. Behav. Nutr. Phys. Act.* **2017**, *14*, 90. [CrossRef] [PubMed]
14. Ojiambo, R.M.; Easton, C.; Casajús, J.A.; Konstabel, K.; Reilly, J.J.; Pitsiladis, Y. Effect of Urbanization on Objectively Measured Physical Activity Levels, Sedentary Time, and Indices of Adiposity in Kenyan Adolescents. *J. Phys. Act. Health* **2012**, *9*, 115–123. [CrossRef] [PubMed]
15. IDF (International Diabetes Federation). *Diabetes Atlas*, 10th ed.; International Diabetes Federation: Brussels, Belgium, 2021.
16. WHO, (World Health Organization). The Mysteries of Type 2 Diabetes in Developing Countries. *Bull. World Health Organ.* **2016**, *94*, 241–242. [CrossRef] [PubMed]
17. Cusack, L.; Del Mar, C.; Chalmers, I.; Gibson, E.; Hoffman, T. Educational Interventions to Improve People's Understanding of Key Concepts in Assessing the Effects of Health Interventions: A Systematic Review. *Syst. Rev.* **2018**, *7*, 68. [CrossRef]
18. MoH, (Ministry of Health). *National Clinical Guidelines for Management of Diabetes Mellitus*; Ministry of Health: Nairobi, Kenya, 2010.
19. MoH, (Ministry of Health). *Kenya National Strategy for The Prevention And Control Of Non-Communicable Diseases (2015–2020)*; Ministry of Health: Nairobi, Kenya, 2015.
20. Torres-Ruiz, M.; Robinson-Ector, K.; Attinson, D.; Trotter, J.; Anise, A.; Clauser, S. A Portfolio Analysis of Culturally Tailored Trials to Address Health and Healthcare Disparities. *Int. J. Environ. Res. Public Health* **2018**, *15*, 1859. [CrossRef]
21. Kupolati, M.D.; MacIntyre, U.E.; Gericke, G.J. A Theory-Based Contextual Nutrition Education Manual Enhanced Nutrition Teaching Skill. *Front. Public Health* **2018**, *6*, 157. [CrossRef]
22. Levitt, N.S.; Steyn, K.; Lambert, E.V.; Reagon, G.; Lombard, C.J.; Fourie, J.M.; Rossouw, K.; Hoffman, M. Modifiable Risk Factors for Type 2 Diabetes Mellitus in a Peri-Urban Community in South Africa. *Diabet. Med.* **1999**, *16*, 946–950. [CrossRef]
23. Muchiri, J.W.; Gericke, G.J.; Rheeder, P. Impact of Nutrition Education on Diabetes Knowledge and Attitudes of Adults with Type 2 Diabetes Living in a Resource-Limited Setting in South Africa: A Randomised Controlled Trial. *J. Endocrinol. Metab. Diabetes South Afr.* **2016**, *21*, 26–34. [CrossRef]
24. Bennett, B.J.; Hall, K.D.; Hu, F.B.; McCartney, A.L.; Roberto, C. Nutrition and the Science of Disease Prevention: A Systems Approach to Support Metabolic Health. *Ann. N. Y. Acad. Sci.* **2015**, *1352*, 1–12. [CrossRef]
25. UCLA. Statistical Consulting Group Introduction to Power Analysis. Available online: https://stats.oarc.ucla.edu/other/mult-pkg/seminars/intro-power/ (accessed on 3 October 2022).
26. ADA, A.D.A. Lifestyle Management: Standards of Medical Care in Diabetes—2019. *Diabetes Care* **2019**, *42*, S46–S60. [CrossRef]
27. VUMC Educational Toolkit Materials | Center for Effective Health Communication. Available online: https://www.vumc.org/cehc/educational-toolkit-materials (accessed on 13 June 2020).
28. USDA Meal Planning, Shopping, and Budgeting. Available online: https://snaped.fns.usda.gov/nutrition-education/nutrition-education-materials/meal-planning-shopping-and-budgeting (accessed on 10 June 2020).
29. UMHS Michigan Diabetes Research Center: Pilot and Feasibility. Available online: http://diabetesresearch.med.umich.edu/Tools_SurveyInstruments.php (accessed on 25 March 2020).
30. Tan, M.Y. The Relationship of Health Beliefs and Complication Prevention Behaviors of Chinese Individuals with Type 2 Diabetes Mellitus. *Diabetes Res. Clin. Pract.* **2004**, *66*, 71–77. [CrossRef] [PubMed]
31. Kartal, A.; Özsoy, S.A. Validity and Reliability Study of the Turkish Version of Health Belief Model Scale in Diabetic Patients. *Int. J. Nurs. Stud.* **2007**, *44*, 1447–1458. [CrossRef] [PubMed]
32. Schwarzer, R.; Renner, B. *Risk and Health Behaviors—Documentation of the Scales of the Research Project: "Risk Appraisal Consequences in Korea" (RACK)*; Freie Universität Berlin: Berlin, Germany, 2005.
33. Willet, W.; Harvard, T.H. Chan School of Public Health Nutrition Department's File Download Site. Available online: https://regepi.bwh.harvard.edu/health/nutrition.html (accessed on 10 May 2020).
34. IPAQ Downloadable Questionnaires—International Physical Activity Questionnaire. Available online: https://sites.google.com/site/theipaq/questionnaire_links (accessed on 8 May 2020).
35. Chawla, S.P.S.; Kaur, S.; Bharti, A.; Garg, R.; Kaur, M.; Soin, D.; Ghosh, A.; Pal, R. Impact of Health Education on Knowledge, Attitude, Practices and Glycemic Control in Type 2 Diabetes Mellitus. *J. Family Med. Prim. Care* **2019**, *8*, 261–268. [CrossRef] [PubMed]

36. Shiferaw, W.S.; Akalu, T.Y.; Desta, M.; Kassie, A.M.; Petrucka, P.M.; Aynalem, Y.A. Effect of Educational Interventions on Knowledge of the Disease and Glycaemic Control in Patients with Type 2 Diabetes Mellitus: A Systematic Review and Meta-Analysis of Randomised Controlled Trials. *BMJ Open* **2021**, *11*, e049806. [CrossRef] [PubMed]
37. Nguyen, B.; Murimi, M. *A Theory-Based Nutrition Education Intervention to Improve Calcium Intake in Hanoi, Vietnam*; Texas Tech University: Lubbock, TX, USA, 2020.
38. Suratman, S.; Ross, K.E.; Babina, K.; Edwards, J.W. The Effectiveness of an Educational Intervention to Improve Knowledge and Perceptions for Reducing Organophosphate Pesticide Exposure among Indonesian and South Australian Migrant Farmworkers. *RMHP* **2016**, *9*, 1–12. [CrossRef] [PubMed]
39. Ashton, L.M.; Hutchesson, M.J.; Rollo, M.E.; Morgan, P.J.; Collins, C.E. Motivators and Barriers to Engaging in Healthy Eating and Physical Activity. *Am. J. Mens. Health* **2017**, *11*, 330–343. [CrossRef]
40. Boyle, M. *Community Nutrition in Action*, 8th ed.; CENGAGE Learning: Belmont, CA, USA, 2021; ISBN 0-357-36808-8.
41. Muyanga, M.; Jayne, T.S.; Argwings-Kodhek, G.; Ariga, J. *Staple Food Consumption Patterns in Urban Kenya: Trends And Policy Implications*; Egerton University: Tegemeo Institute of Agricultural Policy and Development: Njoro, Kenya, 2019.
42. Sawicki, C.M.; Jacques, P.F.; Lichtenstein, A.H.; Rogers, G.T.; Ma, J.; Saltzman, E.; McKeown, N.M. Whole- and Refined-Grain Consumption and Longitudinal Changes in Cardiometabolic Risk Factors in the Framingham Offspring Cohort. *J. Nutr.* **2021**, *151*, 2790–2799. [CrossRef]
43. McKiernan, F.; Hollis, J.H.; Mattes, R.D. Short-Term Dietary Compensation in Free-Living Adults. *Physiol. Behav.* **2008**, *93*, 975–983. [CrossRef]
44. *USDA Dietary Guidelines for Americans, 2020–2025*; United States Department of Agriculture: Washington, DC, USA, 2020.
45. Nyanchoka, A.M.; Stuijvenberg, M.E.V.; Tambe, A.B.; Mbhenyane, X.G. Fruit and Vegetables Consumption Patterns and Risk of Chronic Disease of Lifestyle among University Students in Kenya. *Proc. Nutr. Soc.* **2021**, *80*. [CrossRef]
46. Golden, S.D.; Earp, J.A.L. Social Ecological Approaches to Individuals and Their Contexts: Twenty Years of Health Education & Behavior Health Promotion Interventions. *Health Educ. Behav.* **2012**, *39*, 364–372. [CrossRef]
47. Hall, K.D.; Kahan, S. Maintenance of Lost Weight and Long-Term Management of Obesity. *Med. Clin. N. Am.* **2018**, *102*, 183–197. [CrossRef] [PubMed]

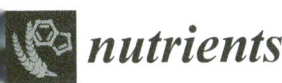

Article

Padres Preparados, Jóvenes Saludables: A Randomized Controlled Trial to Test Effects of a Community-Based Intervention on Latino Father's Parenting Practices

Aysegul Baltaci [1,*], Ghaffar Ali Hurtado Choque [2], Cynthia Davey [3], Alejandro Reyes Peralta [4], Silvia Alvarez de Davila [4], Youjie Zhang [5], Abby Gold [4], Nicole Larson [1] and Marla Reicks [6]

[1] School of Public Health, University of Minnesota, Minneapolis, MN 55455, USA
[2] School of Public Health, University of Maryland, College Park, MD 20742, USA
[3] Clinical and Translational Science Institute, University of Minnesota, Minneapolis, MN 55455, USA
[4] Center for Family Development, University of Minnesota Extension, Saint Paul, MN 55108, USA
[5] Department of Child and Adolescent Health and Social Medicine, School of Public Health, Medical College of Soochow University, Suzhou 215123, China
[6] Department of Food Science and Nutrition, University of Minnesota, Saint Paul, MN 55108, USA
* Correspondence: balta026@umn.edu

Abstract: Parenting practices have been associated with adolescent lifestyle behaviors and weight status. Evidence is limited regarding the efficacy of interventions to address father influences on adolescent lifestyle behaviors through availability and modeling practices. Therefore, the purpose of this study was to evaluate changes in father parenting practices after Latino families with adolescents participated in the Padres Preparados Jóvenes Saludables (Padres) program. Time-1 (baseline) and Time-2 (post-intervention) data were used from Latino father/adolescent (10–14 years) dyads enrolled in the Padres two-arm (intervention vs. delayed-treatment control group) randomized controlled trial in four community locations. The program had eight weekly, 2.5-h experiential learning sessions on food preparation, parenting practices, nutrition, and physical activity. Two types of parenting practices (role modeling and home food availability) were assessed by father report via questionnaire for each of 7 lifestyle behaviors, for a total of 14 parenting practices. Linear regression mixed models were used to evaluate the intervention effects. A total of 94 father/adolescent dyads completed both Time-1 and Time-2 evaluations. Significant positive intervention effects were found for frequencies of fruit modeling ($p = 0.002$) and screen time modeling ($p = 0.039$). Non-significant results were found for the other 12 father parenting practices.

Keywords: randomized controlled trial; community-based intervention; Latino fathers; father's parenting practices; lifestyle behaviors

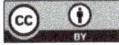

1. Introduction

Many adolescents in the U.S., including Mexican American and other Hispanic adolescents, have poor dietary behaviors [1–3], low levels of physical activity, and frequent screen time [4,5]. These behaviors have been identified as critical behavioral determinants of obesity among adolescents [6]. Childhood obesity increases the risk of developing a variety of health complications and chronic diseases, such as becoming overweight or obese as an adult and developing diabetes, metabolic disorders, and heart disease [7,8]. The current Dietary Guidelines for Americans (DGAs) [9] recommend that U.S adults and adolescents increase their intakes of nutrient-dense foods and a variety of fruits and vegetables while limiting energy-dense foods and beverages to meet the recommended food group and nutrient needs to achieve healthy dietary patterns.

Physical activity is defined as any kind of body movement produced by the skeletal muscles that substantially increases energy expenditure [10]. Adequate physical activity during adolescence may contribute to various short- and long-term benefits for the health and wellbeing of adolescents, including a higher level of cardiorespiratory fitness, stronger muscles and bones, lower body fat, and lower symptoms of depression compared to having an inactive lifestyle [11,12]. On the other hand, screen time is a common sedentary behavior among adolescents in the U.S. [13]. Screen time can contribute to increased risk of adiposity, elevated serum triglyceride concentrations, and metabolic syndrome in adolescents [14].

Parenting practices, which influence these health behaviors, have been defined as intentional or unintentional behaviors/actions by parents that shape their child's attitudes, behaviors, or beliefs [15]. Previous studies have highlighted the positive influence of parenting practices on adolescents' dietary behaviors [16], physical activity, and screen time [17–19]. Several qualitative and cross-sectional studies have shown that Latino parents play a positive role in improving older children and adolescents' lifestyle behaviors [20–26] and weight status [27,28] by engaging in positive food parenting practices. However, these studies have primarily focused on Latino mothers and their adolescents, and little research is available assessing father influences on adolescent lifestyle behaviors and health outcomes.

The limited literature available on the influence of Latino father parenting practices on adolescent behaviors has shown positive findings [20,25,28]. A cross-sectional study with 81 Mexican-origin fathers and children aged 7–13 years who participated in the Entre Familia: Reflejos de Salud study showed that children consumed more fruit and vegetables when their fathers used feeding-related reinforcement of healthy eating more frequently [25]. Another study with 174 mother-father-child triads (8–10 years of age) demonstrated that a father's healthy BMI was related to a child's healthy BMI z-score [28]. Latino fathers of adolescents reported in focus groups that role modeling and making healthy food and physical activity opportunities available were parenting practices that could help adolescents have healthier food and activity behaviors [21]. Therefore, interventions that focus on Latino father parenting practices to promote healthy lifestyles among Latino youth may be beneficial.

The primary goal of the Padres Preparados, Jóvenes Saludables (Padres) (Prepared Parents, Healthy Youth) program was to prevent overweight and obesity among Latino adolescents in low-income households by increasing the frequency of healthy father food and activity parenting practices [29]. The Padres program was adapted from a successful community-based parenting skills education program to prevent substance use among Latino parents and adolescents [30]. The program was grounded in social cognitive theory [31,32] and based on the principles of community-based participatory research [33], with collaboration from community partners in all design and implementation processes [20]. The aims of the current study were 1) to determine baseline (Time-1) to post-intervention (Time-2) changes in father parenting practices (role modeling and making foods and physical activity opportunities available) in a RCT study with intervention and delayed-treatment control groups, and 2) to assess the intervention effect on changes in father parenting practices from Time-1 to Time-2, adjusted for father age and adolescent age and sex.

2. Materials and Methods

2.1. Study Design and Sample

This study used Time-1 (baseline) and Time-2 data (after the 8-week program was conducted for the intervention group) from the Padres program trial [29]. The primary outcomes of the randomized controlled intervention trial (identifier: NCT03641521), which were father and adolescent dietary intake and weight status, are reported elsewhere, as well as intervention details [29]. This paper reports on secondary outcomes regarding the frequency of father parenting practices.

Latino fathers or male caregivers (hereafter referred to as fathers) of adolescents 10–14 years, who identified as Latino, spoke Spanish, and had meals at least three times a week with their adolescents were eligible for the study. Families were recruited using social media, flyers, and announcements at community service centers and churches primarily serving low-income Latino families. Fathers and adolescents completed surveys in person at Time-1 and Time-2. The study protocol was approved by the University of Minnesota Institutional Review Board (project identification code: 1511S80707).

2.2. Intervention

Father/adolescent dyads were randomized to either an intervention or a delayed-treatment control group [29]. The program was implemented in person at four locations (community service centers and churches) in the Minneapolis/St. Paul metropolitan area between September 2017 and December 2019. In-person implementation was discontinued in March 2020 and not resumed because of public health efforts to limit the transmission of COVID-19. During the intervention, fathers and adolescents attended eight weekly, 2.5-h experiential learning sessions facilitated by bilingual Latino educators. In each session, fathers and adolescents participated together in activities to prepare food, be physically active and learn about nutrition and active lifestyles. In separate parts of each session, fathers participated in activities to develop parenting skills and improve frequency of parenting practices, while adolescents participated in activities to reinforce learning about healthy lifestyle behaviors.

2.3. Participation in Evaluation Data Collection

A total of 303 father-adolescent dyads expressed interest in participating in the study (Figure 1). Of those, 266 were screened for eligibility over the telephone and 234 were identified as eligible. Of the 234 dyads, 54 did not attend the Time-1 data collection session, and 20 dyads did not complete the data collection procedures. Time-1 data collection sessions were completed by 147 father/adolescent dyads, with 94 father/adolescent dyads completing both Time-1 and Time-2 data collection.

2.4. Sociodemographic Characteristics

Fathers reported their age, years in the U.S., education, employment status, marital status, family annual income, and language spoken at home via surveys. For ease in describing characteristics, education was categorized as middle school or lower, GED (equivalent to a high school diploma) or high school, and some college or higher. Employment was collapsed into four categories: self-employed, unemployed, employed part-time, and employed full-time. Marital status was categorized as single or married/living with a partner.

Adolescents reported their own birthdates and sex. Adolescent age at Time-1 was calculated by subtracting the birthdate from the date of Time-1 data collection divided by the number of days each year (365; 366 for leap years).

2.5. Anthropometric Measurements

Adolescents' and fathers' body weight and height were measured separately twice in a private space using a digital scale (BWB-800 Scale, Tanita) and a stadiometer by a trained research assistant, according to standardized procedures of the National Health and Nutrition Examination Survey (NHANES) [34]. Two measures of both weight and height were averaged to obtain mean weight and height. Fathers' body mass index (BMI) was calculated using weight (kg) divided by height squared (m^2). Adolescents' BMI percentiles were generated by a SAS program using the 2000 CDC Growth Charts [35].

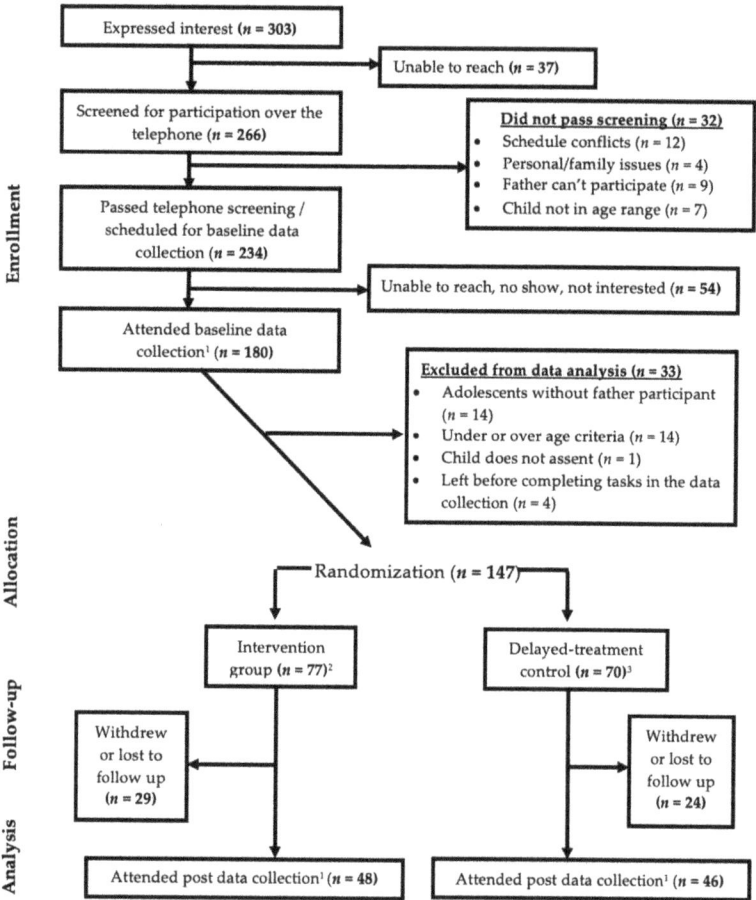

Figure 1. CONSORT diagram (Father/adolescent dyads) [29]. [1] Participants reported frequency of paternal parenting practices; [2] Four participant dyads were randomized to intervention but attended delayed-treatment control group educational sessions; [3] Seven participant dyads were randomized to delayed-treatment control but attended intervention group sessions.

2.6. Father Food and Activity Parenting Practices

The frequency of two types of parenting practices (role modeling and home availability of food or activity opportunities) was assessed by father report via questionnaire for each of seven lifestyle behaviors (fruit, vegetable, sugar-sweetened beverage (SSB), fast food, sweets/salty snack consumption, and frequency of physical activity and screen time) for a total of 14 father food and activity parenting practices. The questionnaire had a total of 33 items, including two items for each of seven role modeling scales, three items for each of six food/activity availability at home scales, and one item for screen time availability at home. Parenting practice questions were developed based on findings from focus groups with Latino fathers [20] and existing validated scales [36–38]. Father food and activity parenting practice items and scales showed adequate criterion validity in a preliminary study and internal consistency for all scales based on Cronbach's α coefficients >0.7 [39].

Fathers were asked two questions about role-modeling frequency, separately, for fruit, vegetable, SSB, fast food, and sweets/salty snack consumption and physical activity and screen time, including (1) how many times fathers were seen by adolescents consuming each type of food or beverage or engaging in physical activity, and (2) how many times fathers consumed each type of food or beverage and engaged in physical activity with adolescents. Response options were almost never or never = 1, <1 time/week = 2, 1–3 times/week = 3, 4–6 times/week = 4, and once a day or more = 5. Responses were coded, summed, and averaged to create a score for each food type or activity.

Fathers were asked three questions about the frequency of practices regarding making fruit, vegetables, SSBs, fast food, sweets/salty snacks, and physical activity available at home. Availability of screen time opportunities was assessed with only one question. Making fruit and vegetables available at home was assessed separately by frequency of fathers (1) buying, (2) preparing, and (3) making sure adolescents had different kinds of fruits and vegetables. Making SSBs, sweets/salty snacks, and fast food available at home was assessed separately for each type of food/beverages by the frequency of fathers (1) buying, (2) preparing, and (3) giving money to adolescents to buy these foods. Making physical activity available was assessed by the frequency of fathers (1) taking their adolescent to a place he/she can be physically active, (2) sending their adolescent outside to be physically active when the weather is nice, and (3) making opportunities available for their adolescent to be physically active. Making screen time available was assessed by the frequency of fathers making screen time opportunities available to their adolescents. Response options for all availability questions were almost never or never = 1, rarely = 2, sometimes = 3, often = 4, and almost always or always = 5. The responses to the three questions for each lifestyle behavior, except for screen time, were coded, summed, and averaged to create an availability score.

2.7. Data Analysis

Initial sample size and power calculations were completed based on expected primary program outcomes as described elsewhere [29]. Post hoc power calculations were completed using nQuery sample size software (Version 4.0.0.0) to determine the power available to detect the observed between-group differences in parenting practice outcomes as significant at alpha = 0.05, using the study sample size in each group.

All fathers who had both Time-1 and Time-2 data were included in the analysis of parenting practice frequency. The first aim of the analysis was to describe observed changes in parenting practices. Descriptive statistics for Time-1 sociodemographic characteristics and Time-1-to-Time-2 changes for parenting practices for intervention and delayed-treatment control groups were assessed using independent two-sample t-tests, Chi-square and Fisher's exact tests.

Linear regression mixed models were used to address the second aim, which was to assess adjusted differences in mean change from Time-1 to Time-2 in father parenting practices outcomes between the intervention and delayed-treatment control groups. The mixed models were adjusted for father age and adolescent sex and age. Additionally, the models included a random intercept for sites and a random intercept for fathers nested within sites to account for clustering of fathers within sites.

All analysis was performed using SAS software version 9.4 (Cary, NC, USA, 2002–2012) with statistical significance defined as $p < 0.05$.

3. Results

The retention rate was 64% for father/adolescent dyads based on withdrawal from the study because of relocation, scheduling conflicts, or loss to follow-up. Mean BMI for the fathers who completed Time-1 and Time-2 data collection (n = 94) was 29.7 vs. 28.3 for the fathers who only completed Time-1 data collection (p = 0.041). Adolescent sex (p = 0.013) was significantly different between those whose fathers completed both Time-1 and Time-2 data collections and those whose fathers only completed Time-1 data collection.

Of 147 father/adolescent dyads, 77 were randomized into the intervention group, and 70 were randomized into the delayed-treatment control group. Random assignment was not followed correctly by 11 father/adolescent dyads (4 father/adolescent dyads randomized to intervention attended the delayed-treatment control group educational sessions, while 7 father/adolescent dyads randomized to the delayed-treatment control group attended the intervention group). Therefore, there were 80 father/adolescent dyads in the intervention group educational sessions, and 67 father/adolescent dyads in the delayed-treatment control group educational sessions. Of the 94 fathers/adolescent dyads who completed both Time-1 and Time-2 data, 48 were in the intervention group, and 46 were in the delayed-treatment control group.

Overall, the demographic characteristics of fathers and adolescents in the intervention and delayed-treatment control groups were similar at Time-1 (Table 1). The mean father age was 42.1 (7.4) years. Most fathers reported having a yearly household income of ≤$49,999 (87%), completing high school or less (77%), being employed full-time (72%), speaking exclusively to primarily Spanish at home (81%), being married (86%), and having lived in the U.S. for more than 10 years (98%). The mean BMI of all the fathers was 29.7 kg/m^2. The mean age of the adolescents was 12.2 (1.4) years, with 62% being male and 38% female. The mean BMI percentile of all adolescents was 77.6.

Table 1. Time-1 father and adolescent demographic characteristics (n = 94).

Demographic Characteristics	All n = 94	Intervention n = 48	Delayed Treatment Control n = 46	p-Values
Father demographics				
Age, mean (SD [1])	42.1 (7.4)	43.1 (7.1)	41.1 (7.7)	0.195 [2]
Annual income, n (%)				
<$25,000	38 (41.8)	23 (48.9)	15 (34.1)	0.229 [3]
$25,000–<$50,000	41 (45.0)	20 (42.6)	21 (47.7)	
≥$50,000	12 (13.2)	4 (8.5)	8 (18.2)	
Marital status, n (%)				
Married	78 (85.7)	41 (87.2)	37 (84.1)	0.674 [4]
Living with partner	6 (6.6)	2 (4.3)	4 (9.1)	
Single/widowed/divorced/separated	7 (7.7)	4 (8.5)	33 (6.8)	
Education, n (%)				
Middle school or less	33 (35.9)	20 (41.7)	13 (29.6)	0.410 [3]
HS [1] grad or GED [1]	38 (41.3)	17 (35.4)	21 (47.7)	
College (any) or technical school	21 (22.8)	11 (22.9)	10 (22.7)	
Employment, n (%)				
Self-employed	10 (11.1)	5 (10.6)	5 (11.6)	0.643 [4]
Unemployed/homemaker	5 (5.6)	3 (6.4)	2 (4.7)	
Part-time employment	8 (8.9)	6 (12.8)	2 (4.7)	
Full-time employment	67 (74.4)	33 (70.2)	34 (79.1)	
Years in the US, n (%)				
<10	2 (2.2)	1 (2.1)	1 (2.3)	0.834 [4]
10–<20	52 (57.1)	29 (61.7)	23 (52.3)	
20–<30	33 (36.3)	15 (31.9)	18 (40.9)	
≥30	4 (4.4)	2 (4.3)	2 (4.6)	
Language, n (%)				
More Spanish than English	76 (81.7)	37 (77.1)	39 (86.7)	0.515 [4]
Equal Spanish and English	15 (16.1)	10 (20.8)	5 (11.1)	
More English than Spanish	2 (2.2)	1 (2.1)	1 (2.2)	
Father BMI [1] (kg/m^2), mean (SD [1])	29.7 (3.7)	29.5 (4.0)	29.8 (3.4)	0.728 [2]
Adolescent demographics				
Age, mean (SD [1])	12.2 (1.4)	12.2 (1.5)	12.1 (1.3)	0.778 [2]
Sex, n (%)				
Male	58 (61.7)	33 (68.8)	25 (54.3)	0.151 [3]
Female	36 (38.3)	15 (31.2)	21 (45.7)	
BMI [1] percentile [5], mean (SD [1])	77.6 (23.8)	80.3 (21.2)	74.7 (26.2)	0.260 [2]

[1] SD = Standard Deviation, HS = High School, GED = General Educational Development test, BMI = body mass index; [2] Two sample t-test; [3] Chi-square test; [4] Fisher's exact test; [5] Adolescent BMI percentiles for age and sex were calculated from SAS codes based on the 2000 CDC Growth Charts; p-value < 0.05.

The means and standard deviations of Time-1 parenting practices were reported for the treatment groups in Table 2. The Time-1 intervention fathers' frequency of fruit role modeling was significantly lower than that of the fathers in the delayed-treatment control group ($p = 0.020$). Also, the Time-1 frequency of screen time role modeling was significantly higher in the intervention fathers compared to the delayed-treatment control group fathers ($p = 0.047$). From Time-1 to Time-2, the intervention fathers reported an increased mean for fruit role modeling frequency (Mean = 0.44, SD = 0.97, $p = 0.001$) and a decreased mean for screen time modeling frequency (Mean = −0.22, SD = 1.18, $p = 0.028$) compared to the fathers in the delayed-treatment control group, based on unadjusted tests for paired data (Table 3).

Table 2. Father-reported paternal parenting practices: Time-1 means and standard deviations for the intervention and delayed-treatment control groups ($n = 94$).

Paternal Parenting Practices	N [1]	All n = 94	Intervention n = 48	Control n = 46	p-Values
Role modeling [3] times/week, mean (SD [2])					
Fruit intake	88	3.19 (0.93)	2.95 (0.97)	3.41 (0.97)	0.020 *
Vegetable intake	91	3.21 (0.98)	3.15 (0.98)	3.27 (0.99)	0.549
SSBs [2] intake	94	2.32 (1.03)	2.36 (1.04)	2.27 (1.02)	0.663
Sweets/salty snack intake	94	1.87 (0.86)	1.89 (0.89)	1.86 (0.84)	0.882
Fast food intake	92	1.85 (0.70)	1.75 (0.71)	1.95 (0.69)	0.183
Physical activity	90	2.75 (1.13)	2.82 (1.19)	2.67 (1.06)	0.516
Screen time	93	2.82 (1.10)	3.04 (1.14)	2.59 (1.02)	0.047 *
Make available [4], mean (SD [2])					
Fruit	94	4.06 (0.74)	4.09 (0.63)	4.03 (0.83)	0.672
Vegetables	93	3.96 (0.84)	4.03 (0.82)	3.88 (0.86)	0.370
SSBs [2]	93	1.77 (0.60)	1.80 (0.60)	1.75 (0.60)	0.660
Sweets/salty snacks	94	1.81 (0.66)	1.88 (0.63)	1.74 (0.68)	0.306
Fast food	94	1.90 (0.66)	1.93 (0.71)	1.86 (0.61)	0.323
Physical activity	93	3.77 (0.93)	3.78 (0.86)	3.77 (1.00)	0.970
Screen time	92	3.10 (1.09)	3.23 (1.15)	2.96 (1.02)	0.223

[1] N reported for each outcome; [2] SSB = Sugar-sweetened beverages, SD = Standard Deviation; [3] Role modeling frequency for fruit, vegetable, SSB, fast food, and sweets/salty snack consumption and physical activity and screen time was based on the average of two items with response options: almost never or never, <1 time/week, 1–3 times/week, 4–6 times/week, and once a day or more; [4] Frequency of making fruit, vegetable, SSB, fast food, and sweets/salty snack consumption and physical activity and screen time available at home was based on the average of three items with response options: almost never or never = 1, not often = 2, sometimes = 3, often = 4, and almost always or always = 5. * Indicates significant differences between groups. p-value < 0.05.

Table 3. Time-1 to Time-2 changes in paternal food and activity parenting practices outcomes.

Paternal Parenting Practices [1]	N [2]	All n = 94	Intervention n = 48	Control n = 46	p Values
Role modeling times/week, mean (SD [3])					
Fruit intake	82	0.12 (0.95)	0.44 (0.97)	−0.23 (0.80)	0.001 *
Vegetable intake	88	0.10 (1.07)	0.20 (0.98)	0.00 (1.17)	0.396
SSBs [3] intake	91	−0.36 (1.02)	−0.45 (1.07)	−0.27 (0.98)	0.407
Sweets/salty snack intake	94	−0.09 (0.85)	−0.19 (0.87)	0.01 (0.81)	0.258
Fast food intake	90	−0.12 (0.65)	−0.16 (0.65)	−0.08 (0.67)	0.575
Physical activity	90	0.01 (0.97)	0.14 (0.97)	−0.14 (0.96)	0.175
Screen time	91	0.04 (1.21)	−0.22 (1.18)	0.33 (1.18)	0.028 *
Make available, mean (SD [3])					
Fruit	93	−0.00 (0.68)	0.06 (0.69)	−0.06 (0.68)	0.405
Vegetables	93	0.02 (0.84)	0.05 (0.88)	−0.00 (0.81)	0.766

Table 3. Cont.

Paternal Parenting Practices [1]	N [2]	All n = 94	Intervention n = 48	Control n = 46	p Values
SSBs [3]	93	−0.04 (0.78)	−0.05 (0.88)	−0.04 (0.81)	0.934
Sweets/salty snacks	94	−0.12 (0.99)	−0.25 (0.90)	0.01 (1.07)	0.204
Fast food	94	0.10 (0.81)	−0.03 (0.82)	0.24 (0.79)	0.108
Physical activity	92	0.02 (0.78)	0.02 (0.79)	0.02 (0.79)	0.991
Screen time	92	−0.05 (1.22)	−0.04 (1.37)	−0.07 (1.05)	0.925

[1] Two-sample t-test of difference in means; [2] N reported for each outcome; [3] SSB = Sugar-sweetened beverages, SD = Standard Deviation; * Indicates significant differences between groups. p-value < 0.05.

After adjusting for covariates (Table 4), the intervention fathers had a significantly increased adjusted mean for fruit modeling frequency and decreased adjusted mean for screen time modeling frequency compared to the delayed-treatment fathers [group*time (SE) = 0.63 (0.19), p = 0.002 for fruit modeling; group*time (SE) = −0.49 (0.24), p = 0.039 for screen time modeling] based on linear regression mixed models (Table 4).

Table 4. Adjusted group differences for Time-1 to Time-2 change in paternal food and activity parenting practice outcomes.

Positive [2] Paternal Parenting Practices (Time-1 to Time-2 Change)	Estimate (SE [1]) and p-Value for Fixed Effects from Mixed Model [2] with Random Intercept for Site and Random Intercept for Father Nested Within Site			
	Group [3] (Ref = Control)	Time [4] (Ref = Time-1)	Group * Time [5] (Ref = Control Time-1 to Time-2 Change)	p Values for Group * Time
Role modeling				
Fruit intake	−0.31 (0.16)	−0.18 (0.14)	0.63 (0.19)	0.002 *
Vegetable intake	−0.12 (0.17)	0.05 (0.15)	0.18 (0.21)	0.414
SSBs [1] intake	−0.03 (0.17)	−0.33 (0.15)	−0.11 (0.21)	0.598
Sweets/salty snack intake	0.01 (0.14)	0.00 (0.12)	−0.17 (0.17)	0.298
Fast food intake	−0.07 (0.12)	−0.09 (0.09)	−0.11 (0.13)	0.395
Physical activity	0.04 (0.18)	−0.11 (0.14)	0.29 (0.20)	0.142
Screen time	0.38 (0.19)	0.28 (0.17)	−0.49 (0.24)	0.039 *
Make Available				
Fruit	−0.07 (0.14)	−0.05 (0.10)	0.16 (0.14)	0.254
Vegetables	0.01 (0.15)	0.02 (0.12)	0.10 (0.17)	0.566
SSBs [1]	−0.04 (0.12)	−0.11 (0.11)	0.03 (0.16)	0.854
Sweets/salty snacks	0.11 (0.12)	0.01 (0.13)	−0.25 (0.18)	0.174
Fast food	0.02 (0.12)	0.19 (0.11)	−0.22 (0.16)	0.160
Physical activity	−0.21 (0.15)	0.01 (0.11)	0.07 (0.16)	0.672
Screen time	0.13 (0.17)	−0.16 (0.17)	0.09 (0.24)	0.700

[1] Abbreviations: SE = standard error, SSB = sugar-sweetened beverages; [2] Models were adjusted for father age, adolescent age and sex; [3] Group effect estimates the adjusted difference between intervention and control means across both times; [4] Time effect estimates the adjusted difference between Time-1 and Time-2 means across both groups; [5] Group*time estimates the adjusted difference in mean change from Time-1 to Time-2 for intervention compared to control; * Indicates significant differences in adjusted Time-1 to Time-2 changes between intervention and control at p < 0.05.

4. Discussion

This randomized controlled trial examined the effects of the Padres program on Latino fathers' food and activity parenting practices. Compared to the delayed treatment control group fathers, the intervention group fathers reported a higher adjusted mean change for fruit modeling frequency and a lower adjusted mean change for screen time modeling frequency from Time-1 to Time-2. Overall, this study identified a moderate positive intervention effect for 2 of 14 parenting practices (adjusted models), including fruit and screen time role modeling. In other studies, role modeling behaviors were associated with greater healthy food consumption [16] and with sedentary activity [40,41] among children and adolescents.

A limited number of studies have examined improvements in Latino food parenting practices in community-based programs, resulting in few studies available for comparison to the current study. One study with primarily low-income Hispanic parents (95% mothers) and children (3–11 years) showed Time-1 to Time-2 intervention improvements in two parenting practices involving food availability [42] but not in frequency of food intake role modeling. This finding was in contrast to the current study, where the intervention group fathers had a mean increase in fruit modeling frequency and a mean decrease in screen time modeling frequency compared to the delayed-treatment control group fathers. The previous intervention was a pilot study [42] with primarily mothers and did not include a control group; therefore, the results were not directly comparable to the results of the current study.

The current study demonstrated no intervention effects for most of the parenting practices, which could be related to ceiling effects. The majority of the fathers in both groups reported a high frequency of healthful food and activity practices and a low frequency of most of the unhealthful food and activity practices at Time-1, except for screen time modeling and availability. For example, intervention fathers reported role modeling screen time more than 1–3 times a week and role modeling sweets/salty snacks and fast food intake less than once a week. Thus, fathers who reported a high frequency of unhealthful food and activity practices before the intervention may have been better able to apply what they learned during the intervention to improve the frequency of some parenting practices.

Another possible explanation for not observing improvements for most parenting practices in the current study could be associated with social determinants of health. Evidence from previous studies demonstrates that being part of a low-income household and having lower educational attainment are two key social factors associated with poor health in the United States [43]. Racial and ethnic minorities with low socioeconomic status, including the Hispanic/Latino population, often experience health disparities [43,44]. The majority of fathers in this study had a high school diploma or less (79%) and had lower-incomes (87%), even though most had full-time employment. The role of fathers as family providers with busy work schedules may have kept fathers from implementing parenting practices. For example, limited resources to purchase healthy foods may have restricted the ability to make healthy foods available at home and/or role model healthy food intake. Also, fathers who work long hours may have limited time to interact with adolescents and apply parenting practices; thus, a longer period of time from post-intervention to the completion of evaluation surveys might have allowed fathers to better apply the practices promoted in the program.

This study had several limitations. The COVID-19 pandemic did not allow for continued in-person program implementation after March 2020, thus limiting the sample size. The low retention rate and smaller sample size than expected resulted in the study being underpowered to detect significant changes in most of the parenting practice comparisons. The Padres program was only implemented in community centers and churches in the Minneapolis/St. Paul metropolitan area and only with low-income families, which limited the generalizability of study findings to the broader Latino/Hispanic population. Defining groups by randomization (not by group assignments) might cause bias in the group comparisons, since the randomization assignments were not followed correctly for eleven dyads. Not correctly following assignments may have occurred because participants in some locations may have known each other and preferred to attend sessions with relatives or friends or needed to share transportation. However, similar results were obtained from a sensitivity analysis when the group comparisons were defined by participation instead of randomization. Another potential limitation is that delayed-treatment control participants may have been exposed to the intervention, since participants may have known each other. Also, participants may have enrolled in this study because of an interest in nutrition and health and/or financial compensation, which could have biased the intervention data.

5. Conclusions

The current study showed positive adjusted Time-1 to Time-2 change in two parenting practices between groups, including an adjusted mean increase in fruit role modeling frequency and an adjusted mean decrease in screen time modeling frequency among intervention group participants compared to delayed-treatment control group participants. Overall, only 2 of 14 Latino father parenting practices were reported to be improved after the intervention. The lack of significant findings for other parenting practices may be associated with the limited sample size, low family socioeconomic status, and possible ceiling effects of baseline paternal parenting practices. Future studies could consider social determinants of health and family strengths when developing interventions to support an increase in healthy Latino father parenting practices.

Author Contributions: Conceptualization, A.B., G.A.H.C., S.A.d.D., Y.Z. and M.R.; methodology, G.A.H.C., A.R.P., A.G. and N.L.; software, C.D.; formal analysis, A.B. and C.D.; investigation, A.B., A.R.P., S.A.d.D., Y.Z. and M.R.; writing—original draft preparation, A.B.; writing—review and editing, A.B., G.A.H.C., C.D., A.R.P., S.A.d.D., Y.Z., A.G., N.L. and M.R.; visualization, A.B.; supervision, M.R.; project administration, M.R.; funding acquisition, G.A.H.C. and M.R. All authors have read and agreed to the published version of the manuscript.

Funding: This research was funded by the Agriculture and Food Research Initiative, grant number 2016-68001-24921, from the USDA National Institute of Food and Agriculture.

Institutional Review Board Statement: The study was conducted in accordance with the Declaration of Helsinki and approved by the Institutional Review Board of the University of Minnesota Institutional Review Board (project identification code: 1511S80707) for studies involving humans.

Informed Consent Statement: Informed consent was obtained from all subjects involved in the study.

Data Availability Statement: The de-identified data and SAS codes used in this study are available on request from the corresponding author. The data are not publicly available because the data analysis phase of the study is still currently being completed, while the intervention and all data collection have been completed.

Acknowledgments: The authors thank the participants, community partners, and organizations for their participation and support; and graduate and undergraduate students for their help in the development of the program, facilitating the program, and collecting evaluation data. Research reported in this publication was supported by the National Center for Advancing Translational Sciences of the National Institutes of Health Award Number UL1-TR002494. The content is solely the responsibility of the authors and does not necessarily represent the official views of the National Institutes of Health.

Conflicts of Interest: The authors declare no conflict of interest. The funders had no role in the design of the study; in the collection, analyses, or interpretation of data; in the writing of the manuscript; or in the decision to publish the results.

References

1. Dunford, E.; Popkin, B. 37 year snacking trends for US children 1977–2014. *Pediatr. Obes.* **2018**, *13*, 247–255. [CrossRef]
2. Vikraman, S.; Fryar, C.D.; Ogden, C.L. *Caloric Intake from Fast Food among Children and Adolescents in the United States, 2011–2012*; NCHS Data Brief, no 213; National Center for Health Statistics: Hyattsville, MD, USA, 2015.
3. Kim, S.A.; Moore, L.V.; Galuska, D.; Wright, A.P.; Harris, D.; Grummer-Strawn, L.M.; Merlo, C.L.; Nihiser, A.J.; Rhodes, D.G. Vital signs: Fruit and Vegetable Intake among Children—United States, 2003–2010. *Morb. Mortal. Wkly. Rep.* **2014**, *63*, 671–676. Available online: https://www.cdc.gov/mmwr/preview/mmwrhtml/mm6331a3.htm (accessed on 3 November 2020).
4. National Physical Activity Plan Alliance. *The 2018 United States Report Card on Physical Activity for Children and Youth*; National Physical Activity Plan Alliance: Washington, DC, USA, 2018; Available online: https://paamovewithus.org/wp-content/uploads/2020/06/2018-US-Report-Card-Summary_WEB.pdf (accessed on 13 August 2020).
5. Yang, L.; Cao, C.; Kantor, E.D.; Nguyen, L.H.; Zheng, X.; Park, Y.; Giovannucci, E.L.; Matthews, C.E.; Colditz, G.A.; Cao, Y. Trends in sedentary behavior among the US population, 2001–2016. *J. Am. Med. Assoc.* **2019**, *321*, 1587–1597. [CrossRef]
6. Rennie, K.L.; Johnson, L.; Jebb, S.A. Behavioural determinants of obesity. *Best Pr. Res. Clin. Endocrinol. Metab.* **2005**, *19*, 343–358. [CrossRef]

7. Gordon-Larsen, P.; The, N.S.; Adair, L.S. Longitudinal trends in obesity in the United States from adolescence to the third decade of life. *Obesity* **2010**, *18*, 1801–1804. [CrossRef] [PubMed]
8. Bösch, S.; Lobstein, T.; Brinsden, H.; Ralston, J.; Bull, F.; Willumsen, J.; Branca, F.; Engesveen, K.; Grummer-Strawn, L.; Nishida, C.; et al. *Taking Action on Childhood Obesity*; World Health Organization: Geneva, Switzerland; World Obesity: London, UK, 2018; Available online: https://apps.who.int/iris/bitstream/handle/10665/274792/WHO-NMH-PND-ECHO-18.1-eng.pdf?ua=1 (accessed on 30 October 2018).
9. U.S. Department of Agriculture; U.S. Department of Health and Human Services. *2020–2025 Dietary Guidelines for Americans*, 9th ed.; U.S. Department of Agriculture: Washington, DC, USA; U.S. Department of Health and Human Services: Washington, DC, USA, 2020. Available online: https://www.dietaryguidelines.gov/ (accessed on 6 August 2021).
10. World Health Organization. Physical Activity. 2018. Available online: https://www.who.int/news-room/fact-sheets/detail/physical-activity (accessed on 13 August 2020).
11. Wu, X.Y.; Han, L.H.; Zhang, J.H.; Luo, S.; Hu, J.W.; Sun, K. The influence of physical activity, sedentary behavior on health-related quality of life among the general population of children and adolescents: A systematic review. *PLoS ONE* **2017**, *12*, e0187668. [CrossRef] [PubMed]
12. U.S. Department of Health and Human Services. *Physical Activity Guidelines for Americans*, 2nd ed.; U.S. Department of Health and Human Services: Washington, DC, USA, 2018. Available online: https://health.gov/sites/default/files/2019-09/Physical_Activity_Guidelines_2nd_edition.pdf (accessed on 15 July 2019).
13. Pearson, N.; Biddle, S.J.H. Sedentary behavior and dietary intake in children, adolescents, and adults: A systematic review. *Am. J. Prev. Med.* **2011**, *41*, 178–188. [CrossRef] [PubMed]
14. Barnett, T.A.; Kelly, A.S.; Rohm Young, D.; Perry, C.K.; Pratt, C.A.; Edwards, N.M.; Rao, G.; Vos, M.B.; on behalf of American Heart Association Obesity Committee of the Council on Lifestyle; Cardiometabolic Health; et al. Sedentary behaviors in today's youth: Approaches to the prevention and management of childhood obesity. *Circulation* **2018**, *138*, e142–e159. [CrossRef] [PubMed]
15. Vaughn, A.E.; Ward, D.S.; Fisher, J.O.; Faith, M.S.; Hughes, S.O.; Kremers, S.P.J.; Musher-Eizenman, D.R.; O'Connor, T.M.; Patrick, H.; Power, T.G. Fundamental constructs in food parenting practices: A content map to guide future research. *Nutr. Rev.* **2016**, *74*, 98–117. [CrossRef]
16. Yee, A.Z.H.; Lwin, M.O.; Ho, S.S. The influence of parental practices on child promotive and preventive food consumption behaviors: A systematic review and meta-analysis. *Int. J. Behav. Nutr. Phys. Act.* **2017**, *14*, 1–14. [CrossRef]
17. Hutchens, A.; Lee, R.E. Parenting practices and children's physical activity: An integrative review. *J. Sch. Nurs.* **2018**, *34*, 68–85. [CrossRef]
18. Xu, H.; Wen, L.M.; Rissel, C. Associations of parental influences with physical activity and screen time among young children: A systematic review. *J. Obes.* **2015**, *2015*, 546925. [CrossRef]
19. Ramirez, E.R.; Norman, G.J.; Rosenberg, D.E.; Kerr, J.; Saelens, B.E.; Durant, N.; Sallis, J.F. Adolescent screen time and rules to limit screen time in the home. *J. Adolesc. Health* **2011**, *48*, 379–385. [CrossRef]
20. Zhang, Y.; Hurtado, G.A.; Flores, R.; Alba-Meraz, A.; Reicks, M. Latino fathers' perspectives and parenting practices regarding eating, physical activity, and screen time behaviors of early adolescent children: Focus group findings. *J. Acad. Nutr. Diet.* **2018**, *118*, 2070–2080. [CrossRef]
21. Flores, G.; Maldonado, J.; Durán, P. Making tortillas without lard: Latino parents' perspectives on healthy eating, physical activity, and weight-management strategies for overweight Latino children. *J. Acad. Nutr. Diet.* **2012**, *112*, 81–89. [CrossRef]
22. Santiago-Torres, M.; Adams, A.K.; Carrel, A.L.; LaRowe, T.L.; Schoeller, D.A. Home food availability, parental dietary intake, and familial eating habits influence the diet quality of urban Hispanic children. *Child. Obes.* **2014**, *10*, 408–415. [CrossRef]
23. Ayala, G.X.; Baquero, B.; Arredondo, E.M.; Campbell, N.; Larios, S.; Elder, J.P. Association between family variables and Mexican American children's dietary behaviors. *J. Nutr. Educ. Behav.* **2007**, *39*, 62–69. [CrossRef]
24. Springer, A.E.; Kelder, S.H.; Barroso, C.S.; Drenner, K.L.; Shegog, R.; Ranjit, N.; Hoelscher, D.M. Parental influences on television watching among children living on the Texas—Mexico border. *Prev. Med.* **2010**, *51*, 112–117. [CrossRef]
25. Parada, H.; Ayala, G.X.; Horton, L.A.; Ibarra, L.; Arrendondo, E.M. Latino fathers' feeding-related parenting strategies on children's eating. *Ecol. Food Nutr.* **2016**, *55*, 292–307. [CrossRef]
26. LeCroy, M.N.; Siega-Riz, A.M.; Albrecht, S.S.; Ward, D.S.; Cai, J.; Perreira, K.M.; Isasi, C.R.; Mossavar-Rahmani, Y.; Gallo, L.C.; Castañeda, S.F.; et al. Association of food parenting practice patterns with obesogenic dietary intake in Hispanic/Latino youth: Results from the Hispanic Community Children's Health Study/Study of Latino Youth (SOL Youth). *Appetite* **2019**, *140*, 277–287. [CrossRef]
27. Tschann, J.M.; Martinez, S.M.; Penilla, C.; Gregorich, S.E.; Pasch, L.A.; de Groat, C.L.; Flores, E.; Deardorff, J.; Greenspan, L.C.; Butte, N.F. Parental feeding practices and child weight status in Mexican American families: A longitudinal analysis. *Int. J. Behav. Nutr. Phys. Act.* **2015**, *12*, 1–10. [CrossRef]
28. Penilla, C.; Tschann, J.M.; Deardorff, J.; Flores, E.; Pasch, L.A.; Butte, N.F.; Gregorich, S.E.; Greenspan, L.C.; Martinez, S.M.; Ozer, E. Fathers' feeding practices and children's weight status in Mexican American families. *Appetite* **2017**, *117*, 109–116. [CrossRef] [PubMed]
29. Baltaci, A.; Hurtado Choque, G.A.; Davey, C.; Reyes Peralta, A.; Alvarez de Davila, S.; Zhang, Y.; Gold, A.; Larson, N.; Reicks, M. Padres Preparados, Jóvenes Saludables: Intervention impact and dose effects of a randomized controlled trial on Latino father and adolescent energy balance-related behaviors. *BMC Public Health* **2022**, *22*, 1–14. [CrossRef]

30. Allen, M.L.; Garcia-Huidobro, D.; Hurtado, G.A.; Allen, R.; Davey, C.S.; Forster, J.L.; Hurtado, M.; Lopez-Petrovich, K.; Marczak, M.; Reynoso, U.; et al. Immigrant family skills-building to prevent tobacco use in Latino youth: Study protocol for a community-based participatory randomized controlled trial. *Trials* **2012**, *13*, 242. [CrossRef] [PubMed]
31. Bandura, A.; Cliffs, N.J. *Social Foundations of Thought and Action: A Social Cognitive Theory*; First printing; Prentice-Hall: Englewood, CL, USA, 1986; p. 376.
32. McAlister, A.L.; Perry, C.L.; Parcel, G.S. How individuals, environments, and health behaviors interact: Social Cognitive Theory. In *Health Behaviors and Health Education: Theory, Research, and Practice*, 4th ed.; Glanz, K., Rimer, B.K., Viswanath, K., Eds.; Jossey-Bass: San Francisco, CA, USA, 2008; pp. 169–188.
33. Arroyo-Johnson, C.; Allen, M.L.; Colditz, G.A.; Hurtado, G.A.; Davey, C.S.; Thompson, V.L.S.; Drake, B.F.; Svetaz, M.V.; Rosas-Lee, M.; Goodman, M.S. A table of two community networks program centers: Operationalizing and assessing CBPR principles and evaluating partnership outcomes. *Prog. Community Health Partn.* **2015**, *9*, 61–69. [CrossRef] [PubMed]
34. Centers for Disease Control and Prevention. *National Health and Nutrition Examination Survey (NHANES), Anthropometric Procedures Manual*; Centers for Disease Control and Prevention: Atlanta, GA, USA, 2017. Available online: https://wwwn.cdc.gov/nchs/data/nhanes/2017-2018/manuals/2017_Anthropometry_Procedures_Manual.pdf (accessed on 21 September 2020).
35. Centers for Disease Control and Prevention. *Growth Chart Training- A SAS Program for the 2000 CDC Growth Chart (Ages 0 to <20 Years)*; Centers for Disease Control and Prevention: Atlanta, GA, USA, 2022. Available online: https://www.cdc.gov/nccdphp/dnpao/growthcharts/resources/sas.htm#print (accessed on 8 September 2020).
36. Pinard, C.A.; Yaroch, A.L.; Hart, M.H.; Serrano, E.L.; McFerren, M.M.; Estabrooks, P.A. The validity and reliability of the Comprehensive Home Environment Survey (CHES). *Health Promot. Pract.* **2014**, *15*, 109–117. [CrossRef]
37. Singh, A.S.; Chinapaw, M.J.; Uijtdewilligen, L.; Vik, F.N.; van Lippevelde, W.; Fernández-Alvira, J.M.; Stomfai, S.; Manios, Y.; van der Sluijs, M.; Terwee, C.; et al. Test-retest reliability and construct validity of the ENERGY-parent questionnaire on parenting practices, energy balance-related behaviours and their potential behavioural determinants: The ENERGY-project. *BMC Res. Notes* **2012**, *5*, 434. [CrossRef]
38. Matthews-Ewald, M.R.; Posada, A.; Wiesner, M.; Olvera, N. An exploratory factor analysis of the Parenting strategies for Eating and physical Activity Scale (PEAS) for use in Hispanic mothers of adolescent and preadolescent daughters with overweight. *Eat Behav.* **2015**, *19*, 193–199. [CrossRef]
39. Zhang, Y.; Reyes Peralta, A.; Arellano Roldan Brazys, P.; Hurtado, G.A.; Larson, N.; Reicks, M. Development of a survey to assess Latino fathers' parenting practices regarding energy balance–related behaviors of early adolescents. *Health Educ. Behav.* **2020**, *47*, 123–133. [CrossRef]
40. Gebremariam, M.K.; Henjum, S.; Terragni, L.; Torheim, L.E. Correlates of screen time and mediators of differences by parental education among adolescents. *Food Nutr. Res.* **2016**, *60*, 32512. [CrossRef]
41. Bassul, C.; Corish, C.A.; Kearney, J.M. Associations between Home Environment, Children's and Parents' Characteristics and Children's TV Screen Time Behavior. *Int. J. Environ. Res. Public Health* **2021**, *18*, 1589. [CrossRef]
42. Otterbach, L.; Mena, N.Z.; Greene, G.; Redding, C.A.; Groot A de Tovar, A. Community-based childhood obesity prevention intervention for parents improves health behaviors and food parenting practices among Hispanic, low-income parents. *BMC Obes.* **2018**, *5*, 11. [CrossRef]
43. Braveman, P.; Egerter, S.; Williams, D.R. The social determinants of health: Coming of age. *Annu Rev. Public Health* **2011**, *32*, 381–398. [CrossRef]
44. Thornton, R.L.J.; Glover, C.M.; Cené, C.W.; Glik, D.C.; Henderson, J.A.; Williams, D.R. Evaluating strategies for reducing health disparities by addressing the social determinants of health. *Health Aff.* **2016**, *35*, 1416–1423. [CrossRef]

Article

Feasibility of a Theory-Based, Online Tailored Message Program to Motivate Healthier Behaviors in College Women

Patrice A. Hubert, Holly Fiorenti and Valerie B. Duffy *

Department of Allied Health Sciences, University of CT, Storrs, CT 06269-1101, USA
* Correspondence: valerie.duffy@uconn.edu; Tel.: +1-860-486-1997

Abstract: We aimed to test the feasibility of an online survey and tailored message program in young women. Recruited from college campuses, women (n = 189) completed an online survey assessing preference for and behaviors toward diet and physical activity as well as theory-based influencers of these behaviors (knowledge/information, motivation, and confidence). Health messages were tailored to the participant's survey responses and learning style to address misconceptions and motivate or reinforce healthy physical activity and dietary behaviors. Most women reported the survey as relevant (92%) and useful for reflecting on their health (83%), with survey responses variable in level of nutrition and physical activity knowledge, motivation, and confidence. Each woman received four tailored messages—most reported the messages as relevant (80%) and learning new information (60%). Across all messages, nearly half of the participants (~48%) reported willingness to try or maintain healthier behaviors and confidence in their ability. Body size discrepancy and dietary restraint had small effects message responses of information learned, and the motivation and confidence in trying healthier behaviors. In summary, these data support the feasibility of this online tailored message program. The college women found the tailored message program acceptable and useful to motivate healthier behaviors. The findings provide direction for behaviorally focused interventions to improve dietary and physical activity behaviors.

Keywords: mhealth; physical activity; diet; tailored intervention; behavior change theory; Information-Motivation-Behavioral Skills Model; women; young adults; college students; brief intervention

1. Introduction

For young adults, the college years present many challenges to the maintenance or development of healthy behaviors (e.g., regular physical activity, high quality diets) [1–4]. Of particular concern are college women, who face barriers such as lack of knowledge, misinformation, poor body image, social pressures, and time obligations that may cause strain on their motivation and self-efficacy for appropriate and healthy engagement in physical activity and dietary habits [3,5–8]. These barriers in tandem with the COVID-19 pandemic have caused further negative effects, with more college women reporting significant changes to their physical activity and dietary intake [9–13]. The 2019–2021 American College Health Association surveys found that only 37% of women identifying students engaged in regular physical activity that would qualify them as active adults, 66% reported drinking ≥1 sugar sweetened beverage(s) a day, and only 18% and 32% met the recommended guidelines of consuming 3 servings of vegetables and fruit a day, respectively [14–16]. Furthermore, college women may be more apt to have extreme physical activity behaviors to compensate for poor dietary behaviors and vice versa [17–21]. However, failure to develop appropriate and sustainable behaviors can lead to decreased adherence to physical activity guidelines and an overall poor diet quality [7,8,22]. Thus, successful health interventions that provide appropriate information and motivation in this population are warranted.

There has been demonstrated short-term improvements in behaviors in response to health interventions targeting college-aged individuals, however, refinement in methodology and personalization are necessary to improve program quality and outcomes [23,24]. A systematic review found that college students are not engaged with general health promotion messaging, thereby limiting their usability and impact [25]. Personalized approaches, which can involve the tailoring of health information to one's phenotype, learning preferences, psychosocial characteristics, activity, and environment, are suggested to improve individual effects of health programming [25,26]. Tailoring health information incorporates methods that personalize communication for the intended receiver, assisting in the reading, remembering, and relevancy of information to the participant [27,28]. Tailored communications, versus generalized and generic communications, have demonstrated greater participant benefit to promote and support health behavior change through increased intention and motivation [28–32]. Tailoring of health information to college women may be key in successful marketing of physical activity and dietary messages to motivate healthier behaviors.

The COVID-19 pandemic has highlighted the importance and normalization of online health care and interventions [33,34]. As online interventions in young adults, incorporating tailoring health information into an internet-based program could improve interest, increase accessibility, reduce participant burden, and offer support/feedback [25,30,35,36]. Computer-generated programs offer an efficient way to tailor health messaging [37] and motivate individuals to improve their physical activity and dietary behaviors by automating delivery of messages via text message, email, or social platforms [30,38–40]. Automating these methods allows messages to be tailored in response to participant's self-reported behaviors versus general goals and recommendations to produce greater changes in physical activity and diet [41]. However, due to poor recall and misreporting of physical activity and dietary intake [42], better measures of self-reported behaviors to tailor physical activity and diet messages are warranted [37].

Assessment of individual food preferences and physical activity though surveying likes/dislikes is a feasible way to measure behavior in young adults/college students as it is cognitively simple, less biased by misreporting [43–46], and has a low time burden [47]. Messages can be tailored to participant reported preferences to help encourage or motivate behavior change. Acknowledging preference and incorporating tailoring into physical activity and nutrition interventions has helped to encourage physical activity engagement [48–51], increase preference of healthy foods [44,52–55], and decrease preference for less healthy foods [56,57]. Acceptability and usability of liking surveys with evidenced based tailored messages has been demonstrated in promoting behavior change in children and adolescents [31,32].

The Informational Motivational Behavioral Skills (IMB) Model has been identified as a supportive framework for tailored messages to participant's behaviors. The IMB Model suggests that each construct (information, motivation, behavioral skills) has a direct effect on behavior; however, behavioral skills mediate the effect of information and motivation on the resulting health behavior [58,59]. This model is commonly used to understand predictive factors for health behavior and outcomes [59,60]. Previous literature supports its use in predicting many different health behaviors, including physical activity and diet [58,60–71]. Thus, the IMB model was used to guide further survey development and creation of tailored messages [72].

Our team has used intervention mapping to develop physical activity and diet messages for college students and young adults based on the IMB model [72]. Included in this approach was examination of literature, assessment of previous survey results, and key informant interviews [72]. The messages were designed with simple language and imagery aligned with IMB model to provide information, motivate, and encourage confidence (i.e., behavioral skills) by either reinforcing or motivating behavior change [72]. As these messages were delivered anonymously and one time, confidence was used to operationalize behavioral skills. Messages were evaluated for participant's response to information, motivation, and confidence as it pertained to the targeted behavior in the message.

Although preliminary feasibility of the survey and tailored messages suggested promising results [72], additional evaluation of feasibility in women is required, as well as testing of information, motivation, and confidence (i.e., behavioral skills) in the survey, response variability, and message usability. Factors such as body size perception and dietary restraint influence women's health behaviors [17–21] and may influence their response to the messages and impact their motivation or confidence for behavior change [3,5–8]. Evidence suggests intersecting relationships between body size perception, dietary restraint, diet quality and physical activity in young women, where body size perception or dietary restraint influence eating behaviors, diet quality and physical activity [21,46,73–81].

Thus, this study aimed to explore the feasibility of an online tailored message program for young adult college women that aligns with changes in information, motivation, and confidence (IMB constructs). Feasibility was defined as variability in responses to baseline knowledge, information learned, motivation, and confidence as well as acceptability and usefulness of the messages to promote healthier behaviors. Secondly, this study aimed to test the effect of body size discrepancy and dietary restraint on participant responses to the behavioral survey and message evaluation measures. It was hypothesized that body size perception and dietary restraint may influence women's responses to the tailored messages. The results from this study address the ability of the survey and participant's response to the messages to provide direction for future health promotion efforts to improve physical activity and diet quality in young women.

2. Materials and Methods

2.1. Participants

This was an observational, cross-sectional study with a convenience sample of 189 female-identifying college students from multiple campuses of one New England University. The survey was open to all students regardless of gender identity, however for purposes of this study, analysis was limited to participants who identified as female. Participants were recruited virtually to complete an online survey and tailored message program from February–April 2021.

A key focus of our marketing plan was recruitment of a diverse student population. We employed a comprehensive marketing strategy and outreach with key stakeholders to recruit students of diverse academic interests, demographics, and campus involvement [72]. Key stakeholders for participant recruitment included academic programs and colleges throughout the University main campus and branches, student health and wellness services, student support services, as well as off-campus and commuter student services. Additionally, the research team created a list and contact information of 250 student-run organizations/clubs, with focus on culturally centered groups. A white paper was created that highlighted the study's purpose, goals, and pictures with brief bios of members of the research team. Prior to initiation of recruitment, research team members reached out to stakeholders and contact persons for each organization to supply them with the white paper, the option to schedule a virtual informational meeting, and identify interest in recruitment assistance efforts. Recruitment information, including the flyer and materials created for social media postings, was sent to the key stakeholders, and interested student groups. In addition, participants were recruited through consistent postings in the online student newsletter throughout the recruitment months [72].

The study received IRB approval from the University Board (X17-084). The online survey began with an information sheet, followed by a yes/no consent to participate. Participation was voluntary, and students could end the online program at any point. After completing, students had the opportunity to enter their email into a raffle for a $25 gift card.

2.2. Procedure

This online tailored message program utilized the IMB framework to adapt an evidence-based program, originally conducted with children their parents/caregivers [31] or children in a middle school setting [32], for college students. The program consisted of a validated survey assessing liking/disliking of usual diet and physical activity behaviors [46,82,83], questions assessing current health knowledge and behaviors [72,84–88], and tailored messages driven by response to the liking survey (food and physical activity), intuitive eating, stress, and sleep. Following the IMB framework, the program assessed knowledge/information of participants through: (1) baseline knowledge related to message Information and responses to each message; (2) reported Information learned; (3) Motivation on how much they would like to try/continue targeted behavior; and (4) Behavioral Skills by assessing confidence/self-efficacy to try/continue the targeted behavior.

The program was designed to be conducted online in a single session via an anonymous Qualtrics platform (Provo, UT, USA). After an online assent to participate, students were asked to report demographic information, liking/disliking of foods and activities, health, and diet related questions (including body size perception, dietary restraint, intuitive eating, food insecurity, weight stigma and perception, stress, and sleep), and the usefulness and acceptance of the survey. Students then received their health messages tailored to their responses and responded to a series of usefulness and acceptance questions for the messages individually and collectively.

2.3. Socio-Demographic and Health Characteristics

Students were asked to report their year in college, gender identity, age, ethnicity, race, self-reported weight, and height (used to calculate BMI), and current/ideal body size (Figure Rating Scale [84], self-reported eating disorder (yes/no), school or college, and device used to take the survey. Additional health questions surveyed frequency of physical activity, food group consumption, and level of dietary restraint.

Body Size Discrepancy: Participants responded twice to Figure Rating Scale [84,89] to choose which figure represented what they consider their current and then ideal body. The Scale consists of 9 figures (males and females) representing underweight to obese body types [84,89], including figures 1–2 as underweight, 3–4 as normal weight, 5–6 as overweight, and 7–9 as obese. The body size discrepancy variable used in the analysis was ideal body figure subtracted from current figure as a proxy of body dissatisfaction [73,74,90,91]. The variable was treated continuously to test relationships with responses to information, motivation, confidence and categorical as Body Discrepancy (scores greater or less than 1) versus No Body Discrepancy (scores 0 or ±1) to describe the sample and test survey and message feasibility.

Dietary Restraint: Participants responded to 6 questions in the Concern for Dieting Subscale from the Dietary Restraint Scale [85]. Scores could range from 0–19. The dietary restraint score was tested for reliability using Cronbach's Coefficient alpha ($\alpha = 0.83$). The score was split at the median (8) for analyses examining differences in survey and message evaluation responses based on level of restraint to indicate young adult woman who were high or low in dietary restraint.

Knowledge Scores: Participants responded to 11 questions on knowledge of physical activity and diet. These questions were based on predetermined health misconceptions and misinformation of college students found in the literature [72], and the concepts were addressed in the in the tailored messages. For each question, the participant selected their level of agreement, scored as −2 (Strongly Disagree) to +2 (Strongly Agree). True/False questions were scored so the correct answers received a value of 1, and incorrect a value of 0. Scores were summed to create a knowledge score, with a maximum score of 15.

2.4. Liking Survey and Tailored Message Program

A proxy of physical activity and dietary behaviors was captured using a previously validated, online liking survey for college-aged individuals [46,82,83]. Each activity, food or beverage item was each shown as an image and text label to the left of a horizontal, hedonic scale with five faces and corresponding descriptors of "love it", "like it", "it's okay", "dislike it", and "hate it", and a slider allowing a continuous rating from ±100. Students were able to move the marker anywhere on the slider containing five faces: "love it"/"hate it" had a midpoint value of ±80, "like it"/"dislike it" a midpoint value of ±40, and "it's okay" as 0. Students were able to select "never tried or done" for any of the activities, foods, and beverages.

Students were oriented to the liking survey by reporting their liking/disliking for generally pleasant and unpleasant experiences (seeing family and friends, receiving a compliment, going on vacation, taking an exam, zoom class, and being caught in a lie). Following orientation, students rated liking/disliking of physical activities (19 items), sedentary activities (5 items), and foods and beverages (47 items). The physical activities represented four categories: aerobic training, resistance training, flexibility training, behavioral inclinations. Behavioral inclinations included general habits related to physical activity preferences such as working up a sweat, exercising alone/with a partner, taking the stairs, going to the gym, attending group classes, and playing sports. Reported liking of physical activities and behavioral inclinations were averaged together to create an overall liking of physical activity score. The foods and beverages represented major food groups (vegetable, fruit, whole grains, heathy fat, low-fat dairy, refined grains, high fat protein, unhealthy fat, salty foods/snacks, sweets, and sugar-sweetened beverages), with at least three items per group.

The messages were tailored to the average liking/disliking of activity and food groups and the responses to intuitive eating, stress, and sleep questions to be motivating or reinforcing as shown in Table 1 [72]. All messages were pilot tested with a small group of college students and were edited based on their feedback [72]. The criteria for receiving a tailored messages as motivating or reinforcing were based on liking responses following our previous studies with young adults [46,82,83], our tailored message program [31,32], and the literature [86–88]. For example, participants who reported a high liking of a healthy item or low liking of a less healthy item received a reinforcing message encouraging the participant to continue the behavior. Participants who reported a low liking of a healthy item or high liking of a less healthy item received a motivating message. The health behavior messages (intuitive eating, stress, sleep) were tailored using participant response to validated questionnaires by criteria reported previously [86–88]. The motivating messages also were tailored to the participant's preferred learning style [92] for either autonomous support or directive support. Two generic health messages were also created to serve as comparison with the tailored messages [72]. Algorithms were embedded within Qualtrics to assure each participant received 5 messages, including 4 tailored messages (reinforcing or motivating), and 1 generic message (randomly assigned from 2 possible). Two of the tailored messages were food-based messages (vegetable, fruit, whole grains, lean protein, fats, hydration, sweets, salt), one physical activity-based, and one health behavior-based (intuitive eating, stress, sleep).

Table 1. Tailored Message Categories and Examples.

Category	Composite Group	Items	Message Category	Message Example
Physical Activities	Aerobic Training	Walking, running, sprinting, high intensity interval training, playing sports, biking, circuit training	Physical Activity	Keep up with the great movement you're doing! Setting timers to do quick stretches or air squats can help to increase physical activity levels. (Reinforcing)
	Resistance Training	Barbell exercises (squat, deadlift, bench press), free weights, cable exercises		
	Flexibility Training	Pilates, yoga, flexibility training		
	Behavioral Inclinations	Exercising alone, exercising with others, going to the gym, taking the stairs, instructor-based classes, working up a sweat		

Table 1. Cont.

Category	Composite Group	Items	Message Category	Message Example
Sedentary Activities	Sedentary	Watching TV/Streamed channels, scrolling through phone/social media, playing video games, using computer, reading	Physical Activity	Try creating a habit of setting a timer to get up and move. Small movements like squats or doing a fun activity help to increase physical activity. (Autonomous Motivating)
Foods	Vegetables	Broccoli, carrots, greens, tomatoes, sweet potato, mushroom	Vegetables	Vegetables are a great source of fiber. Try using the salad bar to add vegetables to meals to eat at least 2 cups a day. (Autonomous Motivating)
	Fruit	Melon, strawberries, blueberries, pineapple	Fruit	Choose Fruit! Fruits are packed with vitamins and minerals that make your skin glow. Eat at least 2 cups or piece of fruit a day. (Directive Motivating)
	Whole Grains	Whole wheat bread, oatmeal, granola, shredded wheat cereal	Whole Grains	Great job! Whole grains are a great source of dietary fiber and B vitamins, which support a healthy digestive system and energy metabolism. Try a whole grain bowl with quinoa or brown rice and your favorite add ins. (Reinforcing)
	Healthy Fat	Tuna, baked white fish, olive oil	Heart Healthy Fat	Great job on choosing heart healthy fats. Foods like nuts, avocado, salmon, & olive oil nourish your body. (Reinforcing)
	Refined Grains	White rice, bagels/rolls, spaghetti/pasta, snack crackers, pizza	Whole Grains	Whole grains are a great source of dietary fiber and B vitamins, which support a healthy digestive system and energy metabolism. Make a whole grain bowl with quinoa or brown rice and your favorite add ins. (Directive Motivating)
	High Fat Protein Foods	Hot dog, fried chicken, bacon, fast food	Lean Protein	Try to select a variety of lean protein foods to improve nutrient intake. Sources like chicken, fish, eggs, and beans, help to build a strong body. (Autonomous Motivating)
	Unhealthy Fat	Cheddar cheese, mayonnaise, full fat dressing, whole milk	Heart Healthy Fat	Healthy fats are good for your heart. Select foods like nuts, avocado, salmon, & olive oil to nourish your body. (Directive Motivating)
	Salty Foods/Snacks	Salty snacks, noodle soups, French fries	Salt	Reading a nutrition label is a great way to reduce salt intake. Continue limiting salt by choosing foods ≤ 140 mg of sodium.
	Sweets	Ice cream, cookies/cake/pastries, cake icing/frosting, cheesecake	Sweets	Feel like you have a sweet tooth? When enjoying sweets, try to make each bite satisfying by taking your time and enjoying every bite! (Autonomous Motivating)

Table 1. Cont.

Category	Composite Group	Items	Message Category	Message Example
Foods	Sugar Sweetened Beverages	Chocolate milk, soda, flavored coffee drinks	Hydration (Water)	Sugary beverages can lead to dehydration which can cloud our thinking and make us tired. Drink a glass of water every hour to stay hydrated. (Directive Motivating)
Health Behaviors	Intuitive Eating	7 Questions from Intuitive Eating Scale (Scored from Strongly Disagree to Agree) [86]	Intuitive Eating	Your body knows best! Continue to eat intuitively by listening to your body's hunger and fullness cues to stay within the green areas for most meals and snacks. (Reinforcing)
	Stress	Within the last 30 days, how would you rate the overall level of stress you have experienced? [87]	Stress	In times of high stress, try to take a few deep breaths. Deep breathing has proven to be effective in calming oneself. (Autonomous Motivating)
	Sleep	4 questions from the Pediatric Daytime Sleepiness Scale (adapted to College Students) [88]	Sleep	Sleep is important for your mental and physical health. Before bed, stretch, reflect, and shut off all screens to improve your sleep. (Directive Motivating)

2.5. Feasibility Measures

Participants rated the feasibility of the survey and the overall acceptability and usefulness of all the messages collectively, as well as provided responses to each message following the IMB model.

Prior to receiving their tailored messages, participants used the sliding hedonic scale to report their level of agreement/disagreement to the survey acceptability and usability questions [93]. Acceptability questions included: (1) I could answer the questions quickly and (2) I would recommend this survey to a friend. Usability questions included: "The survey was helpful in reflecting on my current behaviors", and "The survey questions were relevant to me as a college student". The hedonic scale was labeled with five faces with corresponding descriptors of "strongly agree", "agree", "neutral", "disagree", and "strongly disagree", with ability to slide the marker anywhere to produce a value ± 100.

Following each tailored message, participants completed four questions assessing the IMB constructs to the message and target behavior of the message: (1) interesting and specific Information learned (2 questions); (2) Motivation; and (3) Behavioral Skill (i.e., confidence) for the targeted behavior. Participants responded on the same hedonic scale with facial label (± 100) specific to the displayed tailored message/behavior and text to indicate information agreement, motivation, and behavioral skills as shown in Table 2. Due to participant responses pooling around the scale labels, they were compressed to the label value, creating a 5-point scale (Table 2), and then used to create composite scores of Information, Motivation, and Behavioral Skills constructs. First, responses to the message target behaviors, including food, physical activity, other health behaviors, were averaged separately (e.g., average information for food-based messages, average motivation for physical activity message, average behavior skill for health behavior messages, etc.) and then together to create an overall information, motivation, and behavioral skill variable. For example, the average response to information for food, physical activity, and health behavior messages was averaged to create a composite information variable. Reliability of each composite variable was tested using Cronbach's Coefficient alpha and produced sufficient reliability (<0.6–0.9's).

Table 2. Information, Motivation, behavioral skills (confidence) message response recodes.

Information Labels	Motivation Labels	Behavioral Skills Labels	Original Ranges	Compressed Scale	Interval Range (for Means)
I learned a new or interesting fact from this message. I learned [insert targeted specific fact]	How much would you like to engage in/continue [targeted behavior]?	How confident are you that you can engage/continue [targeted behavior]?			
strongly disagree	hate to	Not all confident	−61 to −100	1	1–1.80
disagree	dislike to	Somewhat confident	−21 to −60	2	1.81–2.60
neutral	neutral	Moderately confident	−21 to 20	3	2.61–3.40
agree	like to	very confident	21 to 60	4	3.41 to 4.20
Strongly agree	Love to	completely confident	61 to 100	5	4.20 to 5.0

Following the individual display and evaluation of messages for information, motivation, and behavioral skills, participants reported the general impressions of all 5 messages using a 5-point rating from strongly agree to strongly disagree. These questions served as on overall evaluation of participants' agreement to learning new information about food and exercise, motivation to make a behavior change, and ability to accomplish behavior change after reading the messages. In addition, participants reported their agreement in relevancy of the messages to their experience as a college student.

2.6. Statistical Analysis

Data were analyzed using SPSS statistical software (Version 28, Chicago, IL, USA) with a significance criterion at $p < 0.05$. Descriptive statistics were used to analyze participant demographics and variability in IMB-based variables (knowledge scores, information, motivation, and behavioral skills measurements). Composite variables were tested for reliability using Cronbach's alpha (diet restraint, information, motivation, behavior skills). Descriptive statistics and were used to examine responses to liking/disliking of food and physical activity items, other health behavior questions, and feasibility measures. Pearson Chi-Square statistics were used to examine differences in survey and message feasibility between participants with and without body size discrepancy, high/low levels of dietary restraint, and differences in IMB constructs between the message types. Linear regression analysis was used to test the influence of body size perception and dietary restraint on participant responses to information, motivation and behavioral skills for both message types combined, reinforcing, and motivating messages. Covariates (where appropriate) included age, race/ethnicity, and self-reported history of diagnosed eating disorder.

3. Results

3.1. Participant Characteristics

Table 3 displays the characteristics of the 189 college women who completed the online tailored health messaging program. The sample was mostly young and normal weight with an average age of 20.8 ± 0.18 and reported BMI of 23.6 ± 0.37. Most women identified as White (69.3%) and not Hispanic/Latino (83.1%). There was good representation across academic year (student status). Participant body size perception fell within the normal weight body figure range [84], with 65.1% reporting little to no body size discrepancy. Average dietary restraint was 8.1 (0–19), indicating that most of the participants had moderate level of dietary restraint.

3.2. Variability in Responses

The sample had good variability in liking/disliking ratings across the food and activity groups (Figure 1). Pleasant activities and being caught in a lie (i.e., unpleasant item) were included to provide context for the liking responses. Refined grains were the most liked, while high fat protein the least liked (Figure 1). Physical activity was generally rated as "It's Okay" to "Like it". Overall, the less healthy food items (e.g., refined grains, sweets, salty foods/snacks, unhealthy fats, sugar sweetened beverages) were liked more than the healthier food items (e.g., physical activity, vegetables, whole grains) and sedentary activities were liked more than physical activities. Internal reliability of the individual food groups and activity groups ranged from below acceptable (alpha < 0.6, $n = 7$) to acceptable (alpha ≥ 0.6, $n = 5$).

Table 3. Characteristics of 189 Young Adult Women.

Category		%
Age	17–20	52.4
	21–24	40.2
	25+	7.4
BMI Categories *	Underweight	6.3
	Normal Weight	62.4
	Overweight	17.5
	Obese Class I	4.8
	Obese Class II	3.7
	Obese Class III	0.5
Race	Asian	15.3
	Black/African American	6.3
	White	69.3
	Other	9
Ethnicity	Hispanic/Latino	16.9
	Not Hispanic/Latino	83.1
Student Status	First-year student	19.0
	Sophomore	17.5
	Junior	21.2
	Senior	27.5
	Graduate Student	13.2
	Other	1.6
Body Size Perception [+]	No Body Size Discrepancy	65.1
	Body Size Discrepancy	34.9

* Calculated using self-reported height and weight. BMI Categories are as follows: Underweight ≤ 18.5; Normal Weight = 18.5–24.9; Overweight = 25.0–29.9; Obese Class I = 30.0–34.9; Obese Class II = 35.0–39.9; Obese Class III = >40; [+] Participants selected which labeled figure matched their current and ideal body size from 1 (smallest) to 9 (largest); Body Size Perception (BSP) was defined by current-ideal body image. Body Size Discrepancy present if BSP > 1 or < −1.

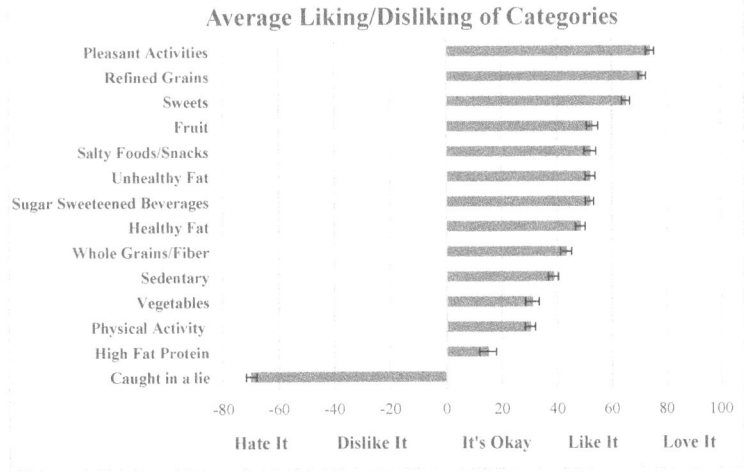

Figure 1. Average reported liking/disliking of foods and activities ranked most to least in young adult college women ($n = 189$).

Intuitive eating responses were variable within the sample, with an average score of 22.5 ± 0.3 (range 11–34), suggesting a moderate amount of intuitive eating behaviors within this sample of young adult women. Additionally, this sample experienced moderate to high stress (91.5%) and inadequate sleep, with an average scores of 11.8 ± 0.19 (range 6–18).

Knowledge Scores: Figure 2 displays the variability in knowledge scores, showing a negative skewness impacted by 3 outliers (low knowledge scores). Examination of the quartiles revealed that many participant's knowledge scores ranged between 10–13 (25th–75th quartile), suggesting an overall low variability in the sample.

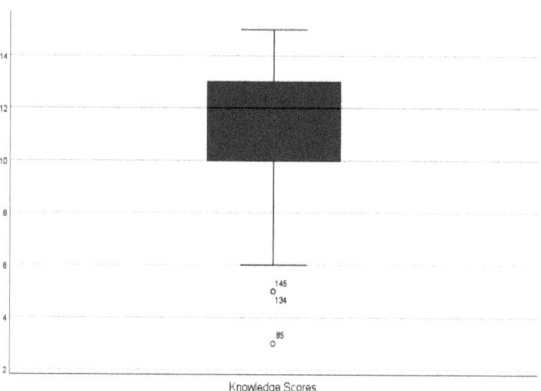

Figure 2. Box Plot of knowledge scores.

3.3. Survey Evaluation (Acceptability and Usefulness)

The study sample of college women found the online survey acceptable and useful. Nearly all (92%) reported at least agree that they could answer questions quickly and found survey questions to be relevant to them as a college student. Slightly fewer women (82.6%) at least agreed the survey was helpful in reflecting on current behaviors and 80% with recommending the survey to a friend. No significant differences were found in survey acceptability and usefulness among women with/without body size discrepancy and high/low levels of dietary restraint.

3.4. Responses to Information, Motivation, and Behavioral Skills

Descriptive statistics are displayed for responses to information, motivation, and behavioral skills (IMB constructs) for all messages (Table 4). Each construct ranged from acceptable to very good internal reliability and good range. With both message types combined, average response to information measures (both interesting and specific) categorized as "agree" to learning interesting information and specific information from messages. Average response to motivation measures categorized as "love to" continue or try behaviors suggested in messages. Average response to measures categorized as "very confident" in continuing or trying behaviors suggested in message. Similar ratings were seen in reinforcing or motivating messages.

Table 4. Descriptive Statistics of IMB Construct Responses for All Messages [†].

Construct	Min	Max	Mean	St Dev	St Error	Cronbach's Alpha
Interesting Information	1	5	3.46	0.98	0.071	0.82
Specific Information	1	5	3.87	0.89	0.064	0.87
Motivation	2	5	4.47	0.57	0.041	0.71
Behavioral Skills	1.33	5	3.99	0.82	0.06	0.66

[†] Mean values between 2.61–3.40 = "neutral", "moderately confident"; 3.41–4.20 = "agree", "like to", "very confident"; 4.20–5.0 = "strongly agree", "love to", "completely confident".

As shown in Table 5, there was variability in response to the messages for each IMB construct (information, motivation, behavioral skills). Frequency in responses to interesting information and specific information learned were similar between reinforcing and motivating types of messages, with 60–74% responses in agreement to learning interesting or specific information. For motivation, there was an overall significant difference between responses to reinforcing and motivational messages. Reinforcing messages had higher (87%) agreement/strongly agree (willingness) than motivational messages (66%). A slightly higher percentage (13%) of responses were neutral in motivational compared to reinforcing messages ($x^2(2, N = 189) = 23.51, p < 0.001$). For behavioral skills, there was a significant difference between responses to reinforcing and motivational messages ($x^2(2, N = 189) = 3.91, p < 0.05$). Very few (<4%) participants reported lack of confidence to try or continue the behavior, with 90% reporting at least confident. Higher percentage was seen in reports of high confidence to reinforcing (68%) compared to motivational messages (53%).

Table 5. Number of participants ($n = 189$) who fell into each response category for message types that were reinforcing or motivation according to information, motivation, and behavioral skills.

Interesting Information	Strongly Disagree	Disagree	Neutral	Agree	Strongly Agree
Reinforcing	14	30	29	76	40
Motivational	15	30	34	80	30
Specific Information					
Reinforcing	11	13	21	87	57
Motivational	6	17	27	89	50
Motivation [†]	Hate to	Dislike to	Neutral	Like to	Love to
Reinforcing	3	6	15	61	104
Motivational	9	17	39	64	60
Behavioral Skills [†]	Not at all confident	Somewhat confident	Moderately confident	Very confident	Completely confident
Reinforcing	1	5	5	49	129
Motivational	0	6	17	66	100

[†] Sum of the highlighted categories significantly different than unhighlighted categories within a message type by chi square testing.

3.5. Message Evaluation

This sample of young adult women rated the overall messages as generally acceptable and relevant to them as college students, with 60% reporting "agree" or higher to learning new information and 80% "agree" or higher to message relevancy. Slightly less than half of the sample of young adult women reported agree or higher to being motivated to and confident in their abilities to accomplish the behaviors in the messages, 48.7% and 47.1%, respectively. There were no significant differences in overall collective message evaluation among participants with/without body discrepancy or with high/low level of dietary restraint.

3.6. Influence of Body Discrepancy and Dietary Restraint on IMB Construct Responses

Body discrepancy did not have a significant relationship with the knowledge scores acroos the sample. However, dietary restraint was a significant predictor of knowledge scores ($F(1, 187) = 4.144, p < 0.05$), where a slight increase in dietary restraint was associated with increases in knowledge scores. Higher dietary restraint scores correlated significantly but weakly with knowledge scores (Pearson $r = 0.147, p < 0.05$). Visual analysis of the relationship showed a group of women who reported a higher diet restraint and higher knowledge scores.

Neither body size discrepancy nor dietary restraint showed significant relationships with the information measurements (i.e., interesting/specific information learned) for both types of messages combined. However, dietary restraint trended on significance to predict specific information learned ($F(1, 187) = 2.550$, $p = 0.07$). Further examination of reinforcing and motivating messages separately also did not result in significant associations with information, yet motivating messages trended on significance with dietary restraint positively predicting motivation measures ($F(1, 174) = 2.512$, $p = 0.081$).

Body size discrepancy ($F(1, 187) = 4.921$, $p < 0.05$) and dietary restraint ($F(1, 187) = 3.93$, $p < 0.05$) were significant predictors of motivation responses across reinforcing and motivating messages. A slight increase in either body size perception or dietary restraint predicted an increase in motivation. However, these factors only accounted for 2.1 to 2.6% of variability in the responses. When examining reinforcing and motivating messages separately, the relationship between body size discrepancy and motivation only was seen for reinforcing messages $F(1, 154) = 6.767$, $p < 0.05$, and accounted for 4.2% of variability (adjusted $R^2 = 3.6\%$). There was no significant relationship seen between body size perception and motivating messages. In motivating messages, dietary restraint trended on significance to positively predict motivation ($F(1, 174) = 3.96$, $p = 0.067$). There was no significant relationship seen between dietary restraint and reinforcing messages.

In both message types combined, body size discrepancy was a significant predictor of behavioral skills responses ($F(1, 187) = 4.283$, $p < 0.05$), accounting for 2.2% of variability (adjusted $R^2 = 1.7$). No relationship was seen between dietary restraint and behavioral skills for both message types combined. Neither body size perception nor dietary restraint significantly predicted behavioral skills responses in motivating messages. In reinforcing messages, body size discrepancy was a significant predictor for behavioral skills ($F(1, 154) = 6.730$, $p < 0.01$), and accounted for 6.1% of variability in responses (adjusted $R^2 = 5.4\%$). No significant relationship was seen between dietary restraint and behavioral skills in reinforcing messages.

Overall, these results suggest that body size discrepancy and dietary restraint have a small influence on some response measures (mainly motivation and behavioral skills). Accordingly, it can be inferred that the survey and response measures are able to capture variability in responses, partially supporting the hypothesis.

4. Discussion

Findings from the present study, conducted during the COVID-19 pandemic, demonstrated the feasibility of an online tailored messaging program (survey and tailored messages) aligned with behavior change theory in 189 young adult college women. The survey and tailored messages were deemed acceptable and useful, evidenced by the women reporting high agreement to learning new information, being motivated, and confident in their abilities to accomplish behaviors targeted in messages. Variability was displayed in the baseline knowledge scores of participants, information learned, motivation, and confidence responses to both motivating and reinforcing messages. Body size discrepancy and level of dietary restraint had only small effects on the participants' level of knowledge, motivation, and confidence. Overall, this program demonstrated applicability for use in communicating tailored health recommendations for general health promotion efforts for college women, especially during a stressful period that was found to impact many health behaviors [9–11].

Despite our comprehensive marketing strategy for diverse recruitment, the sample predominantly identified as White, with an average age of 20 years. Height and weight were self-reported to calculate an average BMI of 23.6 kg/m^2, which is similar to a UConn sample of young adult college women recruited prior to the pandemic [46]. Most of the women did not have a large discrepancy in their body size perception, contrary to the expected higher body size discrepancies reported in the literature [73,74]. The sample displayed a moderate level of dietary restraint, which is similar to a pre-pandemic sample but with a different dietary restraint measure [46]. Thus, the results from the present study may only be generalizable to college women who do not have high risk of excessive adiposity or disordered eating and should be considered as primary or secondary prevention efforts to promote healthier physical activity, diet quality, and other behaviors such as stress and sleep.

The acceptability and usefulness of the survey with tailored messages were equivalent to previous online tailored messaging programs in children alone in a school setting [32] and with their parents/caregivers in a clinical setting [31]. Liking of food items resembled dietary intakes observed in college adults, with higher liking of unhealthier food items suggesting higher intake of nutrient dense foods and risk of not meeting dietary guidelines [94–97]. Physical Activity was generally not liked with scores averaging between "It's okay" and "like it", suggesting that available activities or environment for these activities may be insufficient to be liked enough to compel physical activity behavior in college women [1,8–11]. Responses to intuitive eating, stress, and sleep resemble what is expected in college students [98–101].

The baseline knowledge scores in this sample of college women suggested a range in misinformation and ability of questions to capture variability in response. However, most women (75th quartile) had scores > 10, suggesting higher health behavior knowledge compared to previous literature reports [5,102–104]. Participants with low knowledge scores were considered outliers, and if removed would decrease the range, thus limiting the variability seen. It is possible that participants who elected to take the survey were health seeking with good health behavior knowledge, indicating that questions may have been too easy. However, evidence suggests that though participants may have knowledge and understanding of the importance of healthy behaviors; it does not always translate into behavioral skill and action [6,102,105–107], further supporting need for tailored health interventions.

The variability in responses to the information measures (i.e., interesting and specific) are consistent with past study findings assessing health behavior knowledge. The high agreement to learning information seen in women who received reinforcing messages suggests that, although one may be practicing a behavior, information can be improved [5,6,102,105] and motivate them to continue the behavior, as theorized in the Information Motivation Behavior Skills Theory [59]. The observed agreement to interesting and specific information learned to the motivating messages support the underlying structure of this theory. Information has an influencing relationship on motivation and behavior [59], thus can be inferred that if an individual received a motivating message due to low engagement in targeted behavior, lack of information could be a contributing factor. Although not significant, specific information had slightly higher response agreement than interesting information, suggesting acquisition of the intended information of the message [72]. Based on these results, asking if specific information was learned was the best method to measure the information construct.

Previous literature suggests challenges to assessing the information construct of the Information Motivation Behavioral Skills model. Traditional and common measures have included knowledge questions to specific behaviors [61,64,65,69] or a single general information measure [62]. The present study employed both specific and general information measures. More novel methods of the information construct include cognitive function [58] or qualitative evaluation [66,71]. Alternate measures, such as "food literacy" may increase precision as they measure proficiency in nutrition knowledge, and employing the use of functional knowledge tests to assess behavioral skills [108]. Measuring health promotion literacy, including food literacy, has demonstrated associations with healthy eating habits [109].

The higher frequency of neutral ratings in the motivating type messages, indicative of participant willingness (i.e., motivation) to try the targeted behavior, suggests the need for intervention to move people along the stages of change [110]. Higher willingness (i.e., motivation) ratings in response to the reinforcing messages support that participants were likely practicing the healthy behaviors and were eager to continue them. Within the IMB Model, motivation influences both behavior and behavior skills [59]. Reinforcing feedback can encourage motivation and continued liking of and engagement in healthy behaviors [111,112]. Willingness to try a healthier behavior in response to a motivating message can be the focus of an intervention beyond the tailored message program, including goal setting and follow-up to support achievement of the goal.

The present study observed a higher percentage of neutral confidence ratings for motivational messages than reinforcing. The high confidence observed for reinforcing messages may be indicative that the participant has the confidence or self-efficacy to continue the healthy behavior [111–115]. Conversely, if an individual was not engaging in a behavior, self-efficacy or low confidence could be likely a barrier [113–116]. Other behavioral techniques may be necessary to help increase confidence [110,116] through goal setting and addressing barriers to behavior change.

Though dietary restraint and body size discrepancy had limited influence on knowledge scores, motivation, and behavioral skills in the present study, our findings are consistent with previous literature reports. For example, higher dietary restraint, or cognitive control of eating, appears to associate with a greater level of nutrition knowledge [117–119], consistent with the present study. Body size perception has been found to influence motivation for eating and physical activity behaviors [21,73–81], aligned with the significant associations seen in our sample between higher body size discrepancy and increased motivation to try or continue healthier behaviors. Our study finding of higher body size discrepancy in association with increased confidence in behavior skills adds to the mixed findings of body size effects on self-efficacy in the literature. Some studies report higher body sizes are associated with less engagement in healthy behaviors [120,121] due to low self-efficacy related to body size, experienced weight stigma/bias, discouragement, or fear of failure [19,79–81]. Consequently, high discrepancies can lead to maladaptive behaviors, or compensatory behaviors in young women where over exercise or undereating becomes common [17–21,78]. However, in our sample higher body size discrepancy was significantly associated with increased confidence only in responses to reinforcing messages, further supporting the feedback relationships of motivation, skill, and successful engagement discussed earlier [111–115]. Nevertheless, the significant relationships observed between dietary restraint and body discrepancy with the IMB constructs only accounted for a small percentage of variability in responses. These findings support the feasibility of our survey with tailored messages program for college women who report low risk of excessive adiposity or disordered eating to encourage health promoting physical activity and diet quality.

The study does present several limitations. Due to this being a feasibility study of a smaller sample size, it was not powered to make inferences from the statistical analyses. Although, we implemented a comprehensive marketing plan, recruitment methods were solely virtual due to the University COVID-19 precautions and may have limited our ability to obtain a diverse sample as evidenced by the limited racial/ethnic and body size diversity seen. In person methods may assist in developing trustworthy relationships that can enhance communication and recruitment of less represented populations [122–124]. Although sample characteristics were reflective of many University demographics [16], lack of adequate representations of racial/ethnic minority populations cautions generalizability of findings. Results should only be applied for consideration in health promotion programs targeted for a low-risk groups. Future methods in stakeholder development/communication, recruitment, tailoring of information, and inclusion of multilevel interventions may be necessary to improve program delivery [123–125]. The survey relied on self-reported data, which always presents risk of bias. Nonetheless, utilizing liking as a proxy of behavior has been demonstrated to limit bias in response [43–46]. Another limitation was the degree of randomization for the message delivery. While messages were initially randomized, the algorithms were set for each participant to receive one general message, one physical activity message, 2 food-based messages and one other health behavior message. This is a potential limitation as a participant could have had a higher need to address another behavior over the behavioral message they received. For example, the participant may have had a higher need to address multiple food behaviors over a physical activity behavior. Lastly, although responses to information, motivation, and behavioral skills were combined for each message to equate to 4 responses for each measure for 1 participant, only 1 question was used to measure the constructs. This could limit comparability to other studies that use various validated scales to measure the constructs.

Despite the limitations, there are several strengths to the study. Only using 1 question to measure each construct can strengthen results as the questions were specific to the intended information/behavior versus generalized in many previous studies. Secondly, using liking to measure and trigger the tailored behavior strengthened methods and study results. Differences seen in responses to motivational and behavioral skill measures in the two types of tailored messages (reinforcing, motivational) support the use in liking as a proxy of behavior. Another strength is the ease and accessibility of the online delivery of the survey and messages. The online delivery allowed participants to complete the survey on their own time and at their own pace with relatively low time commitment. This was especially important during the online nature of university classes and programs during COVID-19 and assisted greatly with the distribution of the program during this time. Online delivery also allows for further reach to students in different academic programs. The online program allowed for immediate delivery of information to the participants and researchers. In addition, the online nature allowed for rapid adaptation of the survey and tailored health messages. Although the length of the online program averaged 25 min, it provided participants with information consistent with a nutrition professional as tailored recommendations were provided. This length is shorter than the typical 1 h duration of initial appointments and 30 min follow up appointments with nutrition and physical activity professionals. This demonstrates the future applicability of this program in a counseling setting. The program can be adapted for use as a pre-appointment tool, in between appointments for support, or even in place of appointments for patients who may only need general healthy eating and behavior recommendations. Additionally, the program can be adapted for used as a wide scale campus effort to survey and improve the general health behaviors of student populations. The focus of tailoring in this program can help to increase relevancy to health information, decreasing previous barriers found to traditional health promotion efforts in young adults [25].

5. Conclusions

The results supported the feasibility of the online survey and tailored message program to promote healthier diet and physical activity for college women. The program aligned with a theoretical framework focused on the information, motivation, and confidence needed to follow healthier behaviors. College women found the survey and messages acceptable and useful. There was variability in response to each message for information learned as well as motivation and confidence to follow healthier behaviors, with minimal effects of the participant's body size perception and level of dietary restraint on these responses. The information gained from the responses to the survey and tailored messages can provide direction for further individualized interventions as well as broader campus efforts to promote healthier diets and physical activity.

Author Contributions: Conceptualization, P.A.H., H.F. and V.B.D.; methodology, P.A.H., H.F. and V.B.D.; formal analysis, P.A.H.; investigation, P.A.H. and H.F.; resources, V.B.D., data curation, P.A.H. and H.F.; writing—original draft preparation, P.A.H. and H.F.; writing—review and editing, P.A.H. and V.B.D.; visualization, P.A.H.; supervision. V.B.D.; project administration, V.B.D.; funding acquisition, V.B.D. All authors have read and agreed to the published version of the manuscript.

Funding: This research was funded by the United States Department of Agriculture National Institute of Food and Agriculture, Hatch project 1001056.

Institutional Review Board Statement: The study was conducted in accordance with the Declaration of Helsinki and approved by the Institutional Review Board (or Ethics Committee) of The University of Connecticut (protocol code Exemption #X17-085 and 17 February 2021.

Informed Consent Statement: This study is exempt under 45 CFR 46.101 (b) (2). An approved, validated information sheet was used to consent each subject; participants consented online by agreeing to participate.

Data Availability Statement: The data presented in this study are available on request from the corresponding author.

Conflicts of Interest: The authors declare no conflict of interest. The funders had no role in the design of the study; in the collection, analyses, or interpretation of data; in the writing of the manuscript; or in the decision to publish the results.

References

1. Corder, K.; Winpenny, E.; Love, R.; Brown, H.E.; White, M.; Sluijs, E.V. Change in physical activity from adolescence to early adulthood: A systematic review and meta-analysis of longitudinal cohort studies. *Br. J. Sports Med.* **2019**, *53*, 496. [CrossRef] [PubMed]
2. Munt, A.E.; Partridge, S.R.; Allman-Farinelli, M. The barriers and enablers of healthy eating among young adults: A missing piece of the obesity puzzle: A scoping review. *Obes. Rev.* **2017**, *18*, 1–17. [CrossRef]
3. Kapinos, K.A.; Yakusheva, O.; Eisenberg, D. Obesogenic environmental influences on young adults: Evidence from college dormitory assignments. *Econ. Hum. Biol.* **2014**, *12*, 98–109. [CrossRef] [PubMed]
4. Caso, D.; Miriam, C.; Rosa, F.; Mark, C. Unhealthy eating and academic stress: The moderating effect of eating style and BMI. *Health Psychol. Open.* **2020**, *7*, 2055102920975274. [CrossRef] [PubMed]
5. Werner, E.; Betz, H.H. Knowledge of physical activity and nutrition recommendations in college students. *J. Am. Coll. Health* **2022**, *70*, 340–346. [CrossRef] [PubMed]
6. Guseman, E.H.; Whipps, J.; Howe, C.A.; Beverly, E.A. First-Year Osteopathic Medical Students' Knowledge of and Attitudes Toward Physical Activity. *J. Am. Osteopath. Assoc.* **2018**, *118*, 389–395. [CrossRef] [PubMed]
7. Arigo, D.; Butryn, M.L.; Raggio, G.A.; Stice, E.; Lowe, M.R. Predicting Change in Physical Activity: A Longitudinal Investigation among Weight-Concerned College Women. *Ann. Behav. Med.* **2016**, *50*, 629–641. [CrossRef] [PubMed]
8. Sun, H.; Vamos, C.A.; Flory, S.S.B.; DeBate, R.; Thompson, E.L.; Bleck, J. Correlates of long-term physical activity adherence in women. *J. Sport Health Sci.* **2017**, *6*, 434–442. [CrossRef] [PubMed]
9. Romero-Blanco, C.; Rodríguez-Almagro, J.; Onieva-Zafra, M.D.; Parra-Fernández, M.L.; Prado-Laguna, M.D.C.; Hernández-Martínez, A. Physical Activity and Sedentary Lifestyle in University Students: Changes during Confinement Due to the COVID-19 Pandemic. *Int. J. Environ. Res. Public Health* **2020**, *17*, 6567. [CrossRef] [PubMed]
10. Nienhuis, C.P.; Lesser, I.A. The Impact of COVID-19 on Women's Physical Activity Behavior and Mental Well-Being. *Int. J. Environ. Res. Public Health* **2020**, *17*, 9036. [CrossRef] [PubMed]
11. Wilson, O.W.A.; Holland, K.E.; Elliott, L.D.; Duffey, M.; Bopp, M. The Impact of the COVID-19 Pandemic on US College Students' Physical Activity and Mental Health. *J. Phys. Act. Health* **2021**, *18*, 272–278. [CrossRef] [PubMed]
12. Sidebottom, C.; Ullevig, S.; Cheever, K.; Zhang, T. Effects of COVID-19 pandemic and quarantine period on physical activity and dietary habits of college-aged students. *Sports Med. Health Sci.* **2021**, *3*, 228–235. [CrossRef] [PubMed]
13. Bertrand, L.; Shaw, K.A.; Ko, J.; Deprez, D.; Chilibeck, P.D.; Zello, G.A. The impact of the coronavirus disease 2019 (COVID-19) pandemic on university students' dietary intake, physical activity, and sedentary behaviour. *Appl. Physiol. Nutr. Metab.* **2021**, *46*, 265–272. [CrossRef] [PubMed]
14. American College Health Association, *American College Health Association-National College Health Assessment III: Reference Group Executive Summary Fall 2019*; American College Health Association: Silver Spring, MD, USA, 2020. Available online: https://www.acha.org/documents/ncha/NCHA-III_Fall_2019_Reference_Group_Executive_Summary_updated.pdf (accessed on 5 September 2022).
15. American College Health Association, *American College Health Association-National College Health Assessment III: Reference Group Executive Summary Spring 2020*; American College Health Association: Silver Spring, MD, USA, 2020. Available online: https://www.acha.org/documents/ncha/NCHA-III_SPRING-2020_REFERENCE_GROUP_EXECUTIVE_SUMMARY-updated.pdf (accessed on 5 September 2022).
16. American College Health Association, *American College Health Association-National College Health Assessment III: Reference Group Executive Summary Spring 2021*; American College Health Association: Silver Spring, MD, USA, 2021. Available online: https://www.acha.org/documents/ncha/NCHA-III_SPRING-2021_REFERENCE_GROUP_EXECUTIVE_SUMMARY_updated.pdf (accessed on 5 September 2022).
17. Lepage, M.L.; Crowther, J.H.; Harrington, E.F.; Engler, P. Psychological correlates of fasting and vigorous exercise as compensatory strategies in undergraduate women. *Eat. Behav.* **2008**, *9*, 423–429. [CrossRef] [PubMed]
18. Petersen, J.M.; Prichard, I.; Kemps, E.; Tiggemann, M. The effect of snack consumption on physical activity: A test of the Compensatory Health Beliefs Model. *Appetite* **2019**, *141*, 104342. [CrossRef] [PubMed]
19. Radwan, H.; Hasan, H.A.; Ismat, H.; Hakim, H.; Khalid, H.; Al-Fityani, L.; Mohammed, R.; Ayman, A. Body Mass Index Perception, Body Image Dissatisfaction and Their Relations with Weight-Related Behaviors among University Students. *Int. J. Environ. Res. Public Health* **2019**, *16*, 1541. [CrossRef] [PubMed]

20. Lawless, M.; Shriver, L.H.; Wideman, L.; Dollar, J.M.; Calkins, S.D.; Keane, S.P.; Shanahan, L. Associations between eating behaviors, diet quality and body mass index among adolescents. *Eat. Behav.* **2020**, *36*, 101339. [CrossRef] [PubMed]
21. Schaumberg, K.; Anderson, D.A.; Anderson, L.M.; Reilly, E.E.; Gorrell, S. Dietary restraint: What's the harm? A review of the relationship between dietary restraint, weight trajectory and the development of eating pathology. *Clin. Obes.* **2016**, *6*, 89–100. [CrossRef] [PubMed]
22. Finlayson, G.; Cecil, J.; Higgs, S.; Hill, A.; Hetherington, M. Susceptibility to weight gain. Eating behaviour traits and physical activity as predictors of weight gain during the first year of university. *Appetite* **2012**, *58*, 1091–1098. [CrossRef] [PubMed]
23. Brace, A.M.; De Andrade, F.C.; Finkelstein, B. Assessing the effectiveness of nutrition interventions implemented among US college students to promote healthy behaviors: A systematic review. *Nutr. Health* **2018**, *24*, 171–181. [CrossRef] [PubMed]
24. Maselli, M.; Ward, P.B.; Gobbi, E.; Carraro, A. Promoting Physical Activity among University Students: A Systematic Review of Controlled Trials. *Am. J. Health Promot.* **2018**, *32*, 1602–1612. [CrossRef] [PubMed]
25. Berry, E.; Aucott, L.; Poobalan, A. Are young adults appreciating the health promotion messages on diet and exercise? *Z. Gesundh. Wiss.* **2018**, *26*, 687–696. [CrossRef] [PubMed]
26. NIH Nutrition Research Task Force. 2020–2030 Strategic Plan for NIH Nutrition Research. 2020. Available online: https://dpcpsi.nih.gov/onr/strategic-plan (accessed on 5 September 2022).
27. Brug, J.; Campbell, M.; van Assema, P. The application and impact of computer-generated personalized nutrition education: A review of the literature. *Patient Educ. Couns.* **1999**, *36*, 145–156. [CrossRef]
28. Hawkins, R.P.; Kreuter, M.; Resnicow, K.; Fishbein, M.; Dijkstra, A. Understanding tailoring in communicating about health. *Health Educ. Res.* **2008**, *23*, 454–466. [CrossRef]
29. Noar, S.M.; Benac, C.N.; Harris, M.S. Does tailoring matter? Meta-analytic review of tailored print health behavior change interventions. *Psychol. Bull.* **2007**, *133*, 673–693. [CrossRef] [PubMed]
30. Lustria, M.L.; Noar, S.M.; Cortese, J.; Van Stee, S.K.; Glueckauf, R.L.; Lee, J. A meta-analysis of web-delivered tailored health behavior change interventions. *J. Health Commun.* **2013**, *18*, 1039–1069. [CrossRef] [PubMed]
31. Chau, S.; Oldman, S.; Smith, S.R.; Lin, C.A.; Ali, S.; Duffy, V.B. Online Behavioral Screener with Tailored Obesity Prevention Messages: Application to a Pediatric Clinical Setting. *Nutrients* **2021**, *13*, 223. [CrossRef] [PubMed]
32. Hildrey, R.; Karner, H.; Serrao, J.; Lin, C.A.; Shanley, E.; Duffy, V.B. Pediatric Adapted Liking Survey (PALS) with Tailored Nutrition Education Messages: Application to a Middle School Setting. *Foods* **2021**, *10*, 579. [CrossRef] [PubMed]
33. Mouratidis, K.; Papagiannakis, A. COVID-19, internet, and mobility: The rise of telework, telehealth, e-learning, and e-shopping. *Sustain. Cities Soc.* **2021**, *74*, 103182. [CrossRef] [PubMed]
34. Alzahrani, A.I.; Al-Samarraie, H.; Eldenfria, A.; Dodoo, J.E.; Alalwan, N. Users' intention to continue using mHealth services: A DEMATEL approach during the COVID-19 pandemic. *Technol. Soc.* **2022**, *68*, 101862. [CrossRef] [PubMed]
35. Goldstein, S.P.; Forman, E.M.; Butryn, M.L.; Herbert, J.D. Differential Programming Needs of College Students Preferring Web-Based Versus In-Person Physical Activity Programs. *Health Commun.* **2018**, *33*, 1509–1515. [CrossRef] [PubMed]
36. Pope, Z.C.; Gao, Z. Feasibility of smartphone application- and social media-based intervention on college students' health outcomes: A pilot randomized trial. *J. Am. Coll. Health* **2022**, *70*, 89–98. [CrossRef] [PubMed]
37. Broekhuizen, K.; Kroeze, W.; van Poppel, M.N.; Oenema, A.; Brug, J. A systematic review of randomized controlled trials on the effectiveness of computer-tailored physical activity and dietary behavior promotion programs: An update. *Ann. Behav. Med.* **2012**, *44*, 259–286. [CrossRef] [PubMed]
38. Napolitano, M.A.; Hayes, S.; Bennett, G.G.; Ives, A.K.; Foster, G.D. Using Facebook and text messaging to deliver a weight loss program to college students. *Obesity* **2013**, *21*, 25–31. [CrossRef]
39. Solenhill, M.; Grotta, A.; Pasquali, E.; Bakkman, L.; Bellocco, R.; Trolle Lagerros, Y. The Effect of Tailored Web-Based Feedback and Optional Telephone Coaching on Health Improvements: A Randomized Intervention among Employees in the Transport Service Industry. *J. Med. Internet Res.* **2016**, *18*, e158. [CrossRef]
40. Smeets, T.; Brug, J.; de Vries, H. Effects of tailoring health messages on physical activity. *Health Educ. Res.* **2008**, *23*, 402–413. [CrossRef]
41. Celis-Morales, C.; Livingstone, K.M.; Marsaux, C.F.; Macready, A.L.; Fallaize, R.; O'Donovan, C.B.; Woolhead, C.; Forster, H.; Walsh, M.C.; Navas-Carretero, S.; et al. Effect of personalized nutrition on health-related behaviour change: Evidence from the Food4Me European randomized controlled trial. *Int. J. Epidemiol.* **2017**, *46*, 578–588. [CrossRef]
42. Bel-Serrat, S.; Julián-Almárcegui, C.; González-Gross, M.; Mouratidou, T.; Börnhorst, C.; Grammatikaki, E.; Kersting, M.; Cuenca-García, M.; Gottrand, F.; Molnár, D.; et al. Correlates of dietary energy misreporting among European adolescents: The Healthy Lifestyle in Europe by Nutrition in Adolescence (HELENA) study. *Br. J. Nutr.* **2016**, *115*, 1439–1452. [CrossRef]
43. Pallister, T.; Sharafi, M.; Lachance, G.; Pirastu, N.; Mohney, R.P.; MacGregor, A.; Feskens, E.J.; Duffy, V.; Spector, T.D.; Menni, C. Food Preference Patterns in a UK Twin Cohort. *Twin Res. Hum. Genet.* **2015**, *18*, 793–805. [CrossRef]
44. Sharafi, M.; Faghri, P.; Huedo-Medina, T.B.; Duffy, V.B. A Simple Liking Survey Captures Behaviors Associated with Weight Loss in a Worksite Program among Women at Risk of Type 2 Diabetes. *Nutrients* **2021**, *13*, 1338. [CrossRef]
45. Sharafi, M.; Rawal, S.; Fernandez, M.L.; Huedo-Medina, T.B.; Duffy, V.B. Taste phenotype associates with cardiovascular disease risk factors via diet quality in multivariate modeling. *Physiol. Behav.* **2018**, *194*, 103–112. [CrossRef] [PubMed]

46. Hubert, P.A.; Mahoney, M.; Huedo-Medina, T.B.; Leahey, T.M.; Duffy, V.B. Can Assessing Physical Activity Liking Identify Opportunities to Promote Physical Activity Engagement and Healthy Dietary Behaviors? *Nutrients* **2021**, *13*, 3366. [CrossRef] [PubMed]
47. Duffy, V.B.; Hayes, J.E.; Sullivan, B.S.; Faghri, P. Surveying food and beverage liking: A tool for epidemiological studies to connect chemosensation with health outcomes. *Ann. N. Y. Acad. Sci.* **2009**, *1170*, 558–568. [CrossRef] [PubMed]
48. Thompson, C.E.; Wankel, L.M. The effects of perceived activity choice upon frequency of exercise behavior. *J. Appl. Soc. Psychol.* **1980**, *10*, 436–443. [CrossRef]
49. Aboagye, E. Valuing Individuals' Preferences and Health Choices of Physical Exercise. *Pain Ther.* **2017**, *6*, 85–91. [CrossRef]
50. Doyle, C.B.; Khan, A.; Burton, N.W. Recreational physical activity context and type preferences among male and female Emirati university students. *Int. Health* **2019**, *11*, 507–512. [CrossRef]
51. Ma, J.K.; Floegel, T.A.; Li, L.C.; Leese, J.; De Vera, M.A.; Beauchamp, M.R.; Taunton, J.; Liu-Ambrose, T.; Allen, K.D. Tailored physical activity behavior change interventions: Challenges and opportunities. *Transl. Behav. Med.* **2021**, *11*, 2174–2181. [CrossRef]
52. Magarey, A.; Mauch, C.; Mallan, K.; Perry, R.; Elovaris, R.; Meedeniya, J.; Byrne, R.; Daniels, L. Child dietary and eating behavior outcomes up to 3.5 years after an early feeding intervention: The NOURISH RCT. *Obesity* **2016**, *24*, 1537–1545. [CrossRef]
53. de Wild, V.W.T.; de Graaf, C.; Jager, G. Use of Different Vegetable Products to Increase Preschool-Aged Children's Preference for and Intake of a Target Vegetable: A Randomized Controlled Trial. *J. Acad. Nutr. Diet* **2017**, *117*, 859–866. [CrossRef]
54. Joseph, L.S.; Gorin, A.A.; Mobley, S.L.; Mobley, A.R. Impact of a Short-Term Nutrition Education Child Care Pilot Intervention on Preschool Children's Intention To Choose Healthy Snacks and Actual Snack Choices. *Child. Obes.* **2015**, *11*, 513–520. [CrossRef]
55. Wall, D.E.; Least, C.; Gromis, J.; Lohse, B. Nutrition education intervention improves vegetable-related attitude, self-efficacy, preference, and knowledge of fourth-grade students. *J. Sch. Health* **2012**, *82*, 37–43. [CrossRef] [PubMed]
56. Ledikwe, J.H.; Ello-Martin, J.; Pelkman, C.L.; Birch, L.L.; Mannino, M.L.; Rolls, B.J. A reliable, valid questionnaire indicates that preference for dietary fat declines when following a reduced-fat diet. *Appetite* **2007**, *49*, 74–83. [CrossRef] [PubMed]
57. Ebneter, D.S.; Latner, J.D.; Nigg, C.R. Is less always more? The effects of low-fat labeling and caloric information on food intake, calorie estimates, taste preference, and health attributions. *Appetite* **2013**, *68*, 92–97. [CrossRef]
58. Kim, C.J.; Kang, H.S.; Kim, J.S.; Won, Y.Y.; Schlenk, E.A. Predicting physical activity and cardiovascular risk and quality of life in adults with osteoarthritis at risk for metabolic syndrome: A test of the information-motivation-behavioral-skills model. *Nurs. Open* **2020**, *7*, 1239–1248. [CrossRef] [PubMed]
59. Fisher, W.A.; Fisher, J.D.; Harman, J. The information-motivation-behavioral skills model: A general social psychological approach to understanding and promoting health behavior. In *Social Psychological Foundations of Health and Illness*; Blackwell Publishing Ltd.: Malden, MA, USA, 2003; pp. 82–106. [CrossRef]
60. Chang, S.J.; Choi, S.; Kim, S.-A.; Song, M. Intervention Strategies Based on Information-Motivation-Behavioral Skills Model for Health Behavior Change: A Systematic Review. *Asian Nurs. Res.* **2014**, *8*, 172–181. [CrossRef]
61. Ferrari, M.; Speight, J.; Beath, A.; Browne, J.L.; Mosely, K. The information-motivation-behavioral skills model explains physical activity levels for adults with type 2 diabetes across all weight classes. *Psychol. Health Med.* **2021**, *26*, 381–394. [CrossRef]
62. Fleary, S.A.; Joseph, P.; Chang, H. Applying the information-motivation-behavioral skills model to explain adolescents' fruits and vegetables consumption. *Appetite* **2020**, *147*, 104546. [CrossRef]
63. Goodell, L.S.; Pierce, M.B.; Amico, K.R.; Ferris, A.M. Parental information, motivation, and behavioral skills correlate with child sweetened beverage consumption. *J. Nutr. Educ. Behav.* **2012**, *44*, 240–245. [CrossRef]
64. Molaifard, A.; Mohamadian, H.; Zadeh, M.H.H. Predicting high school students' health-promoting lifestyle: A test of the information, motivation, behavioral skills model. *Int. J. Adolesc. Med. Health* **2018**, *32*, 20170194. [CrossRef]
65. Osborn, C.Y.; Rivet Amico, K.; Fisher, W.A.; Egede, L.E.; Fisher, J.D. An information-motivation-behavioral skills analysis of diet and exercise behavior in Puerto Ricans with diabetes. *J. Health Psychol.* **2010**, *15*, 1201–1213. [CrossRef]
66. Pollard, R.; Kennedy, C.E.; Hutton, H.E.; Mulamba, J.; Mbabali, I.; Anok, A.; Nakyanjo, N.; Chang, L.W.; Amico, K.R. HIV Prevention and Treatment Behavior Change and the Situated Information Motivation Behavioral Skills (sIMB) Model: A Qualitative Evaluation of a Community Health Worker Intervention in Rakai, Uganda. *AIDS Behav.* **2022**, *26*, 375–384. [CrossRef] [PubMed]
67. Puttkammer, N.; Demes, J.A.E.; Dervis, W.; Chéry, J.M.; Elusdort, J.; Haight, E.; Balan, J.G.; Simoni, J.M. The Situated Information, Motivation, and Behavioral Skills Model of HIV Antiretroviral Therapy Adherence Among Persons Living with HIV in Haiti: A Qualitative Study Incorporating Culture and Context. *J. Assoc. Nurses AIDS Care* **2022**, *33*, 448–458. [CrossRef] [PubMed]
68. Rongkavilit, C.; Naar-King, S.; Kaljee, L.M.; Panthong, A.; Koken, J.A.; Bunupuradah, T.; Parsons, J.T. Applying the information-motivation-behavioral skills model in medication adherence among Thai youth living with HIV: A qualitative study. *AIDS Patient Care STDS* **2010**, *24*, 787–794. [CrossRef] [PubMed]
69. Shrestha, R.; Altice, F.L.; Huedo-Medina, T.B.; Karki, P.; Copenhaver, M. Willingness to Use Pre-Exposure Prophylaxis (PrEP): An Empirical Test of the Information-Motivation-Behavioral Skills (IMB) Model among High-Risk Drug Users in Treatment. *AIDS Behav.* **2017**, *21*, 1299–1308. [CrossRef] [PubMed]
70. Tsamlag, L.; Wang, H.; Shen, Q.; Shi, Y.; Zhang, S.; Chang, R.; Liu, X.; Shen, T.; Cai, Y. Applying the information-motivation-behavioral model to explore the influencing factors of self-management behavior among osteoporosis patients. *BMC Public Health* **2020**, *20*, 198. [CrossRef]

71. Tuthill, E.L.; Butler, L.M.; Pellowski, J.A.; McGrath, J.M.; Cusson, R.M.; Gable, R.K.; Fisher, J.D. Exclusive breast-feeding promotion among HIV-infected women in South Africa: An Information-Motivation-Behavioural Skills model-based pilot intervention. *Public Health Nutr.* **2017**, *20*, 1481–1490. [CrossRef]
72. Fiorenti, H. Development and Feasibility of an Online Tailored Messages Program to Motivate Healthier Diet and Physical Activity Behaviors in College Students. Master's Thesis, University of Connecticut, Storrs, CT, USA, 2021.
73. Anton, S.D.; Perri, M.G.; Riley, J.R., 3rd. Discrepancy between actual and ideal body images; Impact on eating and exercise behaviors. *Eat. Behav.* **2000**, *1*, 153–160. [CrossRef]
74. Nomura, K.; Itakura, Y.; Minamizono, S.; Okayama, K.; Suzuki, Y.; Takemi, Y.; Nakanishi, A.; Eto, K.; Takahashi, H.; Kawata, Y.; et al. The Association of Body Image Self-Discrepancy with Female Gender, Calorie-Restricted Diet, and Psychological Symptoms Among Healthy Junior High School Students in Japan. *Front. Psychol.* **2021**, *12*, 576089. [CrossRef]
75. Mahat, G.; Zha, P. Body weight perception and physical activity among young adults: Analysis from the national longitudinal study of adolescent to adult health. *J. Am. Coll. Health* **2022**, *70*, 1257–1264. [CrossRef] [PubMed]
76. Xu, F.; Cohen, S.A.; Greaney, M.L.; Greene, G.W. The Association between US Adolescents' Weight Status, Weight Perception, Weight Satisfaction, and Their Physical Activity and Dietary Behaviors. *Int. J. Environ. Res. Public Health* **2018**, *15*, 1931. [CrossRef]
77. MacNeill, L.P.; Best, L.A. Perceived current and ideal body size in female undergraduates. *Eat. Behav.* **2015**, *18*, 71–75. [CrossRef] [PubMed]
78. Prioreschi, A.; Wrottesley, S.V.; Cohen, E.; Reddy, A.; Said-Mohamed, R.; Twine, R.; Tollman, S.M.; Kahn, K.; Dunger, D.B.; Norris, S.A. Examining the relationships between body image, eating attitudes, BMI, and physical activity in rural and urban South African young adult females using structural equation modeling. *PLoS ONE* **2017**, *12*, e0187508. [CrossRef]
79. Robinson, E.; Haynes, A.; Sutin, A.; Daly, M. Self-perception of overweight and obesity: A review of mental and physical health outcomes. *Obes. Sci. Pract.* **2020**, *6*, 552–561. [CrossRef] [PubMed]
80. Lucibello, K.M.; Sabiston, C.M.; O'Loughlin, E.K.; O'Loughlin, J.L. Mediating role of body-related shame and guilt in the relationship between weight perceptions and lifestyle behaviours. *Obes. Sci. Pract.* **2020**, *6*, 365–372. [CrossRef] [PubMed]
81. Mensinger, J.L.; Meadows, A. Internalized weight stigma mediates and moderates physical activity outcomes during a healthy living program for women with high body mass index. *Psychol. Sport Exerc.* **2017**, *30*, 64–72. [CrossRef]
82. Xu, R.; Blanchard, B.E.; McCaffrey, J.M.; Woolley, S.; Corso, L.M.L.; Duffy, V.B. Food Liking-Based Diet Quality Indexes (DQI) Generated by Conceptual and Machine Learning Explained Variability in Cardiometabolic Risk Factors in Young Adults. *Nutrients* **2020**, *12*, 882. [CrossRef]
83. Blanchard, B.; McCaffery, J.; Woolley, S.; Corso, L.; Duffy, V. Diet Quality Index and Health Behavior Index Generated from a Food Liking Survey Explains Variability in Cardiometabolic Factors in Young Adults (P08-027-19). *Curr. Dev. Nutr.* **2019**, *3*, nzz044.P008-027-019. [CrossRef]
84. Stunkard, A.J.; Sørensen, T.; Schulsinger, F. Use of the Danish Adoption Register for the study of obesity and thinness. *Res. Publ. Assoc. Res. Nerv. Ment. Dis.* **1983**, *60*, 115–120. [PubMed]
85. Herman, C.P.; Polivy, J. Restrained Eating. In *Obesity*; Standard, A.J., Ed.; W.B. Saunders: Philadelphia, PA, USA, 1980; pp. 208–225.
86. Tylka, T.L.; Van Diest, A.M.K. The Intuitive Eating Scale-2: Item refinement and psychometric evaluation with college women and men. *J. Couns. Psychol.* **2013**, *60*, 137–153. [CrossRef] [PubMed]
87. Cohen, S.; Kamarck, T.; Mermelstein, R. A global measure of perceived stress. *J. Health Soc. Behav.* **1983**, *24*, 385–396. [CrossRef]
88. Drake, C.; Nickel, C.; Burduvali, E.; Roth, T.; Jefferson, C.; Pietro, B. The pediatric daytime sleepiness scale (PDSS): Sleep habits and school outcomes in middle-school children. *Sleep* **2003**, *26*, 455–458. [PubMed]
89. Thompson, J.K.; Altabe, M.N. Psychometric qualities of the Figure Rating Scale. *Int. J. Eat. Disord.* **1991**, *10*, 615–619. [CrossRef]
90. Williamson, D.A.; Gleaves, D.H.; Watkins, P.C.; Schlundt, D.G. Validation of self-ideal body size discrepancy as a measure of body dissatisfaction. *J. Psychopathol. Behav. Assess.* **1993**, *15*, 57–68. [CrossRef]
91. Hernández-López, M.; Quiñones-Jiménez, L.; Blanco-Romero, A.L.; Rodríguez-Valverde, M. Testing the discrepancy between actual and ideal body image with the Implicit Relational Assessment Procedure (IRAP). *J. Eat. Disord.* **2021**, *9*, 82. [CrossRef] [PubMed]
92. Resnicow, K.; Davis, R.E.; Zhang, G.; Konkel, J.; Strecher, V.J.; Shaikh, A.R.; Tolsma, D.; Calvi, J.; Alexander, G.; Anderson, J.P.; et al. Tailoring a fruit and vegetable intervention on novel motivational constructs: Results of a randomized study. *Ann. Behav. Med.* **2008**, *35*, 159–169. [CrossRef] [PubMed]
93. Lund, A.M. Measuring Usability with the USE Questionnaire. Usability and User Experience. *Usabil. Interface* **2001**, *8*, 3–6.
94. Anding, J.D.; Suminski, R.R.; Boss, L. Dietary Intake, Body Mass Index, Exercise, and Alcohol: Are College Women Following the Dietary Guidelines for Americans? *J. Am. Coll. Health* **2001**, *49*, 167–171. [CrossRef] [PubMed]
95. González-Torres, S.; González-Silva, N.; Pérez-Reyes, Á.; Anaya-Esparza, L.M.; Sánchez-Enríquez, S.; Vargas-Becerra, P.N.; Villagrán, Z.; García-García, M.R. Food Consumption and Metabolic Risks in Young University Students. *Int. J. Environ. Res. Public Health* **2021**, *19*, 449. [CrossRef] [PubMed]
96. Beaudry, K.M.; Ludwa, I.A.; Thomas, A.M.; Ward, W.E.; Falk, B.; Josse, A.R. First-year university is associated with greater body weight, body composition and adverse dietary changes in males than females. *PLoS ONE* **2019**, *14*, e0218554. [CrossRef] [PubMed]

97. Thompson, N.R.; Asare, M.; Millan, C.; Umstattd Meyer, M.R. Theory of Planned Behavior and Perceived Role Model as Predictors of Nutrition and Physical Activity Behaviors Among College Students in Health-Related Disciplines. *J. Commun. Health* **2020**, *45*, 965–972. [CrossRef] [PubMed]
98. Belon, K.E.; Serier, K.N.; VanderJagt, H.; Smith, J.E. What Is Healthy Eating? Exploring Profiles of Intuitive Eating and Nutritionally Healthy Eating in College Women. *Am. J. Health Promot.* **2022**, *36*, 823–833. [CrossRef] [PubMed]
99. Amanvermez, Y.; Zhao, R.; Cuijpers, P.; de Wit, L.M.; Ebert, D.D.; Kessler, R.C.; Bruffaerts, R.; Karyotaki, E. Effects of self-guided stress management interventions in college students: A systematic review and meta-analysis. *Internet Interv.* **2022**, *28*, 100503. [CrossRef]
100. Dietrich, S.K.; Francis-Jimenez, C.M.; Knibbs, M.D.; Umali, I.L.; Truglio-Londrigan, M. Effectiveness of sleep education programs to improve sleep hygiene and/or sleep quality in college students: A systematic review. *JBI Database System Rev. Implement. Rep.* **2016**, *14*, 108–134. [CrossRef]
101. Musaiger, A.O.; Awadhalla, M.S.; Al-Mannai, M.; AlSawad, M.; Asokan, G.V. Dietary habits and sedentary behaviors among health science university students in Bahrain. *Int. J. Adolesc. Med. Health* **2017**, *29*, 20150038. [CrossRef] [PubMed]
102. Matthews, J.I.; Doerr, L.; Dworatzek, P.D.N. University Students Intend to Eat Better but Lack Coping Self-Efficacy and Knowledge of Dietary Recommendations. *J. Nutr. Educ. Behav.* **2016**, *48*, 12–19.e11. [CrossRef] [PubMed]
103. Dolatkhah, N.; Aghamohammadi, D.; Farshbaf-Khalili, A.; Hajifaraji, M.; Hashemian, M.; Esmaeili, S. Nutrition knowledge and attitude in medical students of Tabriz University of Medical Sciences in 2017–2018. *BMC Res. Notes* **2019**, *12*, 757. [CrossRef]
104. Yahia, N.; Wang, D.; Rapley, M.; Dey, R. Assessment of weight status, dietary habits and beliefs, physical activity, and nutritional knowledge among university students. *Perspect. Public Health* **2016**, *136*, 231–244. [CrossRef] [PubMed]
105. Loprinzi, P.D.; Darnell, T.; Hager, K.; Vidrine, J.I. Physical activity-related beliefs and discrepancies between beliefs and physical activity behavior for various chronic diseases. *Physiol. Behav.* **2015**, *151*, 577–582. [CrossRef] [PubMed]
106. Worsley, A. Nutrition knowledge and food consumption: Can nutrition knowledge change food behaviour? *Asia Pac. J. Clin. Nutr.* **2002**, *11* (Suppl. S3), S579–S585. [CrossRef] [PubMed]
107. Jezewska-Zychowicz, M.; Plichta, M. Diet Quality, Dieting, Attitudes and Nutrition Knowledge: Their Relationship in Polish Young Adults-A Cross-Sectional Study. *Int. J. Environ. Res. Public Health* **2022**, *19*, 6533. [CrossRef]
108. Truman, E.; Lane, D.; Elliott, C. Defining food literacy: A scoping review. *Appetite* **2017**, *116*, 365–371. [CrossRef] [PubMed]
109. Lee, Y.; Kim, T.; Jung, H. The Relationships between Food Literacy, Health Promotion Literacy and Healthy Eating Habits among Young Adults in South Korea. *Foods* **2022**, *11*, 2467. [CrossRef] [PubMed]
110. Hardcastle, S.J.; Hancox, J.; Hattar, A.; Maxwell-Smith, C.; Thøgersen-Ntoumani, C.; Hagger, M.S. Motivating the unmotivated: How can health behavior be changed in those unwilling to change? *Front. Psychol.* **2015**, *6*, 835. [CrossRef]
111. Flack, K.D.; Johnson, L.; Roemmich, J.N. The reinforcing value and liking of resistance training and aerobic exercise as predictors of adult's physical activity. *Physiol. Behav.* **2017**, *179*, 284–289. [CrossRef] [PubMed]
112. Carr, K.A.; Epstein, L.H. Choice is relative: Reinforcing value of food and activity in obesity treatment. *Am. Psychol.* **2020**, *75*, 139–151. [CrossRef] [PubMed]
113. Hibbard, J.H.; Greene, J. What the evidence shows about patient activation: Better health outcomes and care experiences; fewer data on costs. *Health Aff.* **2013**, *32*, 207–214. [CrossRef]
114. Oman, R.F.; King, A.C. Predicting the adoption and maintenance of exercise participation using self-efficacy and previous exercise participation rates. *Am. J. Health Promot.* **1998**, *12*, 154–161. [CrossRef] [PubMed]
115. Strecher, V.J.; DeVellis, B.M.; Becker, M.H.; Rosenstock, I.M. The role of self-efficacy in achieving health behavior change. *Health Educ. Q.* **1986**, *13*, 73–92. [CrossRef]
116. Blake, H.; Stanulewicz, N.; McGill, F. Predictors of physical activity and barriers to exercise in nursing and medical students. *J. Adv. Nurs.* **2017**, *73*, 917–929. [CrossRef] [PubMed]
117. Korinth, A.; Schiess, S.; Westenhoefer, J. Eating behaviour and eating disorders in students of nutrition sciences. *Public Health Nutr.* **2010**, *13*, 32–37. [CrossRef]
118. Mahn, H.M.; Lordly, D. A Review of Eating Disorders and Disordered Eating amongst Nutrition Students and Dietetic Professionals. *Can. J. Diet Pract. Res.* **2015**, *76*, 38–43. [CrossRef] [PubMed]
119. Poínhos, R.; Alves, D.; Vieira, E.; Pinhão, S.; Oliveira, B.M.; Correia, F. Eating behaviour among undergraduate students. Comparing nutrition students with other courses. *Appetite* **2015**, *84*, 28–33. [CrossRef] [PubMed]
120. Sampasa-Kanyinga, H.; Hamilton, H.A.; Willmore, J.; Chaput, J.P. Perceptions and attitudes about body weight and adherence to the physical activity recommendation among adolescents: The moderating role of body mass index. *Public Health* **2017**, *146*, 75–83. [CrossRef] [PubMed]
121. Atlantis, E.; Barnes, E.H.; Ball, K. Weight status and perception barriers to healthy physical activity and diet behavior. *Int. J. Obes.* **2008**, *32*, 343–352. [CrossRef]
122. Whatnall, M.C.; Hutchesson, M.J.; Sharkey, T.; Haslam, R.L.; Bezzina, A.; Collins, C.E.; Tzelepis, F.; Ashton, L.M. Recruiting and retaining young adults: What can we learn from behavioural interventions targeting nutrition, physical activity and/or obesity? A systematic review of the literature. *Public Health Nutr.* **2021**, *24*, 5686–5703. [CrossRef]
123. Carr, L.T.B.; Bell, C.; Alick, C.; Bentley-Edwards, K.L. Responding to Health Disparities in Behavioral Weight Loss Interventions and COVID-19 in Black Adults: Recommendations for Health Equity. *J. Racial Ethn. Health Disparities* **2022**, *9*, 739–747. [CrossRef]

124. Stevens, J.; Pratt, C.; Boyington, J.; Nelson, C.; Truesdale, K.P.; Ward, D.S.; Lytle, L.; Sherwood, N.E.; Robinson, T.N.; Moore, S.; et al. Multilevel Interventions Targeting Obesity: Research Recommendations for Vulnerable Populations. *Am. J. Prev. Med.* **2017**, *52*, 115–124. [CrossRef]
125. Kumanyika, S. Overcoming Inequities in Obesity: What Don't We Know That We Need to Know? *Health Educ. Behav.* **2019**, *46*, 721–727. [CrossRef]

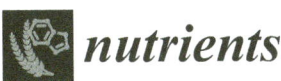

Article

The Effectiveness of a Combined Healthy Eating, Physical Activity, and Sleep Hygiene Lifestyle Intervention on Health and Fitness of Overweight Airline Pilots: A Controlled Trial

Daniel Wilson [1,2,*], Matthew Driller [3], Paul Winwood [2,4], Tracey Clissold [2], Ben Johnston [5] and Nicholas Gill [1,6]

1. Te Huataki Waiora School of Health, The University of Waikato, Hamilton 3216, New Zealand; nicholas.gill@waikato.ac.nz
2. Faculty of Health, Education and Environment, Toi Ohomai Institute of Technology, Tauranga 3112, New Zealand; paul.winwood@toiohomai.ac.nz (P.W.); tracey.clissold@toiohomai.ac.nz (T.C.)
3. Sport and Exercise Science, School of Allied Health, Human Services and Sport, La Trobe University, Melbourne 3086, Australia; m.driller@latrobe.edu.au
4. Sports Performance Research Institute New Zealand, Auckland University of Technology, Auckland 1010, New Zealand
5. Aviation and Occupational Health Unit, Air New Zealand, Auckland 1142, New Zealand; ben.johnston@otago.ac.nz
6. New Zealand Rugby, Wellington 6011, New Zealand
* Correspondence: daniel.wilson@toiohomai.ac.nz; Tel.: +64-7557-6035

Abstract: (1) Background: The aim of this study was to evaluate the effectiveness of a three-component nutrition, sleep, and physical activity (PA) program on cardiorespiratory fitness, body composition, and health behaviors in overweight airline pilots. (2) Methods: A parallel group study was conducted amongst 125 airline pilots. The intervention group participated in a 16-week personalized healthy eating, sleep hygiene, and PA program. Outcome measures of objective health (maximal oxygen consumption (VO_{2max}), body mass, skinfolds, girths, blood pressure, resting heart rate, push-ups, plank hold) and self-reported health (weekly PA, sleep quality and duration, fruit and vegetable intake, and self-rated health) were collected at baseline and post-intervention. The wait-list control completed the same assessments. (3) Results: Significant group main effects in favor of the intervention group were found for all outcome measures ($p < 0.001$) except for weekly walking ($p = 0.163$). All objective health measures significantly improved in the intervention group when compared to the control group ($p < 0.001$, $d = 0.41–1.04$). Self-report measures (moderate-to-vigorous PA, sleep quality and duration, fruit and vegetable intake, and self-rated health) significantly increased in the intervention group when compared to the control group ($p < 0.001$, $d = 1.00–2.69$). (4) Conclusion: Our findings demonstrate that a personalized 16-week healthy eating, PA, and sleep hygiene intervention can elicit significant short-term improvements in physical and mental health outcomes among overweight airline pilots. Further research is required to examine whether the observed effects are maintained longitudinally.

Keywords: weight loss; nutrition; fruit and vegetable intake; aerobic capacity; moderate-to-vigorous physical activity; lifestyle medicine

1. Introduction

Adverse health outcomes promoted by occupational demands of airline pilots including shift and irregular work schedules, circadian disruption, sedentary activity, and high fatigue [1] may be mitigated through attainment of health guidelines for lifestyle behaviors: healthy diet, physical activity (PA), and sleep [2,3]. Non-communicable diseases (NCDs) including cardiovascular disease (CVD), stroke, type 2 diabetes, and their major risk factors are among leading causes of mortality and morbidity worldwide [4]. The presence of

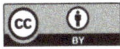

modifiable behavioral NCD risk factors including obesity, hypertension, physical inactivity, low cardiorespiratory fitness, unhealthy dietary patterns, short sleep, depression, high perceived stress levels, and high fatigue are each associated with adverse outcomes to acute and chronic health [4–6]. Obesity is a complex, widespread, yet modifiable NCD risk factor that poses a significant public health threat [7]. The obesity prevalence worldwide was estimated as 13% in 2015, which is nearly double the prevalence from 1980 [7]. In 2020, 67% of male airline pilots in New Zealand were classified as overweight or obese with hypertension affecting 27% of the population [8]. Moreover, this study reported the prevalence of insufficient fruit and vegetable intake, physical inactivity, and <7 h sleep per night among airline pilots as 68%, 48%, 33.5%, respectively [8].

The global economic burden associated with NCDs is estimated as $47 trillion between 2010 and 2030 [4]. Previous research has demonstrated evidence of significantly reduced longitudinal health care cost utilization following diet and exercise lifestyle interventions [9]. Relevantly, airline pilots undergo annual or biannual medical examinations, results of which influence flight certification status [10]. Ongoing health care costs associated with the presence of NCDs and their risk factors present economic implications for aviation medical care [4,10].

Better health status is generally associated with enhanced productivity and work performance [11]. In the context of commercial aviation, pilot work performance is imperative to flight operation safety. As established in the International Civil Aviation Organization's Annex 1, aviation medicine providers are required to implement appropriate health promotion for license holders (pilots) to reduce future medical risks to flight safety [10]. Thus, interventions that promote positive health of pilots, mitigate health risk factors for NCDs, and reduce longitudinal health care costs of employees are of importance to aviation medicine, health practices, and policies.

Limited studies have investigated the efficacy of health promotion interventions among airline pilots, and no studies to date have reported on cardiorespiratory fitness or body fat percentage among this occupational group [1]. Based on the findings of our recent preliminary research [2,12], we found a personalized three-component healthy eating, sleep hygiene, and PA intervention produced favorable outcomes in subjective health and reductions in body mass and blood pressure among airline pilots. Utilizing a different sample of pilots, the aim of the present study was to evaluate the effects of a three-component healthy eating, sleep hygiene, and PA program on cardiorespiratory fitness, body composition, and health behaviors in overweight airline pilots. It was hypothesized that the intervention group would have significantly greater improvements in physical fitness, body composition and health behaviors compared to the wait-list control group at four months.

2. Materials and Methods

2.1. Design

A parallel controlled study (intervention and control) with pre- and post-testing was conducted to evaluate the effectiveness of a personalized three-component, 16-week lifestyle intervention for enhancing subjective and objective health indices in airline pilots. This study was approved by the Human Research Ethics Committee of the University of Waikato in New Zealand; reference number 2020#07. The trial protocol is registered at The Australian New Zealand Clinical Trials Registry (ACTRN12622000233729).

2.2. Participants

The participants comprised of self-selected airline pilots who were recruited from a large international airline in New Zealand. Invitations to participate in the study were distributed to all airline pilots within the company through internal communication networks. Group allocation was determined by a first in, first serve basis due to intervention implementation capacity. Accordingly, pilots who expressed interest to participate in the study early and satisfied the eligibility criteria were allocated to the intervention group

(n = 86) and subsequent enrolments that exceeded initial capacity were allocated to the wait-list control (n = 80). Participants involved pilots from short-haul (regional flights) and long-haul (international flights) rosters. The participants allocated to the wait-list control group received no intervention and were invited to participate in the intervention after the study period.

Potentially eligible pilots who volunteered to participate were screened according to the following eligibility criteria: (a) aged >18 years, (b) pilots with a valid commercial flying license, (c) working on a full-time basis, (d) having a body mass index (BMI) of $\geq$25 (overweight), and (e) a resting blood pressure of >120/80 (systolic/diastolic). Pilots were excluded if medical clearance was deemed necessary prior to engagement in a PA program after completion of the 2020 Physical Activity Readiness Questionnaire for Everyone (PAR-Q+) [13].

Informed consent was obtained from participants prior to commencement of participation in the study and participants were notified that they were permitted to withdraw at any time during the study if they wish to do so. To encourage data blinding and anonymity during data analysis, participants were allocated a unique identifier code on their informed consent form and were instructed to input this into their online health survey in lieu of their name.

2.3. Intervention

At baseline the intervention group completed an individual face-to-face 60-min consultation session with an experienced health coach practitioner located at the airline occupational health facility, followed by provision of a personalized health program. Participants also received weekly educational content emails throughout the intervention and a mid-intervention follow-up phone call with a health coach to discuss progress and support adherence. Health coaching advice delivered to pilots was evidence-based and derived from experts in the fields of dietetics, physical activity, and sleep science.

For extended details of the procedures associated with the three-component intervention, readers are referred to the study of Wilson and colleagues [12]. In brief, the intervention incorporated seven behavior change techniques (BCT) including collaborative goal setting, action planning, problem solving, information about health consequences, self-monitoring, feedback on behaviors, and reviewing of outcomes. The intervention utilized 35 participant interactions: including two face-to-face consultations (baseline and post-intervention), one mid-intervention telephone call, 16 weekly emails, and 16 weekly self-monitoring surveys.

Between the participant and health coach, personalized collaborative outcome, process, and performance goals [12] were established at baseline for (a) sleep hygiene, (b) healthy eating, and (c) PA. Healthy eating goals were defined based on a healthy eating resource (see Appendix A, adapted from Beeken and colleagues [14] with amendments derived from Cena and Calder [15]). Sleep goals were set based on a Sleep Hygiene Checklist (see Appendix B) which was derived from previous sleep hygiene and stimulus control studies [12]. Physical activity prescription goals were established based on assessment of individual barriers and facilitators to physical activity, implementation of the frequency, intensity, time, and type principles [16], and progression to fulfillment of sufficient moderate-to-vigorous-intensity physical activity (MVPA) to meet World Health Organization health guidelines [17] according to individual capabilities. Sufficient physical activity was defined as $\geq$150 min moderate-intensity, or $\geq$75 min vigorous-intensity, or an equivalent combination MVPA per week [17].

2.4. Outcome Measures

Objective measures of health (maximal oxygen consumption (VO_{2max}), body mass, skinfolds, girths, blood pressure, resting heart rate, pushups, plank hold) and self-report measures (weekly PA, sleep quality and duration, fruit and vegetable intake, and self-rated health) were collected at baseline and 4 months (post-intervention). Self-report measures (weekly MVPA, sleep duration, fruit, and vegetable intake) were also collected weekly to monitor intervention adherence via an online survey delivered through Qualtrics software (Qualtrics, Provo, UT, USA).

Participants were instructed to avoid large quantities of food, stimulants such as caffeine, and strenuous exercise 4 h prior to measurement of physiological outcome measures. Outcome measurement protocols for body mass, blood pressure, and subjective health have been previously described in detail [2,12]. In brief, at the start of the consultation session, participants completed an electronic questionnaire via an iPad (Apple, California, CA, USA) to provide data for self-report measures. Using standardized methods previously described [2], resting heart rate was measured utilizing a Rossmax pulse oximeter SB220 (Rossmax Taipei, Taiwan, China), height was recorded with SECA 206 height measures, body mass was measured with SECA 813 electronic scales (SECA, Hamburg, Germany), and blood pressure was measured with an OMRON HEM-757 device (Omron Corporation, Kyoto, Japan).

Skinfold measurements were collected following standardized procedures of the International Society for the Advancement of Kinanthropometry (ISAK) [18]. The skinfold sum was determined by measurements obtained for eight locations: biceps, triceps, subscapular, abdominal, supraspinale, iliac crest, mid-thigh, and medial calf. All skinfold measurements were taken from the right side of the body twice, with a third measurement taken if the difference between recordings were greater than 4%. The anthropometrical technical errors were under the recommended limits [18] for all final recorded measurements. Skinfold measurements were conducted by an accredited ISAK anthropometrist, using Harpenden calipers (British Indicators, Hertfordshire, UK) which were sufficiently calibrated as per the manufacturers' guidelines. Body fat percentage was derived from skinfold assessments and was calculated using updated sex and ethnicity specific equations reported elsewhere [19]. Girth measurements for the waist and hip locations were measured with a thin-line metric tape measure (Lufkin; Apex Tool Group, Sparks, MD, USA) congruent with standardized technique [20].

Push-ups and the plank isometric hold were utilized as assessments of musculoskeletal fitness, using previously reported standardized methods [21,22]. For push-ups, the hand release technique was utilized, where participants were instructed to keep their torso tight so that the shoulders, hips, knees, and ankles were aligned throughout the range of motion. At the bottom position, the hands were lifted from the floor between each push-up. Push-up cadence was coordinated by a metronome and participants completed maximum full range of motion repetitions until the onset of failure to maintain correct form [21]. The basic plank isometric hold technique was utilized, consisting of the participant holding a prone bridge position supported by their feet and forearms. Elbows were below the shoulders with the forearms and fingers extending forward. The neck was maintained in a neutral position so that the body remained straight from the head to the heels. Time was recorded from initiation of the position until the loss of the plank position [22].

For quantification of aerobic fitness, estimated VO_{2max} was obtained by participants performing a previously validated [23,24] 3-min aerobic test (3mAT) on a Wattbike (Woodway USA, Waukesha, WI, USA) electro-magnetically and air-braked cycle ergometer. Participants were given a full explanation of the protocol, safety procedures, the Wattbike seat and handle were fitted appropriately for the participant, who was also fitted with a Polar H10 heart rate strap (Polar Electro, Kempele, Finland). Full details on the procedure have been detailed elsewhere [23]. Participants completed a 10-min warmup consisting of self-paced cycling at 70–90 rpm with two 6-s sprints within that timeframe, as suggested by the manufacturer. The goal of the 3mAT was to maintain the highest power output possible for 3 full minutes. Verbal encouragement was provided, and participants were allowed to adjust the resistance and pedal cadence as needed throughout the test. Each participant's customized setup was noted, and the same procedures were carried out for the retest at 4 months.

Prior to baseline testing, the Wattbike was calibrated by the manufacturer, and a between session reliability assessment was conducted with the Wattbike utilizing a convenience sample of seven untrained airline pilots (aged = 42 ± 12 years, body mass = 80 ± 11 kg, height = 173 ± 4 cm, mean ± standard deviation (SD), 5 males, 2 females). Following standardized procedures [23,24], participants of the reliability trial performed the 3mAT twice separated by >48 h between assessments. For measurement of estimated VO_{2max}, the reliability trial produced a coefficient of variation (CV) of 4.3% and an intraclass correlation coefficient (ICC) of 0.98 (0.90–0.99), denoting acceptable CV [25] and excellent ICC reliability [26].

Self-report measures (PA, sleep quality and duration, fruit and vegetable intake, and self-rated health) have been previously described in detail [12]. In brief, self-rated health (physical and mental) were measured utilizing the Short Health Form 12v2 (SF-12v2) [27]. The International Physical Activity Questionnaire Short Form (IPAQ) was utilized to quantify self-report MVPA [28]. Self-report subjective sleep quality and duration were measured with the Pittsburgh Sleep Quality Index (PSQI) [29]. Daily fruit and vegetable intake were measured using dietary recall questions derived from the New Zealand Health Survey [28].

2.5. Statistical Analyses

G-Power software was utilized to calculate sample size required to detect a clinically significant change in primary outcome measures of ≥5% weight loss and a change of 3.5 mL/kg/min for VO_{2max} [30]. Our sample size power calculation suggested 65 pilots were required in each group to achieve 90% power and a 5% significance criterion to detect relevant differences between the intervention and wait-list control groups. To account for 20% dropout observed in a similar study [2], our target sample size was 156.

Statistical Package for the Social Sciences (SPSS, version 28; IBM Corp., Armonk, NY, USA) was utilized for all analyses. Listwise deletion (i.e., entire case record removal) was applied if individual datasets had missing values or for participants who did not complete post-tests. Stem and leaf plots were inspected to ascertain whether there were any outliers in the data for each variable. A Shapiro–Wilk test ($p > 0.05$) and its histograms, Q–Q plots, and box plots were analyzed for the normality of data distribution for all variables. Levene's test was used to test homogeneity of variance.

Independent *t*-tests were utilized to calculate whether any significant differences existed between groups at baseline. For categorical variables (long haul and short haul) the Chi square test was used. Between group analysis of pre-test and post-test were assessed using paired *t*-tests and analysis of covariance (ANCOVA) (respectively). To control for baseline differences between groups, baseline data were included as a covariate in the ANCOVA [31], in addition to inclusion of age and sex. Effect sizes were calculated using Cohen's d to quantify between-group effects from pre-test to post-test. Effect size thresholds were set at >1.2, >0.6, >0.2, and <0.2, which were classified as large, moderate, small, and trivial, respectively [32]. The α level was set at a p value of less than 0.05.

3. Results

3.1. Characteristics of the Study Population

Two-hundred twelve airline pilots were considered for eligibility and 148 were recruited to participate (Figure 1). Of them, 84% ($n = 125$) of recruits provided data for both timepoints, which comprised a combination of short-haul and long-haul rosters ($n = 60$ and 65, respectively). The dropout rates from baseline to post-intervention were 12% (time commitment $n = 5$; ceased employment $n = 3$; testing not fully completed $n = 1$) and 19% (time commitment $n = 8$; ceased employment $n = 4$) for the intervention and wait-list control groups, respectively. As displayed in Table 1, at baseline both groups demonstrated similar characteristics for most health parameters, yet the wait-list control group had lower SBP ($t(123) = 1.191$, $p = 0.03$, $d = 0.39$) and lower MAP ($t(123) = 2.113$, $p = 0.03$, $d = 0.38$). No significant differences were observed between groups for sex and fleet type.

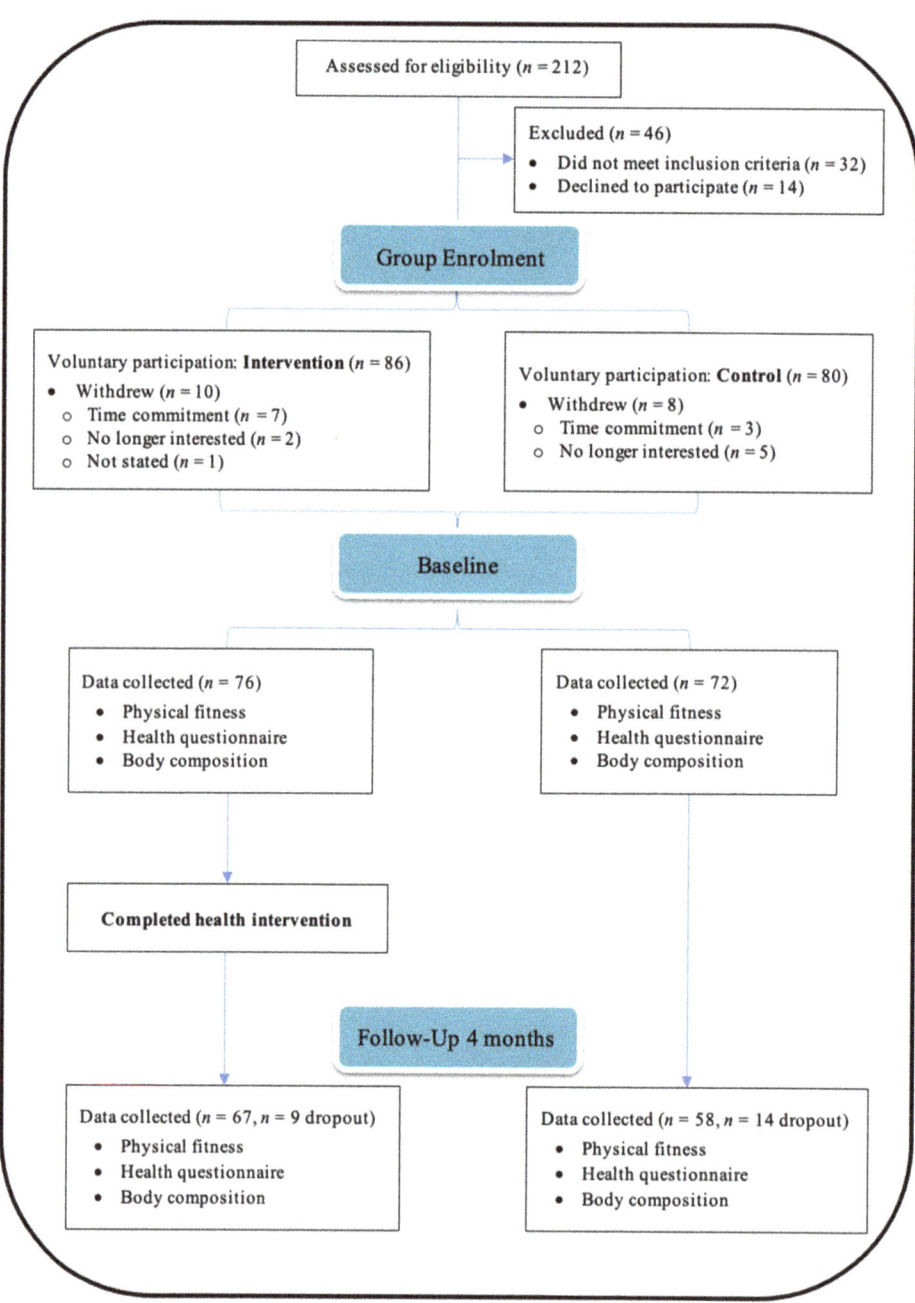

Figure 1. Flow diagram of participant recruitment and data collection.

Table 1. Baseline characteristics of participants.

Parameters	All subjects (n = 125)	Intervention (n = 67)	Control (n = 58)
Sex (female/male)	12/113	6/61	6/52
Age (years)	44.5 ± 10.7	43.7 ± 10.0	45.6 ± 11.4
Short haul (n)	60	34	26
Long haul (n)	65	33	32
Height (cm)	178.4 ± 7.4	179.2 ± 6.9	177.4 ± 7.8
Systolic BP (mmHg)	132.3 ± 5.6	133.3 ± 6.0	131.1 ± 4.9 *
Diastolic BP (mmHg)	85.6 ± 3.8	86.0 ± 3.9	85.0 ± 3.6
MAP (mmHg)	101.1 ± 3.8	101.8 ± 3.8	100.4 ± 3.6 *
Pulse (bpm)	66.9 ± 6.6	67.4 ± 6.1	66.4 ± 7.2
Body mass (kg)	90.5 ± 9.2	91.1 ± 8.0	89.8 ± 10.5
BMI (kg/m^2)	28.4 ± 2.0	28.3 ± 1.7	28.5 ± 3.4
Skinfold sum × 8 sites (mm)	136.5 ± 24.1	138.3 ± 17.7	134.4 ± 29.9
Bodyfat (%)	24.3 ± 3.6	24.7 ± 3.2	23.9 ± 4.0
Waist girth (cm)	96.6 ± 7.6	97.8 ± 8.1	95.2 ± 6.8
Waist to hip ratio	0.93 ± 0.07	0.94 ± 0.07	0.93 ± 0.08
VO$_{2max}$ (mL/kg/min)	36.3 ± 5.4	35.6 ± 5.8	37.0 ± 4.8
Push-ups (repetitions)	17.2 ± 7.3	16.4 ± 6.8	18.1 ± 7.7
Plank hold (s)	79.7 ± 24.7	77.2 ± 25.5	82.5 ± 23.7
Walking per week (min)	73.8 ± 42.5	70.5 ± 32.2	77.7 ± 52.0
MVPA per week (min)	141.8 ± 41.1	138.0 ± 41.6	146.2 ± 40.3
Fruit intake (serve/day)	1.3 ± 0.7	1.5 ± 0.8	1.0 ± 0.6
Vegetable intake (serve/day)	2.0 ± 0.7	1.8 ± 0.7	2.4 ± 0.5
F&V intake (serve/day)	3.3 ± 0.7	3.3 ± 0.7	3.4 ± 0.7
Sleep per day (h)	7.0 ± 0.5	7.0 ± 0.4	7.0 ± 0.6
Global PSQI (score)	6.3 ± 2.1	6.4 ± 2.2	6.1 ± 1.9
MCS-12 (score)	48.9 ± 4.6	48.6 ± 5.8	49.3 ± 2.8
PCS-12 (score)	46.7 ± 3.4	46.3 ± 3.8	47.2 ± 2.8

Note: Mean ± SD reported for all subjects, intervention and control. Abbreviations: SD = Standard deviation; BMI = body mass index; VO$_{2max}$ = maximal oxygen consumption; BP = blood pressure; MAP = mean arterial pressure; MVPA = moderate-to-vigorous physical activity; F&V = fruit and vegetable intake; MCS-12 = Short Health Form 12v2 mental component summary scale; PCS-12 = Short Health Form 12v2 physical health component summary scale; PSQI = Pittsburgh Sleep Quality Index. * Indicates statistical significance ($p < 0.05$).

3.2. Intervention Adherence

For the intervention group, compliance was measured mid-intervention for health behaviors, including self-report weekly MVPA, daily fruit and vegetable intake and average sleep duration per night. Sixty-four (97%) were achieving ≥5 serves of fruit and vegetables per day, 94% reported sleeping ≥7 h sleep per night, and 97% were obtaining ≥150 MVPA (min) per week. Comparatively, 36% of the wait-list control group were achieving ≥5 serves of fruit and vegetables per day, 71% were sleeping ≥7 h per night, and 53% were obtaining ≥150 MVPA (min) per week.

3.3. Body Mass, Skinfolds, Waist Girth, Bodyfat Percentage, Blood Pressure and Pulse

Significant group main effects ($p < 0.001$) in favor of the intervention group were found for all variables. Small to large effect size differences were observed from baseline to post-intervention (Table 2). The within-group analysis revealed that the intervention elicited significant improvements ($p < 0.001$) in all measures at post-intervention associated with moderate to large effect sizes (Table 2; Figure 2). The wait-list control group reported a significantly lower body mass (t(57) = 2.538, $p = 0.014$, d = 0.33) and reduced waist girth (t(57) = 2.358, $p = 0.022$, d = 0.31), yet no significant changes were observed in other measures.

Table 2. Changes in objective and self-report health measures from baseline to post-intervention at 4-months.

	Time (Months)	Intervention (n = 67)			Control (n = 58)			ANCOVA (Group Main Effects)	Between Group ES
		M	SD	Follow Up Change (95% CI)	M	SD	Follow Up Change (95% CI)	p	d
Body mass (kg)	0	91.1	8.0		89.8	10.5			0.14, Trivial
	4	85.6	7.7	5.5 (4.8–6.1)	89.4	85.6	0.4 (0.1–0.7)	<0.001	−0.41, Small
BMI (kg/m²)	0	28.3	1.7		28.5	3.4			0.08, Trivial
	4	26.7	1.6	1.7 (1.5–1.9)	28.4	2.4	0.1 (0.0–0.2)	<0.001	−0.86, Moderate
Systolic BP (mmHg)	0	133.3	6.0		131.1	4.9			0.39, Small
	4	125.2	5.8	8.1 (7.3–8.9)	132.5	5.9	1.3 (0.1–2.8)	<0.001	−1.25, Large
Diastolic BP (mmHg)	0	86.0	3.9		85.0	3.6			0.27, Small
	4	80.8	5.4	5.2 (4.2–6.2)	84.8	4.7	0.2 (0.9–1.4)	<0.001	−0.77, Moderate
MAP (mmHg)	0	101.8	3.8		100.4	3.6			0.38, Small
	4	95.6	5.0	6.2 (5.4–6.9)	100.7	4.7	0.3 (0.8–1.4)	<0.001	−1.04, Moderate
Pulse (bpm)	0	67.4	6.1		66.4	7.2			0.15, Trivial
	4	61.0	6.5	6.3 (4.8–7.8)	67.0	8.8	0.6 (1.0–2.2)	<0.001	−0.78, Moderate
Skinfold sum (mm)	0	138.3	17.7		134.4	29.9			0.16, Trivial
	4	110.1	14.5	28.2 (26–30.5)	133.0	29.8	1.5 (0.5–3.4)	<0.001	−1.00, Moderate
Bodyfat (%)	0	24.7	3.2		23.9	4.0			0.21, Small
	4	21.0	2.8	3.6 (3.3–4.0)	23.7	4.1	0.2 (0.1–0.4)	<0.001	−0.79, Moderate
Waist (cm)	0	97.8	8.1		95.2	6.8			0.35, Small
	4	91.8	7.9	6.0 (5.3–6.8)	94.3	6.9	1.0 (0.1–1.8)	<0.001	−0.34, Small
Waist to hip ratio	0	0.94	0.07		0.93	0.08			0.09, Trivial
	4	0.90	0.07	0.03 (0.02–0.04)	0.92	0.07	0.1 (0.0–0.2)	<0.001	−0.22, Small
VO₂max (mL/kg/min)	0	35.6	5.8		37.0	4.8			−0.26, Small
	4	40.2	5.9	4.5 (4.0–5.0)	37.3	5.1	0.2 (0.1–0.6)	<0.001	0.52, Small
Push-ups (repetitions)	0	16.4	6.8		18.1	7.7			−0.22, Small
	4	24.3	7.1	7.8 (6.5–9.1)	19.9	8.1	1.9 (1.2–2.6)	<0.001	0.57, Small
Plank hold (s)	0	77.2	25.5		82.5	23.7			−0.21, Small
	4	120.0	39.6	42.8 (34.4–51.3)	92.1	32.1	9.5 (3.8–15.1)	<0.001	0.77, Moderate
Hours slept (h/day)	0	7.0	0.4		7.0	0.6			−0.17, Trivial
	4	7.6	0.5	0.7 (0.6–0.8)	7.1	0.5	0.1 (0.0–0.2)	<0.001	1.00, Moderate
PSQI Global (score)	0	6.4	2.2		6.1	1.9			0.14, Trivial
	4	4.0	1.3	2.4 (2.0–2.8)	5.8	1.8	0.3 (0.1–0.5)	<0.001	−1.16, Moderate
IPAQ-walk (min)	0	70.5	32.2		77.7	52.0			−0.17, Trivial
	4	97.0	30.0	26.5 (18.1–34.9)	95.4	49.0	17.8 (8.0–27.6)	0.163	0.04, Trivial
IPAQ-MVPA (min)	0	138.0	41.6		146.2	40.3			−0.20, Small
	4	210.3	44.3	72.4 (60.0–84.8)	156.9	46.4	10.8 (5.0–16.5)	<0.001	1.18, Moderate
F&V Intake (serve/day)	0	3.3	0.7		3.4	0.7			−0.17, Trivial
	4	6.9	1.3	3.6 (3.3–4.0)	3.8	0.9	0.4 (0.1–0.7)	<0.001	2.69, Large
PCS-12 (score)	0	46.3	3.8		47.2	2.8			−0.28, Small
	4	51.5	3.4	5.2 (4.4–5.9)	47.9	2.8	0.7 (0.3–1.1)	<0.001	1.14, Moderate
MCS-12 (score)	0	48.6	5.8		49.3	2.8			−0.15, Trivial
	4	53.3	3.6	4.7 (3.7–5.8)	49.5	2.9	0.2 (0.2–0.7)	<0.001	1.15, Moderate

Note: Mean ± SD reported for all participants, intervention and control. Abbreviations: M = mean; SD = standard deviation; CI = Confidence interval; ES = effect size; BMI = body mass index. BP = blood pressure. MAP = mean arterial pressure. MVPA = moderate-to-vigorous physical activity. PSQI = Pittsburgh Sleep Quality Index. IPAQ = International Physical Activity Questionnaire. F&V = fruit and vegetable intake. PCS-12 = Short Health Form 12v2 physical component summary score. MCS-12 = Short Health Form 12v2 mental component summary score.

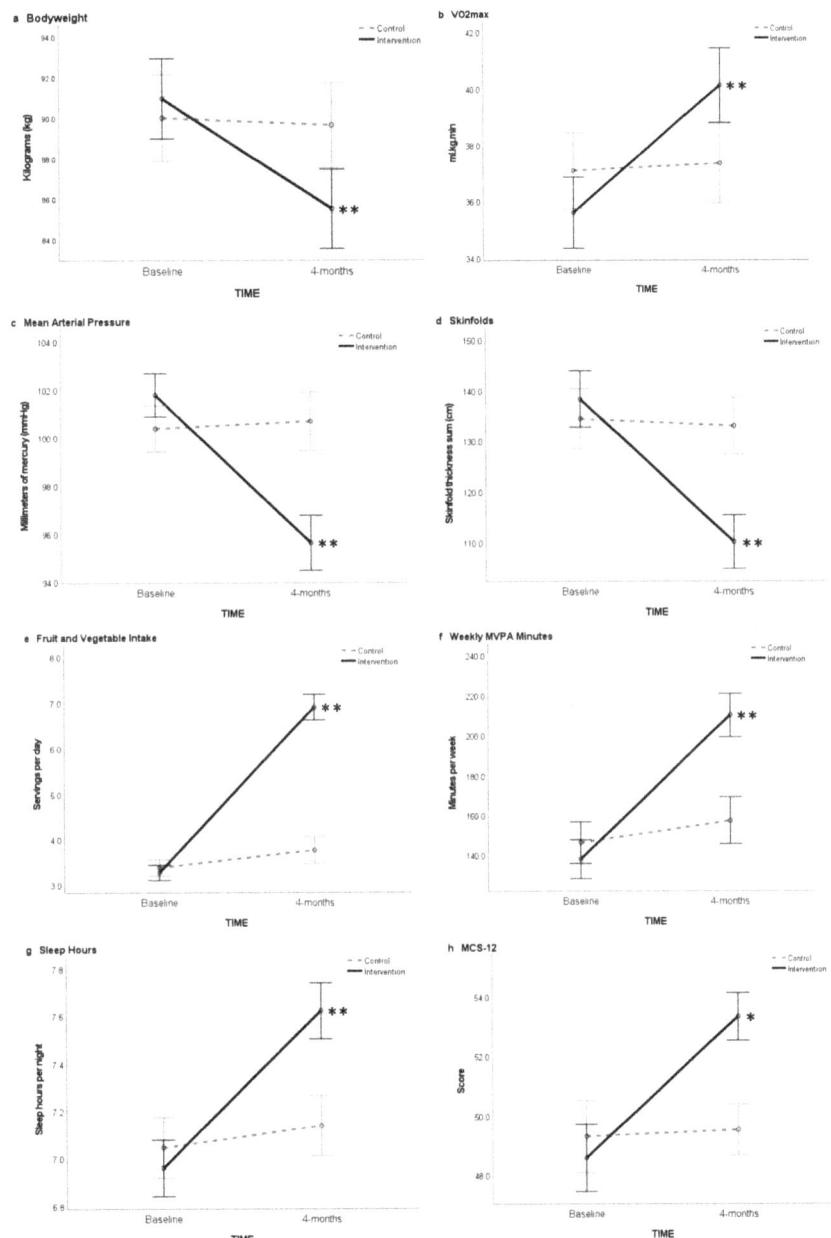

Figure 2. Mean values for health outcomes across time (baseline and 4-months), showing 95% confidence intervals ((**a**), bodyweight; (**b**), VO$_{2max}$; (**c**), Mean Arterial Pressure; (**d**), Skinfolds; (**e**), Fruit and Vegetable Intake; (**f**), Weekly MVPA Minutes; (**g**), Sleep Hours; (**h**), MCS-12). Abbreviations: VO$_{2max}$ = maximal oxygen consumption; MVPA = moderate-to-vigorous physical activity; MCS-12 = Short Health Form 12v2 mental component summary score. Notes: * indicates moderate within group effect size from baseline to 4-months. ** indicates large within group effect size from baseline to 4-months.

3.4. VO$_{2max}$, Pushups and Plank Hold

Significant group main effects were found for all measures ($p < 0.001$) in favor of the intervention group. The within-group analysis reported significantly greater improved changes from baseline to post-intervention for all physical performance measures in the intervention group ($p < 0.001$), associated with large effect sizes (Table 2; Figure 2). In contrast, the wait-list control group significantly increased push-ups (t(57) = 5.323, $p < 0.001$, $d = 0.69$) and plank hold (t(57) = 3.365, $p = 0.001$, $d = 0.44$), yet no significant change was observed for VO$_{2max}$.

3.5. Health Behaviors and Self-Rated Health

Significant group main effects in favor of the intervention group were found for all self-report health measures ($p < 0.001$) except for weekly walking minutes ($p = 0.163$). The within-group analysis reported significantly greater improved health changes from baseline to post-intervention for all self-report health measures in the intervention group ($p < 0.001$), associated with moderate to large effect sizes (see Table 2; Figure 2). Further, the wait-list control group significantly improved weekly walking, weekly MVPA, global PSQI score, and Short Health Form 12v2 physical component summary scale score (PCS-12, $p < 0.001$), enhanced fruit and vegetable intake ($p = 0.008$), and increased sleep hours ($p = 0.020$). The significant changes observed within the wait-list control group from baseline to post-intervention were associated with trivial to small effect sizes (see Table 2).

4. Discussion

To our knowledge, this study is the first clinical trial that has explored the effects of a lifestyle intervention on physical fitness and body composition measures among airline pilots. This study aimed to promote enhancement in cardiorespiratory and musculoskeletal fitness, body composition, and health behaviors through a personalized intervention on healthy eating, sleep hygiene, and PA.

For most outcome measures, in support of our initial hypothesis the controlled trial revealed significantly higher improvements in the intervention group compared to the wait-list control group. Our findings suggest that a face-to-face health assessment alone with no provision of an intervention may promote small short-term effects for improvements in health behaviors and weight management among airline pilots. Furthermore, the provision of a personalized multicomponent lifestyle intervention may facilitate moderate to large short-term effects for promoting healthy changes in physical fitness, body composition, and health behaviors among airline pilots.

These findings are important for health care professionals and researchers to provide insight regarding the efficacy of lifestyle interventions for promoting health, and to inform practices relating to disease prevention, health promotion, and public health policymaking. Furthermore, in relation to the limited literature base pertaining to three-component sleep, nutrition, and PA interventions and the insufficient depth of health behavior intervention research among airline pilots, our findings provide novel contributions to this field.

Excessive adiposity is evidently associated with higher all-cause mortality and elevated risk of cardiometabolic NCDs [33]. Counteractively, clinically significant improvements in NCD risk factors have been reported with as little as 2–3% of weight loss among those with high BMI [34]. A meta-analysis of 59 lifestyle weight loss interventions reported a pooled mean weight loss range of 5–8.5 kg (5–9% body mass) within the initial six months, and among studies exceeding 48 months a mean weight loss range of 3–6 kg (3–6% body mass) [35]. Comparatively, in our intervention group we observed 6% weight loss and 1.6 reduction in BMI at four months. Weight loss and BMI alone as assessments of body composition change are inherently limited due to their inability to precisely measure central adiposity, fat distribution, bone density, and lean mass [36].

In the present study we assessed additional body composition metrics with girth and skinfold measures. Waist circumference has been reported as being strongly associated with all-cause and cardiovascular mortality, with or without adjustment for BMI [36]. Further, skinfold thickness has been reported as a better predictor of body fatness compared to BMI [37]. We found the intervention elicited a decrease of 6 cm waist circumference and 28 mm skinfold thickness sum reduction, which were associated with an overall 3.7% reduction in predicted body fat percentage and a decrease of 8.1 mmHg for systolic blood pressure (SBP). These findings are consistent, yet of higher magnitude than a previous meta-analysis which reported exercise training programs were associated with pooled mean reductions of 5.1 mmHg SBP and 2.2 cm waist girth [38]. This study also reported that reductions in blood pressure (BP) and waist circumference were associated with reduced high-density lipoprotein (HDL) cholesterol and metabolic syndrome risk reduction [38]. Thus, interventions which induce these adaptations are of importance for risk reduction of these well-established NCD risk factors [4].

To our knowledge, our study is the first to report on objective measures of cardiorespiratory capacity among airline pilots. Prospective cohort research suggests exercise capacity is an authoritative predictor of mortality among adults, and an increase of 1 MET (3.5 mL/kg/min) is associated with a 12% CVD risk reduction [30]. A meta-analysis of aerobic exercise training interventions among adults (aged 41 ± 5 y) reported a pooled mean increase in VO_{2max} of 3.5 mL/kg/min (1.9–5.2, 95% confidence interval (CI)), associated with a moderate effect size of 0.6 [39]. In comparison, we observed an increase of 4.5 mL/kg/min within our intervention group, associated with a large effect size which exceeds previously suggested thresholds for clinical relevance [26]. However, future research is required to determine whether these acute adaptations are longitudinally maintained after the brief 16-week intervention.

The intervention promoted significant positive health outcomes for health behaviors and self-rated health, associated with moderate to large effect sizes. Sleep duration increased by 0.6 h in the intervention group, which is a lower magnitude compared with a recent meta-analysis of behavioral interventions to extend sleep length, which reported a pooled increase of 0.8 h per night (0.28–1.31, 95% CI) [40]. In part, this variance may be related to the different nature of interventions, where the present intervention targeted multiple-behavior modification for nutrition, sleep, and PA simultaneously, compared with the individual component focus in other studies (i.e., targeting sleep modification alone) [40].

For weekly MVPA we found the intervention elicited an increase of 72 min/week, which is notably higher than a previous meta-analysis which reported a mean increase of 24 min/week from PA interventions implemented in primary care settings [41]. Similarly, a meta-analysis of behavior interventions to increase fruit and vegetable intake reported a pooled mean increase of 1.1 servings per day [42], which was a lower magnitude of change compared to the increase of 3.6 servings following the present intervention. Notably, a meta-analysis of effective BCTs for promoting PA and healthy eating in overweight and obese adults highlighted the use of goal setting and self-monitoring of behavior as strong predictors of positive short and long-term health behavior change [43]. Congruently, our intervention implemented these components in addition to five other BCTs, which may have contributed to the observed effect sizes of change.

Strengths and Limitations

A strength of this study is our findings add valuable contribution to a small global literature base pertaining to interventions that include components for each healthy eating, PA, and sleep hygiene. The magnitude of effect sizes for positive health change observed in the intervention may be at least partly attributable to; (a) the implementation of seven BCTs including collaborative goal setting, (b) the personalized multiple-component nutrition, PA and sleep approach, (c) the multimodal intra-intervention communication administered via face-to-face consultations, a telephone call, and regular educational emails, and (d) the potential underlying motivation of airline pilots to improve their health to maintain their aviation medical license.

Potential limitations of this study need to be considered in the interpretation of our findings. Firstly, pilots voluntarily participated in the study via self-selection. Thus, those who enrolled may have exhibited higher readiness and motivation for health behavior change than the general population, which may limit the generalizability of our findings. Secondly, for feasibility of implementation and to minimize participant burden, self-report measures for health behaviors were utilized which inherently possess inferior validity to more invasive objective methods. Accordingly, future research, including measures such as a food frequency questionnaire or photo meal logging for dietary behaviors and actigraphy coupled with heart rate monitoring (e.g., smart watches) for PA and sleep monitoring, would be valuable contributions to increase the validity of findings. Third, although the sex characteristics of our sample are congruent with the general airline pilot population [8], the lack of female participants limits the generalizability of our findings to female populations. Thus, future research should evaluate the effects of the intervention among an ample sample size of females. Finally, the intervention was delivered by an experienced health coach, which presents a barrier to intervention adoption at scale. Future research should evaluate the delivery of interventions using similar procedures via cost-effective and scalable methods, such as online modes of delivery (i.e., smartphone application).

5. Conclusions

The personalized 16-week healthy eating, sleep hygiene, and PA intervention implemented in this study elicited significant positive changes associated with moderate to large effects sizes in all main outcome measures at four months follow-up, relative to the wait-list control group. Our findings suggest that the achievement of these three guidelines promotes physical and mental health among overweight airline pilots and these outcomes may be transferrable to other populations. However, there is a need for future research to examine whether the observed effects are longitudinally maintained following the intervention.

Author Contributions: D.W. and N.G. participated in conceptualization of the study and data collection; D.W., M.D., B.J., P.W., T.C. and N.G. contributed to the design of the study, data analysis, interpretation of the results, and manuscript writing. All authors have read and agreed to the published version of the manuscript.

Funding: This research received no external funding.

Institutional Review Board Statement: This study was approved by the Human Research Ethics Committee of the University of Waikato in New Zealand; reference number 2020#07. The trial protocol is registered at The Australian New Zealand Clinical Trials Registry (ACTRN12622000233729).

Informed Consent Statement: Informed consent was obtained from all subjects involved in the study.

Data Availability Statement: Not applicable.

Acknowledgments: The authors wish to thank the pilots for providing their time to voluntarily participate in this study.

Conflicts of Interest: The authors declare no conflict of interest.

Appendix A

TOP TEN TIPS FOR HEALTHY EATING

A system of habits to support a healthier you.

1. Emphasize whole foods

   Choose unprocessed natural foods.
   As food processing increases, nutrient density decreases. The more ingredients that are listed on a food, the more processed the food will likely be.

2. Reduce sugar where possible

Limit foods with added sugar (cookies, cakes, sugar sweetened beverages etc.) where you can. Read labels to avoid hidden sugars (sauces, cereals, dairy products etc.). Aim for less than 10% of daily energy from sugar or under 5% for better health.

3. Eat a rainbow of foods

Eat a variety of fruit and vegetables each day. Try those with rich colors of red, blue, green and orange. The more color in your day the more antioxidant, vitamins and minerals you will be getting.

4. Reduce white

Try to avoid the energy dense white foods like pasta, rice, bread, and potato. Use MyFitnessPal to understand other options. For example, 2 cups of broccoli with a curry is a healthier meal and some would say tastier than 2 cups of rice, and far fewer calories! Also consider having more vegetables that grow above the ground than those that grow below the ground.

5. Eat lean protein with each meal

Protein foods such as lean meat, chicken, fish, eggs, low fat dairy foods, bean, nuts, seeds, legumes and lentils aid in muscle repair and support lean body mass.

6. Caution with your portions

Do not heap food on your plate (except vegetables). Use the hand portion sizing guide to make good meal size decisions. Think twice before having second helpings.

7. Eat slowly and mindfully

Set aside adequate time for your meal so you're not rushed and chew your food well. While eating try to avoid watching TV or eating on the go. Pay attention to your food. Eat until you feel 80% full.

8. Think about your drinks

Drink 2 L of fluids a day. Choose mainly water. Unsweetened fruit juice contains natural sugar so limit to one glass a day (200 mL/one third pint). Alcohol is high in calories; limit to one unit a day for women and two for men.

9. Choose good fats

Choose fats that enhance your recovery and immune system not those that break it down. Some good sources of are nuts and seeds, nut butters, avocado, fatty fish, olive oil, and flaxseed oils.

10. Setup your healthy environment

If a food is in your house or possession, either you or someone you love, will eat it. If you remove the temptation of unhealthy foods from your surroundings and add more healthy options, you will set yourself up for success.

Appendix B

Sleep Hygiene Strategies for Enhancing Sleep	YES Achieving	NOT Achieving
1. Sleep at least 7 h		
2. Sleep routine or depower hour		
3. Regular sleep and wake time		
4. Dim lights near bedtime and turn off electronics >30 min before bed		
5. Avoid sleep disruptors 4–6 h before bed e.g., caffeine, large meals, alcohol		
6. Have a dark, cool, quiet sleep environment		
7. Exercise every day, not too close to bedtime		
8. Use the bedroom only for sleeping and intimacy		
9. Do a brain dump on paper before bed		
10. Early morning light exposure		

References

1. Wilson, D.; Driller, M.; Johnston, B.; Gill, N. The Prevalence of Cardiometabolic Health Risk Factors among Airline Pilots: A Systematic Review. *Int. J. Environ. Res. Public Health* **2022**, *19*, 4848. [CrossRef] [PubMed]
2. Wilson, D.; Driller, M.; Winwood, P.; Johnston, B.; Gill, N. The Effects of a Brief Lifestyle Intervention on the Health of Overweight Airline Pilots during COVID-19: A 12-Month Follow-Up Study. *Nutrients* **2021**, *13*, 4288. [CrossRef] [PubMed]
3. Van Drongelen, A.; Boot, C.R.; Hlobil, H.; Twisk, J.W.; Smid, T.; van der Beek, A.J. Evaluation of an mHealth intervention aiming to improve health-related behavior and sleep and reduce fatigue among airline pilots. *Scand. J. Work. Environ. Health* **2014**, *40*, 557–568. [CrossRef] [PubMed]
4. Miranda, J.J.; Barrientos-Gutiérrez, T.; Corvalan, C.; Hyder, A.A.; Lazo-Porras, M.; Oni, T.; Wells, J.C.K. Understanding the rise of cardiometabolic diseases in low- and middle-income countries. *Nat. Med.* **2019**, *25*, 1667–1679. [CrossRef] [PubMed]
5. Marmot, M.; Bell, R. Social determinants and non-communicable diseases: Time for integrated action. *BMJ* **2019**, *364*, l251. [CrossRef] [PubMed]
6. Lasserre, A.M.; Strippoli, M.P.; Glaus, J.; Gholam-Rezaee, M.; Vandeleur, C.L.; Castelao, E.; Marques-Vidal, P.; Waeber, G.; Vollenweider, P.; Preisig, M. Prospective associations of depression subtypes with cardio-metabolic risk factors in the general population. *Mol. Psychiatry* **2017**, *22*, 1026–1034. [CrossRef]
7. Chooi, Y.C.; Ding, C.; Magkos, F. The epidemiology of obesity. *Metab.—Clin. Exp.* **2019**, *92*, 6–10. [CrossRef] [PubMed]
8. Wilson, D.; Driller, M.; Johnston, B.; Gill, N. The prevalence and distribution of health risk factors in airline pilots: A cross-sectional comparison with the general population. *Aust. N. Z. J. Public Health* **2022**. [CrossRef]
9. Klatt, M.D.; Sieck, C.; Gascon, G.; Malarkey, W.; Huerta, T. A healthcare utilization cost comparison between employees receiving a worksite mindfulness or a diet/exercise lifestyle intervention to matched controls 5 years post intervention. *Complementary Ther. Med.* **2016**, *27*, 139–144. [CrossRef]
10. International Civil Aviation Authority. *Manual of Civil Aviation Medicine*, 3rd ed.; International Civil Aviation Authority: Montreal, QC, Canada, 2012; p. 580.
11. Keyes, C.L.M.; Grzywacz, J.G. Health as a Complete State: The Added Value in Work Performance and Healthcare Costs. *J. Occup. Environ. Med.* **2005**, *47*, 523–532. [CrossRef]
12. Wilson, D.; Driller, M.; Johnston, B.; Gill, N. The effectiveness of a 17-week lifestyle intervention on health behaviors among airline pilots during COVID-19. *J. Sport Health Sci.* **2021**, *10*, 333–340. [CrossRef] [PubMed]
13. Warburton, D.E.R.; Jamnik, V.; Bredin, S.S.; Shephard, R.J.; Gledhill, N. The 2020 Physical Activity Readiness Questionnaire for Everyone (PAR-Q+) and electronic Physical Activity Readiness Medical Examination (ePARmed-X+): 2020 PAR-Q+. *Health Fit. J. Can.* **2019**, *12*, 58–61.
14. Beeken, R.J.; Croker, H.; Morris, S.; Leurent, B.; Omar, R.; Nazareth, I.; Wardle, J. Study protocol for the 10 Top Tips (10TT) Trial: Randomised controlled trial of habit-based advice for weight control in general practice. *BMC Public Health* **2012**, *12*, 667. [CrossRef]
15. Cena, H.; Calder, P.C. Defining a Healthy Diet: Evidence for the Role of Contemporary Dietary Patterns in Health and Disease. *Nutrients* **2020**, *12*, 334. [CrossRef] [PubMed]
16. Barisic, A.; Leatherdale, S.T.; Kreiger, N. Importance of Frequency, Intensity, Time and Type (FITT) in physical activity assessment for epidemiological research. *Can. J. Public Health* **2011**, *102*, 174–175. [CrossRef] [PubMed]
17. World Health Organization. *Global Recommendations on Physical Activity for Health*; World Health Organization: Geneva, Switzerland, 2010.
18. Esparza-Ros, F.; Vaquero-Cristobal, R.; Marfell-Jones, M. *International Standards for Anthropometric Assessment (2019)*; The International Society for the Advancement of Kinanthropometry: Murcia, Spain, 2019.
19. Davidson, L.E.; Wang, J.; Thornton, J.C.; Kaleem, Z.; Silva-Palacios, F.; Pierson, R.N.; Heymsfield, S.B.; Gallagher, D. Predicting Fat Percent by Skinfolds in Racial Groups: Durnin and Womersley Revisited. *Med. Sci. Sports Exerc.* **2011**, *43*, 542. [CrossRef]
20. World Health Organization. *Waist Circumference and Waist-Hip Ratio: Report of a WHO Expert Consultation*; World Health Organization: Geneva, Switzerland, 2008.
21. Clemons, J. Construct Validity of Two Different Methods of Scoring and Performing Push-ups. *J. Strength Cond. Res.* **2019**, *33*, 2971–2980. [CrossRef]
22. Tong, T.K.; Wu, S.; Nie, J. Sport-specific endurance plank test for evaluation of global core muscle function. *Phys. Ther. Sport* **2014**, *15*, 58–63. [CrossRef]
23. Hanson, N.J.; Scheadler, C.M.; Katsavelis, D.; Miller, M.G. Validity of the Wattbike 3-Minute Aerobic Test: Measurement and Estimation of VO_{2max}. *J. Strength Cond. Res.* **2022**, *36*, 400–404. [CrossRef]
24. Storer, T.W.; Davis, J.A.; Caiozzo, V.J. Accurate prediction of VO2max in cycle ergometry. *Med. Sci. Sports Exerc.* **1990**, *22*, 704–712. [CrossRef]
25. Atkinson, G.; Nevill, A.M. Statistical methods for assessing measurement error (reliability) in variables relevant to sports medicine. *Sports Med.* **1998**, *26*, 217–238. [CrossRef] [PubMed]
26. Koo, T.K.; Li, M.Y. A Guideline of Selecting and Reporting Intraclass Correlation Coefficients for Reliability Research. *J. Chiropr. Med.* **2016**, *15*, 155–163. [CrossRef] [PubMed]
27. Ware, J.E.; Keller, S.D.; Kosinski, M. *SF-12: How to Score the SF-12 Physical and Mental Health Summary Scales*; Health Institute, New England Medical Center: Boston, MA, USA, 1995.

28. Ministry of Health. Methodology Report 2017/18: New Zealand Health Survey. 2019. Available online: https://www.health.govt.nz/publication/methodology-report-2017-18-new-zealand-health-survey (accessed on 1 January 2020).
29. Buysse, D.J.; Reynolds, C.F., III; Monk, T.H.; Berman, S.R.; Kupfer, D.J. The Pittsburgh Sleep Quality Index: A new instrument for psychiatric practice and research. *Psychiatry Res.* **1989**, *28*, 193–213. [CrossRef]
30. Myers, J.; Prakash, M.; Froelicher, V.; Do, D.; Partington, S.; Atwood, J.E. Exercise Capacity and Mortality among Men Referred for Exercise Testing. *N. Engl. J. Med.* **2002**, *346*, 793–801. [CrossRef] [PubMed]
31. Egbewale, B.E.; Lewis, M.; Sim, J. Bias, precision and statistical power of analysis of covariance in the analysis of randomized trials with baseline imbalance: A simulation study. *BMC Med. Res. Methodol.* **2014**, *14*, 49. [CrossRef]
32. Cohen, J. *Statistical Power Analysis for the Behavioral Sciences*, 2nd ed.; Taylor & Francis Group: Florence, Italy, 1988.
33. Di Angelantonio, E.; Bhupathiraju, S.N.; Wormser, D.; Gao, P.; Kaptoge, S.; de Gonzalez, A.B.; Cairns, B.J.; Huxley, R.; Jackson, C.L.; Joshy, G.; et al. Body-mass index and all-cause mortality: Individual-participant-data meta-analysis of 239 prospective studies in four continents. *Lancet* **2016**, *388*, 776–786. [CrossRef]
34. Donnelly, J.E.; Blair, S.N.; Jakicic, J.M.; Manore, M.M.; Rankin, J.W.; Smith, B.K. Appropriate Physical Activity Intervention Strategies for Weight Loss and Prevention of Weight Regain for Adults. *Med. Sci. Sports Exerc.* **2009**, *41*, 459–471. [CrossRef]
35. Franz, M.J.; VanWormer, J.J.; Crain, A.L.; Boucher, J.L.; Histon, T.; Caplan, W.; Bowman, J.D.; Pronk, N.P. Weight-Loss Outcomes: A Systematic Review and Meta-Analysis of Weight-Loss Clinical Trials with a Minimum 1-Year Follow-Up. *J. Am. Diet. Assoc.* **2007**, *107*, 1755–1767. [CrossRef]
36. Ross, R.; Neeland, I.J.; Yamashita, S.; Shai, I.; Seidell, J.; Magni, P.; Santos, R.D.; Arsenault, B.; Cuevas, A.; Hu, F.B.; et al. Waist circumference as a vital sign in clinical practice: A Consensus Statement from the IAS and ICCR Working Group on Visceral Obesity. *Nat. Rev. Endocrinol.* **2020**, *16*, 177–189. [CrossRef]
37. Nooyens, A.C.J.; Koppes, L.L.; Visscher, T.L.; Twisk, J.W.; Kemper, H.C.; Schuit, A.J.; van Mechelen, W.; Seidell, J.C. Adolescent skinfold thickness is a better predictor of high body fatness in adults than is body mass index: The Amsterdam Growth and Health Longitudinal Study. *Am. J. Clin. Nutr.* **2007**, *85*, 1533–1539. [CrossRef]
38. Lemes, Í.R.; Turi-Lynch, B.C.; Cavero-Redondo, I.; Linares, S.N.; Monteiro, H.L. Aerobic training reduces blood pressure and waist circumference and increases HDL-c in metabolic syndrome: A systematic review and meta-analysis of randomized controlled trials. *J. Am. Soc. Hypertens.* **2018**, *12*, 580–588. [CrossRef] [PubMed]
39. Huang, G.; Gibson, C.A.; Tran, Z.V.; Osness, W.H. Controlled Endurance Exercise Training and VO2max Changes in Older Adults: A Meta-Analysis. *Prev. Cardiol.* **2005**, *8*, 217–225. [CrossRef] [PubMed]
40. Baron, K.G.; Duffecy, J.; Reutrakul, S.; Levenson, J.C.; McFarland, M.M.; Lee, S.; Qeadan, F. Behavioral interventions to extend sleep duration: A systematic review and meta-analysis. *Sleep Med. Rev.* **2021**, *60*, 101532. [CrossRef] [PubMed]
41. Kettle, V.E.; Madigan, C.D.; Coombe, A.; Graham, H.; Thomas, J.J.C.; Chalkley, A.E.; Daley, A.J. Effectiveness of physical activity interventions delivered or prompted by health professionals in primary care settings: Systematic review and meta-analysis of randomised controlled trials. *BMJ* **2022**, *376*, e068465. [CrossRef] [PubMed]
42. Thomson, C.A.; Ravia, J. A Systematic Review of Behavioral Interventions to Promote Intake of Fruit and Vegetables. *J. Am. Diet. Assoc.* **2011**, *111*, 1523–1535. [CrossRef]
43. Samdal, G.B.; Eide, G.E.; Barth, T.; Williams, G.; Meland, E. Effective behaviour change techniques for physical activity and healthy eating in overweight and obese adults; systematic review and meta-regression analyses. *Int. J. Behav. Nutr. Phys. Act.* **2017**, *14*, 42. [CrossRef]

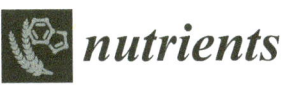

Article

Improving Willingness to Try Fruits and Vegetables and Gross Motor Skills in Preschool Children in Guam

Tanisha F. Aflague [1,*], Grazyna Badowski [1], Hyett Sanchez [1], Dwight Sablan [2], Catherine M. Schroeder [3], Eloise Sanchez [4] and Rachael T. Leon Guerrero [2]

1. College of Natural and Applied Sciences, University of Guam, Mangilao, GU 96923, USA; gbadowski@triton.uog.edu (G.B.); sanchezh@triton.uog.edu (H.S.)
2. Office of Research & Sponsored Programs, University of Guam, Mangilao, GU 96923, USA; sabland9706@triton.uog.edu (D.S.); rachaeltlg@triton.uog.edu (R.T.L.G.)
3. Guam Head Start Program, Guam Department of Education, Barrigada, GU 96913, USA; cmschroeder@gdoe.net
4. Division of Curriculum & Instruction, Guam Department of Education, Barrigada, GU 96913, USA; esanchez@gdoe.net
* Correspondence: taflague@triton.uog.edu; Tel.: +1-671-735-2026

Abstract: Early childhood interventions have the potential to promote long-term healthy eating and physical activity habits to prevent obesity. However, research studies including indigenous young children are lacking. This study examined the effectiveness of the Food Friends®: Fun with New Foods™ and Get Movin' with Mighty Moves™ (FFMM) curricula on willingness to try fruits and vegetables (FV) and gross motor (GM) skills among preschoolers in Guam. A pre-post community-based study included preschoolers from Head Start (HS), gifted and talented education (Pre-GATE), and Pre-Kindergarten programs during school years (SY) 2017–2018 and 2018–2019. In SY2017–2018, the intervention group had a significant increase in imported FV when compared with the other three groups. No significant differences between groups were found on the other FV scales. Regarding gross motor skills, no significant differences between groups were found. In SY2018–2019, the intervention group had a significant increase in all FV scales except imported FV when compared with the enhanced intervention group. With gross motor skills, no significant differences were found between groups on its progress. These results warrant FFMM adaptations for the prevention of obesity among Guam preschoolers.

Keywords: preschool children; motor skills; fruit and vegetable intake; Guam

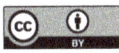

1. Introduction

Early childhood overweight and obesity (OWOB) increases the risk for adult OWOB and associated chronic diseases, which are high among indigenous children [1]. The prevalence of early childhood overweight and obesity (OWOB) in 2011–2012 was 22.8% among 2–5 years old in the US [2]. In 2013, the OWOB prevalence among children 2–8 years old in Guam was 27.4% [3]. Early childhood obesity prevalence was also higher in Guam (13.2%) than the US (8.4%) during the same time and among similar ages [2,3]. Successful obesity interventions for young indigenous and/or socioeconomically disadvantaged children (0–5 years), employed a dual focus on obesity prevention and school readiness, engaged children and parents in educational activities related to nutrition and physical activity, and physical activity sessions that focused on the development of gross motor skills [4].

A recent community randomized environmental childhood obesity intervention in Guam and other jurisdictions in the US Affiliated Pacific region, known as the Children's Healthy Living (CHL) project, found a decrease in OWOB and acanthosis nigricans prevalence in young children after the intervention [5]. One component of the multi-level CHL intervention was the implementation of Food Friends®: Fun with New Foods™ and Get

Movin' with Mighty Moves™ curricula, referred to as "Food Friends and Mighty Moves" or FFMM, in childcare centers [6,7]. Although the outcomes of FFMM were not evaluated independently, the feasibility and implementation in Guam expanded the reach into preschool programs that provide school readiness support and family engagement.

FFMM aims to improve diet quality, such as increasing fruits and vegetables (FV) and physical activity in early childhood by addressing food neophobia and developing gross motor skills, respectively [8,9]. There are limited diet data among young children in Guam, yet one study revealed the mean intake of FV among 2–8-year-olds was 0.88 and 0.61 cups per day, respectively, which does not meet the recommendations [3]. Additionally, the majority of young children exceeded the recommended, 2 h or less, for screen-time with a mean duration of 5.29 h per day [3], which consequently decreases the chance to be physically active.

Early childhood interventions show a great potential to promote the development of long-term healthful habits, such as regular physical activity and healthy eating to prevent obesity [10–12]. One study in Guam found children's willingness to try FV improved after receiving nutrition education [13]. In addition to knowledge, preference is another personal factor that determines children's FV intake. Early food likes and dislikes are influenced by preferences, yet modifiable through repeated exposures to novel and disliked foods in a positive, supportive environment [14,15]. Despite the growing body of childhood obesity research, there is still a lack of research including indigenous young children. Guam is a US territory located in the northwestern Pacific region of Micronesia and the southernmost island of the Mariana Islands where 37% of the population are CHamoru, the indigenous people of Guam; 12% are other Pacific islanders, 26% are Filipino and 7% are other Asian [16].

The Food Friends®: Fun with New Foods™ and Get Movin' with Mighty Moves™, or FFMM, are research-based nutrition and physical activity curricula developed by researchers in Colorado State University. During the CHL program, FFMM was implemented in childcare centers without adaptation and evaluation. For this study, we will examine the effectiveness of the FFMM curricula on willingness to try fruits and vegetables (FV) and gross motor (GM) skills among preschool children in Guam during two school years (i.e., SY2017–2018 and SY2018–2019) as part of a research project to determine the best practices for obesity prevention in Guam.

2. Materials and Methods

2.1. Study Design

This study was a pre-post community-based study design targeting preschool children, 3–5 years old, from three (3) Guam Department of Education (GDOE) preschool programs: Guam Head Start (HS) Program, gifted and talented education pre-Kindergarten (Pre-GATE), and Pre-Kindergarten (Pre-K). "Head Start" is a comprehensive program funded by the U.S. Department of Health & Human Services that promotes school readiness of preschool children, 3–5 years, from low-income families by enhancing their cognitive, social, and emotional development. HS supports children's growth and development in a positive learning environment through comprehensive services in the areas of education and child development, health, and family and community engagement. Locally, the Guam Department of Education is the grantee for Head Start. The GATE pre-K program, referred to as Pre-GATE, implements a curriculum specifically designed for 4 year old gifted children that includes acceleration and enrichment activities to ensure their physical, social, emotional, and intellectual needs are met without pressure and unnecessary structure. The Pre-Kindergarten (Pre-K) program follows the Guam Early Learning Guidelines for young children 3–5 years that focuses on five areas—physical development, health and safety; self-concept and social-emotional development; cognitive development; communication, language development and literacy, and creative development.

During SY2017–2018, preschool programs that were prepared and willing to implement the Food Friends®: Fun with New Foods and Get Movin' with Mighty Moves™

(FFMM) curricula were pre-K (4 classrooms) and Guam HS (7 classrooms). Other preschool programs that participated in this study in SY2017–2018, were half-day Guam HS sites (7 classrooms) and the pre-GATE program (4 classrooms) from the same villages that did not receive FFMM. For the Guam HS Program a standard curriculum implemented in all HS classrooms was "I Am Moving, I Am Learning (IMIL)", which has similar components to FFMM. IMIL was a curriculum used in previous years for all Guam Head Start Program classrooms which includes a flexible framework of strategies to promote movement skills, healthy eating, parent engagement, and a healthy workplace and community [17]. Among the Guam HS Program: (1) classrooms that were transitioning to full-day schedules and, therefore, had the need for additional classroom activities implemented FFMM plus IMIL (classified for this study as "Enhanced Intervention"); (2) classrooms that had a half-day schedule implemented only IMIL (classified for this study as "Standard"). Pre-K program classrooms that only implemented FFMM were classified as "Intervention" and Pre-GATE program classrooms that did not receive either FFMM or IMIL were the "Control". During SY2018–2019, all HS classrooms (i.e., half-day and full-day) implemented both FFMM and IMIL (classified for this study as "Enhanced Intervention") and Pre-GATE and Pre-K implemented FFMM only (considered for this study as "Intervention").

Child participants were recruited from study sites (i.e., preschool classrooms) during orientation or the first week of school. Research staff conducted study presentations at orientation or distributed recruitment packets (e.g., recruitment flyer and study forms) to parents. Parents provided consent for their child (ren) to participate and completed the About My Child (i.e., age, sex, ethnicity/race) and healthy behavior forms. The data from the behavior forms were not used in this study. Child assent was obtained for pre- and post-assessments. Child participants were provided a USD 10 gift card after completing each assessment. The University of Guam (UOG) Institutional Review Board (CHRS 17-139) and Guam Department of Education approved the study protocols.

2.2. Study Participants

There were a total of 316 children recruited from all sites during SY2017–2018, where 110 received the enhanced intervention, 63 received the intervention, 92 received the standard, and 51 were in the control group. All study sites (i.e., enhanced intervention, intervention, standard, and control) received the FFMM curricula the following year, SY2018–2019, where 355 children participated in the study activities, specifically the pre- and post-assessments. Notably, all children received FFMM in intervention sites no matter if they participated in the study or not in both study years.

2.3. Intervention

The intervention was implemented by trained teachers and teachers' aides working within the study sites (i.e., preschool classrooms). FFMM teacher training was conducted prior to classroom implementation by one of the FFMM developers and/or trained research staff. A major component of the curricula are the eight (8) Food Friends (stuffed puppets) characters that are incorporated in lesson activities and featured in lesson materials for both children and parents [18], which was a component of training. Food service provider training was also conducted by trained research staff prior to the implementation of the FF on food preparation and delivery schedule to support taste tests.

The Food Friends®: Fun with New Foods™ (FF) curriculum was implemented in September until December of each school year. Teachers preferred to implement FF a few weeks after the start of the school year for preschoolers to acclimate. The FF intervention program lasted 12 weeks, with two lessons per week, for a total of 24 lessons. Each week children participated in hands-on food and nutrition activities, story time, and/or taste tests that lasted about 15–20 min. Children were given repeated exposures to the same new foods (i.e., Gouda cheese and raw daikon radish) for eight weeks followed by weekly opportunities to try new foods (foods varied based on seasonality/availability) [8]. During these months, lesson foods were most available, which also informed the FF curriculum implementation timeline.

The Get Movin' with Mighty Moves™ (MM) curriculum was implemented each school year from January to May, which was ideal for implementing all 18-weeks of the curriculum. Teachers had up to four (4) lessons per week to select from and were asked to implement at least two (2) lessons each week, for a total of 36–72 lessons. Children participated in activities that focused on one of the gross motor skill categories each week: stability (e.g., trunk strength), locomotor (e.g., running, hopping, skipping), or manipulation (e.g., ball skills) and described in detail elsewhere [9].

2.4. Evaluations

Data collection was conducted at each study site before and after the implementation of both curricula, FFMM, which was within two weeks after the start and before the end of the school year, respectively. This aligned with program assessments that are a regular part of each preschool program. Study assessments did not take away from instructional time and did not appear to be different from ongoing school day activities.

Children's willingness to try new foods and FV were assessed using the validated *Adapted WillTry* tool for children 3–11 years in Guam [13,19,20]. Only FV data will be reported in this study, which were captured in one of four FV scales in the *Adapted WillTry* tool: local novel (6 items), local common (4 items), imported (3 items), and total FV (14 items) [19]. Trained research staff conducted one-to-one interviews with children, where children self-reported their willingness to try new foods and FV. These methods have been tested in a similar population in Guam and described elsewhere [13].

Gross motor skills were observed and recorded using the Get Movin' with Mighty Moves™ Pre- and Post- Program Evaluation Tool and Guidelines (provided with the curriculum) [9], which consists of five (5) items assessing: (1) standing on one foot (dominant and non-dominant leg), (2) standing on tiptoes, (3) walking line backward, (4) tossing ball underhand (distance), and (5) tossing ball with or without opposition. Each gross motor skill was assigned a score to determine proficiency (i.e., 1) or levels (i.e., 1, 2, or 3) based on the age-appropriate criteria outlined in the Get Movin' with Mighty Moves™ Pre- and Post- Program Evaluation Tool and referenced in standard assessment tools used in Guam preschool programs, such as Brigance® Early Childhood Screen III and Developmental Indicators for the Assessment of Learning (DIAL-4). Standing on one foot (dominant) and the other (non-dominant) was given a score of "1" if held for 5 s or more for 3-year-olds and 10 s or more for 4- and 5-year-olds. Similarly, "1" was scored if a child could stand on tiptoes for 4 s or more for 3-year-olds or 8 s or more for 4- and 5-year-olds. Durations less than the criteria for these skills were assigned a score of "0". All children were scored "1" for less than 2 steps, "2" for 2–4 steps, and "3" for 5 steps or more when they were observed walking line backward (toe-to-heel). Any child that tossed the ball underhand more than 10-feet was scored with "1" and less than 10-feet was scored "0". While observing the same child toss the ball underhand, research staff also observed whether the child used opposition "1" or no opposition "0". The Pre- and Post-Program Evaluation Tool describes opposition as tossing the ball underhand, rotating upper body, moving arms in opposition to legs, and beginning toss by moving arms down and back.

2.5. Data Analysis

All data collection forms were created in Qualtrics and used for data entry, then exported as an Excel file that was imported into SPSS (version 27). Double-data entry procedures were used. Two-way mixed ANOVAs were used to examine between (group) and within subjects (pre- and post-assessment) program effects for all *Adapted WillTry* FV scores and both study years. For SY2017–2018, groups were defined as enhanced intervention (i.e., FFMM and IMIL), intervention (i.e., FFMM only), standard (i.e., IMIL only), and control. For SY2018–2019, intervention groups were categorized as enhanced intervention (i.e., Head Start) and intervention (i.e., pre-GATE and pre-K). Simple main effect analyses were conducted when ANOVA revealed significant interactions. The Bonferroni correction was used to adjust for multiple comparisons. *Adapted WillTry* FV pre- and post-means with standard deviations (SDs) were reported for local novel, local common, imported categories, and total FV scales.

Once proficiency was calculated for each gross motor skill the number of children that were proficient in each skill was calculated and reported in percent for each study year, except walking line backward for which means were reported. An exact McNemar's test was used to examine the difference in the proportion of children proficient in each skill pre- and post-intervention. A Wilcoxon test was conducted to determine the effect of the intervention on walking line backward performance. Multiple logistic regression was used to examine the differences in post-percentages between groups and adjusted for pre-percentages, sex, age and ethnicity. p-values < 0.05 were considered statistically significant.

3. Results

Demographic characteristics of the child participants are presented in Table 1. The majority of children were CHamoru or Filipino and 4–6 years old in both study years.

Table 1. Characteristics of child study participants in Guam preschool programs that received FFMM, IMIL, both, or none during two school years (i.e., SY2017–2018 and SY2018–2019).

Child Characteristics	SY2017–2018 (n = 316)				SY2018–2019 (n = 355)	
	Enhanced Intervention [1]	Intervention [2]	Standard [3]	Control [4]	Enhanced Intervention [1]	Intervention [2]
Sex [a]						
Female	51 (46.4)	26 (41.3)	44 (47.8)	29 (56.9)	102 (43.8)	63 (51.6)
Male	59 (53.6)	37 (58.7)	48 (52.2)	22 (43.1)	131 (56.2)	59 (48.4)
Age [1] **(years)**						
2–3	11 (11.1)	0 (0.0)	18 (22.5)	0 (0.0)	35 (15.6)	2 (1.7)
4–6	88 (88.9)	60 (100.0)	62 (77.5)	51 (100.0)	189 (84.4)	116 (98.3)
Ethnicity [a]						
CHamoru	44 (40.0)	21 (33.9)	56 (61.5)	15 (29.4)	117 (50.0)	31 (27.2)
Filipino	27 (24.5)	23 (37.1)	14 (15.4)	20 (39.2)	40 (17.1)	38 (33.3)
Other Asian	2 (1.8)	7 (11.3)	2 (2.2)	4 (7.8)	9 (3.8)	10 (8.8)
Other Pacific Islander	22 (20.0)	1 (1.6)	12 (13.2)	1 (2.0)	51 (21.8)	5 (4.4)
2+ race/ethnic groups and other [b]	15 (13.6)	10 (16.1)	7 (7.7)	11 (21.6)	17 (7.3)	30 (26.3)

[1] Preschool children received Food Friends®: Fun with New Foods and Get Movin' with Mighty Moves™ (FFMM) and I am Moving, I am Learning (IMIL) lessons. [2] Preschool children received Food Friends®: Fun with New Foods and Get Movin' with Mighty Moves™ (FFMM) lessons. [3] Preschool children received I am Moving, I am Learning (IMIL) lessons. [4] Preschool children with no intervention. [a] Not all parents reported child participant characteristics; therefore, n is different for sex, age group, and ethnicity. [b] Child participants that identified as Black, White, American Indian or Alaska Native or with two (2) or more race/ethnic groups.

Four (4) individual two-way mixed ANOVAs were performed for each school year separately. The *Adapted WillTry* FV scores for local novel, local common, imported, and total FV were the dependent variables. In SY2017–2018, the interaction between time and group were not significant for local novel, local common, and total *Adapted WillTry* FV scores, but there was a significant interaction between time and groups on the imported *Adapted WillTry* FV score. Post-hoc test using the Bonferroni correction revealed that the intervention group had a significant increase in imported *Adapted WillTry* FV score when compared with the other three groups (Table 2).

In SY2018–2019, there was a significant interaction between the group and time on all *Adapted WillTry* FV scores except imported *Adapted WillTry* FV. The intervention group (i.e., non-HS) had significantly lower total, local novel and local common *Adapted WillTry* pre-scores than the enhanced intervention group. After completing FFMM, the intervention group showed a significant increase for all *Adapted WillTry* FV scores. The mean *Adapted WillTry* FV scores did not change over time in the enhanced intervention group and both groups had similar post-scores (Table 2).

Table 2. Means, standard deviations (SD), and mixed ANOVAs interaction effects between time and group for all Adapted WillTry fruit and vegetable (FV) pre- and post-scores by study group in both school years [a].

Adapted WillTry FV Scales	SY2017–2018								p	η^2_p
	Enhanced Intervention [1]		Intervention [2]		Standard [3]		Control [4]			
	Pre	Post	Pre	Prost	Pre	Post	Pre	Post		
	Mean ± SD		Mean ± SD		Mean ± SD		Mean ± SD			
Total FV	2.52 ± 0.69	2.40 ± 0.66	2.16 ± 0.74	2.31 ± 0.56	2.46 ± 0.66	2.40 ± 0.64	2.3 ± 0.72	2.20 ± 0.61	0.220	0.023
Local Novel	2.45 ± 0.78	2.25 ± 0.75	2.04 ± 0.83	2.16 ± 0.66	2.36 ± 0.78	2.21 ± 0.79	2.17 ± 0.85	2.06 ± 0.77	0.242	0.020
Local Common	2.47 ± 0.75	2.42 ± 0.71	2.21 ± 0.77	2.25 ± 0.67	2.34 ± 0.77	2.36 ± 0.74	2.37 ± 0.75	2.19 ± 0.76	0.517	0.011
Imported	2.72 ± 0.52	2.68 ± 0.56	2.41 ± 0.73	2.75 ± 0.5 [a]	2.74 ± 0.44	2.70 ± 0.5	2.62 ± 0.53	2.50 ± 0.53	0.001 [b]	0.072

	SY2018–2019				p	η^2_p
	Enhanced Intervention [1]		Intervention [2]			
	Pre	Post	Pre	Post		
	Mean ± SD		Mean ± SD			
Total FV	2.49 ± 0.63	2.49 ± 0.55	2.22 ± 0.61	2.47 ± 0.54 [a]	0.012	0.029
Local Novel	2.41 ± 0.72	2.37 ± 0.68	2.03 ± 0.76	2.31 ± 0.72 [a]	0.011	0.030
Local common	2.49 ± 0.73	2.51 ± 0.63	2.29 ± 0.68	2.52 ± 0.55 [a]	0.041	0.019
Imported	2.67 ± 0.54	2.72 ± 0.49	2.62 ± 0.47	2.79 ± 0.37 [a,b]	0.131	0.011

p: p-value of the time x group interaction effect determined by two-way mixed ANOVA. η^2_p: partial eta squared. [1] Preschool children received Food Friends®: Fun with New Foods and Get Movin' with Mighty Moves™ (FFMM) and I am Moving, I am Learning (IMIL) lessons. [2] Preschool children received Food Friends®: Fun with New Foods and Get Movin' with Mighty Moves™ (FFMM) lessons. [3] Preschool children received I am Moving, I am Learning (IMIL) lessons. [4] Preschool children with no intervention. [a] $p < 0.05$ versus pre-score. [b] The intervention group had a significant increase on imported FV values when compared with the other 3 groups as determined by Bonferroni test.

For SY2017–2018, it was hypothesized that the intervention groups (i.e., enhanced intervention and intervention) would have higher levels of proficiency for all motor skills than other groups. To examine this hypothesis, multiple logistic regression of the post-scores for each motor skill were conducted. There were no significant differences ($p < 0.05$) between any of the groups for all gross motor skills post-scores, even after adjusting for sex, age, ethnicity and pre-scores. Within-group comparisons of changes in skills over time were examined using McNemar's and Wilcoxon tests. The enhanced intervention group was the only one that improved all stability gross motor skills ($p < 0.05$), that is standing on one leg (either leg) and standing on tiptoes. The intervention group significantly increased two stability gross motor skills ($p < 0.05$) and significantly decreased one gross motor skill (tossing ball underhand—opposition). The standard group only improved one stability gross motor skill and the control group improved in two stability gross motor skills. None of the groups improved in tossing a ball (distance) (Table 3).

In SY2018–2019 no significant differences were found in all gross motor skills post-scores between the two groups even after adjusting for sex, age, ethnicity and pre-scores. Within-group analyses revealed a significant improvement in all GM skills ($p < 0.05$), except tossing ball underhand (opposition) in the enhanced intervention group, and tossing ball underhand (distance) and tossing a ball underhand (opposition) in the intervention group (Table 4).

Table 3. Percent of preschool child participants that met gross motor (GM) skill proficiency and mean scale score for walking line backgrounds at pre- and post-study period during school year (SY) 2017–2018.

	SY2017–2018											
	Enhanced Intervention [1] (n = 53)			Intervention [2] (n = 48)			Standard [3] (n = 45)			Control (n = 33)		
Gross Motor Skill	Pre (%)	Post	p-Value	Pre (%)	Post	p-Value	Pre (%)	Post	p-Value	Pre (%)	Post	p-Value
Standing on 1 foot (dominant Leg)	34.0	58.5	0.011 [a]	41.7	66.7	0.017 [a]	37.8	60.0	0.031 [a]	39.4	63.6	0.057 [a]
Standing on 1 foot (non-dominant leg)	30.2	58.5	0.001 [a]	35.4	62.5	0.021 [a]	35.6	51.1	0.143 [a]	33.3	57.6	0.039 [a]
Standing on tiptoes	30.2	56.6	0.014 [a]	45.8	62.5	0.152 [a]	42.2	60.0	0.115 [a]	42.2	81.8	<0.001 [a]
Tossing ball-underhand (distance)	37.5	36.8	>0.999 [a]	48.0	30.0	0.093 [a]	45.5	48.9	>0.999 [a]	37.5	33.3	>0.999 [a]
Tossing ball-underhand (opposition)	83.8	73.7	0.18 [a]	96.0	66.0	<0.001 [a]	88.9	75.6	0.146 [a]	87.5	72.7	0.180 [a]
	Means			Means			Means			Means		
Walking line backward (toe-to-heel) [b]	2.21	1.96	0.062 [b]	2.18	2.08	0.539 [b]	2.02	1.8	0.174 [b]	2.09	2.13	0.875 [b]

[1] Preschool children received Food Friends®: Fun with New Foods and Get Movin' with Mighty Moves™ (FFMM) and I am Moving, I am Learning (IMIL) lessons. [2] Preschool children received Food Friends®: Fun with New Foods and Get Movin' with Mighty Moves™ (FFMM) lessons. [3] Preschool children received I am Moving, I am Learning (IMIL) lessons. [a] Based on McNemar's test. [b] Means for the scale is reported. p-values are based on Wilcoxon test.

Table 4. Percent of preschool child participants that met gross motor (GM) skill proficiency and mean scale score for walking line backgrounds at pre- and post-intervention during school year (SY) 2018–2019.

	SY2018–2019					
	Enhanced Intervention [1] (n = 150 to 162)			Intervention [2] (n = 93 to 104)		
Gross Motor Skill	Pre (%)	Post	p-Value	Pre (%)	Post	p-Value
Standing on 1 foot (dominant leg)	37.0	56.0	0.001 [a]	50.0	66.7	0.006 [a]
Standing on 1 foot (non-dominant leg)	24.1	50.0	<0.001 [a]	34.0	55.9	0.002 [a]
Standing on tiptoes	34.6	55.0	<0.001 [a]	35.0	57.0	0.001 [a]
Tossing ball-underhand (distance)	39.3	58.0	0.008 [a]	37.5	44.7	0.201 [a]
Tossing ball-underhand (opposition)	61.8	65.8	0.457 [a]	61.5	67.0	0.243 [a]
	Means		p-value	Means		p-value
Walking line backward (toe-to-heel) [b]	1.56	1.78	0.008 [b]	1.60	1.98	0.018 [b]

[1] Preschool children received Food Friends®: Fun with New Foods and Get Movin' with Mighty Moves™ (FFMM) and I am Moving, I am Learning (IMIL) lessons. [2] Preschool children received Food Friends®: Fun with New Foods and Get Movin' with Mighty Moves™ (FFMM) lessons. [a] Based on McNemar's test. [b] Means for the scale reported. p-values are based on Wilcoxon test.

4. Discussion

In SY2017–2018, there were differences in *Adapted WillTry* FV scores. The intervention group had a significant increase in imported *Adapted WillTry* FV scores when compared with the other three groups. No significant differences between groups were found on the other *Adapted WillTry* FV scores. The post-score of imported *Adapted WillTry* FV in the intervention group was significantly higher than the pre-score. Since the enhanced intervention (i.e., HS) was composed of both the FFMM and the IMIL curricula, it was expected that this group would demonstrate greater improvements in the *Adapted WillTry* FV scores compared to the intervention group; however, this was not the case. The enhanced intervention group actually demonstrated a decrease, although not significant, on all FV scores. The reason for this is unknown, but may be due to the enhanced intervention teachers focusing on implementing their required curriculum, IMIL, and only teaching the FFMM when time allowed. In addition, the intervention group had significantly lower *Adapted WillTry* FV scores (all $p \leq 0.01$) at pre-assessment compared to the enhanced intervention group (i.e., HS). Therefore, FFMM may be more effective in improving willingness to try FV among children that initially have a low willingness to try FV (score). The community-based study design may have also contributed to the lack significant improvements of *Adapted WillTry* FV scores among children who received the enhanced intention in SY2017–2018. FFMM was implemented in the Pre-K program (four classrooms) and only full-day classrooms in the Guam Head Start Program (seven classrooms), which was also the first year (SY2017–2018) to pilot a full-day class schedule in the Guam Head Start Program. To fulfill the day's activities, full-day classrooms continued to implement the curriculum, "I Am Moving, I Am Learning" (IMIL) in addition to implementing the FFMM intervention. Similarly, the Guam Head Start Program half-day classrooms implemented IMIL that has similar components to the FFMM intervention. The effect of the FFMM intervention on willingness to try FV may have been attenuated by the implementation of IMIL in both HS groups.

As mentioned previously, the intervention only demonstrated a significant improvements in imported *Adapted WillTry* FV scores in SY2017–2018. This may be due to several factors. First, the post- *Adapted WillTry* tool was administered at the end of the SY, 5 months after the FF curriculum ended. Therefore, children may have forgotten some of the local common and local novel foods they had been introduced to earlier in the school year. Second, the FFMM curriculum may need to be modified so that it is more culturally relevant and better promotes local FV. Third, previous studies have shown that there is an abundance of imported and processed foods on Guam [21], and a majority of Guam residents consume a high volume of processed foods that are imported [3,22]. Thus, imported foods, including FV, are acceptable and possibly even desirable to Guam residents, including children. The abundance, acceptability, and easy access to imported foods on Guam may have contributed to higher imported *Adapted WillTry* FV scores, especially if the FFML curriculum promoted mainly imported FV.

In SY2017–2018, there were no significant differences in gross motor skills found between groups. The group that had a greater increase in gross motor skills was the enhanced intervention group (i.e., Guam Head Start program), with a significant improvement on all stability gross motor skills. This was expected as the enhanced intervention group was exposed to both the FFML and the IMIL curricula. Unfortunately, authors are uncertain as to the exact number of lessons given to each group as teachers were inconsistent in their intervention fidelity reports. However, having both IMIL and/or FFMM positively influenced gross motor skill development.

In SY2018–2019, the intervention group reported significant increases in all *Adapted WillTry* FV scores except imported FV when compared with the enhanced intervention group (i.e., Guam Head Start program). All *Adapted WillTry* FV scores improved from pre- to post- in the intervention group. The children in the enhanced intervention group may have had a higher willingness to try (score) at pre-assessment related to the family style mealtimes during the school day which supports FV intake [23]. For the enhanced intervention group, most *Adapted WillTry* FV scores were in the expected direction, yet the increase was not significant. Being that the FFMM curricula was developed in Colorado and used food and food characters (stuffed puppets) known to this state (e.g., hamburger puppet), curricula modifications to include local foods and cultural components to be more relevant to Guam residents, predominantly CHamorus and Filipinos, are warranted. Regarding gross motor skills, no significant differences were found between groups during their progression over the school year. Stability gross motor skills improved in both groups and the enhanced intervention group also improved in tossing the ball–underhand (distance) and walking the line backwards.

The actual child eating behavior of trying new foods has been related to children who perceive themselves as more willing to try [24]. In this study children's self-competence to try new foods was assessed immediately followed by observations of willingness to taste novel foods. Although *Adapted WillTry* FV post-scores were assessed approximately 5 months after the FF curriculum ended, which was at the end of the school year after the MM curriculum was completed, the mean *Adapted WillTry* scores for all the FV scales maintained a trend (from high to low) in willingness to try imported, local common, and local novel FV observed in previous studies [11,19]. This was observed for pre- and post-assessment mean scores and for all groups in both study years, demonstrating the robustness of the *Adapted WillTry* tool and FV scales; and indicating that preschool children in Guam are more likely to try (eat) imported FV over local FV, which further justifies the need for a culturally relevant curriculum to promote local FV.

Although the community-based study design may have influenced the study outcomes, this study included new and long-standing preschool programs in Guam that, for the first time, implemented the same curricula in a unified approach to reach young children during SY2018–2019. This study also demonstrated the sustainability of one of the components of the multi-level CHL intervention, and further demonstrating the feasibility and implementation of FFMM in Guam. None of the study activities, including FFMM implementation and assessments, interrupted the regular school day activities. The food tasting activities complemented the family style mealtimes in the Head Start program and were the only food-related activity in the classroom for Pre-GATE and Pre-K. The FFMM curricula addressed the Pre-Kindergarten Curriculum Standards in the areas of health, physical education, fine arts, language arts/reading, math, social science, and science. Overall, this study helps to fill a research gap in the Pacific region as diet and physical activity is not well documented in indigenous peoples, such as CHamorus and other Pacific Islanders, especially young children.

This study is not without limitations. Researchers and staff asked teachers to complete fidelity logs to document the number of lessons completed; however, not all teachers completed or submitted logs. We were unable to assess lesson dose and compare groups. Due to the nature of this community-based study, the number of lessons likely varied related to unplanned events, such as fire drills or seasonal weather disturbances (e.g., tropical depressions). Similarly, restricting the type of activities that took place in the classroom was not possible with regard to lesson plans and/or curriculum. The Guam Head Start Program is required to address health and wellness in the school-day and used IMIL when FFMM was not implemented, such as in the standard group during SY2017–2018. Another limitation was attrition—not all students completed all assessment periods due to being absent or refusal related to competing activities (e.g., children playing, class activity).

5. Conclusions

In SY2017–2018, no differences in GM skills were found among groups; however, there was an improvement in three of six GM skills in enhanced intervention and intervention groups. There was an increase in the willingness to try imported FV in the intervention group. In SY2018–2019, four of six GM skills significantly improved for both groups. Willingness to try FV only improved for children participating in non-HS programs. FFMM adaptations/modifications are needed to be more culturally relevant to Guam, especially in HS programs.

Author Contributions: The following authors contributed the following: conceptualization, T.F.A. and R.T.L.G.; methodology, T.F.A.; data curation, G.B. and D.S.; formal analysis, G.B. and D.S.; investigation, T.F.A. and H.S.; resources, C.M.S. and E.S.; writing—original draft preparation, H.S. and T.F.A.; writing—review and editing, R.T.L.G., T.F.A., E.S., G.B. and H.S.; visualization, R.T.L.G. and T.F.A.; supervision, R.T.L.G., C.M.S. and E.S.; project administration, T.F.A.; funding acquisition, R.T.L.G. and T.F.A. All authors have read and agreed to the published version of the manuscript.

Funding: This research was funded by Hatch, National Institute of Food and Agriculture, United States Department of Agriculture, grant number 1008850.

Institutional Review Board Statement: The study was conducted according to the guidelines of the Declaration of Helsinki, and approved by the Institutional Review Board (Committee on Human Research Subjects) of the University of Guam (CHRS #17-139, 12 September 2017).

Informed Consent Statement: Informed consent and assent was obtained from all subjects involved in the study.

Data Availability Statement: The data presented in this study are available on request from the corresponding author. The data are not publicly available due to privacy restrictions.

Acknowledgments: The authors thank the Guam Head Start, DOE Pre-GATE, and DOE Pre-K programs and the families and children who participated in the study; Laura Bellows and the University of Colorado Food Science and Human Nutrition for permission to use FFMM and training provided; and Sodexo and Guam DOE food services and Pay-Less Super Markets for the support provided for the taste tests.

Conflicts of Interest: The authors declare no conflict of interest. The funders had no role in the design of the study; in the collection, analyses, or interpretation of data; in the writing of the manuscript, or in the decision to publish the results.

References

1. Geserick, M.; Vogel, M.; Gaushe, R.; Lipek, T.; Spielau, U.; Keller, E.; Pfäffle, R.; Kiess, W.; Körner, A. Acceleration of BMI in Early Childhood and Risk of Sustained Obesity. *N. Engl. J. Med.* **2018**, *379*, 1303–1312. [CrossRef]
2. Ogden, C.L.; Carroll, M.D.; Kit, B.K.; Flegal, K.M. Prevalence of childhood and adult obesity in the United States, 2011–2012. *JAMA* **2014**, *311*, 806–814. [CrossRef] [PubMed]
3. Leon Guerrero, R.T.; Barber, L.R.; Aflague, T.F.; Paulino, Y.C.; Hattori-Uchima, M.P.; Acosta, M.; Wilkens, L.R.; Novotny, R. Prevalence and Predictors of Overweight and Obesity among Young Children in the Children's Healthy Living Study on Guam. *Nutrients* **2020**, *12*, 2527. [CrossRef] [PubMed]
4. Laws, R.; Campbell, K.J.; van der Pligt, P.; Russell, G.; Ball, K.; Lynch, J.; David, C.; Taylor, R.; Askew, D.; Denney-Wilson, E. The impact of interventions to prevent obesity or improve obesity related behaviours in children (0–5 years) from socioeconomically disadvantaged and/or indigenous families: A systematic review. *BMC Public Health* **2014**, *14*, 779. [CrossRef]
5. Novotny, R.; Davis, J.; Butel, J.; Boushey, C.J.; Fialkowski, M.K.; Nigg, C.R.; Braun, K.L.; Leon Guerrero, R.T.; Coleman, P.; Bersamin, A.; et al. Effect of the Children's Healthy Living Program on Young Child Overweight, Obesity, and Acanthosis Nigricans in the US-Affiliated Pacific Region: A Randomized Clinical Trial. *JAMA Netw. Open* **2018**, *1*, e183896. [CrossRef] [PubMed]
6. Wilken, L.R.; Novotny, R.; Fialkowski, M.K.; Boushey, C.J.; Nigg, C.; Paulino, Y.; Leon Guerrero, R.; Bersamin, A.; Vargo, D.; Kim, J.; et al. Children's Healthy Living (CHL) Program for remote underserved minority populations in the Pacific region: Rationale and design of a community randomized trial to prevent early childhood obesity. *BMC Public Health* **2013**, *13*, 944. [CrossRef]
7. Fialkowski, M.K.; DeBaryshe, B.; Bersamin, A.; Nigg, C.; Leon Guerrero, R.; Rojas, G.; Areta, A.R.; Vargo, A.; Belyeu-Camacho, T.; Castro, R.; et al. A community engagement process identifies environmental priorities to prevent early childhood obesity: The Children's Healthy Living (CHL) program for remote underserved populations in the US Affiliated Pacific Islands, Hawaii and Alaska. *Matern. Child Health J.* **2014**, *18*, 2261–2274. [CrossRef] [PubMed]
8. Young, L.; Anderson, J.; Beckstrom, L.; Bellows, L.; Johnson, S.L. Making new foods fun for kids. *J. Nutr. Edu. Behav.* **2003**, *35*, 337–338. [CrossRef]
9. Bellows, L.L.; Daivies, P.L.; Anderson, J.; Kennedy, C. Effectiveness of a Physical Activity Intervention for Head Start Preschoolers: A randomized Intervention Study. *Am. J. Occup. Ther.* **2013**, *67*, 28–36. [CrossRef]

10. Pandita, A.; Sharma, D.; Pandita, D.; Pawar, S.; Tariq, M.; Kaul, A. Childhood obesity: Prevention is better than cure. *Diabetes Metab. Syndr. Obes.* **2016**, *9*, 83–89. [CrossRef]
11. Foster, B.A.; Farragher, J.; Parker, P.; Sosa, E.T. Treatment interventions for early childhood obesity: A systematic review. *Acad. Pediatr.* **2015**, *15*, 353–361. [CrossRef] [PubMed]
12. Gubbels, J.S.; Kremmers, S.P.; Stafleu, A.; Goldbohn, A.R.; de Vris, N.K.; Thijs, C. Clustering of energy balance-related in 5 years old children: Lifestyle patterns and their longitudinal association with weight status development in early childhood. *Int. J. Behav. Nutr. Phys. Act.* **2012**, *9*, 77. [CrossRef] [PubMed]
13. Aflague, T.F.; Leon Guerrero, R.T.; Delormier, T.; Novotny, R.; Wilkens, L.R.; Boushey, C.J. Examining the Influence of Cultural Immersion on Willingness to Try Fruits and Vegetables among Children in Guam: The Traditions Pilot Study. *Nutrients* **2019**, *12*, 18. [CrossRef] [PubMed]
14. Rasmussen, M.; Krølner, R.; Klepp, K.I.; Lytle, L.; Brug, J.; Due, P. Determinants of fruit and vegetable consumption among children and adolescents: A review of the literature. Part I: Quantitative studies. *Int. J. Behav. Nutr. Phys. Act.* **2006**, *3*, 22. [CrossRef]
15. Ventura, A.K.; Worobey, J. Early influences on the development of food preferences. *Curr. Biol.* **2013**, *23*, R401–R408. [CrossRef]
16. US Census Bureau. Guam State Data Center Bureau of Statistics and Plans. 2010 Census of Population Housing Guam. Demographic Profile Summary File. 2012. Available online: http://bsp.guam.gov/index.php?option=com_content&view=artcile&id=166%3A2010-census-demographic-profile-summary-file&catid=1&Itemid=100008 (accessed on 30 August 2021).
17. SNAP-Ed Toolkit. I Am Moving, I Am Learning (IMIL). Available online: https://snapedtoolkit.org/interventions/programs/i-am-moving-i-am-learning-imil/ (accessed on 27 September 2021).
18. Johnson, S.L.; Bellows, L.; Beckstrom, L.; Anderson, J. Evaluation of a social marketing campaign targeting preschool children. *Am. J. Health Behav.* **2007**, *31*, 44–55. [CrossRef]
19. Aflague, T.F.; Leon Guerrero, R.T.; Boushey, C.J. Adaptation and evaluation of the WillTry tool to assess willingness to try fruits and vegetables among children 3–11y in Guam. *Prev. Chronic. Dis.* **2014**, *11*, E142. [CrossRef]
20. Thomson, J.L.; McCabe-Sellers, B.J.; Strickland, E.; Lovera, D.; Nuss, H.J.; Yadrick, K.; Duke, S.; Bogle, M.L. Development and evaluation of WillTry. An instrument for measuring children's willingness to try fruits and vegetables. *Appetite* **2010**, *54*, 465–472. [CrossRef]
21. Snowdon, W.; Raj, A.; Reeve, E.; LeonGuerrero, R.; Fesaitu, J.; Cateine, K.; Guignet, C. Processed foods available in the Pacific Islands. *Global Health* **2013**, *9*, 53. [CrossRef]
22. Leon Guerrero, R.; Paulino, Y.; Novotny, R.; Murphy, S. Diet and obesity among Chamorro and Filipino adults on Guam. *Asia Pac. J. Clin. Nutr.* **2008**, *17*, 216–222.
23. Harnack, L.J.; Oakes, J.M.; Fench, S.A.; Rydell, S.A.; Farah, F.M.; Taylor, G.L. Results from an experimental trial at head starts center to evaluate two meal service appropriate to increase fruit and vegetable intake of preschool aged children. *Int. J. Behav. Nutr. Phys. Act.* **2012**, *9*, 51. [CrossRef] [PubMed]
24. Johnsson, S.L.; Moding, K.J.; Maloney, K.; Bellows, L.L. Development of the Trying New Foods Scale: A preschooler self-assessment of willingness to try new foods. *Appetite* **2018**, *128*, 21–31. [CrossRef] [PubMed]

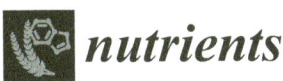

Article

The Effects of a Brief Lifestyle Intervention on the Health of Overweight Airline Pilots during COVID-19: A 12-Month Follow-Up Study

Daniel Wilson [1,2,*], Matthew Driller [3], Paul Winwood [2], Ben Johnston [4] and Nicholas Gill [2,5]

1. Te Huataki Waiora School of Health, The University of Waikato, Hamilton 3216, New Zealand
2. Faculty of Health, Education and Environment, Toi Ohomai Institute of Technology, Tauranga 3112, New Zealand; paul.winwood@toiohomai.ac.nz (P.W.); nicholas.gill@waikato.ac.nz (N.G.)
3. Sport and Exercise Science, School of Allied Health, Human Services and Sport, La Trobe University, Melbourne 3086, Australia; m.driller@latrobe.edu.au
4. Aviation and Occupational Health Unit, Air New Zealand, Auckland 1142, New Zealand; ben.johnston@otago.ac.nz
5. New Zealand Rugby, Wellington 6011, New Zealand
* Correspondence: daniel.wilson@toiohomai.ac.nz; Tel.: +64-75576035

Abstract: The aim of this study was to perform a 12-month follow-up of health parameters after a 17-week lifestyle intervention in overweight airline pilots. A parallel-group (intervention and control) study was conducted amongst 72 overweight airline pilots (body mass index > 25) over a 12-month period following the emergence of COVID-19. The intervention group ($n = 35$) received a personalized dietary, sleep, and physical activity program over a 17-week period. The control group ($n = 37$) received no intervention. Measurements for subjective health (physical activity, sleep quality and quantity, fruit and vegetable intake, and self-rated health) via an electronic survey, and objective measures of body mass and blood pressure were taken at baseline and at 12 months. Significant interactions for group × time from baseline to 12-months were found for all outcome measures ($p < 0.001$). Body mass and mean arterial pressure significantly decreased in the intervention group when compared to the control group ($p < 0.001$). Outcome measures for subjective health (physical activity, sleep quality and quantity, fruit and vegetable intake, and self-rated health) significantly increased in the intervention group when compared to the control group ($p < 0.001$). Results provide preliminary evidence that a brief three-component healthy sleep, diet and physical activity intervention can elicit and sustain long-term improvements in body mass and blood pressure management, health behaviors, and perceived subjective health in pilots and may support quality of life during an unprecedented global pandemic.

Keywords: healthy eating; weight loss; moderate-to-vigorous physical activity; sleep; lifestyle medicine

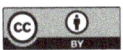

1. Introduction

The COVID-19 pandemic has impacted operations of numerous industries, including the aviation industry which has been significantly disrupted by global travel restrictions, causing a substantial economic decline within the industry [1]. Following the World Health Organization's characterization of COVID-19 as a pandemic on 11 March 2020, the global commercial airline industry experienced an approximate 60–80% decrease in flight operations during the proceeding months [2]. Accordingly, airline pilots have been affected by decreased work availability [1], job security, financial concerns, increased time spent confined to the indoors due to self-isolation requirements during travel [3], and limited control over food choices during hotel self-isolation after flying internationally. The consequent psychosocial impacts of these conditions may adversely affect the engagement in health promoting behaviors [4].

The COVID-19 pandemic has influenced considerable changes to behavior, and subsequent physical and mental health related outcomes [4]. Authorities in countries worldwide have implemented strict control strategies in attempt to limit the spread of the virus [5]. Consequently, these viral spread mitigation measures in the community pose significant barriers to engagement with health promoting behaviors [6]. For example, financial insecurity, elevated psychosocial stress, and emotional dysregulation may lower motivation and limit accessibility to healthful dietary behaviors [7,8]. Further, stay at home isolation and lockdown measures present an inhibitory effect on engagement in physical activity [4,9].

Negative effects on physical [10] and mental wellbeing, along with elevated levels of psychosocial stress [11] have been reported in research exploring the effects of COVID-19 environmental conditions, such as social distancing and lockdown confinement in adults. Decreases in physical and mental health during COVID-19 have shown associations with unhealthy lifestyle behaviors; sedentary behavior, physical inactivity, poor sleep quality, and unhealthy dietary intake [11]. Prospective cohort studies exploring health behavior status during lockdowns have reported increased sedentary behavior and physical inactivity [12], decreased fruit and vegetable intake [13], increased alcohol intake [8], and increased sleep problems [14], yet little evidence has been reported regarding the prolonged effects after lockdown.

Overweight, obesity and hypertension are independently associated with unhealthy lifestyle behaviors; insufficient sleep, poor diet, and physical inactivity [15–18]. Widespread societal and economic implications of COVID-19 present perturbations to these health behaviors [3,4,8,10]. Unhealthy lifestyle risk factors synonymous with an elevated risk of non-communicable disease are a risk factor for COVID-19 complications and severity of health outcomes following infection [6]. Markedly, obesity is associated with chronic low-grade inflammation, impaired innate immunity and immunologic compromise [19]. Indeed, recent studies report increased morbidity and mortality risk from COVID-19 in those with obesity [20]. Overweight and obesity are also major risk factors for essential hypertension, of which emerging evidence denotes as a risk factor strongly associated with adverse outcomes from COVID-19 [21].

Behavioral countermeasures for individuals are vital determinants to health resilience amongst exposure to unprecedented environmental events such as the COVID-19 pandemic and its widespread implications [7]. Obtaining seven to nine hours of sleep per night [22], consuming $\geq$400 g of fruit and vegetables per day fruits and vegetables [23], and engaging in $\geq$150 min of moderate-to-vigorous physical activity intensity per week are three protective lifestyle behaviors that significantly reduce all-cause mortality [23–25], and have a positive effect on physical and mental health [26,27], support healthy bodyweight and blood pressure management [15], and support immune system function [28]. Given the evidence for physical activity, healthy nutrition and sleep quality in promoting health outcomes, it is of public health importance that effective evidence-based interventions targeting the promotion of these behaviors are established for intervention preventive measures to mitigate the adverse health effects of future lockdowns [7].

Our previous research investigated the use of a personalized three-component healthy eating, physical activity and sleep hygiene intervention for promoting health during a COVID-19 lockdown in New Zealand [29]. The intervention's effectiveness at four-months has been reported [29], which revealed significant improvements in health behavior and subjective health. The aim of the current study is to report on the longer-term outcomes of the intervention; specifically, to evaluate the effects on weight loss and blood pressure. Further, to evaluate what health behavioral changes are sustained or decayed over a period of 12-months and what influence they have on health parameters. It was hypothesized that the intervention group would have significantly greater improvements in health behaviors and health parameters compared to the control group at 12-months. It was also hypothesized that some decay in health behaviors and parameters would be evident in the intervention group from post intervention (4 months) to 12 months.

2. Materials and Methods

2.1. Design

A two-arm, parallel, controlled design was utilized to evaluate the effectiveness of a brief three-component lifestyle intervention for enhancing and maintaining health behaviors, body mass, and blood pressure management during the COVID-19 pandemic in New Zealand. The acute (17-week) effects of this lifestyle intervention on subjective measures for physical activity, sleep duration, and fruit and vegetable intake have been previously reported [29]. Therefore, the purpose of the present study was to complete a 12-month follow-up to that study [29].

This study was approved by the Human Research Ethics Committee of the University of Waikato in New Zealand; reference number 2020#07. The trial protocol is registered at The Australian New Zealand Clinical Trials Registry (ACTRN12621001105831).

2.2. Intervention Timing

After baseline testing, the first five weeks of the intervention period preceded the New Zealand (NZ) Government's implementation of a four-tier response system to COVID-19 on 21 March 2020 [30]. Thereafter, five weeks were at highest alert level 4, two and a half weeks were at alert level 3, and two weeks were at alert level 2. Thereafter, NZ returned to alert level 1 [31]. Restrictions associated with each alert level is defined elsewhere [29]. Pre-testing occurred between 14 February and 9 March 2020 and follow-up testing was carried out during February and March 2021.

2.3. Participants

The study population for both groups consisted of commercial pilots from a large international airline. Inclusion criteria were (a) pilots with a valid commercial flying license, (b) working on a full-time basis, (c) having a body mass index (BMI) of ≥ 25 (overweight), and (d) a resting blood pressure of >120/80 (systolic/diastolic).

Control group participants consisted of airline pilot volunteers recruited at the time of completing their routine aviation medical examinations located at the airline medical unit during the time of the pre-test period. The intervention group volunteered to participate in the lifestyle intervention by responding to an invitation delivered to all pilots within the company via internal organization communication channels. Participants consisted of pilot rosters including long haul (international flights), short haul (regional flights), and mixed-fleet (variable schedule of regional and short international flights).

All participants provided informed consent prior to participation in the study and were made aware that they could withdraw from the study at any time should they wish to do so. Participants were provided with a unique identification code on their informed consent form, which they were instructed to input into their electronic health survey instead of their name at each data collection timepoint, in order to support anonymity and dataset blinding during data analysis.

The sample size was based on previous research with congruent outcome measures [29]. Clinically significant weight loss is defined as at least a 5% reduction in body mass from the baseline level [32]. Our power calculation suggested that 37 participants were required in each group to achieve an 80% power and 5% significance criterion to detect a 4 kg body mass reduction difference between the intervention and the control. To account for 20% attrition [33], we recruited 89 participants.

2.4. Intervention Group

The intervention group participated in a 17-week health intervention consisting of individualized goal setting for physical activity, healthy eating, and sleep hygiene. The intervention commenced with a one-hour individual face-to-face consultation session with an experienced health coach at the airline medical unit. For the intervention group, all participants conducted consultations with the same health coach. In this initial consultation session, the pilots' barriers and facilitators to health behavior change were assessed with methods outlined elsewhere [34], which were factored into the development of an individualized health program. Further, personalized collaborative goal setting was carried out for the pilot with assistance from the health coach, establishing appropriate outcome, performance, and process goals [35] for (a) sleep hygiene, (b) healthy eating, and (c) physical activity. A mid-intervention phone call was utilized to support adherence, monitor progress and measure compliance to health behaviors. The intervention utilized 20 participant contacts; including 2 face-to-face consultations (baseline and follow-up), 1 telephone call and 17 intra-intervention emails. For full detail of the procedures associated with the intervention readers are referred to the study of Wilson and colleagues [29].

2.5. Control Group

The participants in the control group received no intervention or instruction regarding health behaviors during the study timeframe. Pilots were invited to voluntarily complete an electronic survey and consent to providing records of their cardiovascular disease risk factor data from their aviation medical examinations. Pilots who volunteered to participate during the previously defined baseline testing period were sent an invitation via email to voluntarily complete the electronic survey again during the post intervention period and then finally again at the completion of their proceeding annual aviation medical examination to provide insight into the effects of COVID-19 on their health. The control group were invited to participate in the intervention after follow-up testing.

2.6. Outcome Measures

Measurements for subjective health (physical activity, sleep quality and quantity, fruit and vegetable intake, and self-rated health) via an electronic survey, and objective measures of body mass and blood pressure were taken at baseline and 12-month follow-up (see Figure 1).

Prior to attending data collection sessions, participants were instructed to avoid any strenuous exercise, stimulants (for example, caffeine or energy drinks), or large meals 4 h before testing. Height was recorded with a SECA 206 height measures and body mass was measured with SECA 813 electronic scales (SECA, Hamburg, Germany). For body mass measurement, participants were wearing clothes with emptied pockets and footwear removed. Blood pressure was measured with an OMRON HEM-757 device (Omron Corporation, Kyoto, Japan), which has been successfully validated independently against international criteria [36]. Measurements of blood pressure were conducted according to the standardized aviation medicine protocol [37]. Systolic blood pressure (SBP) and diastolic blood pressure (DBP) readings were used to calculate mean arterial pressure (MAP) with the following formula: $DP + 1/3(SP-DP)$ [38]. Resting pulse was measured using a Rossmax pulse oximeter SB220 (Rossmax Taipei, Taiwan, China) after a 5-min period of sitting in a chair quietly. All measurement instruments were calibrated prior to data collection.

Outcome measures for subjective health (physical activity, sleep quality and quantity, fruit and vegetable intake, and self-rated health) have been previously described in detail [29]. In brief, moderate-to-vigorous physical activity was determined using the International Physical Activity Questionnaire Short Form (IPAQ) [39]. To measure subjective sleep quality and quantity, the Pittsburgh Sleep Quality Index (PSQI) [40] was utilized. Daily fruit and vegetable intake were measured using dietary recall questions derived from the New Zealand Health Survey [39], and self-rated health was determined using the Short Health Form 12v2 (SF-12v2) [41].

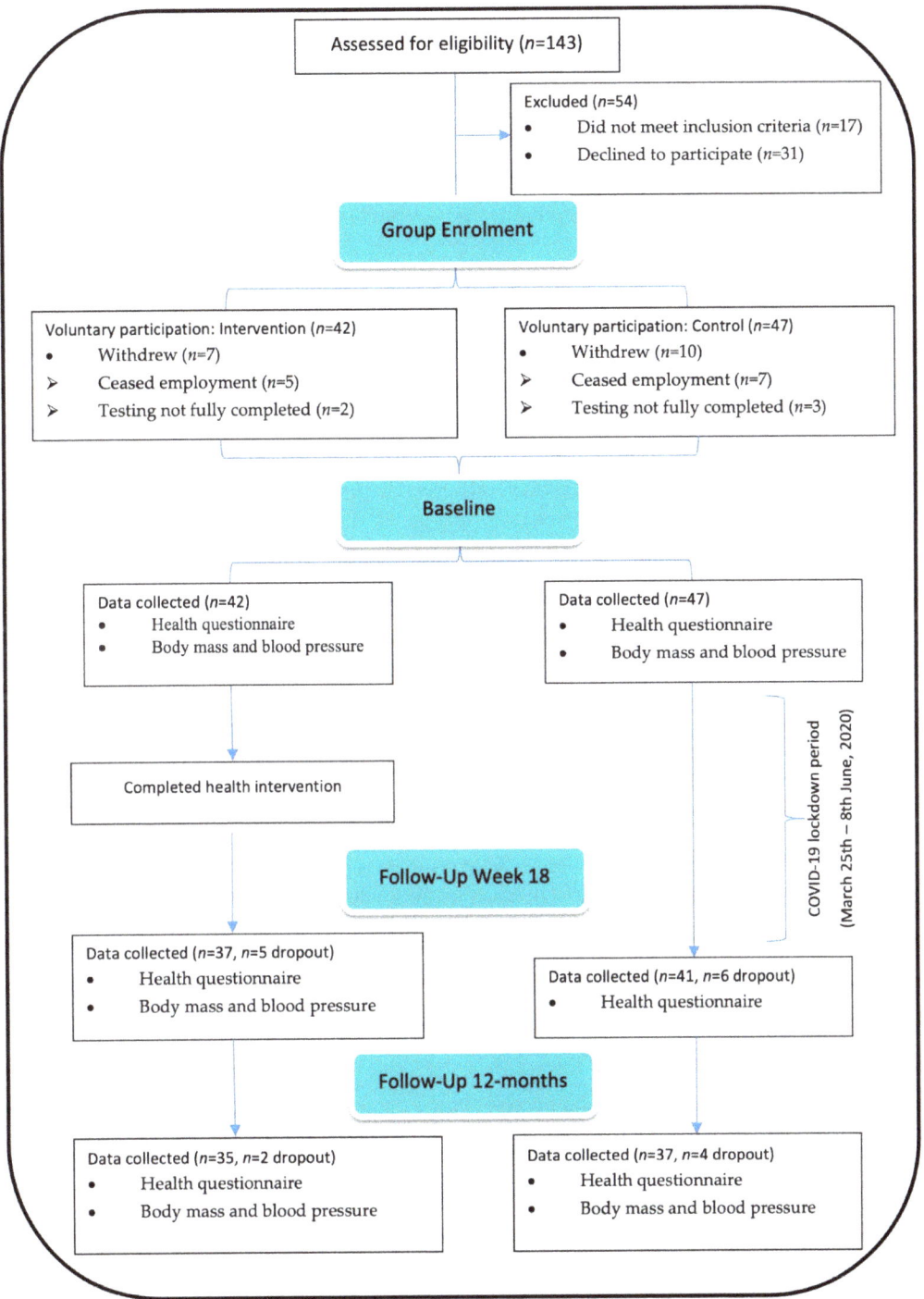

Figure 1. Flow diagram of participant recruitment and data collection.

2.7. Statistical Analysis

Raw data was extracted from the Qualtrics online survey software (Qualtrics, Provo, UT, USA), entered into an Excel spreadsheet (Microsoft, Seattle, WA, USA) and then imported into the Statistical Package for the Social Sciences (SPSS, version 27; IBM, New York, NY, USA) for all statistical analyses. All variables were assessed using the Shapiro–Wilk's test ($p > 0.05$) and its histograms, Q-Q plots and box plots for inspection for data normality. Levene's test was used to test homogeneity of variance. Listwise deletion was applied for individual datasets with missing values or participants who did not complete post-testing.

t-Tests were utilized to explore baseline differences between groups. A Chi-squared test was utilized to calculate whether any significant differences exist between fleet types at baseline. A one-way analysis of variance (ANOVA) was utilized to calculate whether any significant differences exist between fleet type for flight frequency and flight hours. Repeated-measures ANOVA using the General Linear Modelling function in SPSS was utilized test for group x time interactions, group effects, and time effects (baseline to 12-months). Age, sex, and flights were included as covariates in the ANOVA. As an additional analysis utilizing paired t-test, we examined change in health parameters within the intervention group from post intervention at 4-months to 12-months follow-up. Effect sizes were calculated using Cohen's d to quantify between group effects from pre-testing to post-testing. Effect sizes thresholds were set at >1.2, >0.6, >0.2, <0.2 were classified as *large, moderate, small,* and *trivial* [42]. The alpha level was set at $p < 0.05$.

3. Results

3.1. Baseline Characteristics of the Study Population

A total of 143 airline pilots were initially assessed for eligibility and 89 were recruited to participate (see Figure 1). Moreover, 72/89 (81%) pilots (mean ± SD, age; 46 ± 11 year, 11 females, 61 males) provided outcome measure data at all data collection timepoints, which consisted of a combination of short haul, long haul, and mixed fleet rosters (n = 28, 35, and 9, respectively). The dropout rates from baseline to 12-months were 17% (ceased employment n = 4; testing not fully completed n = 3) and 21% (testing not fully completed n = 7; ceased employment n = 3) for the intervention and control group, respectively.

As displayed in Table 1, at baseline the control and intervention group were of similar height, body mass, DBP, resting pulse, and flight hours. The control group were of advanced age (t(70) = 2.342, p = 0.02, d = 0.55), consumed more fruit and vegetables (t(70) = 4.570, p = <0.001, d = 1.08), performed more walking (t(70) = 5.650, p = <0.001, d = 1.33), higher PCS-12 and MCS-12 scores (t(70) = 7.751, p = <0.001, d = 1.82, and t(70) = 4.798, p = <0.001, d = 1.13, respectively), achieved greater sleep duration (t(70) = 3.012, p = 0.004, d = 0.71), and had a lower MAP (t(70) = −2.598, p = 0.011, d = 0.61). No significant differences were observed between groups for flights during lockdown and flight hours after lockdown.

Table 1. Baseline characteristics of participants.

Parameters	All Participants (n = 72)	Intervention (n = 35)	Control (n = 37)
Sex (f/m)	11/61	7/28	4/33
Age (year)	45.8 ± 11.1	42.8 ± 10.4	48.7 ± 11.2 *
Height (cm)	178.6 ± 7.2	178.5 ± 8.1	178.6 ± 6.3
Body mass (kg)	90.4 ± 13.9	91.7 ± 13.5	89.2 ± 14.5
BMI (kg·m^2)	28.3 ± 3.3	28.7 ± 3.3	27.9 ± 2.8
Systolic BP (mmHg)	134.4 ± 11.8	138.4 ± 10.6	130.6 ± 11.7
Diastolic BP (mmHg)	84.8 ± 8.3	86.7 ± 8.1	83.1 ± 8.2
MAP (mmHg)	101.3 ± 8.5	103.9 ± 8.0	98.9 ± 8.5 *
Pulse (bpm)	68.7 ± 9.5	69.2 ± 7.8	68.1 ± 10.9
Hours slept (h/day)	7.3 ± 0.9	7.0 ± 0.8	7.6 ± 0.8 *
IPAQ-walk (min)	102.4 ± 58.5	69.0 ± 37.9	134.0 ± 57.2 *
IPAQ-MVPA (min)	144.5 ± 89.0	125.9 ± 79.7	162.1 ± 94.7
F&V Intake (serve/day)	3.5 ± 1.4	2.8 ± 1.3	4.1 ± 1.1 *

Table 1. *Cont.*

Parameters	All Participants (n = 72)	Intervention (n = 35)	Control (n = 37)
PCS-12 (score)	46.7 ± 6.6	42.1 ± 4.1	51.1 ± 5.5 *
MCS-12 (score)	49.1 ± 7.5	45.3 ± 8.2	52.7 ± 4.5 *
Short Haul (n, %)	28 (39%)	20 (57%)	8 (22%) *
Long Haul (n, %)	35 (49%)	13 (37%)	22 (59%)
Mixed Fleet (n, %)	9 (12%)	2 (6%)	7 (19%)
Flights during lockdown (n)	8.0 ± 7.4	7.9 ± 7.7	8.1 ± 7.2
Flight hours after lockdown (h)	152.1 ± 71.9	153.9 ± 63.8	150.5 ± 79.7

Mean ± SD reported for all participants, intervention and control. Abbreviations: SD = standard deviation. BMI—body mass index. BP = blood pressure. MAP = mean arterial pressure. IPAQ = International Physical Activity Questionnaire. MVPA = moderate-to-vigorous physical activity. F&V = fruit and vegetable intake. PCS-12 = physical component summary score. MCS-12 = mental component summary score. * indicates statistical significance between groups ($p < 0.05$). Flight hours after lockdown = flight hours during the 6-months prior to 12-months follow-up testing.

3.2. Intervention Adherence

For the intervention group, compliance was measured mid-intervention for health behaviors, including average sleep hours, weekly MVPA and daily fruit and vegetable consumption. Thirty-two (91%) were achieving ≥7 h sleep per night and three (9%) were obtaining ≤6.9 h per night. For fruit and vegetable servings per day, 33 (94%) were achieving ≥5 serves of fruit and vegetables per day, whereas two (6%) were eating two to four serves per day. Thirty were achieving ≥150 min MVPA (86%), and five (14%) were completing ≤149 min MVPA per week.

3.3. Body Mass, BMI, BP, and Pulse

Group changes from baseline to 12-months are presented in Table 2. Significant interactions for group x time were found for all variables (p = <0.001), associated with *small* to *large* effect size differences between groups from baseline to 12-months (see Table 2). The within-group analysis revealed that the intervention elicited significant improvements ($p < 0.001$) in all physical metrics at 12-months, associated with *large* effect sizes (see Table 2). The control group reported a significantly higher body mass and BMI ($p < 0.001$) at 12-months, yet no significant changes were observed in other physical metrics.

3.4. Health Behaviors and Self-Rated Health

Significant interactions for group × time were found for all subjective health measures (p = <0.001). The within-group analysis reported significantly greater improved health changes from baseline to 12-months for all subjective health measures in the intervention group ($p < 0.001$), associated with *moderate* to *large* effect sizes (see Table 2; Figure 2). In contrast, the control group experienced significant decreases in all outcome measures: sleep duration ($t(36) = -2.589$, $p = 0.014$, $d = -0.42$), PSQI global score ($t(36) = 3.853$, p = <0.001, $d = 0.63$), and MCS-12 scores ($t(36) = -2.300$, $p = 0.027$, $d = -0.38$). No significant group differences were reported in other health metrics.

Table 2. Changes in objective and subjective health metrics from baseline and follow-up at 12-months.

	Time (Months)	Intervention (n = 35) M	SD	Follow-Up Change (95% CI)	Control (n = 37) M	SD	Follow-Up Change (95% CI)	ANOVA (Time × Group Interaction) p	Between Group ES d
Body mass (kg)	0	91.7	13.5		89.2	14.5			0.2, Trivial
	12	86.8	11.3	−4.9 (−3.5—−6.3)	90.5	14.5	1.3 (0.6–1.9)	<0.001	−0.3, Small
BMI (kg/m²)	0	28.7	3.3		27.9	2.8			0.2, Trivial
	12	27.1	2.7	−1.6 (−1.1—−2.0)	28.3	3.7	0.4 (0.2–0.6)	<0.001	−0.4, Small
Systolic BP (mmHg)	0	138.4	10.6		130.6	11.7			0.7 *, Moderate
	12	128.1	10.3	−10.3 (−7.2—−13.5)	134.4	9.9	3.8 (0.0–7.6)	<0.001	−0.6 *, Moderate
Diastolic BP (mmHg)	0	86.7	8.1		83.1	8.2			0.4, Small
	12	78.9	8.0	−7.8 (−5.0—−10.6)	83.2	7.0	0.1 (−2.6–2.8)	<0.001	−0.6 *, Moderate
MAP (mmHg)	0	103.9	8.0		98.9	8.5			0.6 *, Moderate
	12	95.3	7.6	−8.6 (−6.0—−11.3)	100.2	7.2	1.3 (−1.2–4.0)	<0.001	−0.7 *, Moderate
Pulse (bpm)	0	69.2	7.8		68.1	10.9			0.1, Trivial
	12	63.4	8.5	−5.8 (−3.8—−8.2)	69.2	12.2	1.1 (−0.7–5.6)	<0.001	−0.7 *, Moderate
Hours slept (h/day)	0	7.0	0.8		7.6	0.8			−0.7 *, Moderate
	12	7.7	0.7	0.7 (0.4–1.1)	7.5	0.7	−0.1 (0.0—−0.3)	<0.001	0.4, Small
PSQI Global (score)	0	6.4	2.8		4.5	2.6			0.7 *, Moderate
	12	4.1	1.5	−2.3 (−1.7—−3.2)	5.0	2.7	0.5 (0.2–0.7)	<0.001	−0.5 *, Small
IPAQ-walk (min)	0	69.0	37.9		134.0	57.2			−1.3 **, Large
	12	102.3	69.2	33.3 (22.1–49.6)	122.6	77.6	−11.4 (−16.2–9.4)	<0.001	−0.6 *, Moderate
IPAQ-MVPA (min)	0	125.9	79.7		162.1	94.7			−0.4, Small
	12	227.0	83.0	101.1 (62.2–126.0)	159.0	99.8	−3.1 (−16.9–11.1)	<0.001	0.8 *, Moderate
F&V Intake (serve/day)	0	2.8	1.3		4.1	1.1			−1.1 **, Moderate
	12	5.5	1.7	2.7 (2.0–3.2)	3.9	1.3	−0.2 (−0.5—−0.1)	<0.001	1.1 **, Moderate
PCS-12 (score)	0	42.1	4.1		51.1	5.5			−1.8 **, Large
	12	51.7	4.0	9.6 (7.1–10.8)	50.7	4.9	−0.4 (−1.3—−0.2)	<0.001	0.1, Trivial
MCS-12 (score)	0	45.3	8.2		52.7	4.5			−1.1 **, Moderate
	12	51.1	4.9	5.8 (3.6–8.0)	51.8	4.7	−0.9 (−0.1—−1.7)	<0.001	0.2, Trivial

Mean ± SD reported for all participants, intervention, and control. Abbreviations: SD = standard deviation. BMI = body mass index. BP = blood pressure. MAP = mean arterial pressure. PSQI = Pittsburgh Sleep Quality Index. IPAQ = International Physical Activity Questionnaire. F&V = fruit and vegetable intake. PCS-12 = physical component summary score. MCS-12 = mental component summary score. * indicates statistical significance between groups ($p < 0.05$). ** indicates statistical significance between groups ($p < 0.001$).

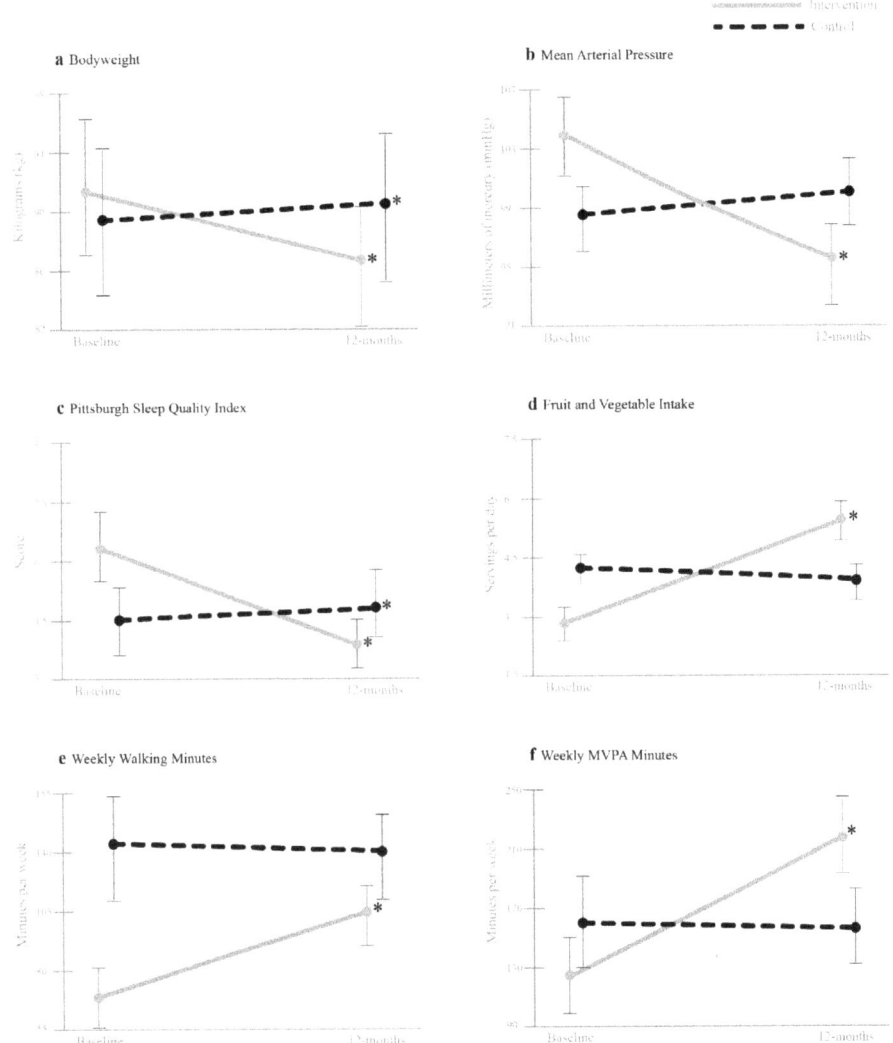

Figure 2. *Cont.*

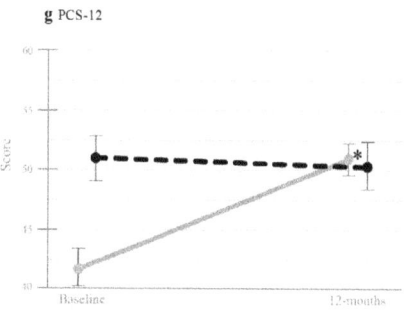
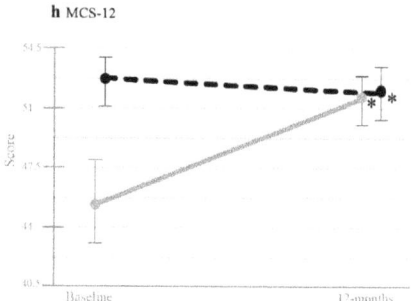

Figure 2. Mean values on objective and subjective health outcomes measured across time (Baseline and 12-months), showing 95% confidence intervals. (**a**), Bodyweight; (**b**), Mean Arterial Presurre; (**c**), Pittsburgh Sleep Quality Indx; (**d**), Fruit and Vegetable Intake, (**e**) Weekly Waliking Minuters; (**f**), Weekly MVPA Minutes; (**g**) PCS-12; (**h**), MCS-12. MVPA = moderate-to-vigorous physical activity. PCS-12 = physical component summary score. MCS-12 = mental component summary score. * indicates a significant difference compared to Baseline.

3.5. Additional Analysis: Four-Month Post-Intervention to 12-Month Follow-Up Change

Table 3 presents changes within the intervention group between four-months (post-intervention) and 12-months follow-up. There were significant within group differences reported for body mass, BMI, MAP, weekly MVPA (p = < 0.05), and DBP (p = < 0.001), which were associated with *small* to *moderate* effect sizes towards positive health change. Conversely, a decay of *small* magnitude was observed for health parameters average sleep hours (d = −0.23), PCS-12 score (d = −0.22), and MCS-12 score (d = −0.20). No significant differences were observed for other health parameters.

Table 3. Additional analysis: Changes in objective and subjective health metrics from post intervention at 4-months to follow-up at 12-months in the intervention group.

	Time (Months)	Intervention (n = 35)			Effect Size
		M	SD	Post-Follow-Up Change (95% CI)	d
Body mass (kg)	4	87.7	12.8	-	-
	12	86.8	11.3	−0.97 (−1.81–0.1)	−0.47, *small* *
BMI (kg/m²)	4	27.5	3.1	-	-
	12	27.1	2.7	−0.32 (−0.58–0.07)	−0.44, *small* *
Systolic BP (mmHg)	4	130.9	11.1	-	-
	12	128.1	10.3	−2.89 (−6.09–0.32)	−0.31, *small*
Diastolic BP (mmHg)	4	83.8	9.7	-	-
	12	78.9	8.0	−4.86 (−7.56−−2.15)	−0.62, *moderate* **
MAP (mmHg)	4	99.5	9.4	-	-
	12	95.3	7.6	−4.11 (−6.77−−1.46)	−0.53, *small* *
Pulse (bpm)	4	62.6	7.2	-	-
	12	63.4	8.5	0.74 (−2.0–3.5)	0.09, *trivial*
Hours slept (h/day)	4	7.8	1.0	-	-
	12	7.7	0.7	−0.11 (−0.27–0.05)	−0.23, *small*
PSQI Global (score)	4	4.1	1.8	-	-
	12	4.1	1.5	−0.09 (−0.31–0.14)	−0.13, *trivial*
IPAQ-walk (min)	4	94.3	96.5	-	-
	12	102.3	69.2	8.0 (−10.4–26.4)	0.15, *trivial*

Table 3. Cont.

	Time (Months)	Intervention (n = 35)			Effect Size
		M	SD	Post-Follow-Up Change (95% CI)	d
IPAQ-MVPA (min)	4	207.6	79.0	-	-
	12	227.0	82.6	19.7 (5.57–33.74)	0.48, small *
F&V Intake (serve/day)	4	5.6	1.9	-	-
	12	5.5	1.7	−0.13 (−0.49–0.23)	0.12, trivial
PCS-12 (score)	4	52.3	4.5	-	-
	12	51.7	4.0	−0.54 (−1.38–0.29)	−0.22, small
MCS-12 (score)	4	54.5	5.7	-	-
	12	51.1	4.9	−0.52 (−1.41–0.36)	−0.20, small

Mean ± SD reported for the intervention group. Abbreviations: SD = standard deviation. BMI = body mass index. BP = blood pressure. MAP = mean arterial pressure. PSQI = Pittsburgh Sleep Quality Index. IPAQ = International Physical Activity Questionnaire. F&V = fruit and vegetable intake. PCS-12 = physical component summary score. MCS-12 = mental component summary score. * indicates statistical significance ($p < 0.05$). ** indicates statistical significance ($p < 0.001$).

4. Discussion

This is the first 12-month follow-up study after a lifestyle health intervention during the COVID-19 pandemic. The present intervention aimed to improve health-related behaviors and promote healthy changes in bodyweight and blood pressure within overweight pilots through a personalized intervention on healthy eating, sleep hygiene and physical activity. The controlled trial showed that at 12-months follow-up, there appeared to be a significant improvement on health parameters from being provided the 17-week intervention [29], relative to our control group which supports our initial hypothesis. These results are important for researchers and health care professionals to provide insight into prolonged health and quality of life perturbations resulting from COVID-19 that may have potential implications to flight safety. Furthermore, given the dearth of published data pertaining to health behavior interventions during a pandemic and the limited availability of preventive lifestyle-based interventions in pilots, these findings provide novel contributions to this field.

Poor long-term maintenance of weight loss and health behavior change achieved from lifestyle diet and exercise interventions is frequently reported [43]. In our intervention group we observed sustained positive change in health behaviors at 12-months follow-up, relative to baseline characteristics. Further, body mass, blood pressure, and weekly MVPA continued to improve at 12-months compared to post-intervention, whereas other health parameter improvements demonstrated non-significant *trivial* to *small* magnitudes of decay from post intervention. These findings support our secondary hypothesis and are consistent with other health behavior research reporting reduced magnitude of change in health parameters at longitudinal follow-up, compared to post-intervention [44]. A contributing factor that has been proposed is the discontinuation of health care professional support, following intervention completion [45]. Thus, highlighting the importance of ongoing care to facilitate additional health outcome improvements after a brief intervention.

Prospective cohort studies have reported significant increases in body mass within four-months after the onset of the initial COVID-19 lockdown [46,47], yet limited studies have evaluated whether body mass gain is sustained longitudinally after lockdown conditions are lifted. In the present study, participants in the intervention group lost 4.9 kg (↓5.4%), while the control group gained 1.2 kg (↑1.3%) at 12-months, resulting in a 6.1 kg difference in body mass change between groups. Existing literature of lifestyle interventions targeting combined diet, physical activity, and sleep with longitudinal follow-up measures are scarce, limiting comparison accuracy of the present findings to existing research. Airline pilot populations are often male dominant [48]; indeed, our participant sample reflected this demographic. Contrarily, a recent meta-analysis reported the majority of participants in diet and exercise weight management interventions were women [49]. Thus, our study provides important evidence regarding the effectiveness of lifestyle interventions within males.

The intervention utilized 20 participant contacts; including two face-to-face consultations, one telephone call, and 17 intra-intervention emails. Comparatively, a recent review indicated a mean body mass reduction of 2.5 kg at one year follow-up within dietary interventions consisting of 13–24 intra-intervention participant contacts [50]. Another review reported a higher mean body mass reduction of 6.7 kg at one year follow-up pertaining to intensive combined diet and exercise interventions [33]. However, the average length of treatment of these interventions were 37 weeks [33], which is considerably higher than our 17-week intervention [29].

Another gap in the literature base is whether body mass gain observed during lockdown conditions is associated with increased blood pressure, which remains largely unexplored. The body mass gain evident in our control group was associated with a 3.8 mmHg increase in SBP at 12-months, compared to a reduction of 10.3 mmHg observed in the intervention group. The SBP reduction observed in the intervention group is comparable with previous research, which reported a 9.5 mmHg reduction in SBP at 12-months following an intensive diet and exercise lifestyle intervention [51]. Correspondingly, in our intervention group we observed a DBP reduction of 2.9 mmHg, and a further 4.9 mmHg at four-months and 12-months, respectively. Compared with our present findings, a similar longitudinal relationship between body mass and blood pressure following intentional weight loss has been reported [52]. Stevens and colleagues reported participants who succeeded at weight loss maintenance at 36 months post-intervention also maintained blood pressure reduction obtained after the intervention, whereas participants who gained weight also experienced increased blood pressure [52].

We discovered a significantly reduced MCS-12 score and increased PSQI global score (denoting worse sleep) at 12-months follow-up in our control group, with no significant change in other subjective measures. Indeed, previous studies have demonstrated associations between sleep and mental health [53]. Further, negative changes in sleep quality during the pandemic have been associated with negative affect, worry and elevated psychosocial stress [54,55]. These findings may be contributed to by additional factors acting on the pilot population during the time of this study, including decreased work availability [1], job security, financial concerns, increased time spent confined to the indoors due to self-isolation requirements during travel [3], and limited control over food choices during hotel self-isolation after flying internationally.

The magnitude of change observed in the present intervention may be at least partly attributable to; (a) the three-component diet, exercise, and sleep approach, (b) behavioral approaches including collaborative goal setting, face-to-face coaching, telephone call and regular emails, and (c) the potential active interest of the pilot population in enhancing their health to support their aviation medical license. Weight loss factors such as restrictive diets and restrictive caloric patterns have been suggested as effective in the short term, but often have a poor long term success rate, leading to weight regain [56]. Whereas the methods utilized in the present study supported a physically active lifestyle, managing life stress with health behaviors, accountability, and facilitation of autonomy via self-determined goal setting, all of which are associated with successful weight loss maintenance [57]. Airline pilots have been reported to exhibit higher personality scores for maturity, emotional stability, and intelligence when compared to general population norms [58]. These characteristics may positively influence intervention engagement and adherence, thus presenting an important consideration when generalizing our findings to the general population.

Potential limitations of the current study need to be considered in the interpretation of our findings. Firstly, although the sample size provided adequate power to distinguish statistically significant effects in the key outcome variables, the differential recruitment strategies and participant self-selection may have contributed to the differences which were observed at baseline for age, fruit and vegetable intake, weekly walking minutes, PCS-12 and MCS-12 scores, sleep duration, and MAP, with healthier characteristics in favor of the control group. Further, those who voluntarily participated in the intervention may have had strong motivation to engage in healthy change, which may have supported the magnitude of intervention effects observed. Thus, it is advisable that future research implements a randomization design, assigning conditions to participants. Secondly, for feasibility purposes the present study utilized self-report measures for health behaviors, which inherently produce lower accuracy to more invasive objective measures. To enhance outcome measure validity and reliability, utilization of objective methods would be preferential such as actigraphy to monitor sleep and physical activity, and photo logging of dietary behaviors to quantify health behavior metrics; however, this would be somewhat difficult to achieve over a period of 12-months.

5. Conclusions

In conclusion, the individualized 17-week healthy eating, physical activity, and sleep hygiene intervention implemented in this study elicited sustained positive change in all outcome measures at 12-months follow-up, relative to baseline characteristics. Further, body mass, blood pressure, and weekly MVPA continued to improve at 12-months compared to post-intervention, whereas other health parameter improvements demonstrated non-significant *trivial* to *small* magnitudes of decay from post intervention. These findings suggest that achievement of these three guidelines promote physical and mental health and improves quality of life among pilots during a global pandemic, yet more regular monitoring post intervention may further strengthen behavior change maintenance. Our study provides preliminary evidence that a multi-behavior intervention may be efficacious during a pandemic and that similar outcomes may be transferrable to other populations.

Author Contributions: D.W. and N.G. participated in conceptualization of the study, data collection and contributed to the design of the study, data analysis, interpretation of the results, and manuscript writing; M.D., P.W. and B.J. contributed to the design of the study, data analysis, interpretation of the results, and manuscript writing. All authors have read and agreed to the published version of the manuscript.

Funding: This research received no external funding.

Informed Consent Statement: Informed consent was obtained from all subjects involved in the study. Written informed consent has been obtained from the patient(s) to publish this paper.

Acknowledgments: The authors wish to thank the pilots for providing their time to voluntarily participate in this study.

Conflicts of Interest: The authors declare no conflict of interest.

References

1. Dube, K.; Nhamo, G.; Chikodzi, D. COVID-19 pandemic and prospects for recovery of the global aviation industry. *J. Air Transp. Manag.* **2021**, *92*, 102022. [CrossRef]
2. Sobieralski, J.B. COVID-19 and airline employment: Insights from historical uncertainty shocks to the industry. *Transp. Res. Interdiscip. Perspect.* **2020**, *5*, 100123. [CrossRef]
3. Parmet, W.E.; Sinha, M.S. Covid-19—The law and limits of quarantine. *N. Engl. J. Med.* **2020**, *382*, e28. [CrossRef]
4. McBride, E.; Arden, M.A.; Chater, A.; Chilcot, J. The impact of COVID-19 on health behaviour, well-being, and long-term physical health. *Br. J. Health Psychol.* **2021**, *26*, 259–270. [CrossRef] [PubMed]
5. Douglas, M.; Katikireddi, S.V.; Taulbut, M.; McKee, M.; McCartney, G. Mitigating the wider health effects of covid-19 pandemic response. *BMJ* **2020**, *369*, m1557. [CrossRef]
6. Hamer, M.; Kivimäki, M.; Gale, C.R.; Batty, G.D. Lifestyle risk factors, inflammatory mechanisms, and COVID-19 hospitalization: A community-based cohort study of 387,109 adults in UK. *Brain Behav. Immun.* **2020**, *87*, 184–187. [CrossRef] [PubMed]
7. Naja, F.; Hamadeh, R. Nutrition amid the COVID-19 pandemic: A multi-level framework for action. *Eur. J. Clin. Nutr.* **2020**, *74*, 1117–1121. [CrossRef]
8. Naughton, F.; Ward, E.; Khondoker, M.; Belderson, P.; Marie Minihane, A.; Dainty, J.; Hanson, S.; Holland, R.; Brown, T.; Notley, C. Health behaviour change during the UK COVID-19 lockdown: Findings from the first wave of the C-19 health behaviour and well-being daily tracker study. *Br. J. Health Psychol.* **2021**, *26*, 624–643. [CrossRef] [PubMed]
9. Herle, M.; Smith, A.D.; Bu, F.; Steptoe, A.; Fancourt, D. Trajectories of eating behavior during COVID-19 lockdown: Longitudinal analyses of 22,374 adults. *Clin. Nutr. ESPEN* **2021**, *42*, 158–165. [CrossRef] [PubMed]

10. Fernández-Abascal, E.G.; Martín-Díaz, M.D. Longitudinal study on affect, psychological well-being, depression, mental and physical health, prior to and during the COVID-19 pandemic in Spain. *Pers. Individ. Differ.* **2021**, *172*, 110591. [CrossRef] [PubMed]
11. Ammar, A.; Trabelsi, K.; Brach, M.; Chtourou, H.; Boukhris, O.; Masmoudi, L.; Bouaziz, B.; Bentlage, E.; How, D.; Ahmed, M.; et al. Effects of home confinement on mental health and lifestyle behaviours during the COVID-19 outbreak: Insight from the ECLB-COVID19 multicenter study. *Biol. Sport* **2021**, *38*, 9–21. [CrossRef]
12. Stockwell, S.; Trott, M.; Tully, M.; Shin, J.; Barnett, Y.; Butler, L.; McDermott, D.; Schuch, F.; Smith, L. Changes in physical activity and sedentary behaviours from before to during the COVID-19 pandemic lockdown: A systematic review. *BMJ Open Sport Exerc. Med.* **2021**, *7*, e000960. [CrossRef]
13. Litton, M.; Beavers, A. The Relationship between Food Security Status and Fruit and Vegetable Intake during the COVID-19 Pandemic. *Nutrients* **2021**, *13*, 712. [CrossRef]
14. Jahrami, H.; Bahammam, A.S.; Bragazzi, N.L.; Saif, Z.; Faris, M.; Vitiello, M.V. Sleep problems during the COVID-19 pandemic by population: A systematic review and meta-analysis. *J. Clin. Sleep Med.* **2021**, *17*, 299–313. [CrossRef]
15. Valenzuela, P.L.; Carrera-Bastos, P.; Gálvez, B.G.; Ruiz-Hurtado, G.; Ordovas, J.M.; Ruilope, L.M.; Lucia, A. Lifestyle interventions for the prevention and treatment of hypertension. *Nat. Rev. Cardiol.* **2021**, *18*, 251–275. [CrossRef]
16. Broussard, J.L.; Van Cauter, E. Disturbances of sleep and circadian rhythms: Novel risk factors for obesity. *Curr. Opin. Endocrinol. Diabetes Obes.* **2016**, *23*, 353–359. [CrossRef] [PubMed]
17. Drewnowski, A. Obesity and the food environment: Dietary energy density and diet costs. *Am. J. Prev. Med.* **2004**, *27*, 154–162. [CrossRef]
18. Cecchini, M.; Sassi, F.; Lauer, J.A.; Lee, Y.Y.; Guajardo-Barron, V.; Chisholm, D. Tackling of unhealthy diets, physical inactivity, and obesity: Health effects and cost-effectiveness. *Lancet* **2010**, *376*, 1775–1784. [CrossRef]
19. Michalakis, K.; Panagiotou, G.; Ilias, I.; Pazaitou-Panayiotou, K. Obesity and COVID-19: A jigsaw puzzle with still missing pieces. *Clin. Obes.* **2021**, *11*, e12420. [CrossRef] [PubMed]
20. Popkin, B.M.; Du, S.; Green, W.D.; Beck, M.A.; Algaith, T.; Herbst, C.H.; Alsukait, R.F.; Alluhidan, M.; Alazemi, N.; Shekar, M. Individuals with obesity and COVID-19: A global perspective on the epidemiology and biological relationships. *Obes. Rev.* **2020**, *21*, e13128. [CrossRef]
21. Tadic, M.; Saeed, S.; Grassi, G.; Taddei, S.; Mancia, G.; Cuspidi, C. Hypertension and COVID-19: Ongoing Controversies. *Front. Cardiovasc. Med.* **2021**, *8*, 639222. [CrossRef] [PubMed]
22. Hirshkowitz, M.; Whiton, K.; Albert, S.M.; Alessi, C.; Bruni, O.; DonCarlos, L.; Hazen, N.; Herman, J.; Adams Hillard, P.J.; Katz, E.S.; et al. National Sleep Foundation's updated sleep duration recommendations: Final report. *Sleep Health* **2015**, *1*, 233–243. [CrossRef] [PubMed]
23. Bellavia, A.; Larsson, S.; Bottai, M.; Wolk, A.; Orsini, N. Fruit and vegetable consumption and all-cause mortality: A dose-response analysis. *Am. J. Clin. Nutr.* **2013**, *98*, 454–459. [CrossRef]
24. Cappuccio, F.P.; D'Elia, L.; Strazzullo, P.; Miller, M.A. Sleep Duration and All-Cause Mortality: A Systematic Review and Meta-Analysis of Prospective Studies. *Sleep* **2010**, *33*, 585–592. [CrossRef]
25. Lear, S.A.A.; Hu, W.; Rangarajan, S.; Gasevic, D.; Leong, D.; Iqbal, R.; Casanova, A.; Swaminathan, S.; Anjana, R.M.; Kumar, R.; et al. The effect of physical activity on mortality and cardiovascular disease in 130 000 people from 17 high-income, middle-income, and low-income countries: The PURE study. *Lancet* **2017**, *390*, 2643–2654. [CrossRef]
26. Mozaffarian, D.; Wilson, P.W.; Kannel, W.B. Beyond established and novel risk factors: Lifestyle risk factors for cardiovascular disease. *Circulation* **2008**, *117*, 3031–3038. [CrossRef] [PubMed]
27. Mandolesi, L.; Polverino, A.; Montuori, S.; Foti, F.; Ferraioli, G.; Sorrentino, P.; Sorrentino, G. Effects of Physical Exercise on Cognitive Functioning and Wellbeing: Biological and Psychological Benefits. *Front. Psychol.* **2018**, *9*, 509. [CrossRef]
28. Walsh, N.P.; Gleeson, M.; Shephard, R.J.; Gleeson, M.; Woods, J.A.; Bishop, N.C.; Fleshner, M.; Green, C.; Pedersen, B.K.; Hoffman-Goetz, L.; et al. Position statement. Part one: Immune function and exercise. *Exerc. Immunol. Rev.* **2011**, *17*, 6–63. [PubMed]
29. Wilson, D.; Driller, M.; Johnston, B.; Gill, N. The effectiveness of a 17-week lifestyle intervention on health behaviors among airline pilots during COVID-19. The effectiveness of a 17-week lifestyle intervention on health behaviors among airline pilots during COVID-19. *J. Sport Health Sci.* **2021**, *10*, 333–340. [CrossRef]
30. Baker, M.G.; Kvalsvig, A.; Verrall, A.J.; Telfar-Barnard, L.; Wilson, N. New Zealand's elimination strategy for the COVID-19 pandemic and what is required to make it work. *N. Z. Med. J.* **2020**, *133*, 10–14. [PubMed]
31. Ministry of Health. COVID-19 (Novel Coronavirus). 2020 2 July 2020 [Cited 2020 2 July 2020]. Available online: https://www.health.govt.nz/our-work/diseases-and-conditions/covid-19-novel-coronavirus?mega=Our%20work&title=COVID-19 (accessed on 27 April 2021).
32. Donnelly, J.E.; Blair, S.N.; Jakicic, J.M.; Manore, M.M.; Rankin, J.W.; Smith, B.K.; American College of Sports Medicine. American College of Sports Medicine Position Stand. Appropriate Physical Activity Intervention Strategies for Weight Loss and Prevention of Weight Regain for Adults. *Med. Sci. Sports Exerc.* **2009**, *41*, 459–471. [CrossRef]
33. Curioni, C.C.; Lourenço, P.M. Long-term weight loss after diet and exercise: A systematic review. *Int. J. Obes.* **2005**, *29*, 1168–1174. [CrossRef] [PubMed]

34. Kulavic, K.; Hultquist, C.N.; McLester, J.R. A Comparison of Motivational Factors and Barriers to Physical Activity Among Traditional Versus Nontraditional College Students. *J. Am. Coll. Health* **2013**, *61*, 60–66. [CrossRef]
35. Weinberg, R. Making Goals Effective: A Primer for Coaches. *J. Sport Psychol. Action* **2010**, *1*, 57–65. [CrossRef]
36. El Assaad, M.A.; Topouchian, J.A.; Asmar, R.G. Evaluation of two devices for self-measurement of blood pressure according to the international protocol: The Omron M5-I and the Omron 705IT. *Blood Press. Monit.* **2003**, *8*, 127–133. [CrossRef]
37. Civil Aviation Authority. Medical Manual Part 3—Clinical Aviation Medicine. 2021 [cited 2021 27/04/2021]. Available online: https://www.aviation.govt.nz/assets/publications/medical-manual/Med_Man_Part-3.pdf (accessed on 27 April 2021).
38. Sesso, H.D.; Stampfer, M.J.; Rosner, B.; Hennekens, C.H.; Gaziano, J.M.; Manson, J.E.; Glynn, R.J. Systolic and Diastolic Blood Pressure, Pulse Pressure, and Mean Arterial Pressure as Predictors of Cardiovascular Disease Risk in Men. *Hypertension* **2000**, *36*, 801–807. [CrossRef] [PubMed]
39. Ministry of Health. Methodology Report 2017/18: New Zealand Health Survey 2019 [Cited 2020 1/1/2020]. Available online: https://www.health.govt.nz/publication/methodology-report-2017-18-new-zealand-health-survey (accessed on 27 April 2021).
40. Buysse, D.J.; Reynolds, C.F., III; Monk, T.H.; Berman, S.R.; Kupfer, D.J. The Pittsburgh sleep quality index: A new instrument for psychiatric practice and research. *Psychiatry Res.* **1989**, *28*, 193–213. [CrossRef]
41. Ware, J.E.; Keller, S.D.; Kosinski, M. *SF-12: How to Score the SF-12 Physical and Mental Health Summary Scales*; Health Institute, New England Medical Center: Boston, USA, 1995.
42. Cohen, J. *Statistical Power Analysis for the Behavioral Sciences*, 2nd ed.; Taylor & Francis Group: Florence, Italy, 1988.
43. Marchesini, G.; Montesi, L.; El Ghoch, M.; Brodosi, L.; Calugi, S.; Grave, R.D. Long-term weight loss maintenance for obesity: A multidisciplinary approach. *Diabetes Metab. Syndr. Obesity Targets Ther.* **2016**, *9*, 37–46. [CrossRef]
44. Varkevisser, R.D.M.; Van Stralen, M.M.; Kroeze, W.; Ket, J.C.; Steenhuis, I. Determinants of weight loss maintenance: A systematic review. *Obes. Rev.* **2019**, *20*, 171–211. [CrossRef]
45. Middleton, K.R.; Anton, S.D.; Perri, M. Long-Term Adherence to Health Behavior Change. *Am. J. Lifestyle Med.* **2013**, *7*, 395–404. [CrossRef]
46. Lin, A.L.; Vittinghoff, E.; Olgin, J.E.; Pletcher, M.J.; Marcus, G.M. Body Weight Changes During Pandemic-Related Shelter-in-Place in a Longitudinal Cohort Study. *JAMA Netw. Open* **2021**, *4*, e212536. [CrossRef]
47. Bakaloudi, D.R.; Barazzoni, R.; Bischoff, S.C.; Breda, J.; Wickramasinghe, K.; Chourdakis, M. Impact of the first COVID-19 lockdown on body weight: A combined systematic review and a meta-analysis. *Clin. Nutr.* **2021**. [CrossRef]
48. Houston, S.; Mitchell, S.; Evans, S. Prevalence of cardiovascular disease risk factors among UK commercial pilots. *Eur. J. Cardiovasc. Prev. Rehabil.* **2011**, *18*, 510–517. [CrossRef] [PubMed]
49. Johns, D.J.; Hartmann-Boyce, J.; Jebb, S.A.; Aveyard, P. Diet or Exercise Interventions vs Combined Behavioral Weight Management Programs: A Systematic Review and Meta-Analysis of Direct Comparisons. *J. Acad. Nutr. Diet.* **2014**, *114*, 1557–1568. [CrossRef] [PubMed]
50. Singh, N.; Stewart, R.A.H.; Benatar, J.R. Intensity and duration of lifestyle interventions for long-term weight loss and association with mortality: A meta-analysis of randomised trials. *BMJ Open* **2019**, *9*, e029966. [CrossRef] [PubMed]
51. Elmer, P.J.; Obarzanek, E.; Vollmer, W.M.; Simons-Morton, D.; Stevens, V.J.; Young, D.R.; Lin, P.-H.; Champagne, C.; Harsha, D.W.; Svetkey, L.P.; et al. Effects of Comprehensive Lifestyle Modification on Diet, Weight, Physical Fitness, and Blood Pressure Control: 18-Month Results of a Randomized Trial. *Ann. Intern. Med.* **2006**, *144*, 485–495. [CrossRef]
52. Stevens, V.J.; Obarzanek, E.; Cook, N.R.; Lee, I.-M.; Appel, L.J.; West, D.S.; Milas, N.C.; Mattfeldt-Beman, M.; Belden, L.; Bragg, C.; et al. Long-Term Weight Loss and Changes in Blood Pressure: Results of the Trials of Hypertension Prevention, Phase II. *Ann. Intern. Med.* **2001**, *134*, 1–11. [CrossRef] [PubMed]
53. Freeman, D.; Sheaves, B.; Goodwin, G.M.; Yu, L.-M.; Nickless, A.; Harrison, P.J.; Emsley, R.; Luik, A.I.; Foster, R.G.; Wadekar, V.; et al. The effects of improving sleep on mental health (OASIS): A randomised controlled trial with mediation analysis. *Lancet Psychiatry* **2017**, *4*, 749–758. [CrossRef]
54. Kocevska, D.; Blanken, T.F.; Van Someren, E.J.; Rösler, L. Sleep quality during the COVID-19 pandemic: Not one size fits all. *Sleep Med.* **2020**, *76*, 86–88. [CrossRef] [PubMed]
55. Franceschini, C.; Musetti, A.; Zenesini, C.; Palagini, L.; Scarpelli, S.; Quattropani, M.C.; Lenzo, V.; Freda, M.F.; Lemmo, D.; Vegni, E.; et al. Poor Sleep Quality and Its Consequences on Mental Health During the COVID-19 Lockdown in Italy. *Front. Psychol.* **2020**, *11*, 574475. [CrossRef]
56. MacLean, P.S.; Bergouignan, A.; Cornier, M.; Jackman, M.R. Biology's response to dieting: The impetus for weight regain. *Am. J. Physiol.-Regul. Integr. Comp. Physiol.* **2011**, *301*, R581–R600. [CrossRef]
57. Elfhag, K.; Rossner, S. Who succeeds in maintaining weight loss? A conceptual review of factors associated with weight loss maintenance and weight regain. *Obes. Rev.* **2005**, *6*, 67–85. [CrossRef]
58. Wakcher, S.; Cross, K.; Blackman, M.C. Personality Comparison of Airline Pilot Incumbents, Applicants, and the General Population Norms on the 16PF. *Psychol. Rep.* **2003**, *92*, 773–780. [CrossRef]

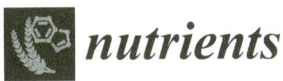

Article

Evaluation of Latent Models Assessing Physical Fitness and the Healthy Eating Index in Community Studies: Time-, Sex-, and Diabetes-Status Invariance

Scott B. Maitland [1,*], Paula Brauer [1], David M. Mutch [2], Dawna Royall [1], Doug Klein [3], Angelo Tremblay [4,5], Caroline Rheaume [6], Rupinder Dhaliwal [7] and Khursheed Jeejeebhoy [8]

1. Department of Family Relations & Applied Nutrition, University of Guelph, 50 Stone Road E, Guelph, ON N1G 2W1, Canada; pbrauer@uoguelph.ca (P.B.); phcnutr@uoguelph.ca (D.R.)
2. Department of Human and Health Nutritional Sciences, University of Guelph, Guelph, ON N1G 2W1, Canada; dmutch@uoguelph.ca
3. Department of Family Medicine, University of Alberta, Edmonton, AB T6G 1C9, Canada; doug.klein@ualberta.ca
4. Department of Kinesiology, Faculty of Medicine, Université Laval, Quebec City, QC G1V 0A6, Canada; angelo.tremblay@kin.ulaval.ca
5. Centre de recherche Nutrition, Santé et Société (NUTRISS), INAF, Quebec City, QC G1V 0A6, Canada
6. Department of Family Medicine and Emergency Medicine, Faculty of Medicine, Université Laval, Quebec City, QC G1V 0A6, Canada; Caroline.Rheaume@fmed.ulaval.ca
7. Canadian Nutrition Society, Ottawa, ON K1C 6A8, Canada; rupinder@cns-scn.ca
8. Departments of Nutritional Sciences and Physiology, University of Toronto, Toronto, ON M5S 1A8, Canada; khushjeejeebhoy@hotmail.com
* Correspondence: smaitlan@uoguelph.ca

Abstract: Accurate measurement requires assessment of measurement equivalence/invariance (ME/I) to demonstrate that the tests/measurements perform equally well and measure the same underlying constructs across groups and over time. Using structural equation modeling, the measurement properties (stability and responsiveness) of intervention measures used in a study of metabolic syndrome (MetS) treatment in primary care offices, were assessed. The primary study (N = 293; mean age = 59 years) had achieved 19% reversal of MetS overall; yet neither diet quality nor aerobic capacity were correlated with declines in cardiovascular disease risk. Factor analytic methods were used to develop measurement models and factorial invariance were tested across three time points (baseline, 3-month, 12-month), sex (male/female), and diabetes status for the Canadian Healthy Eating Index (2005 HEI-C) and several fitness measures combined (percentile VO$_2$ max from submaximal exercise, treadmill speed, curl-ups, push-ups). The model fit for the original HEI-C was poor and could account for the lack of associations in the primary study. A reduced HEI-C and a 4-item fitness model demonstrated excellent model fit and measurement equivalence across time, sex, and diabetes status. Increased use of factor analytic methods increases measurement precision, controls error, and improves ability to link interventions to expected clinical outcomes.

Keywords: physical fitness; diet quality; factor analysis; structural equation modeling; measurement equivalence/invariance; metabolic syndrome; cardiometabolic health

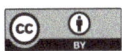

1. Introduction

1.1. Lifestyle Treatment of Cardio-Metabolic Conditions

Significant progress has been made in demonstrating the overall benefits of personalized lifestyle counselling in prevention of cardiometabolic conditions. Cardiometabolic risk (CMR) conditions include various combinations of prediabetes and type 2 diabetes, hypertension, dyslipidemia and higher visceral abdominal fat accumulation, as typically assessed by waist circumference. Several large clinical trials have demonstrated reductions in cardiovascular (CVD) mortality and diabetes incidence, namely the PREDIMED study [1,2] and the Diabetes Prevention Program [3–5] and subsequent studies [6,7]. CMR conditions and diseases are a major and growing health burden in many countries, as obesity continues to increase worldwide [8]. Excess body weight is associated with adverse metabolic effects in a sizable minority and become more prominent in middle age. These adverse effects manifest as the already mentioned conditions, as well as the combination described as metabolic syndrome (MetS). MetS is defined as three or more indicators, including higher waist circumference, higher blood pressure, dyslipidemia characterized by low high-density lipoprotein and elevated triglyceride levels, and elevated glucose levels [9]. The various clinical definitions describe overlapping populations [10], and different combinations of risk factors likely differentially affect CVD risk [11]. For example, people with MetS have approximately double the CVD risk as people without MetS [12].

Worldwide prevalence of some of the risk factors like hypertension, obesity and type 2 diabetes are well documented [13], while prediabetes [14] and MetS have less often been assessed in national surveys [15]. In Canada, 21% of adults 20–79 years old had MetS in the 2012–2013 survey [16], whereas in the United States (US) 33% of adults aged 20 and older met the criteria for the condition in NHANES 2002–2013 [17]. Among people 60 years and older, 39% of Canadians and 46% of Americans from the same analyses had MetS [16,17]. Ongoing costs of CMR are substantial, as confirmed in a 2016 US study of the Medical Expenditure Panel Survey. Among those with three or four risk factors (mostly MetS) compared to those with none of the CMR conditions, health care utilization was 50% higher, days missed from work 75% higher and yearly health care costs more than twice as high [18]. In addition, recent experience with COVID-19 has confirmed increased risk of severe disease in the presence of these CMR conditions, although estimates of excess risk vary [19,20].

1.2. Measurement Issues

All relevant practice guidelines for CMR conditions promote lifestyle change in a general way [21–24]. Effective lifestyle services to treat CMR are not, however, routinely being offered within health care in Canada [25] and elsewhere, and multiple issues are involved, including structural issues like lack of resources and expertise in family medicine practices, and clinician perceptions of poor effectiveness of lifestyle programs in practice (the efficacy-effectiveness gap) [6]. Focusing on the efficacy-effectiveness gap, key challenges for researchers include: (1) measurement challenges in assessing diet and exercise in typical community and healthcare settings, (2) measurement issues in identifying the key aspects of the intervention processes, and (3) linking process indicators to key changes in clinical measures at the individual level.

Better measures of diet and exercise (issue 1) that are relatively simple to collect, reliable and could validly assess the achieved level of diet and fitness status at each time point and over time are a priority. With a focus on improving measures, it may be possible to identify key aspects of interventions and better link them to clinical changes.

Assessment of the measurement properties of diet quality and physical fitness measures is the focus of this secondary analysis of a primary care-based lifestyle study [26]. A 19% reversal of MetS and reduction in CVD risk score, as measured by PROCAM risk score (analogous to the Framingham risk score but for MetS) [27] was seen in this one-year study overall, as previously published [26]. Unpublished data showed changes in individual scores for diet quality and aerobic capacity were not correlated with individual changes in PROCAM scores as was hoped, given the overall group results. Only changes in waist circumference were correlated with PROCAM score. Therefore, we asked if measurement error in the intervention measures could have accounted for the lack of associations, and secondly whether changes in one behavior could have had effects on the other. This latter question came from consideration of the potential for a carry-over effect, as discussed in the multiple behavior change literature [28]. Diet and physical activity interventions are the most commonly studied multiple risk behavior interventions [29]. To explore these possibilities, a detailed structural equation modeling (SEM) analysis was undertaken.

First, the physical activity and diet measures are briefly reviewed, followed by an introduction to SEM, which represents a melding of factor analysis and path analysis into one comprehensive statistical methodology. In general, a structural equation model consists of two parts: (1) the measurement model, which links observed variables to latent variables via a confirmatory factor analysis, and (2) the structural model linking latent variables to each other via systems of simultaneous equations [30]. This measurement analysis uses both exploratory factor analysis (EFA) and confirmatory factor analysis (CFA) with detailed explanations of the modeling process. The analysis for carry-over effects was conducted with the resulting latent variables.

1.3. Fitness Assessment

Fitness assessment in community- or primary care-based studies may include multiple tests to determine measures of some or all of the four main health-related fitness components: cardio-respiratory fitness or aerobic capacity, muscle fitness or strength, flexibility, and body composition, based on a wide range of standardized procedures [31,32]. A key measure of cardiorespiratory fitness employed in many studies is an estimate of maximal oxygen consumption (VO_2 max), providing an indicator of both cardiac and pulmonary functioning. VO_2 max may be expressed as an absolute rate in litres of oxygen per minute (L/min) or in terms of percentiles relative to age-and-sex-based averages. Accurate VO_2 max measurement requires physical effort sufficient in duration and intensity to put the aerobic energy (i.e., cardiorespiratory) system through its range of capacity. A treadmill or exercise bike is used to vary exercise intensity progressively while measuring pulmonary function and the chemical composition of inhalation/exhalation air for the oxygen/carbon dioxide ratio. Accurate assessment of VO_2 max is beyond the capacity of community studies, so many groups have created various sub-maximal exercise-based and non-exercise-based estimation equations for clinical practice [32]. Significant error has been demonstrated using these less accurate methods and research is underway to develop tools that can be used in clinical practice [33]. In the meantime, a variety of approaches have been used.

1.4. Diet Quality Assessment

Assessment of diet in community-based intervention studies remains challenging, given the complexity of diet with many foods eaten daily and the large day-to-day variation in intake. Personalized diet counselling or therapy for CMR conditions, including MetS, involves two main approaches [34]; a weight loss focus as exemplified by the Diabetes Prevention Program [3] versus a focus on diet quality, as exemplified by the PREDIMED study, which promoted a Mediterranean diet [2]. Therefore, multiple diet assessment methods were used to take advantage of the complementary strengths and limitations of different tools, specifically recalls coupled with a food frequency questionnaire (FFQ) approach. In North America, the use of the Healthy Eating Index (HEI) was originally developed for epidemiological studies, as it is scored against the benchmark of the US Dietary Guidelines (the basis of nutrition policy in the US), and has had extensive development, and population data are available for comparison [35]. More recently, its use has been reviewed in CMR intervention studies [36]. Other diet quality tools used in intervention studies include various versions of the Mediterranean Diet Score (MDS) [37], as well as scores based on different aspects of diet (see Miller et al. for recent review [38]). Interest in the use of diet quality scores in lifestyle intervention studies has been growing, as they provide a summary measure that can potentially be linked to clinical outcomes. Therefore, this analysis is timely.

1.5. Structural Equation Modeling and Measurement Equivalence/Invariance (ME/I)

Accurate measurement and representation of summary indices and measures requires assessment of measurement equivalence/invariance (ME/I) to demonstrate that the items/tests/measurements perform equally well and measure the same underlying constructs across groups and/or over time [39–43]. The longitudinal design of the current study allows for analysis of a combination of cross sectional and change models, as well as assessment of ME/I [41]. This requires examining simultaneous relationships between constructs in the SEM framework. Appropriate baseline sampling allowed us to understand the extent (i.e., prevalence) of cardiovascular risk, profiles of dietary behaviors, and the initial and subsequent levels of physical activity/fitness. The repeated measures data allows each participant to serve as their own baseline or control, as well as measuring changes in each of the two areas of concern (i.e., dietary/nutritional behavior, physical activity/exercise). Information garnered from cross-sectional models and the evaluation of appropriate measurement models developed through EFA and CFA methods will help inform models to be used to predict changes within constructs as well as testing structural relationships between constructs. As noted by Hayduk [39] creation of latent variables relies on accurate measurement of observed constructs.

With appropriate conceptual models established and ME/I assessed, relationships between the latent HEI and physical activity/fitness constructs over time were assessed to see if changes in one lifestyle intervention were associated with changes in the other over time, in line with the emerging area of multiple risk behavior interventions. The basic argument is that experiences, skills, knowledge and self-efficacy can be carried-over to different behaviors and domains [28].

2. Methods

2.1. Data from Original Study

The data come from a non-randomized 12-month feasibility study for lifestyle treatment of MetS conducted from 2012–2015 at three Canadian primary care clinics in three different provinces (Edmonton, Alberta, Toronto, Ontario, and Quebec City, Quebec) [26]. All participants were recruited by their primary care physicians. Inclusion criteria included: (1) adults at least 18 years age; (2) a body mass index (BMI) less than 35; and (3) presence of at least 3 out of 5 criteria for MetS [9]. Exclusion criteria included relevant medical, safety or logistic reasons, as described in the primary paper [26]. The study plan is shown in Figure 1. Study data were obtained from the patients' medical charts and entered into a secure online data capture system (Research Electronic Data Capture; REDCap: http://www.projectredcap.org/; accessed on 1 November 2021) by locally designated clinic staff. The current sample was comprised of 293 adults, aged 18–81 years old (mean 59 years), and 52% female.

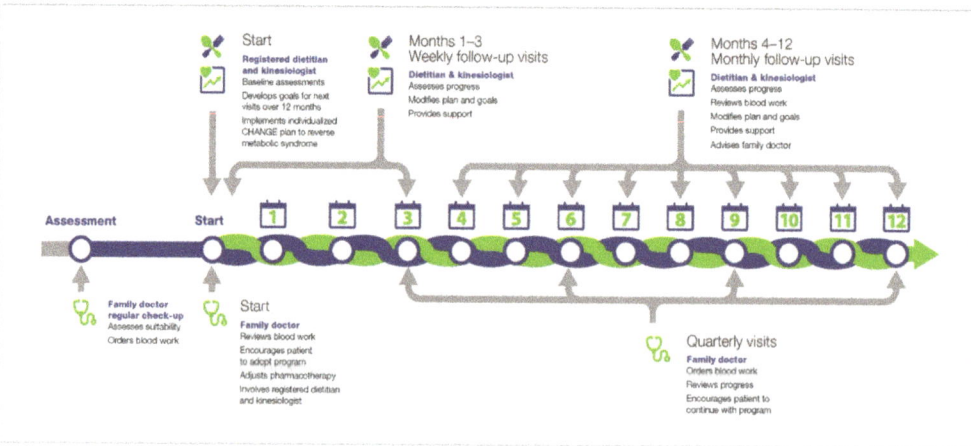

Figure 1. Data collection plan for lifestyle intervention study.

Physician review with participants occurred quarterly. As noted in Figure 1, lifestyle intervention consists of weekly appointments for 12 weeks, followed by monthly appointments and interactions for up to one year by locally employed Registered Dietitians (RD) and kinesiologists. All interventions were personalized, and practitioners were trained and supported by the research team [44,45]. The patient experience was highly positive, as documented by focus groups and a questionnaire [46]. This analysis uses the baseline, 3-month and 12-month data.

2.2. Available Measures

2.2.1. Physical Activity/Fitness

Aerobic fitness of participants was assessed by a methodology described by Ebbeling et al. to estimate maximal oxygen consumption [47], using a submaximal aerobic fitness test that is considered safe and appropriate for low risk, apparently healthy, non-athletic adults 20–59 years of age. A steady state heart rate is established after a warm-up by altering the treadmill speed at a 5% incline for 4 min, as described in detail elsewhere [48]. Both speed (in miles/h) and heart rate (bpm) are required in the calculation of this version of VO_2 max. The measure was further adjusted to create a percentile score relative to others in the same age-sex category. Other measures of exercise output and fitness assessed muscular strength, flexibility, and endurance [45,48]. Each of these measures interacts with and is dependent upon the fitness level of the cardiopulmonary system. These various measures were not combined into an overall fitness score in the original study [48,49].

2.2.2. Diet Quality—HEI-C

To calculate the Canadian version of the HEI (HEI-C) [50,51], a FFQ was developed to assess the average number of servings of food groups eaten over the past month and then scored according to specific age and sex criteria based on Canada's Food Guide (CFG) 2007 recommendations and serving sizes [52] (see Supplement Table S1). The scores for the moderation components, energy (kcal) from saturated fat and other foods (as a percentage of total energy), and sodium (in milligrams) were calculated from the results of two 24-h recalls, done about one week apart, at baseline, 3-months and 12-months, as previously described [50]. The dietary intake data were collected by the RDs at each centre and analyzed centrally to maintain quality control using a comprehensive nutrient analysis program (ESHA Food Processor—Canadian Version 10, Salem, OR, USA) and double data entry.

2.2.3. Other Variables

Many other clinical measures were collected in the dataset, including medical diagnoses and medication usage [26]. While all participants met the criteria for MetS, prevalence of specific features vary in different samples [53], and in the primary study, approximately half of the sample had a formal diagnosis of type 2 diabetes mellitus (DM). As this was a main clinical issue, we assessed by DM status.

2.3. Analytics Plan

Correlation matrices were examined for all items from the HEI-C, physical activity/fitness measures, and the PROCAM scores to confirm previous findings. Test-retest correlations across time points were also examined.

Baseline data were considered the first step to establishing the measurement models for HEI-C and physical activity/fitness. Upon establishing an acceptable fit for the baseline models, longitudinal extensions of measurement models were examined. Females were utilized for model development, with replication/extension to males. For disease status, models were initially tested on the no-DM group (i.e., MetS but no diagnosis of DM), then extended to examine those with DM. The fit of all models was assessed using model chi square (χ^2; non-significant result is desirable but often unlikely in larger samples), Comparative Fit Index, (CFI > 0.90), Non-Normed Fit Index (NNFI, also known as the

Tucker-Lewis Index NNFI > 0.90), Root Mean Square Error of Approximation (RMSEA range 0.05–0.08 accepted, smaller values indicate better fit) (see Tables 1 and 2). The general recommendation is to evaluate model fit through consensus of an array of fit indexes. These fit indices are consistent with recommendations from Bentler [54], Cheung and Rensvold [55], Kline [56], Lai and Green [57], McNeish, An and Hancock [58] and others. Statistically significant χ^2 values are not unusual in larger samples or more complex models, and the model(s) fit may still be acceptable.

Comparisons of the same constructs over time or in different groups assumes the tests/items demonstrate factorial invariance and this has been described as the most important empirical question to address whenever multiple groups or time points are present [59]. Invariance testing involves a series of nested constraints that examine whether the variance/covariance relationships among variables operate similarly across groups/points of measurement. Multiple tests of ME/I were conducted following the strategies described by Hayduk [39], Little [59], Meredith [60], Millsap [61], Vandenberg and Lance [41], and van de Schoot et al. [42].

Configural invariance, weak metric invariance, strong invariance of measurement intercepts, and strict invariance of the uniqueness or error terms were all examined, as indicated in Tables 1 and 2. Configural invariance is also called pattern invariance, meaning the same variables are loading onto the same factors across groups or over time. A lack of configural invariance in the physical activity/fitness model would be demonstrated if a measure like speed was important at baseline but not later in the study (or if it was salient for men but not for women). Configural invariance says nothing about the magnitude of the factor loadings, simply that the same variables load onto the same factors across groups [43]. Weak metric invariance, also called factor loading invariance, is a test of the equivalence of the magnitude or size of the factor loadings across groups or time (Little [59], Meredith [60], Vandenberg and Lance [41]). In addition to the same variables loading onto the same factors across groups (or over time), the relationship or proportionality of the loadings on the factors is demonstrated to be the same (i.e., the rank order and the size of the factor loadings are consistent across comparisons). Tests of weak metric or factor loading invariance are often the highest level of ME/I accomplished and finding this evidence is a sizable accomplishment in complex models. There is some disagreement about how difficult weak invariance is to obtain as Horn, McArdle and Mason [62] suggested that configural invariance is often the best one can hope to obtain in social science data. Physiological measure or laboratory values often demonstrate more precision than self-reported data. Little [59] provided a different perspective, suggesting weak invariance is often attained, whereas invariance of intercepts, is much more important and difficult. Every observed variable/item in the SEM model has an intercept and tests of invariance of these intercepts is important if one hopes to examine mean comparisons between groups or over time (as is implicitly done in analysis of variance models). This is often referred to as strong invariance (also known as scalar invariance or intercept invariance) [59]. Finally, the most restrictive form of invariance, and one that is often impossible to attain, is strict invariance (i.e., demonstrating the equality of the error/residual/uniqueness terms across groups/time—also known as error variance invariance or residual invariance). Little [59] suggests this level is overly restrictive and argues even if found, strict invariance does not ensure a "better" level of invariance. Therefore, testing for strict invariance was undertaken, but models were not rejected based on a lack of strict invariance. All tests of invariance are part of a hierarchy, and these nested models are tested from the least restrictive (configural model) to the more restrictive test (strict invariance).

Model fit was evaluated and the presence or absence of ME/I was determined using the fit indexes and thresholds previously described. Additionally, the model χ^2 is additive and allows for tests of the differences of chi-square values ($\Delta\chi^2$) between nested models to determine whether the tested level of invariance is accepted (i.e., is the inclusion of added restrictions, for example—constraining factor loadings to be equal across groups—acceptable or does it degrade the fit of the model?). The $\Delta\chi^2$ should be a non-significant difference for the test of invariance to be accepted. This indicates that the change from a less restrictive model to a more restrictive model is negligible [59]. One concern with this approach to comparing models is that $\Delta\chi^2$ values are overly sensitive. Additional methods for model comparison include computing differences or delta values for the CFI and RMSEA fit indexes (Tables 1 and 2). The delta values for CFI would be rejected if the model change exceeds 0.005, or if delta for RMSEA exceeds 0.01 [63]. The process was similar for both physical activity/fitness and the HEI-C.

Modeling of associations in latent factors was then completed, to assess possible associations across the interventions.

3. Results
3.1. Physical Activity/Fitness
3.1.1. Exploratory Factor Analysis Model

Pearson correlations were examined among the physical activity/fitness variables (i.e., treadmill speed, percentile VO_2 max, partial curl-ups, push-ups, flexibility). Moderate to high correlations were observed for all but flexibility (range r = 0.36 between speed and push-ups to r = 0.85 between speed and VO_2 max). Baseline reliability and test-retest correlations for the rest of the measures was good (α = 0.65; r_{speed} = 0.74, r_{VO2max} = 0.89, r_{curlup} = 0.66, r_{pushup} = 0.81). Flexibility was dropped from further consideration.

Exploratory Factor Analysis of the physical activity/fitness items, using Maximum Likelihood extraction demonstrated a one-factor model fit the data. The Kaiser–Meyer–Olkin (KMO) measure of sampling adequacy was only moderate with a value of 0.66. The KMO ranges from 0–1.00 with values greater than 0.8 providing evidence that the relationships among examined variables are amenable to factor analytic procedures. Individual items were assessed using the KMO values from the diagonal of the anti-image matrix. KMO values ranged from 0.61 for speed and VO_2 max to 0.83 for partial curl-ups.

There was only one eigenvalue greater than 1.0 and the Scree Plot showed a sharp break between one and two factors, suggesting a one-factor solution. VO_2 max is often used as a "gold-standard" measure of fitness, and our goal was to evaluate whether adding measures of strength would contribute to measuring fitness above and beyond cardiorespiratory measures. Model fit was moderate, with a model χ^2 (2) = 24.12, p = 0.001. The Goodness of Fit Index (GFI) index in EFA should be non-significant, but one also has to interpret the factor loadings, which ranged from moderate to large (i.e., Λpush-ups = 0.44, Λcurl-ups = 0.46, Λspeed = 0.88, and ΛVO_2 max = 0.97). The communalities (i.e., the amount of variance accounted for in each item) were 0.19 for push-ups, 0.21 for curl-ups, 0.77 for speed, and 0.93 for VO_2 max. The overall sum of squared factor loadings or percentage of variance accounted for by the model was 53% utilizing the single-factor solution.

Upon confirmation of this result, we examined CFA utilizing the Analysis of Moments Structures (AMOS) Structural Equation Modeling (SEM) program (Amos Version 26.0. Chicago: IBM SPSS). The results from AMOS are presented below. All factor loadings were statistically significant, and the variance accounted for in the observed indicators varied between 18% and 97% (see Figure 2). These results map onto the EFA results described above. One benefit of the SEM/CFA approach is that AMOS provides numerous measures of model fit not available in EFA statistical packages. Overall model fit was strong and supported the multiple indicator model of fitness (see Figure 2 and Table 1, Models #2 and #3). The only modification of the factor model was correlating the error term between push-ups and curl-ups, as both were indicators of strength.

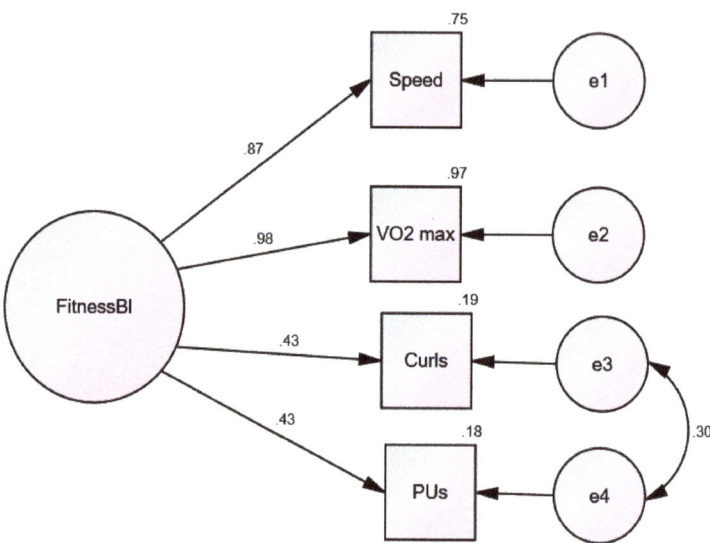

Figure 2. Baseline confirmatory factor analysis model. FitnessBl = latent factor; Speed = treadmill speed; VO$_2$ max = age-sex percentile of VO$_2$ max; Curls = Curl-ups; Pus = Push-ups; e# = error terms. Squares are measured variables; circles are latent variables.

Table 1. Model Comparison for Physical Activity/Fitness Models.

Model #	Model	X^2 (df)	X^2 p-Value	CFI	NNFI	RMSEA [95% CI]	ΔX^2 ΔCFI ΔRMSEA
	Desirable Criterion or Range		NS desirable	>0.9	>0.9	0.05–0.08 acceptable; lower better	ΔX^2 = NS ΔCFI $\leq$ 0.005 ΔRMSEA $\leq$ 0.01
			Longitudinal Invariance				
1	1-Factor Model	0.939 (1)	0.333	1.00	1.00	0.000 0.000–0.153	
2	Longitudinal Configural	139.29 (37)	0.001	0.97	0.94	0.097 0.080–0.115	
3	Longitudinal Metric	159.36 (43)	0.001	0.96	0.93	0.096 0.081–0.112	Reject. Accept Accept
4	Longitudinal Intercepts Only	394.09 (45)	0.001	0.89	0.80	0.157 0.148–0.178	Reject Reject Reject
5	Longitudinal Loadings and Intercepts	415.82 (51)	0.001	0.88	0.82	0.157 0.143–0.171	Reject Reject Reject
6	Longitudinal Model Residuals		Not tested as invariant intercepts not found				
			Sex Models—Female				
7	Female Baseline	0.100 (1)	0.752	1.00	1.00	0.000 0.000–0.148	
8	Female Longitudinal Configural	56.99 (37)	0.019	0.98	0.96	0.060 0.025–0.089	

Table 1. Cont.

Model #	Model	X^2 (df)	X^2 p-Value	CFI	NNFI	RMSEA [95% CI]	ΔX^2 ΔCFI ΔRMSEA
9	Female Longitudinal Metric	66.57 (43)	0.012	0.98	0.96	0.060 0.029–0.088	Accept Accept Accept
10	Female Intercepts Only	171.13 (45)	0.001	0.88	0.80	0.136 0.115–0.158	Reject Reject Reject
11	Female Loadings and Intercepts	180.89 (51)	0.001	0.88	0.82	0.130 0.110–0.151	Accept Accept Accept
12	Female Residuals		Not	tested	as invariant	intercepts not found	
		Sex Models—Male					
13	Male Baseline	3.94 (1)	0.047	0.99	0.90	0.145 0.014–0.307	
14	Males Longitudinal Configural	117.59 (37)	0.001	0.95	0.90	0.125 0.100–0.150	
15	Males Longitudinal Metric	136.59 (43)	0.001	0.95	0.90	0.125 0.102–0.149	Reject Accept Accept
16	Male Intercepts Only	250.41 (45)	0.001	0.88	0.80	0.181 0.159–0.203	Reject Reject Reject
17	Male Loadings and Intercepts	275.94 (51)	0.001	0.87	0.80	0.177 0.157–0.198	Reject Reject Reject
18	Male Residuals		Not	tested	as invariant	intercepts not found	
		Gender Invariance of Longitudinal Fitness Model					
19	Sex Invar. Configural	174.60 (74)	0.001	0.96	0.93	0.068 0.055–0.082	
20	Sex Model Sex Invariant	180.76 (83)	0.001	0.97	0.94	0.064 0.051–0.076	Accept Accept Accept
21	Sex Model Time Invariant	206.58 (89)	0.001	0.96	0.93	0.067 0.055–0.079	Reject Accept Accept
22	Sex Model Intercepts		Not	run based	on previous	intercept models	
23	Sex Model Residuals		Not	run as intercept	models	were not accepted	
		Disease-State Models—No Diabetes					
24	NoDM Baseline	1.12 (1)	0.290	1.00	0.96	0.029 0.000–0.228	
25	NoDM Longitudinal Configural	97.42 (37)	0.001	0.96	0.91	0.108 0.082–0.134	
26	NoDM Longitudinal Metric	106.96 (43)	0.001	0.95	0.91	0.103 0.079–0.128	Accept Accept Accept
27	NoDM Longitudinal Intercepts Only	218.98 (45)	0.001	0.87	0.78	0.166 0.145–0.189	Reject Reject Reject

Table 1. Cont.

Model #	Model	X^2 (df)	X^2 p-Value	CFI	NNFI	RMSEA [95% CI]	ΔX^2 ΔCFI ΔRMSEA
28	NoDM Residuals			Not tested as invariant intercepts not found			
			Disease-State Models—Diabetes				
29	DM Baseline	0.002 (1)	0.968	1.00	1.00	0.000 0.000–0.000	
30	DM Longitudinal Configural	72.57 (37)	0.001	0.98	0.96	0.080 0.052–0.107	
31	DM Longitudinal Metric	89.75 (43)	0.001	0.97	0.95	0.085 0.060–0.110	Reject Accept Accept
32	DM Longitudinal Intercepts Only	215.14 (45)	0.001	0.91	0.84	0.158 0.137–0.180	Reject Reject Reject
33	DM Residuals		Not tested as invariant intercepts not found				
			Disease Invariance of Longitudinal Fitness Model				
34	Disease Model Configural	170.00 (74)	0.001	0.97	0.94	0.067 0.054–0.080	
35	*Disease Model Disease Invariant*	*184.87 (83)*	*0.001*	*0.97*	*0.94*	*0.065 0.052–0.078*	*Accept Accept Accept*
36	*Disease Model Time Invariant*	*201.93 (89)*	*0.001*	*0.96*	*0.94*	*0.066 0.054–0.078*	*Reject Accept Accept*
37	Disease Model Intercepts		Not run based on previous intercept models				
38	Disease Model Residuals		Not run as intercept models were not accepted				

X^2 = Model chi square; CFI = Comparative Fit Index; NNFI = Non-Normed Fit Index; RMSEA = Root Mean Square Error of Approximation; Δ = change. Best model(s) in each hierarchal set of models shown in italics.

3.1.2. Longitudinal Extension of Physical Activity/Fitness Model

Given the results above, we extended the measurement model in AMOS to test a longitudinal (i.e., three time points: baseline, 3-months, 12-months) model [59]. As we measured the same indicators of fitness on each occasion, the AMOS program and standard convention in SEM allows for correlations between the same indicators over time (e.g., speed at baseline is expected to correlate with the subsequent speed measures at 3- and 12-months). Each of the four indicators were treated in this manner, to allow for the autocorrelation of measuring the same indicators on the same participants, over time (see Figure 3). The extended, longitudinal model of fitness (Table 1, Model #2) demonstrated excellent model fit (χ^2 (37) = 139.29, $p < 0.001$, CFI =.97, NNFI = 0.94, RMSEA= 0.097). All factor loadings were statistically significant, with squared multiple correlation or variance accounted for ranging from 8% to 87% (not shown).

The fitness factor created at each measurement point was regressed onto the subsequent measure (i.e., baseline fitness predicting 3-month fitness, 3-month fitness predicting 12-month fitness) and the results showed that 73% of the variance in fitness at 3-months was predicted by baseline fitness, and 84% of variance in fitness at 12-months was explained by fitness level at 3-months of the intervention (see Figure 3 and Table 1, Model #3). The model did not meet criteria for invariance of intercepts however, longitudinal invariance of factor loadings was found (Table 1, Models #4 and #5 compared to Model #3).

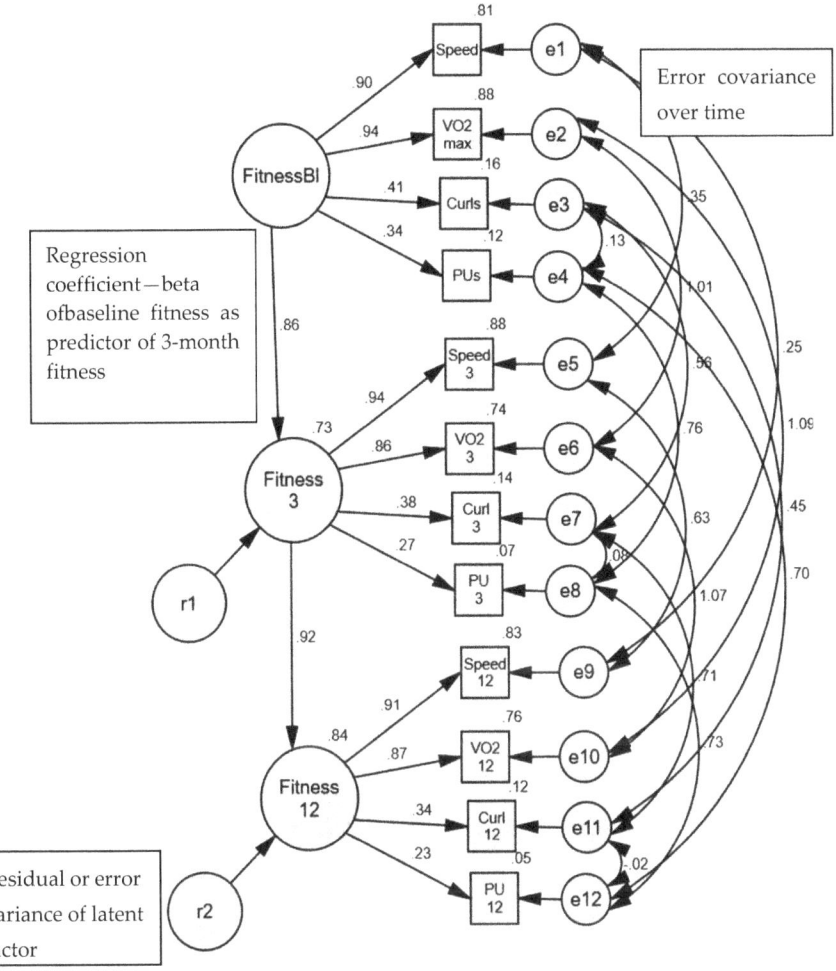

Figure 3. Sex and time invariance. FitnessB1 = baseline; Fitness3 = 3-months; Fitness12 = 12-months Speed = treadmill speed; VO$_2$ max = age-sex percentile; Curls = Curl-ups; PU = Push-ups; e# and r# = error terms. Squares are measured variables; circles are latent variables.

3.1.3. Sex Invariance of Physical Activity/Fitness Model

Invariance testing was conducted for females (cross-sectional/baseline fitness model, longitudinal extension of fitness model (tests of invariance of variable loadings, intercepts, intercepts and loadings, and residuals if appropriate); males (testing the same sequence noted above); then examining the issue of sex invariance for the longitudinal fitness model (i.e., test of invariance of loading across time in a simultaneous model, constraining equality of the longitudinal loadings across sex, tests of equality of intercepts, and tests of residuals, if appropriate). Our results showed that, in addition to the model fitting well for both women (Model #9) and men (Model #15), invariance of the fitness model was demonstrated across the three time points of the intervention as well as across sex (Table 1, Models #20 and #21).

Testing equivalence of the variable intercepts were mixed at best, and based on overall decrement of model fit, it was deemed that invariant intercepts were not accepted (Table 1, Models #10 and #16). Given this result, and that all models are hierarchical regarding their restrictiveness (i.e., if one fails to accept equivalence of loadings, you should not continue with ME/I testing), we concluded that the fitness model demonstrated invariant factor loadings for sex and across time. The final result is shown in Figure 3. The magnitudes of the standardized loadings were identical for males and females, however, as we were unable to accept the constraint of the residual or uniqueness terms, the loadings appear slightly different in size over time (i.e., unstandardized loadings were identical across the three time points). Standardized loadings are presented as they are generally easier to interpret (with values ranging from 0–1, with larger values indicating stronger loadings) and they are similar to correlations for general interpretation purposes. VO_2 max and speed measures contributed more to the physical activity/fitness factor than the strength measures (push-ups, curl-ups), yet all four measures are significant components of the overall factor.

3.1.4. Disease-State Invariance of Physical Activity/Fitness Model

Invariance was tested for participants with noDM (cross-sectional/baseline fitness model, longitudinal extension of fitness model, tests of invariance of variable loadings, intercepts, intercepts and loadings, and residuals if appropriate); those with DM (testing the same sequence noted above); then examining the issue of disease-state invariance for the longitudinal fitness model (i.e., test of invariance of loadings across time in a simultaneous model, constraining equality of the longitudinal loadings across disease-state, tests of equality of intercepts, and tests of residuals, if appropriate). Results showed that, in addition to the model fitting well for participants with noDM (Table 1, Model #26), and those with DM (Model #31), invariance of the fitness model was demonstrated across the three time points of the intervention as well as across disease-states (Table 1, Models #35 and #36). Testing equivalence of the variable intercepts gave mixed results at best, and based on overall decrement of model fit, it was deemed that invariant intercepts were not accepted.

We found that the fitness model demonstrated invariant loadings for disease-states (noDM vs. DM) and across time (baseline, 3-months, 12-months). The results for the disease-state model are shown in Figure 4. The magnitude of the standardized loadings are identical for noDM and DM, however, as we were unable to accept the constraint of the residual or uniqueness terms, the loadings appear slightly different in size over time (i.e., unstandardized loadings were identical across the three time points and across disease-states). As noted in the previous results, VO_2 max and speed measures contributed more to the physical activity/fitness factor than the strength measures (push-ups, curl-ups), yet all four measures are significant components of the overall factor. It was noted that the amount of explained variance in the physical activity/fitness factor was higher in the DM group (73% at 3-months, 91% at 12-months, than the noDM group: 73% at 3-months, 75% at 12-months).

3.2. Healthy Eating Index (HEI-C)
3.2.1. Exploratory Factor Analysis Model

Pearson correlations were examined for the 11 HEI-C items (see Supplement, Table S1). Low to moderate correlations were observed, with some items showing very small correlations (e.g., milk and alternatives, unsaturated fats, total grains, and meat and alternatives showed the lowest correlations). We examined EFA of the full complement of 11 HEI-C items, using Maximum Likelihood extraction, with Promax rotation if the result had more than one resulting factor (i.e., to allow the resulting factors to correlate). The Kaiser-Meyer-Olkin (KMO) measure of sampling adequacy was only moderate with a value of 0.604. Individual items were assessed using the KMO values from the diagonal of the anti-image matrix. Variables with the lowest KMO values (i.e., below 0.6) were: total grains, meat and alternatives, milk and alternatives, raising concern about the inclusion of these items.

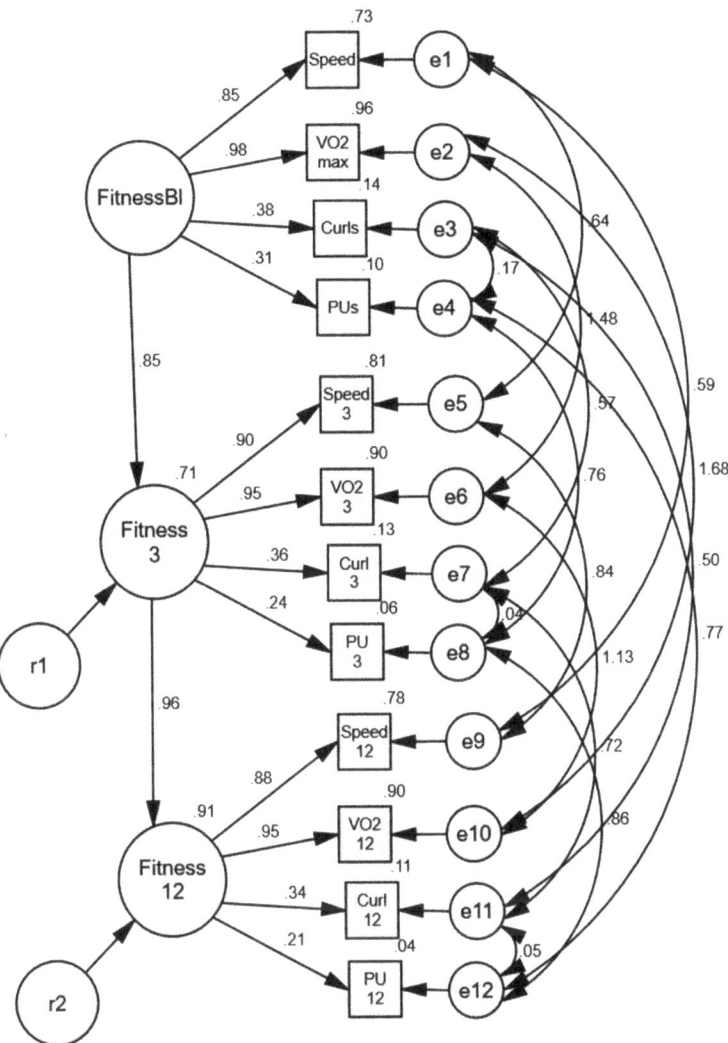

Figure 4. Disease invariance model. FitnessB1 = baseline; Fitness3 = 3-months; Fitness12 = 12-months Speed = treadmill speed; VO$_2$ max = age-sex percentile; Curls= Curl-ups; PU= Push-ups; e# and r# = error terms.

There were four eigenvalues exceeding 1.0, however, the Scree Plot showed a gradual decline without any clear breaks or drop-offs, suggesting a one-factor solution was most likely. Four factors with only 11 items would not be reasonable (i.e., ideally three or more items should result per factor), and the one-factor solution, especially if weak items were going to be removed/deleted, made conceptual sense. We evaluated the four-factor solution (based on eigenvalues greater than 1.0). Model fit was poor, with a model χ^2 (17) = 26.59, p = 0.064 and factor loadings were not conceptually meaningful.

The total score of the HEI-C is most widely used, therefore a one-factor solution would provide evidence whether this is a valid and meaningful approach. We examined a one-factor HEI-C model. The resulting factor loadings for the 11-item HEI-C EFA still reflected the same items noted earlier as being weak in this solution (i.e., milk and alternatives, meat and alternatives, total grains, and unsaturated fats). While many of these items make conceptual sense or might be seen as useful in dietary models, statistical evidence was not supporting retention of these items. We also noted that the communalities (i.e., the amount of variance accounted for in each item) were very low for these four items.

Additional EFA with 7 HEI-C items (i.e., removing the poorly fitting items: milk and alternatives, meat and alternatives, total grains, and unsaturated fats), Maximum Likelihood extraction, and no rotation in one factor was examined. The Kaiser–Meyer–Olkin (KMO) measure of sampling adequacy improved to 0.675 but was still low. Individual items ranged from 0.621–0.780.

There were two eigenvalues exceeding 1.0 (the second values barely exceeded 1.0 at 1.09), the Scree Plot showed a gradual decline without any clear breaks or drop-offs, suggesting a one-factor solution. Model fit was improved from the previous model, but it is still not an ideal model χ^2 (14) = 35.97, p = 0.001. Factor loadings ranged from 0.25–0.85.

3.2.2. Testing the Reduced HEI-C in CFA/SEM

The results of testing the reduced HEI-C model in a single factor solution with seven items in AMOS are presented in Figure 5. All factor loadings were statistically significant (low of 0.34 for whole Grains to a high of 0.50 for total vegetables/Fruit) and the variance accounted for ranged between 12% (whole grains) to 25% (vegetables/fruit), with an average variance of 18%. These results are consistent with the EFA results described above. We added two correlated error/residual terms to the model. Total vegetables/fruits and whole fruits, and also between total vegetables/fruits and dark green and orange vegetables. These variables are conceptually related. Model fit for the 7-item version (Table 2, Model #1) was exceptional with χ^2 (12) = 11.10, p < 0.521, CFI = 1.00, and RMSEA = 0.000. For comparison purposes, the 11-item (full) HEI-C resulted in two items with non-significant factor loadings (i.e., total grains and meat and alternatives), and both milk and alternatives and unsaturated fats had marginal/borderline values and χ^2 (44) = 208.28, p < 0.001, CFI= 0.57, and RMSEA = 0.11, outside the published cut-off values range (0.05 to 0.08).

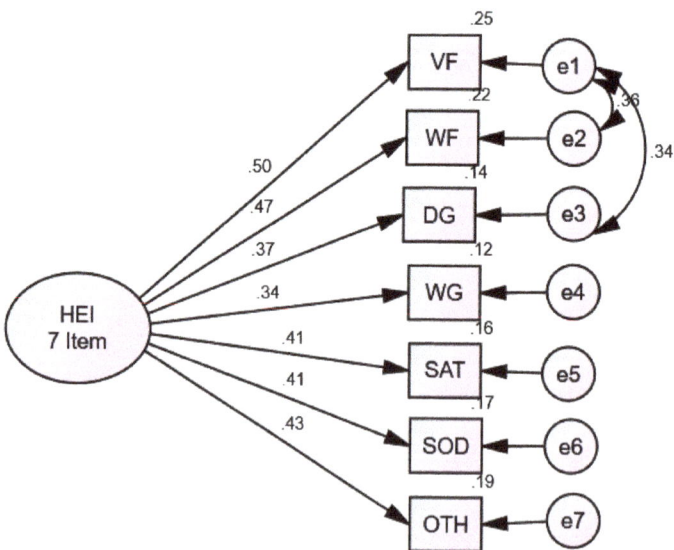

Figure 5. Baseline confirmatory factor analysis model for HEI-C. HEI = total HEI-C; VF = total vegetables and fruit; WF = whole fruit; DG = dark green and orange vegetables; WG = whole grains; SF = saturated fats; SOD = sodium; OTH = Other foods; e# = error terms. Squares are measured variables; circles are latent variables.

The reduced-item HEI-C model was therefore tested for longitudinal invariance in the total sample, as well as for each sex and each disease group (i.e., noDM/DM). The model demonstrated weak metric invariance (i.e., equivalence of the magnitude of the factor loadings over all three measurement points in the intervention—Table 2, Model #3). The model also demonstrated weak invariance of all factor loadings when compared across sex (Model #20) and across disease groups (Model #35).

Table 2. Model Comparison for Reduced (7-Item) HEI-C Models.

Model #	Model	X^2 (df)	X^2 p-value	CFI	NNFI	RMSEA [95% CI]	ΔX^2 ΔCFI $\Delta RMSEA$
	Desirable Criterion or Range		NS desirable	>0.9	>0.9	0.05–0.08 acceptable; lower better	$\Delta X2 = NS$ $\Delta CFI \leq 0.005$ $\Delta RMSEA \leq 0.01$
			Longitudinal Invariance				
1	1-Factor Model	11.10 (12)	0.521	1.00	1.00	0.000 0.000 -0.056	
2	Longitudinal Configural	205.15 (160)	0.009	0.95	0.93	0.031 0.046–0.063	
3	Longitudinal Metric	219.33 (172)	0.009	0.95	0.94	0.031 0.016–0.042	Accept Accept Accept
4	Longitudinal Intercepts Only	371.10 (174)	0.001	0.80	0.74	0.062 0.054–0.071	Reject Reject Reject
5	Longitudinal Loadings and Intercepts	388.17 (186)	0.001	0.80	0.75	0.061 0.052–0.070	Accept Accept Accept
6	Longitudinal Model Residuals		Not tested as invariant intercepts not found				
			Sex Models—Female				
7	Female Baseline	25.39 (12)	0.019	0.90	0.77	0.086 0.038–0.133	
8	Female Longitudinal Configural	200.85 (160)	0.016	0.93	0.89	0.041 0.019–0.058	
9	Female Longitudinal Metric	219.28 (172)	0.009	0.92	0.89	0.043 0.028–0.059	Accept Accept Accept
10	Female Intercepts Only	290.84 (174)	0.001	0.79	0.72	0.067 0.053–0.080	Reject Reject Reject
11	Female Loadings and Intercepts	309.48 (186)	0.001	0.78	0.72	0.066 0.053–0.079	Accept Accept Accept
12	Female Residuals		Not tested as invariant intercepts not found				
			Sex Models—Male				
13	Male Baseline	8.11 (12)	0.777	10.00	10.00	0.000 0.000–0.059	
14	Males Longitudinal Configural	210.31 (160)	0.005	0.90	0.85	0.047 0.027–0.064	
15	Males Longitudinal Metric	219.33 (172)	0.009	0.95	0.94	0.031 0.016–0.042	Accept Accept Accept

Table 2. Cont.

Model #	Model	X^2 (df)	X^2 p-value	CFI	NNFI	RMSEA [95% CI]	ΔX^2 ΔCFI ΔRMSEA
16	Male Intercept Only	310.29 (174)	0.001	0.72	0.63	0.072 0.061–0.088	Reject Reject Reject
17	Male Loadings and Intercepts	324.04 (186)	0.001	0.72	0.65	0.073 0.059–0.086	Reject Reject Reject
18	Male Residuals			Not tested as invariant intercepts not found			
	Sex Invariance of Longitudinal HEI-C Model						
19	Sex Invar. Configural	415.75 (320)	0.001	0.94	0.91	0.026 0.018–0.033	
20	Sex Model Sex Invariant	420.65 (338)	0.001	0.92	0.88	0.030 0.019–0.038	Accept Accept Accept
21	Sex Model Time Invariant	454.23 (350)	0.001	0.90	0.87	0.032 0.023–0.040	Reject Accept Accept
22	Sex Model Intercepts			Not run based on previous intercept models			
23	Sex Model Residuals			Not run as intercept models were not accepted			
	Disease-State Models—No Diabetes						
24	NoDM Baseline	16.12 (12)	0.186	0.96	0.91	0.059 0.000–0.106	
25	NoDM Longitudinal Configural	205.10 (160)	0.009	0.91	0.87	0.045 0.023–0.062	
26	NoDM Longitudinal Metric	224.15 (172)	0.005	0.89	0.86	0.047 0.027–0.063	Accept Accept Accept
27	NoDM Longitudinal Intercepts Only	283.75 (174)	0.001	0.77	0.70	0.067 0.053–0.081	Reject Reject Reject
28	NoDM Residuals			Not tested as invariant intercepts not found			
	Disease-State Models—Diabetes						
29	DM Baseline	9.50 (12)	0.660	1.00	1.00	0.000 0.000–0.068	
30	DM Longitudinal Configural	172.59 (160)	0.235	0.98	0.96	0.023 0.000–0.045	
31	DM Longitudinal Metric	183.88 (172)	0.254	0.98	0.97	0.021 0.000–0.043	Accept Accept Accept
32	DM Longitudinal Intercepts Only	276.63 (174)	0.001	0.80	0.73	0.063 0.048–0.076	Reject Reject Reject
33	DM Residuals			Not tested as invariant intercepts not found			
	Disease Invariance of Longitudinal HEI-C Model						
34	Disease Model Configural	377.70 (320)	0.015	0.95	0.92	0.025 0.012–0.034	

Table 2. Cont.

Model #	Model	X^2 (df)	X^2 p-value	CFI	NNFI	RMSEA [95% CI]	ΔX^2 ΔCFI ΔRMSEA
35	*Disease Model Disease Invariant*	397.95 (338)	0.014	0.94	0.92	0.025 0.012–0.034	*Accept Accept Accept*
36	*Disease Model Time Invariant*	410.90 (350)	0.014	0.94	0.92	0.024 0.012–0.034	*Accept Accept Accept*
37	Disease Model Intercepts	Not run based on previous intercept models					
38	Disease Model Residuals	Not run as intercept models were not accepted					

X^2 = Model chi square; CFI = Comparative Fit Index; NNFI = Non-Normed Fit Index; RMSEA = Root Mean Square Error of Approximation; Δ = change. Best model(s) in each hierarchal set of models shown in italics. This explains why the acceptable model is the longitudinal metric models (Model #3 and #9) and not the loadings and intercepts models (Model #5 and #11).

3.2.3. Longitudinal Extension of Reduced HEI-C Model

Based on the cross-sectional results above, we extended the reduced (7-item) HEI-C model to test the fit longitudinally. As with the physical activity/fitness models previously, we allowed correlations between the same indicators over time (e.g., vegetable/fruit at baseline are expected to correlate with the subsequent vegetable/fruit measures). We also maintained the correlation between the vegetable/fruit variable error terms as described above. The autocorrelation of the same indicators on the same participants over time was evaluated (see Supplement Figure S1). The extended, longitudinal model demonstrated excellent model fit (Table 2, Model #3). All measures of model fit improved for the longitudinal HEI-C model compared to the cross-sectional or baseline model. All factor loadings were statistically significant with the exception of the sodium variable at 3-months, and squared multiple correlations or variance accounted for in each variable, ranging from just over 1% (sodium at 3-months) to 72% for vegetables/fruit at baseline.

The HEI-C factor was regressed onto the subsequent measure (i.e., baseline HEI-C predicting 3-month HEI-C, 3-month HEI-C predicting 12-month HEI-C) and the results showed that 42% of the variance in HEI-C at 3-months was predicted by baseline HEI, and 52% of variance in HEI-C at 12-months was explained by HEI-C at 3-months of the intervention (see Supplement Figure S1).

3.2.4. Sex Invariance of Reduced HEI-C Model

Invariance testing followed the same sequence as for the physical activity/fitness model. Models were examined for females (cross-sectional/baseline HEI-C model, longitudinal extension of HEI-C model (tests of invariance of variable loadings, intercepts, intercepts and loadings, and residuals if appropriate); males (testing the same sequence noted above); then examining the issue of sex invariance for the longitudinal HEI-C model (i.e., test of invariance of loading across time in a simultaneous model, constraining equality of the longitudinal loadings across sex, tests of equality of intercepts, and tests of residuals, if appropriate). Results showed that, in addition to the model fitting well for both men (Model #15) and women (Model #9), invariance of the HEI-C model was demonstrated across the three time points of the intervention as well as across sex (Models #20 and #21). Testing equivalence of the variable intercepts yielded results that were mixed at best, and based on overall decrement of model fit, it was deemed that invariant intercepts were not accepted. The HEI-C model demonstrated invariant loadings for sex and across time. The final result is shown in Supplement Figure S2.

The magnitudes of the standardized loadings are identical for males and females, however, as we were unable to accept the constraint of the residual or uniqueness terms, the loadings appear slightly different in size over time (i.e., unstandardized loadings were identical across the three time points).

3.2.5. Disease State Invariance of Reduced HEI-C Model

Invariance testing participants with and without DM (cross-sectional/baseline HEI-C model, longitudinal extension of HEI-C model, tests of invariance of variable loadings, intercepts, intercepts and loadings, and residuals if appropriate); then examining the issue of disease-state invariance for the longitudinal HEI-C model (i.e., test of invariance of loading across time in a simultaneous model, constraining equality of the longitudinal loadings across disease-state, tests of equality of intercepts, and tests of residuals, if appropriate). Results showed that, in addition to the model fitting well for participants with no DM (Model #26), and those with DM (Model #31), invariance of the HEI-C model was demonstrated across the three time points of the intervention as well as across disease-states (Models #35 and #36). Testing equivalence of the variable intercepts yielded poor results, and invariant intercepts were not accepted. We found that the HEI-C model demonstrated invariant loadings for disease-states (noDM vs DM) and across time (Supplement Figure S3).

3.3. Assessment of Associations between Physical Activity/Fitness and Reduced HEI-C

To test whether diet quality and physical activity/fitness were significantly related over the course of the year-long intervention, structural regression was conducted. For males and females overall, regression paths in green showed significant results, structural regression in red were not statistically significant (Figure 6). The following relationships were significant: fitness-baseline to HEI-C-3month; HEI-C-3-month to fitness-12-month; fitness-3-month to HEI-C-12-months.

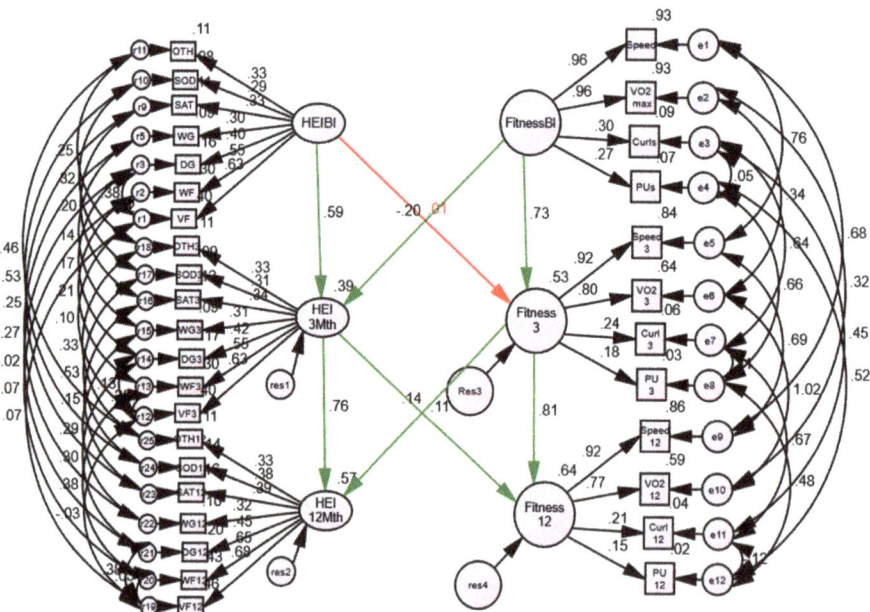

Figure 6. Overall sex and time invariant results showing structural regressions between HEI and Fitness factors. Regression paths in green show significant results, structural regression in red were not statistically significant. FitnessB1 = baseline; Fitness3 = 3-months; Fitness12 = 12-months Speed = treadmill speed; VO$_2$ max = age-sex percentile; Curls = Curl-ups; PU = Push-ups. HEIBl = total HEI-C baseline; HEI3Mth = total HEI-C at 3-months; HEI12Mth = total HEI-C at 12-months; VF = total vegetables and fruit; WF = whole fruit; DG = dark green and orange vegetables; WG = whole grains; SF = saturated fats; SOD = sodium; OTH = Other foods; e# and r# = error terms.

The models were then examined for sex and disease-state comparisons. Previous results suggested that both models were at least weak-metric invariant (i.e., the factor loadings for both physical activity/fitness and HEI-C, demonstrated equivalence across the comparison group and over time). This result was found, with the sex-model demonstrating weak-metric invariance as the highest level χ^2 (935) = 1375.33, CFI = 0.89, NNFI = 0.87, RMSEA = 0.040. Strong auto-regressive relationships were noted for fitness, wherein fitness-baseline predicted 53% of the variance of fitness-3-month, and fitness-3-month predicted 64% of the variance in fitness at 12-months in females, whereas these values were 64% and 84% respectively in males. Regarding HEI-C, baseline to 3-months accounted for 39% variance and 3-month to 12-months accounted for 57% in females, whereas 51% and 40% variance were accounted for in males.

We then examined the relationships separately for women and men (Supplement Figures S4 and S5). For women, the only significant relationship was fitness at baseline was significantly related to HEI-C at 3-months (Supplement Figure S4), while for men HEI-C at 3-months was significantly related to fitness at 12-months and fitness at 3-months predicted HEI-C at 12-months (Supplement Figure S5).

The disease-state model showed invariance through the level of structural variances/covariance (i.e., the only coefficients in the model that were not equivalent were the residual or error terms). Strong auto-regressive relationships were noted for fitness whereby fitness-baseline predicted 70% of the variance of fitness-3-month, and fitness-3-month predicted 91% of the variance in fitness at 12-months in DM, whereas these values were 74% and 78% respectively in participants with noDM. Regarding HEI-C, baseline to 3-months accounted for 44% variance and 3-month to 12-months accounted for 41% in DM, whereas 42% and 67% variance were accounted for in noDM. Model fit: χ^2 (978) = 1261.94, CFI = 0.93, NNFI = 0.92, RMSEA = 0.032. Of note among the structural regressions, only the relationship from HEI-C-3-month to fitness-12-month was statistically significant in participants with noDM and those with DM (see Supplement Figure S6).

4. Discussion

Health behavior change researchers working in community and primary care contexts are interested in the potential for using composite summary scales and measures to describe changes in health behaviors. Scales have typically been developed and validated by researchers within the nutrition and kinesiology disciplines and it is common to adopt validated tools in community intervention studies, as was done in this secondary analysis. To answer our original question, could measurement error have accounted for the lack of association with the CVD risk score? Certainly, the measurement properties of the original HEI-C were poor and could have contributed to a lack of association. Lack of association of changes in percentile VO$_2$ max could also be due to measurement issues with VO$_2$ max, especially given recent documentation of measurement error in similar equations tested by Peterman et al. [33]. The Ebbeling equation was not specifically tested in their validation study on multiple equations against measured VO$_2$ max. Further work on the measurement properties of both diet quality and fitness measures is warranted.

The results of the analysis of the measurement properties of HEI-C were particularly interesting as the concept of using scales to assess overall diet quality has a relatively long history in nutritional epidemiology, with the first HEI published in 1995, based on the work of Kennedy and colleagues [64]. Four measures within the original 11-item HEI-C model did not contribute to the latent HEI-C factor: milk and alternatives, meat and alternatives, total grains, and unsaturated fats. While these food groups are important for general health, if intake did not vary among the participants with low vs. high HEI scores at baseline and did not change with intervention, they will not contribute to the model. Examination of the data from the original study provides indirect evidence to support this interpretation [50]. Mean HEI scores for meat and alternates were high at baseline (8/10 possible points) and remained high throughout the 12-month intervention. Scores for milk and alternates were average at baseline (4.8 of 10 possible points), increased slightly at 3-months and returned to 5.0 at 12-months, reflecting no change attributable to the dietary intervention. Scores for total grains declined from 3.4 of 5 possible points to 3.1 at 12-months, while carbohydrate intake was 48% of kcal throughout. Unsaturated fat intake was confirmed to be low and relatively stable both from the nutrient analysis and HEI-C analysis. The reduced latent HEI-C factor had better measurement properties and it was possible to detect interesting interactions between physical activity and diet change.

Going forward, development of new diet quality tools is needed for the intervention context. Such intervention tools can potentially be adapted from tools already developed in epidemiology. Interesting work is underway to develop an adapted diet quality tool for Canada that is associated with lower risk of MetS markers. Lafreniere et al. have used reduced rank regression to identify food groups associated with MetS markers in a French Canadian sample [65]. Their retained food groups in their modified C-HEI tool were total vegetables and fruit, whole fruit, dark green and orange vegetables, whole grains, yogurt, nuts and legumes, red and processed meat, refined grains, sugar-sweetened beverages, "other foods". While there is substantial overlap with our reduced 7-item HEI-C, namely five of seven items are on both lists (total vegetables and fruit, whole fruit, dark green and orange vegetables, whole grains "other foods") with only saturated fat and sodium retained in our version but not in their version. Interestingly, both our work and Lafreniere et al. use variance as a key criterion for retention of food groups. There is some danger to this data-driven approach, in that food groups that are important to health may be missed. For example, fish may be important; it is a key component of the Mediterranean diet with desirable nutritional properties, yet Canadians do not eat very much fish and it did not emerge as a group in the LaFreniere analysis. For future intervention studies, fish might need to be included as a target food to increase intake. Still, Lafreniere's results are very interesting, and along with our work provide a basis for progress in the development of new diet quality tools for intervention work.

Parallel work in physical activity/fitness is needed but was not reviewed in detail. A one factor model that included cardiorespiratory fitness, treadmill speed, and measures of strength was generalizable across comparison groups, providing stable, reliable measurement of true mean differences in the latent fitness factor. The results confirm the relevance of VO_2 max as a prominent contributor and that muscular strength is also relevant. The flexibility measure did not contribute, yet it may be possible to find other indicators of flexibility which could contribute to a summary measure. The results contribute to ongoing development and validation of summary physical activity/fitness scales suitable for community studies.

The results of the analysis showing that diet quality and physical activity/fitness were associated over time was informative, especially in that the effect was more prominent in men than women, with change in physical activity/fitness more likely to affect later changes in HEI-C, rather than diet changes influencing fitness later in the intervention. No comparable analyses were found in the literature. Recent studies in multiple health behavior change have developed composite summary scores of health behavior change [66], used other analysis methods [67] or focused on associations with other measures such as self-efficacy [68]. These preliminary results do suggest different strategies for programming with men and women and tend to support longer term interventions.

SEM has been used extensively in psychology, given the need to analyze latent constructs and non-independent longitudinal data within and across individuals and use is gradually increasing in nutrition and kinesiology, with the increasing interest in multi-dimensional scales for assessing diet quality and physical fitness change. Expertise is required to do the analysis; hence the process was more thoroughly explained than is typical Most past validation studies in diet and physical fitness have sought to establish means and ranges to be similar to some more accurate standard, with comparison to specific nutrients or physiologic measures, a basic strategy. However, if the other measurement properties (i.e., variances and covariances, variable intercepts, and residuals) addressed by SEM are not invariant, then the likelihood of detecting measurable change decreases dramatically. Further analyses, including structural regressions between latent constructs or development of latent change models, may be conducted with confidence that measurement error has been minimized and observed outcomes or differences are true differences and not driven by inaccurate measurement or imprecise methodology.

SEM is not without limitations [69,70]. There are methodological challenges in dealing with non-normal and missing data, both common in lifestyle intervention studies. Modelling complex phenomena is inherently challenging and use of SEM does not solve the inherent problem of model mis-specification and omitted variables. In addition, study design features such as the number of time points, number of indicators and their reliability will influence the power of SEM analysis. Generally, sample sizes in the range of ~200 are needed. Tomarken and Waller provide a useful introduction to strengths and limitations [70].

Expertise in both the content area and SEM is required to do the analysis; hence the analytical process was more thoroughly explained than is typical. Some invariance papers will not include all tests, however, the sequence should be examined in the appropriate order (i.e., some studies do not test intercept invariance but will test configural, weak, and strict invariance or others will include intercept invariance and stop without testing strict invariance). When the result of an invariance test is rejected or implausible, testing stops (e.g., if weak metric invariance was accepted/plausible, but invariance of intercepts rejected, we revert to the weak metric model as the accepted level for that model). Additional tests of structural (not measurement) invariance exist, when relationships between latent factors are tested for equality across groups/time (i.e., constraining factor variances/covariances or structural regression coefficients between factors). There are often questions of interest in these structural relationships of latent variables, but they are outside the realm of measurement invariance [71,72]. Regardless of the labels applied, demonstration of invariance is critically important in establishing the validity and application of the resulting factor models. Collaborators with expertise in SEM should be brought into the validation process much earlier and could be informing initial development of new diet and physical fitness measures for community intervention studies.

In conclusion, assessment of the measurement properties of diet quality and physical fitness measures was the main focus of this analysis, with an example analysis of possible associations between different lifestyle interventions. The original issue that prompted exploration of SEM; lack of association of intervention measures with disease risk score can now be partially explained. Work is underway to address the "mechanisms of action" for lifestyle programs in CMR conditions and we look forward to meaningful progress to improve effectiveness of lifestyle programs in health care and community settings.

Supplementary Materials: The following are available online at https://www.mdpi.com/article/10.3390/nu13124258/s1, Figure S1: Longitudinal Invariance of Reduced HEI-C Model, Figure S2: Sex Invariance of Reduced HEI-C Model, Figure S3: Disease-State Invariance of Reduced HEI-C Model, Figure S4: Results for women, Figure S5: Results for men, Figure S6: Overall disease and time invariant results, Table S1: Age and sex specific criteria to achieve maximum scores for each HEI-C component.

Author Contributions: K.J. and D.K. were principal investigators of the main study on which this study is based, while D.M.M., P.B., A.T. and C.R. were co-investigators and D.R. and R.D. were involved in overall project management. S.B.M. completed the analyses. All authors contributed to the interpretation of data, critically reviewed the manuscript for important intellectual content. All authors have read and agreed to the published version of the manuscript.

Funding: Funding was provided by Metabolic Syndrome Canada. https://www.metabolicsyndromecanada.ca/ (accessed on 19 November 2021). The funding source played no role in this secondary analysis.

Institutional Review Board Statement: This study was conducted under the World Medical Association's Declaration of Helsinki. Ethics approvals for the study were obtained from Health Research Ethics Board- Biomedical (University of Alberta), Comité d'éthique de la recherche des Centres de santé et de services sociaux de la Vieille-Capitale (Laval University), University of Guelph Research Ethics Board, and Institutional Review Board Services, a Chesapeake IRB Company (Aurora, Ont.).

Informed Consent Statement: Informed consent was obtained from all subjects involved in the study.

Data Availability Statement: The datasets used and/or analysed during the current study are available from the corresponding author on reasonable request.

Conflicts of Interest: The authors declare no conflict of interest.

References

1. Babio, N.; Toledo, E.; Estruch, R.; Ros, E.; Martínez-González, M.A.; Castañer, O.; Bulló, M.; Corella, D.; Arós, F.; Gómez-Gracia, E.; et al. Mediterranean diets and metabolic syndrome status in the PREDIMED randomized trial. *CMAJ* **2014**, *186*, E649–E657. [CrossRef]
2. Estruch, R.; Ros, E.; Salas-Salvado, J.; Covas, M.I.; Corella, D.; Aros, F.; Gomez-Gracia, E.; Ruiz-Gutierrez, V.; Fiol, M.; Lapetra, J.; et al. Primary Prevention of Cardiovascular Disease with a Mediterranean Diet Supplemented with Extra-Virgin Olive Oil or Nuts. *N. Engl. J. Med.* **2018**, *378*, e34. [CrossRef]
3. Knowler, W.C.; Barrett-Connor, E.; Fowler, S.E.; Hamman, R.F.; Lachin, J.M.; Walker, E.A.; Nathan, D.M. Reduction in the incidence of type 2 diabetes with lifestyle intervention or metformin. *N. Engl. J. Med.* **2002**, *346*, 393–403. [CrossRef] [PubMed]
4. Look Ahead Research Group; Wing, R.R.; Bolin, P.; Brancati, F.L.; Bray, G.A.; Clark, J.M.; Coday, M.; Crow, R.S.; Curtis, J.M.; Egan, C.M.; et al. Cardiovascular effects of intensive lifestyle intervention in type 2 diabetes. *N. Engl. J. Med.* **2013**, *369*, 145–154. [CrossRef]
5. Goldberg, R.B.; Mather, K. Targeting the consequences of the metabolic syndrome in the Diabetes Prevention Program. *Arterioscler. Thromb. Vasc. Biol.* **2012**, *32*, 2077–2090. [CrossRef]
6. Galaviz, K.I.; Weber, M.B.; Straus, A.; Haw, J.S.; Narayan, K.M.V.; Ali, M.K. Global Diabetes Prevention Interventions: A Systematic Review and Network Meta-analysis of the Real-World Impact on Incidence, Weight, and Glucose. *Diabetes Care* **2018**, *41*, 1526–1534. [CrossRef]
7. Mudaliar, U.; Zabetian, A.; Goodman, M.; Echouffo-Tcheugui, J.B.; Albright, A.L.; Gregg, E.W.; Ali, M.K. Cardiometabolic Risk Factor Changes Observed in Diabetes Prevention Programs in US Settings: A Systematic Review and Meta-analysis. *PLoS Med.* **2016**, *13*, e1002095. [CrossRef]
8. GBD 2017 Risk Factor Collaborators. Global, regional, and national comparative risk assessment of 84 behavioural, environmental and occupational, and metabolic risks or clusters of risks for 195 countries and territories, 1990–2017: A systematic analysis for the Global Burden of Disease Study 2017. *Lancet* **2018**, *392*, 1923–1994. [CrossRef]
9. Alberti, K.G.; Eckel, R.H.; Grundy, S.M.; Zimmet, P.Z.; Cleeman, J.I.; Donato, K.A.; Fruchart, J.C.; James, W.P.; Loria, C.M.; Smith, S.C., Jr.; et al. Harmonizing the metabolic syndrome: A joint interim statement of the International Diabetes Federation Task Force on Epidemiology and Prevention; National Heart, Lung, and Blood Institute; American Heart Association; World Heart Federation; International Atherosclerosis Society; and International Association for the Study of Obesity. *Circulation* **2009**, *120*, 1640–1645. [CrossRef]
10. Diamantopoulos, E.J.; Andreadis, E.A.; Tsourous, G.I.; Ifanti, G.K.; Katsanou, P.M.; Georgiopoulos, D.X.; Vassilopoulos, C.V.; Dimitriadis, G.; Raptis, S.A. Metabolic syndrome and prediabetes identify overlapping but not identical populations. *Exp. Clin. Endocrinol. Diabetes Off. J. Ger. Soc. Endocrinol. Ger. Diabetes Assoc.* **2006**, *114*, 377–383. [CrossRef]
11. Liu, J.; Grundy, S.M.; Wang, W.; Smith, S.C.; Lena Vega, G.; Wu, Z.; Zeng, Z.; Wang, W.; Zhao, D. Ten-year risk of cardiovascular incidence related to diabetes, prediabetes, and the metabolic syndrome. *Am. Heart J.* **2007**, *153*, 552–558. [CrossRef]
12. Leiter, L.A.; Fitchett, D.H.; Gilbert, R.E.; Gupta, M.; Mancini, G.B.; McFarlane, P.A.; Ross, R.; Teoh, H.; Verma, S.; Anand, S.; et al. Identification and management of cardiometabolic risk in Canada: A position paper by the cardiometabolic risk working group (executive summary). *Can. J. Cardiol.* **2011**, *27*, 124–131. [CrossRef]
13. Roth, G.A.; Mensah, G.A.; Johnson, C.O.; Addolorato, G.; Ammirati, E.; Baddour, L.M.; Barengo, N.C.; Beaton, A.Z.; Benjamin, E.J.; Benziger, C.P.; et al. Global Burden of Cardiovascular Diseases and Risk Factors, 1990–2019: Update From the GBD 2019 Study. *J. Am. Coll. Cardiol.* **2020**, *76*, 2982–3021. [CrossRef] [PubMed]
14. Hostalek, U. Global epidemiology of prediabetes—Present and future perspectives. *Clin. Diabetes Endocrinol.* **2019**, *5*, 5. [CrossRef]
15. Saklayen, M.G. The Global Epidemic of the Metabolic Syndrome. *Curr. Hypertens. Rep.* **2018**, *20*, 12. [CrossRef] [PubMed]
16. Statistics Canada. Metabolic Syndrome in Adults, 2012 to 2013. Available online: https://www150.statcan.gc.ca/n1/pub/82-625-x/2014001/article/14123-eng.htm (accessed on 13 June 2018).
17. Aguilar, M.; Bhuket, T.; Torres, S.; Liu, B.; Wong, R.J. Prevalence of the Metabolic Syndrome in the United States, 2003–2012. *JAMA* **2015**, *313*, 1973. [CrossRef]
18. McQueen, R.; Ghushchyan, V.; Olufade, T.; Sheehan, J.; Nair, K.; Saseen, J. Incremental increases in economic burden parallels cardiometabolic risk factors in the US. *Diabetes Metab. Syndr. Obes. Targets Ther.* **2016**, *9*, 233–241. [CrossRef] [PubMed]

19. Clark, A.; Jit, M.; Warren-Gash, C.; Guthrie, B.; Wang, H.H.X.; Mercer, S.W.; Sanderson, C.; McKee, M.; Troeger, C.; Ong, K.L.; et al. Global, regional, and national estimates of the population at increased risk of severe COVID-19 due to underlying health conditions in 2020: A modelling study. *Lancet Glob. Health* **2020**, *8*, e1003–e1017. [CrossRef]
20. Ghoneim, S.; Butt, M.U.; Hamid, O.; Shah, A.; Asaad, I. The incidence of COVID-19 in patients with metabolic syndrome and non-alcoholic steatohepatitis: A population-based study. *Metab. Open* **2020**, *8*, 100057. [CrossRef]
21. Arnett, D.K.; Blumenthal, R.S.; Albert, M.A.; Buroker, A.B.; Goldberger, Z.D.; Hahn, E.J.; Himmelfarb, C.D.; Khera, A.; Lloyd-Jones, D.; McEvoy, J.W.; et al. 2019 ACC/AHA Guideline on the Primary Prevention of Cardiovascular Disease: Executive Summary: A Report of the American College of Cardiology/American Heart Association Task Force on Clinical Practice Guidelines. *Circulation* **2019**, *140*, e563–e595. [CrossRef]
22. Tobe, S.W.; Stone, J.A.; Anderson, T.; Bacon, S.; Cheng, A.Y.Y.; Daskalopoulou, S.S.; Ezekowitz, J.A.; Gregoire, J.C.; Gubitz, G.; Jain, R.; et al. Canadian Cardiovascular Harmonized National Guidelines Endeavour (C-CHANGE) guideline for the prevention and management of cardiovascular disease in primary care: 2018 update. *CMAJ* **2018**, *190*, E1192–E1206. [CrossRef]
23. National Institute for Health and Care Excellence. NICE Pathway: Cardiovascular Disease Prevention Overview. Available online: https://pathways.nice.org.uk/pathways/cardiovascular-disease-prevention/cardiovascular-disease-prevention-overview (accessed on 19 June 2020).
24. Royal Australian College of General Practitioners. Chap. 8. Prevention of vascular and metabolic disease. In *Guidelines for Preventive Actitivies in General Practice*, 9th ed.; Royal Australian College of General Practitioners Ltd.: East Melbourne, MEL, Australia, 2018.
25. Teoh, H.; Despres, J.P.; Dufour, R.; Fitchett, D.H.; Goldin, L.; Goodman, S.G.; Harris, S.B.; Langer, A.; Lau, D.C.; Lonn, E.M.; et al. Identification and management of patients at elevated cardiometabolic risk in canadian primary care: How well are we doing? *Can. J. Cardiol.* **2013**, *29*, 960–968. [CrossRef]
26. Jeejeebhoy, K.; Dhaliwal, R.; Heyland, D.K.; Leung, R.; Day, A.G.; Brauer, P.; Royall, D.; Tremblay, A.; Mutch, D.M.; Pliamm, L.; et al. Family physician-led, team-based, lifestyle intervention in patients with metabolic syndrome: Results of a multicentre feasibility project. *CMAJ Open* **2017**, *5*, E229–E236. [CrossRef]
27. Assmann, G.; Schulte, H.; Seedorf, U. Cardiovascular risk assessment in the metabolic syndrome: Results from the Prospective Cardiovascular Munster (PROCAM) Study. *Int. J. Obes. (2005)* **2008**, *32* (Suppl. S2), S11–S16. [CrossRef]
28. Geller, K.; Lippke, S.; Nigg, C.R. Future directions of multiple behavior change research. *J. Behav. Med.* **2017**, *40*, 194–202. [CrossRef]
29. Meader, N.; King, K.; Wright, K.; Graham, H.M.; Petticrew, M.; Power, C.; White, M.; Sowden, A.J. Multiple Risk Behavior Interventions: Meta-analyses of RCTs. *Am. J. Prev. Med.* **2017**, *53*, e19–e30. [CrossRef]
30. Kaplan, D. *Structural Equation Modeling (2nd ed.): Foundations and Extensions*, 2nd ed.; SAGE Publications, Inc.: Thousand Oaks, CA, USA, 2009. [CrossRef]
31. Raghuveer, G.; Hartz, J.; Lubans, D.R.; Takken, T.; Wiltz, J.L.; Mietus-Snyder, M.; Perak, A.M.; Baker-Smith, C.; Pietris, N.; Edwards, N.M. Cardiorespiratory Fitness in Youth: An Important Marker of Health: A Scientific Statement From the American Heart Association. *Circulation* **2020**, *142*, e101–e118. [CrossRef] [PubMed]
32. Ross, R.; Blair, S.N.; Arena, R.; Church, T.S.; Després, J.-P.; Franklin, B.A.; Haskell, W.L.; Kaminsky, L.A.; Levine, B.D.; Lavie, C.J.; et al. Importance of Assessing Cardiorespiratory Fitness in Clinical Practice: A Case for Fitness as a Clinical Vital Sign: A Scientific Statement From the American Heart Association. *Circulation* **2016**, *134*, e653–e699. [CrossRef]
33. Peterman, J.E.; Harber, M.P.; Imboden, M.T.; Whaley, M.H.; Fleenor, B.S.; Myers, J.; Arena, R.; Kaminsky, L.A. Accuracy of Exercise-based Equations for Estimating Cardiorespiratory Fitness. *Med. Sci. Sports Exerc.* **2021**, *53*, 74–82. [CrossRef] [PubMed]
34. Castro-Barquero, S.; Ruiz-León, A.M.; Sierra-Pérez, M.; Estruch, R.; Casas, R. Dietary Strategies for Metabolic Syndrome: A Comprehensive Review. *Nutrients* **2020**, *12*, 2983. [CrossRef] [PubMed]
35. Kirkpatrick, S.I.; Reedy, J.; Krebs-Smith, S.M.; Pannucci, T.E.; Subar, A.F.; Wilson, M.M.; Lerman, J.L.; Tooze, J.A. Applications of the Healthy Eating Index for Surveillance, Epidemiology, and Intervention Research: Considerations and Caveats. *J. Acad. Nutr. Diet.* **2018**, *118*, 1603–1621. [CrossRef] [PubMed]
36. Brauer, P.; Royall, D.; Rodrigues, A. Use of the Healthy Eating Index in Intervention Studies for Cardiometabolic Risk Conditions: A Systematic Review. *Adv. Nutr.* **2021**, *12*, 1317–1331. [CrossRef]
37. Zaragoza-Martí, A.; Cabañero-Martínez, M.; Hurtado-Sánchez, J.; Laguna-Pérez, A.; Ferrer-Cascales, R. Evaluation of Mediterranean diet adherence scores: A systematic review. *BMJ Open* **2018**, *8*, e019033. [CrossRef] [PubMed]
38. Miller, V.; Webb, P.; Micha, R.; Mozaffarian, D. Defining diet quality: A synthesis of dietary quality metrics and their validity for the double burden of malnutrition. *Lancet Planet. Health* **2020**, *4*, e352–e370. [CrossRef]
39. Hayduk, L.A. Improving measurement-invariance assessments: Correcting entrenched testing deficiencies. *BMC Med. Res. Methodol.* **2016**, *16*, 130. [CrossRef] [PubMed]
40. Reimer, H.D.; Keller, H.H.; Maitland, S.B.; Jackson, J. Nutrition Screening Index for Older Adults (SCREEN II©) Demonstrates Sex and Age Invariance. *J. Nutr. Elder.* **2010**, *29*, 192–210. [CrossRef]
41. Vandenberg, R.J.; Lance, C.E. A Review and Synthesis of the Measurement Invariance Literature: Suggestions, Practices, and Recommendations for Organizational Research. *Organ. Res. Methods* **2000**, *3*, 4–70. [CrossRef]
42. Van De Schoot, R.; Lugtig, P.; Hox, J. A checklist for testing measurement invariance. *Eur. J. Dev. Psychol.* **2012**, *9*, 486–492. [CrossRef]

43. Maitland, S.B.; Nyberg, L.; Bäckman, L.; Nilsson, L.-G.; Adolfsson, R. On the structure of personality: Are there separate temperament and character factors? *Personal. Individ. Differ.* **2009**, *47*, 180–184. [CrossRef]
44. Royall, D.; Brauer, P.; Bjorklund, L.; O'Young, O.; Tremblay, A.; Jeejeebhoy, K.; Heyland, D.; Dhaliwal, R.; Klein, D.; Mutch, D.M. Development of a Dietary Management Care Map for Metabolic Syndrome. *Can. J. Diet. Pract. Res.* **2014**, *75*, 132–139. [CrossRef]
45. Klein, D.; Jeejeebhoy, K.; Tremblay, A.; Kallio, M.; Rheaume, C.; Humphries, S.; Royall, D.; Brauer, P.; Heyland, D.; Dhaliwal, R.; et al. The CHANGE program: Exercise intervention in primary care. *Can. Fam. Physician* **2017**, *63*, 546–552. [PubMed]
46. Klein, J.; Brauer, P.; Royall, D.; Israeloff-Smith, M.; Klein, D.; Tremblay, A.; Dhaliwal, R.; Rheaume, C.; Mutch, D.M.; Jeejeebhoy, K. Patient experiences of a lifestyle program for metabolic syndrome offered in family medicine clinics: A mixed methods study. *BMC Fam. Pr.* **2018**, *19*, 148. [CrossRef] [PubMed]
47. Ebbeling, C.B.; Ward, A.; Puleo, E.M.; Widrick, J.; Rippe, J.M. Development of a single-stage submaximal treadmill walking test. *Med. Sci. Sports Exerc.* **1991**, *23*, 966–973. [CrossRef]
48. Tremblay, A.; Bélanger, M.P.; Dhaliwal, R.; Brauer, P.; Royall, D.; Mutch, D.M.; Rhéaume, C. Impact of a multidisciplinary intervention on physical fitness, physical activity habits and the association between aerobic fitness and components of metabolic syndrome in adults diagnosed with metabolic syndrome. *Arch. Public Health* **2020**, *78*, 22. [CrossRef]
49. Hayduk, L.A.; Littvay, L. Should researchers use single indicators, best indicators, or multiple indicators in structural equation models? *BMC Med. Res. Methodol.* **2012**, *12*, 159. [CrossRef]
50. Brauer, P.; Royall, D.; Li, A.; Rodrigues, A.; Green, J.; Macklin, S.; Craig, A.; Pasanen, J.; Brunelle, L.; Maitland, S.; et al. Nutrient intake and dietary quality changes within a personalized lifestyle intervention program for metabolic syndrome in primary care. *Appl. Physiol. Nutr. Metab.* **2019**, *44*, 1297–1304. [CrossRef]
51. Garriguet, D. Diet quality in Canada. *Health Rep.* **2009**, *20*, 41–52.
52. Health Canada. Eating Well with Canada's Food Guide. Available online: https://www.canada.ca/en/health-canada/services/canada-food-guides.html (accessed on 19 January 2018).
53. van Vliet-Ostaptchouk, J.V.; Nuotio, M.-L.; Slagter, S.N.; Doiron, D.; Fischer, K.; Foco, L.; Gaye, A.; Gögele, M.; Heier, M.; Hiekkalinna, T.; et al. The prevalence of metabolic syndrome and metabolically healthy obesity in Europe: A collaborative analysis of ten large cohort studies. *BMC Endocr. Disord.* **2014**, *14*, 9. [CrossRef]
54. Bentler, P.M. On tests and indices for evaluating structural models. *Personal. Individ. Differ.* **2007**, *42*, 825–829. [CrossRef]
55. Cheung, G.W.; Rensvold, R.B. Evaluating goodness-of-fit indexes for testing measurement invariance. *Struct. Equ. Modeling* **2002**, *9*, 233–255. [CrossRef]
56. Kline, R.B. *Principles and Practice of Structural Equation Modeling*; Guilford Publications: New York, NY, USA, 2015.
57. Lai, K.; Green, S.B. The Problem with Having Two Watches: Assessment of Fit When RMSEA and CFI Disagree. *Multivar. Behav. Res.* **2016**, *51*, 220–239. [CrossRef]
58. McNeish, D.; An, J.; Hancock, G.R. The Thorny Relation Between Measurement Quality and Fit Index Cutoffs in Latent Variable Models. *J. Pers. Assess* **2018**, *100*, 43–52. [CrossRef]
59. Little, T.D. *Longitudinal Structural Equation Modeling*; Guilford Press: New York, NY, USA, 2013; pp. xxii, 386–xxii, 386.
60. Meredith, W. Measurement invariance, factor analysis and factorial invariance. *Psychometrika* **1993**, *58*, 525–543. [CrossRef]
61. Millsap, R.E. Structural equation modeling made difficult. *Personal. Individ. Differ.* **2007**, *42*, 875–881. [CrossRef]
62. Horn, J.L.; McArdle, J.J.; Mason, R. When is invariance not invarient: A practical scientist's look at the ethereal concept of factor invariance. *South. Psychol.* **1983**, *1*, 179–188.
63. Chen, F.F. Sensitivity of goodness of fit indexes to lack of measurement invariance. *Struct. Equ. Modeling A Multidiscip. J.* **2007**, *14*, 464–504. [CrossRef]
64. Kennedy, E.T.; Ohls, J.; Carlson, S.; Fleming, K. The Healthy Eating Index: Design and applications. *J. Am. Diet. Assoc.* **1995**, *95*, 1103–1108. [CrossRef]
65. Lafrenière, J.; Carbonneau, É.; Laramée, C.; Corneau, L.; Robitaille, J.; Labonté, M.-È.; Lamarche, B.; Lemieux, S. Is the Canadian Healthy Eating Index 2007 an Appropriate Diet Indicator of Metabolic Health? Insights from Dietary Pattern Analysis in the PREDISE Study. *Nutrients* **2019**, *11*, 1597. [CrossRef]
66. Spring, B.; Schneider, K.; McFadden, H.G.; Vaughn, J.; Kozak, A.T.; Smith, M.; Moller, A.C.; Epstein, L.H.; Demott, A.; Hedeker, D.; et al. Multiple behavior changes in diet and activity: A randomized controlled trial using mobile technology. *Arch. Intern. Med.* **2012**, *172*, 789–796. [CrossRef]
67. Chevance, G.; Golaszewski, N.M.; Baretta, D.; Hekler, E.B.; Larsen, B.A.; Patrick, K.; Godino, J. Modelling multiple health behavior change with network analyses: Results from a one-year study conducted among overweight and obese adults. *J. Behav. Med.* **2020**, *43*, 254–261. [CrossRef]
68. Heredia, N.I.; Fernandez, M.E.; van den Berg, A.E.; Durand, C.P.; Kohl, H.W.; Reininger, B.M.; Hwang, K.O.; McNeill, L.H. Coaction Between Physical Activity and Fruit and Vegetable Intake in Racially Diverse, Obese Adults. *Am. J. Health Promot.* **2020**, *34*, 238–246. [CrossRef]
69. Tarka, P. An overview of structural equation modeling: Its beginnings, historical development, usefulness and controversies in the social sciences. *Qual. Quant.* **2018**, *52*, 313–354. [CrossRef] [PubMed]
70. Tomarken, A.J.; Waller, N.G. Structural equation modeling: Strengths, limitations, and misconceptions. *Annu. Rev. Clin. Psychol* **2005**, *1*, 31–65. [CrossRef] [PubMed]

71. Schaie, K.W.; Maitland, S.B.; Willis, S.L.; Intrieri, R.C. Longitudinal invariance of adult psychometric ability factor structures across 7 years. *Psychol Aging* **1998**, *13*, 8–20. [CrossRef] [PubMed]
72. Maitland, S.B.; Intrieri, R.C.; Schaie, W.K.; Willis, S.L. Gender differences and changes in cognitive abilities across the adult life span. *Aging Neuropsychol. Cogn.* **2000**, *7*, 32–53. [CrossRef]

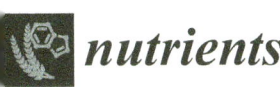

Article

Effectiveness of a Lifestyle Modification Program Delivered under Real-World Conditions in a Rural Setting

Cally Jennings [1,*], Elsie Patterson [1], Rachel G. Curtis [2], Anna Mazzacano [1] and Carol A. Maher [2]

1. Sonder, Edinburgh North, SA 5113, Australia; epatterson@sonder.net.au (E.P.); amazzacano@sonder.net.au (A.M.)
2. Alliance for Research in Exercise, Nutrition and Activity, Allied Health and Human Performance, University of South Australia, Adelaide, SA 5001, Australia; rachel.curtis@unisa.edu.au (R.G.C.); carol.maher@unisa.edu.au (C.A.M.)
* Correspondence: cjennings@sonder.net.au

Abstract: Whilst there is considerable evidence to support the efficacy of physical activity and dietary interventions in disease and death prevention, translation of knowledge into practice remains inadequate. We aimed to examine the uptake, retention, acceptability and effectiveness on physical activity, physical function, sitting time, diet and health outcomes of a Healthy Eating Activity and Lifestyle program (HEAL^{TM}) delivered under real-world conditions. The program was delivered to 430 adults living across rural South Australia. Participants of the program attended weekly 2 h healthy lifestyle education and exercise group-based sessions for 8 weeks. A total of 47 programs were delivered in over 15 communities. In total, 548 referrals were received, resulting in 430 participants receiving the intervention (78% uptake). At baseline, 74.6% of participants were female, the mean age of participants was 53.7 years and 11.1% of participants identified as Aboriginal and/or Torres Strait Islander. Follow-up assessments were obtained for 265 participants. Significant improvements were observed for walking, planned physical activity, incidental physical activity, total physical activity, 30 s chair stand, 30 s arm curl, 6 min walk, fruit consumption and vegetable consumption, sitting time and diastolic blood pressure. Positive satisfaction and favourable feedback were reported. The healthy lifestyle program achieved excellent real-world uptake and effectiveness, reasonable intervention attendance and strong program acceptability amongst rural and vulnerable communities.

Keywords: physical activity; nutrition; health program; lifestyle; weight management; prevention; service evaluation; health service

Citation: Jennings, C.; Patterson, E.; Curtis, R.G.; Mazzacano, A.; Maher, C.A. Effectiveness of a Lifestyle Modification Program Delivered under Real-World Conditions in a Rural Setting. *Nutrients* **2021**, *13*, 4040. https://doi.org/10.3390/nu13114040

Academic Editor: Carlos Vasconcelos

Received: 24 September 2021
Accepted: 11 November 2021
Published: 12 November 2021

Publisher's Note: MDPI stays neutral with regard to jurisdictional claims in published maps and institutional affiliations.

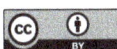

Copyright: © 2021 by the authors. Licensee MDPI, Basel, Switzerland. This article is an open access article distributed under the terms and conditions of the Creative Commons Attribution (CC BY) license (https://creativecommons.org/licenses/by/4.0/).

1. Introduction

Poor diet and insufficient physical activity are leading modifiable causes of death and disease [1]. They increase the risk of developing chronic health conditions, such as cardiovascular disease (CVD), type 2 diabetes, obesity, cancers, depression and anxiety, leading to premature death and reduced quality of life, and massive economic and healthcare burden [2]. In Australia, over ninety percent of adults do not consume the recommended daily intakes of vegetables and fruit [3], and two-thirds do not meet guidelines for 30 min of physical activity per day [4].

International evidence consistently shows that physical inactivity and poor dietary patterns disproportionately affect people residing in rural areas, and those who are socioeconomically disadvantaged [5–8]. People living in rural areas experience poorer health outcomes in comparison to those living in metropolitan areas due to skills shortages and high turnover of healthcare staff, reduced access to and use of preventative health services, as well as disparities in employment, income and education [9]. In addition, lifestyle behaviours and health risks vary based on ethnicity. In particular, Indigenous people tend to have poorer lifestyles and experience worse health outcomes than non-first nation counterparts including an increased risk of chronic disease such as diabetes and shortened life expectancy [10–12]. Clearly, there is an urgent need for effective programs to better support people residing in rural areas and high-risk groups to adopt healthier lifestyles.

There is a great deal of evidence supporting the efficacy of physical activity and dietary interventions among adults in the scientific literature [13–15]. Evidence has supported improvements in total physical activity, cardiorespiratory fitness, reduced caloric intake and consumption of saturated fat, and an increased intake of fruit and vegetables [15,16]. This includes the delivery of interventions across a variety of modalities (e.g., individual, group based, telephone, print, web-based), settings (e.g., communities, workplaces and healthcare settings) and target groups [16,17]. Yet, such programs are typically evaluated under tightly controlled conditions, such as through randomised controlled trials (RCTs), which limits their external validity, and fail to consider the complexities surrounding delivery and adoption in practice within "real-world" settings [18]. These complexities can include differences in uptake among the public, competing demands on staff, organisational processes and priorities, and resourcing considerations [18,19]. Thus, a gap remains in the translation and implementation of research into practice, and the generalisability of these programs and results to real-world conditions is unclear [18,20,21].

Real-world trials are needed to help close this gap. Two evidence-based programs that have been evaluated under real-world conditions and reported in the peer-reviewed literature are studies based on the US Diabetes Prevention Program and the Australian Healthy Eating Activity and Lifestyle (HEAL^{TM}) program. A systematic review of 28 real-world studies of lifestyle programs modelled on the Diabetes Prevention Program, on average, led to 4 percent weight loss [22]. Not surprisingly, the Diabetes Prevention Program-based programs have been heavily targeted at people with pre-diabetes (25 out of 28 studies), so the effectiveness for people with other chronic diseases and risk factors is unclear.

In Australia, the HEAL^{TM} program has been developed as an evidence-based group-delivered healthy lifestyle intervention. A real-world pre–post evaluation among participants (n = 2827) across 67 local government areas suggested the program leads to measurable improvements in physical activity, sitting time, fruit and vegetable consumption, anthropometry, and physical function [23]. However, results were only reported in brief; an overly simplistic statistical approach was used (t-tests) and did not consider or account for differences in program effectiveness based on sex, age, ethnicity, and it is also unclear which settings the program was tested in (e.g., rural or metropolitan).

This study helps to address these gaps in the literature, offering an analysis of the HEAL^{TM} program delivered under real-world conditions in rural and Indigenous settings such as Aboriginal Controlled Community Health Organisations (ACCHOs). In particular, we aimed to: (1) describe the program's uptake, retention and engagement; (2) examine the effectiveness of the program for improving physical activity, sedentary behaviour, diet, health outcomes and physical function; and (3) describe participants' and health professionals' views on program acceptability and satisfaction. Understanding how healthy lifestyle programs work in real-world settings and with rural and vulnerable communities is essential to address chronic disease risk and management.

2. Materials and Methods

2.1. Design

This study uses a mixed quantitative and qualitative methods, pre–post design comprising of the delivery of the HEAL^{TM} program—a group-focused lifestyle program implemented in a 'real world' primary health care setting. The HEAL^{TM} program is an evidence-based program, developed by South Western Sydney Primary Health Network and supported by Exercise & Sport Science Australia (ESSA) [23]. Sonder was funded by the Country South Australia Primary Health Network to implement the HEAL^{TM} program across rural South Australia. A project officer employed by Sonder was responsible for the implementation of the program. This included undertaking regular promotion and engagement activities with local General Practitioners (GPs) and practice nurses to encourage and support referrals into the program. The project officer recruited local allied health professionals who were subsequently trained and certified to deliver the HEAL™ program as facilitators through ESSA. Local facilitators also engaged with local GPs to support referrals and local community engagement. Intervention and data collection took place between 1 July 2018 and 30 September 2019. Participants provided written consent to partake in the program and for their data to be used for program evaluation purposes. This retrospective analysis of quality assurance data was deemed to be exempt from ethics approval by the University of South Australia's Human Research Ethics Committee (application no. 204196).

2.2. Participants and Procedure

To be eligible, participants were required to be referred by a GP or Nurse Practitioner located in one of the following South Australia regions: Gawler, Barossa, Lower North, Mid North, Yorke Peninsula, Far West, Flinders and Port Augusta, Lower Eyre and Upper Eyre. Participants were eligible for referral if they met one of the following criteria: CVD or 2+ CVD risk factors, were diagnosed with Type 2 diabetes, were pre-diabetic, or had a body mass index (BMI) ≥ 30. Further eligibility criteria assessed upon receipt of the referral included aged 18 years or over and completion of pre-exercise screening [24] with appropriate medical practitioner approval, if required.

Participant referrals were sent from the general practice to Sonder, where they were processed and allocated to a HEAL™ facilitator located in their region of residence. Facilitators contacted participants via phone to enrol them into the next available program. Participant anthropometry, blood pressure, and physical function assessments were conducted by facilitators in-person prior to the participants' commencement in the program and immediately following program completion (8 weeks). Participants completed a paper survey assessing their physical activity, sitting time, and diet at baseline and 8 weeks and were invited to complete an online or paper-based satisfaction survey following the completion of the program.

Stakeholders, including program facilitators, referrers and practice/service managers, were invited (n = 30) to complete an online survey to provide feedback about the program in June 2019.

2.3. Intervention

The HEAL™ program is an 8-week, group-based lifestyle program that is targeted towards adults with or at risk of developing chronic diseases. Allied health professionals were trained to deliver the HEAL™ program as a facilitator through a 1-day training course run through ESSA. The intervention is guided by the Transtheoretical Model and Stages of Change theory [4] and includes a focus on self-efficacy to support a self-management approach to encourage autonomy and goal-setting for sustained behaviour change [5]. The HEAL™ program included a weekly 2 h group-based session over an 8-week period. Programs varied in relation to both time of day and day of delivery. Group sessions were delivered face-to-face and included 1 h of supervised exercise and 1 h of lifestyle education focused on promoting physical activity and healthy eating through a modified Mediterranean diet approach [6]. Supervised exercise sessions varied weekly and involved low- to moderate-intensity aerobic and resistance activities, which are modified to suit the needs and interests of the participant group. The most common sessions comprised of gym-based, circuit-style exercises where participants followed a prescribed workout, modified according to their fitness level and needs. This commonly included a 10 min warm-up, followed by the main exercise session (free weights, weight machines and/or cardio) for 30–40 min, with a 10-minute warm down. Facilitators monitored and assessed exercise intensity using the perceived exertion scale provided in HEAL™ program materials and/or clinical judgement. As part of the program, materials consisting of education slides, resources and home-based activities including exercises were provided to all participants. Participants also received one-on-one health consultations to assess current fitness, plan an appropriate exercise program, and measure and monitor ongoing progress during and following the program. A comprehensive overview of the intervention has been previously described [2].

2.4. Measures

Demographic data were collected at the referral stage, which included date of birth, gender, Aboriginal and Torres Strait Islander status, and postcode. Remoteness was derived from postcode using the Accessibility and Remoteness Index of Australia (ARIA+) [25]. Socioeconomic status categories were derived from postcode using the 2016 Socio-Economic Indexes for Australia (SEIFA) index of socioeconomic disadvantage national decile ranking [26].

Physical activity questions were based on the Active Australia Survey [27] and included weekly minutes spent: walking for more than 10 min; completing other physical activity (not walking); or gardening or household chores that made participants breathe hard. The Active Australia Survey has demonstrated acceptable reliability ($r_s = 0.56$–0.64) and validity ($r_s = 0.52$) [28,29] compared with accelerometer data. In addition to summarising the modes of physical activity separately, the three physical activity variables were combined to calculate total weekly physical activity time.

Sitting time was captured by a single item measuring the average number of hours per day in the previous week spent in sedentary activities [30].

Daily fruit and vegetable consumption was assessed by two questions: one which asked the number of servings of fruit per day and another which asked the number of servings of vegetables per day. Each question provided examples and serving size equivalents. These questions were taken from the valid and reliable Fat and Fibre Barometer questionnaire [31].

Height (cm), weight (kg), waist circumference (cm), hip circumference (cm), and blood pressure (mm/Hg) were measured objectively. Stadiometers were used to measure height; digital scales were used to measure weight; and waist/hip circumference were measured using tape measures. Blood pressure was measured once with the participant seated using a clinical grade sphygmomanometer. The brand and model of instruments varied based on facilitators' access to equipment; however, participants' baseline and follow-up assessments were collected using the same instrument. Physical function measures included the 6 min walk test, 30 s arm curl, and 30 s chair rise [32,33].

Weekly program attendance was recorded by the facilitator. The participant program satisfaction survey was delivered in paper form and consisted of 13 items with a mix of Likert scale and open-ended questions [23]. The stakeholder satisfaction survey was delivered via SurveyMonkey and consisted of 15 items with a mix of Likert scale and open-ended questions.

2.5. Statistical Analysis

Baseline participants' characteristics were analysed descriptively. Differences between those who accepted and did not accept their referral, and differences between those who completed and did not complete the 8-week follow-up assessments, were assessed using one-way analysis of variance and chi-square with post hoc Bonferroni-corrected z-test pairwise comparisons. Analyses were conducted in SPSS 25 (IBM Corp., Armonk, NY, USA).

To account for repeated measures and the hierarchical data structure (participants nested within program sites), linear mixed models with restricted maximum likelihood (REML) estimation were used to examine the effectiveness of the program. Random effects were specified to account for the hierarchical structure of the data and time was specified as a fixed effect. Consistent with the principle of intention-to-treat [34], REML allows all available data to contribute to model parameters. Analyses were conducted in Stata15.1 (StataCorp., College Station, TX, USA). An alpha of 0.05 was used to denote statistical significance.

Descriptive statistics for program satisfaction and stakeholder feedback was reflected as percentages of participants responding across the Likert scale items. Open-ended questions were analysed thematically using Microsoft Word.

3. Results

3.1. Uptake and Retention

Forty-seven programs were delivered across more than 15 communities, including the regions of Lower/Mid North, Lower Eyre, Yorke Peninsula, Gawler/Barossa, ACCHOs and Remote/Royal Flying Doctor communities.

Figure 1 shows participant flow through the program. A total of 548 referrals were received with 129 GPs or nurses referring at least one person into the program. A total of 430 people accepted the referral and received the intervention.

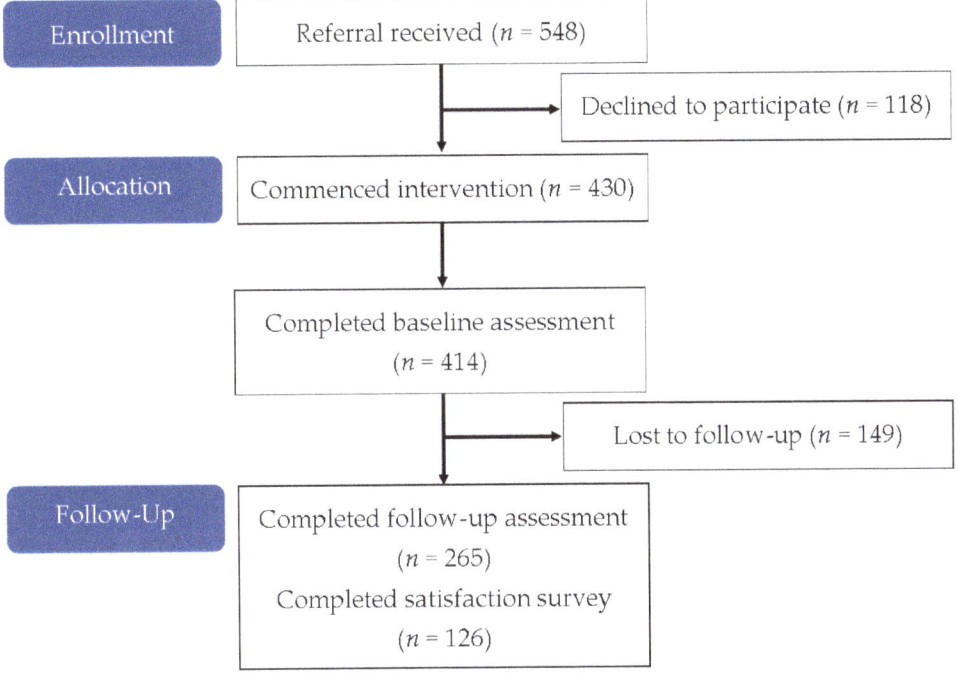

Figure 1. Flow of participants through program.

A comparison was undertaken of those who accepted vs. those who declined the referral (Table S1). A greater proportion of females (81.0%) compared to males (71.1%) accepted the referral ($p = 0.02$). Additionally, a greater proportion of those without a healthcare card (90.9%) compared to those with a healthcare card (81.9%) accepted the referral ($p = 0.01$). Acceptance also differed based on remoteness ($p = 0.01$); rates of acceptance in major cities (57.9%) was similar to inner regional (81.6%), outer regional (73.8%), and remote SA (81.0%), but lower than very remote SA (100.0%). There were no significant differences for age, socioeconomic status, or Aboriginal and/or Torres Strait Islander status for uptake in referrals.

Four hundred and fourteen participants completed baseline assessments. Table 1 shows participant characteristics at baseline.

Table 1. Participant characteristics at baseline (n = 414).

	n	Males (n = 102)	Females (n = 300)	All (n = 414) [a]
Age (years), M (SD)	383	55.3 (12.55)	53.2 (14.4)	53.7 (13.9)
Aboriginal, n (%)	380	12 (12.2)	30 (10.6)	42 (11.1)
Health care card (yes), n (%)	362	53 (55.8)	113 (49.8)	186 (51.4)
Remoteness, n (%)	399			
Major Cities		3 (2.9)	5 (1.7)	8 (2.0)
Inner Regional		30 (29.4)	93 (31.5)	123 (30.8)
Outer Regional		47 (46.1)	99 (33.6)	147 (36.8)
Remote		18 (17.6)	87 (29.5)	106 (26.6)
Very Remote		4 (3.9)	11 (3.7)	15 (3.8)
SES decile, n (%)	399			
1–2		36 (35.3)	71 (24.1)	107 (26.8)
3–4		26 (25.5)	119 (40.3)	146 (36.6)
5–6		28 (27.5)	70 (23.7)	98 (24.6)
7–8		5 (4.9)	28 (9.5)	34 (8.5)
9–10		5 (6.9)	7 (2.4)	14 (3.5)
Completed sessions, M (SD)	290	6.2 (2.3)	6.1 (2.0)	6.1 (2.1)
Walking (min/week), M (SD)	394	91.8 (118.9)	71.6 (99.3)	75.7 (103.9)
Planned PA (min/week), M (SD)	397	66.7 (112.2)	56.1 (96.7)	59.1 (100.2)
Incidental PA (min/week), M (SD)	378	119.7 (170.9)	116.6 (170.5)	116.9 (169.0)
Total PA (min/week), M (SD)	358	277.0 (282.6)	230.2 (227.7)	240.7 (241.5)
Sitting time (h/day), M (SD)	400	6.7 (3.8)	5.8 (2.9)	6.03 (3.15)
Fruit (servings/day), M (SD)	409	1.5 (1.1)	1.6 (1.2)	1.6 (1.1)
Vegetables (servings/day), M (SD)	411	2.4 (1.3)	2.6 (1.4)	2.6 (1.4)
Weight (kg), M (SD)	413	109.9 (26.8)	95.6 (22.3)	99.3 (24.2)
Waist circumference (cm), M (SD)	404	120.4 (16.9)	111.5 (16.8)	113.8 (17.2)
BMI, M (SD)	412	35.8 (7.8)	36.6 (8.0)	36.4 (7.9)
Systolic BP (mmHg), M (SD)	384	139.8 (14.8)	133.3 (15.8)	135.1 (15.7)
Diastolic BP (mmHg), M (SD)	377	81.0 (10.0)	79.0 (10.4)	79.5 (10.3)
30 s chair stand (n), M (SD)	396	10.9 (3.8)	10.9 (3.5)	10.9 (3.5)
30 s arm curl (n), M (SD)	403	23.0 (9.5)	22.2 (9.5)	22.3 (9.4)
6 min walk (m), M (SD)	377	380.0 (127.6)	375.0 (127.8)	376.6 (130.2)

[a] All is more than the sum of Male and Female, due to missing gender data. Note: SES = socioeconomic status, PA = physical activity, BP = blood pressure.

At baseline, 74.6% of the participants were female, the mean age of participants was 53.7 and average weight was 99.3 kg. Additionally, 11.1% of the sample identified as Aboriginal and/or Torres Strait Islander. Most participants lived in inner regional (30.8%) and outer regional (36.8%) areas and were in the lowest two socioeconomic status categories (63.4%). Participants completed an average of six of eight weekly sessions.

Eight-week follow-up assessments were obtained for 265 participants (64%). A comparison was undertaken of those who completed vs. those who did not complete the follow-up assessment (Table S2). Compared with non-completers, participants who completed the 8-week assessment were older (M = 55.0 ± 13.6 vs. M = 51.4 ± 14.3, $p = 0.02$), had a lower weight (M = 95.6 ± 22.1 vs. M = 105.9 ± 26.3, $p < 0.001$), smaller waist circumference (M = 111.5 ± 17.0 vs. M = 117.9 ± 16.8, $p < 0.001$), more 30 s chair stands (M = 11.2 ± 3.5 vs. M = 10.4 ± 3.6, $p = 0.048$), and completed more weekly sessions (M = 6.7 ± 1.5 vs. M = 4.0 ± 2.7, $p < 0.001$). Completion differed by remoteness ($p = 0.003$); rates of completion in major cities (100.0%) were similar to inner regional (57.7%), outer regional (68.0%), and remote SA (70.8%) but higher than very remote SA (33.3%). Completion also differed by socioeconomic status ($p = 0.02$); rates of completion in deciles 5–6 (55.1%) were lower than in deciles 3–4 (74.0%), while deciles 1–2 (59.8%), 3–4 (74.0%), 7–8 (73.5%), and 9–10 (57.1%) were similar. There were no differences in completion based on gender, Aboriginal and/or Torres Strait Islander status, health care card status, systolic blood pressure, diastolic blood pressure, walking, planned physical activity, incidental physical activity, total physical activity, sitting time, servings of fruit, servings of vegetables, 6 min walk test, or 30 s arm curl.

3.2. Program Effectiveness

At 8 weeks, statistically significant increases were shown in walking, planned physical activity, incidental physical activity, total physical activity, 30 s chair stand, 30 s arm curl, 6 min walk, fruit consumption and vegetable consumption. Statistically significant reductions were seen in sitting time, weight, waist circumference, and diastolic blood pressure. There were no changes in systolic blood pressure. Table 2 provides an overview of descriptive statistics and effectiveness results.

Table 2. Descriptive statistics and results from multilevel models examining the effectiveness of the HEAL™ program.

	Baseline		8 Weeks		Estimated Difference
	n	M (SD)	n	M (SD)	B [95% CI]
Walking (min/week)	394	75.7 (103.9)	250	110.7 (116.7)	31.66 [20.77, 42.56] ***
Planned PA (min/week)	397	59.1 (100.2)	251	115.4 (99.9)	58.09 [45.88, 70.30] ***
Incidental PA (min/week)	378	116.9 (169.0)	239	157.2 (204.4)	46.17 [24.24, 68.11] ***
Total PA (min/week)	358	277.0 (282.6)	292	387.5 (277.3)	140.98 [112.87, 169.09] ***
Sitting time (h/day)	400	6.03 (3.15)	252	5.5 (2.7)	−0.36 [−0.59, −0.12] **
Fruit (servings/day)	409	1.6 (1.1)	255	2.0 (1.0)	0.38 [0.27, 0.48] ***
Vegetables (servings/day)	411	2.6 (1.4)	256	3.4 (1.4)	0.81 [0.66, 0.96] ***
Weight (kg)	413	99.27 (24.17)	263	94.45 (22.05)	−1.43 [−2.44, −0.41] **
Waist circumference (cm)	404	113.8 (17.2)	257	110.3 (17.8)	−1.61 [−2.50, −0.72] ***
Systolic BP (mmHg)	384	135.1 (15.7)	245	133.4 (15.4)	−1.63 [−3.42, 0.17]
Diastolic BP (mmHg)	377	79.5 (10.3)	239	78.3 (10.4)	−1.10 [−2.15, −0.05] *
30 s chair stand (n)	396	10.9 (3.5)	250	13.1 (4.9)	2.01 [1.61, 2.42] ***
30 s arm curl (n)	403	22.3 (9.4)	255	24.6 (10.0)	2.61 [2.03, 3.19] ***
6 min walk (m)	377	376.6 (130.2)	234	402.0 (146.9)	24.68 [12.70, 36.66] ***

* $p < 0.05$, ** $p < 0.01$, *** $p < 0.001$; Note: PA = physical activity, BP = blood pressure.

3.3. Satisfaction

Overall, 126 program participants (66% female) completed the satisfaction survey One hundred percent reported that they would recommend the program to family and friends and that the program was run at a convenient place. Most participants reported that the program was run at a convenient time (98%), that the quality of presentation was 'excellent' (89% vs. 'good' 10%, and 'fair' 0.8%), and that they were 'confident' or 'very confident' that they were able to make changes to their lifestyle as a result of the program (98%). Participants reported that the program raised their awareness of the health benefits of healthy eating and physical activity 'a lot' (90%), 'a little' (7%), or 'not much' (3%). Most participants reported that the program increased their healthy eating and physical activity skills by 'a lot' (71%) or 'a little' (26%) and many reported that the program prompted them to want to change their eating and physical activity habits 'a lot' (73%) or 'a little' (25%).

A total of 22 of the 30 stakeholders invited (73%) provided feedback; this included 10 program facilitators, 9 referrers and 3 practice/service managers. A minimum of one stakeholder from each region of delivery responded to the survey. One hundred percent of stakeholders reported that they were 'very satisfied' or 'satisfied' with the program and that they were 'very likely' or 'likely' to recommend the program to potential participants and colleagues/other health professionals. All respondents either 'strongly agreed' or 'agreed' that the program both met the needs of participants and was beneficial for people with chronic disease. Most (90%) reported the program is effective and appropriate for chronic disease management. The majority (82%) 'strongly agreed' or 'agreed' that the referral process was simple and easy, with the remaining 'neither agreeing nor disagreeing' (5%) or 'disagreeing' (14%). 95% 'strongly agreed' or 'agreed' that the program aligned with existing prevention and management programs within their organisation. A total of 60% reported ('a great deal' and 'a lot') that 2 h weekly group sessions for 8 weeks is sufficient for promoting positive behaviour change, with 40% reporting ('a great deal' and 'a lot') that this was sufficient for improving self-management of chronic disease risk factors. Ratings were lower regarding receiving adequate communication, with 40% of respondents reporting that they received adequate communication and updates on the progress of people they had referred. Among facilitators ($n = 13$), 85% reported they received adequate training to deliver HEAL™ and 77% reported that the resources provided were 'extremely' or 'very effective', with the remaining reporting that they were 'somewhat effective' (23%).

4. Discussion

This study set out to determine the uptake, retention, effectiveness and acceptability of a group-based healthy lifestyle intervention delivered in rural and disadvantaged communities under "real-world" conditions. Overall, the results were positive, with strong referral to the program from a large number of health care providers. The program uptake rate was high amongst those referred. On average, participants completed six out of eight program sessions, and around half of participants completed the 8-week follow-up assessments, showing measurable improvements in most behavioural and physiological parameters measured. Participants' feedback was highly favourable. Stakeholder feedback was also generally favourable, although referring clinicians wanted further communication regarding progress of the people they had referred into the program.

Results suggested that the HEAL™ program led to measurable improvement in participants' lifestyle behaviours. On average, program completers reported consuming two servings of fruit per day, which meant that by the program's end, the average participant was meeting the recommended daily intake of fruit as per the Australian dietary guidelines [35]. Vegetable consumption increased substantially (0.8 increase in daily servings), though the average completer still fell short of healthy eating guidelines [35,36]. Self-reported physical activity increased by 140 min per week, representing a very large and clinically meaningful increase. It is important to acknowledge that these are self-reported changes, which are susceptible to social-desirability bias [37]. Previous research has highlighted that significant improvements in self-reported outcomes may not be reflected in significant changes when they are measured objectively [38].

Improvements seen in a variety of objectively measured health outcomes suggest that program participants did make meaningful changes to their lifestyle. In particular, participants, on average, lost approximately 1.4 kg. This degree of weight loss is comparable to, or perhaps slightly better than, one other study based on real-world delivery of the HEAL™ intervention, in which completers lost, on average, 1.0 kg [23]. In contrast, a meta-analysis of the effects on 28 interventions modelling on the Diabetes Prevention Program found they led to 4 percent body weight loss at 12 months (vs. 1.4% loss at 8 weeks in our study) [22]. The comparability of these results is unclear, given their contrasting length of follow-up. The improvements in diastolic blood pressure, 6 min walk test and 30 s chair rise are all in line with improvements previously reported for the HEAL™ intervention.

A particularly important finding from the current study was the high level of intervention uptake and acceptability. This is especially important when viewed in the light that the healthy lifestyle intervention was delivered in high-need communities that are typically hard to reach. Eleven percent of program participants were indigenous Australians (compared with 3.3% percent for the entire Australian population) [39] and SEIFA values indicate that the program was delivered in disadvantaged regions. This contrasts with many research-based health lifestyle programs, which typically reach white, relatively advantaged participants [40,41]. Whilst the program had good penetration in disadvantaged regions, loss to follow up was associated with SEIFA, highlighting the challenges of retaining socioeconomically disadvantaged participants across a prolonged period. Additionally, the current study continued that trend often seen in researcher-led programs, where they both attracted a large proportion of female participants [42].

The key strength of this study was that it evaluated a community-based physical activity and healthy eating program delivered under real-world conditions. Not only did the intervention reach a large number of underserved participants, but it was embedded within the existing health care system, with participants referred through other local health service providers. The reporting of the program's results in the peer-reviewed literature demonstrates a clinician-instigated collaboration between health service providers and health researchers. Such collaborations are vital to support the reporting of real-world outcome data in the peer-reviewed literature [43]. At present, the largest body of peer-reviewed evidence regarding lifestyle interventions comes from researcher-led interventions, which often are discontinued at the end of the research project, and are not delivered under real-world conditions (e.g., participation is incentivised through financial payments, recruitment methods are not embedded in the health system, and participants are provided extensive support to complete the program and assessments).

Limitations must also be acknowledged. As is common for real-world intervention evaluations, a pre–post design was used with no control group. In addition, data relating to reasons for declining participation and attrition and drop-out were not captured Furthermore, physical activity and dietary outcomes were self-reported using simple instruments suited to a clinical setting, with modest validity relative to gold standard research measures. However, the changes in objectively measured health outcomes suggest that behaviour change was achieved. A further limitation was that blood pressure was measured using clinical-grade sphygmomanometers available at each site, but the brand and model were not recorded. However, given that the same sphygmomanometer was used for pre and post measures within participants, this should not have influenced the results, which focused on changes in blood pressure over time. Whilst these limitations might be considered major weaknesses for a traditional efficacy study, the health benefits of physical activity and healthy eating are well established, so the primary contribution of this study relates to implementation outcomes (e.g., uptake and acceptability). A key limitation was that the program was delivered and evaluated over a relatively short period due to funding constraints. Thus, the longer-term impacts are unknown. Ideally, real-world lifestyle programs should embed long-term follow-up assessment procedures to capture long-term impacts.

Overall, results suggest the HEAL™ program was successfully delivered into these underserved rural communities, with strong uptake, reasonable intervention attendance, and excellent program acceptability. In the future, longer-term evidence and cost-effectiveness data would be valuable to support funding for ongoing programming and scale-up. Further work is needed to improve referral of, and program uptake, amongst men, who were under-represented in this study, and are characteristically reticent to partake in preventive health programs. The program may be improved by building in a communication mechanism by which participants' progress is reported back to their referring health care providers.

5. Conclusions

In conclusion, this study evaluated the real-world uptake, retention, effectiveness and acceptability of a group-based healthy lifestyle intervention delivered in rural and underserved communities. The program achieved strong referral from clinicians, and uptake from participants. Around half of participants completed the 8-week program and follow-up assessments, with measurable improvements in behavioural and physiological outcomes. Future collaborative research between health service providers and researchers is warranted to establish the cost-effectiveness of the program and improve participation amongst men.

Supplementary Materials: The following are available online at https://www.mdpi.com/article/10.3390/nu13114040/s1, Table S1: Comparison of individuals who accepted and did not accept the referral to HEAL™, Table S2: Comparison of participants who completed the eight-week follow-up assessment and non-completers.

Author Contributions: Conceptualization, E.P., C.J., R.G.C. and C.A.M.; methodology, C.J. and E.P.; formal analysis, R.G.C. and C.J.; interpretation C.J., R.G.C. and C.A.M.; resources, E.P.; writing—original draft preparation, C.J., C.A.M., R.G.C., A.M. and E.P.; writing—review and editing, C.A.M. and E.P.; supervision, C.A.M.; project administration, E.P.; funding acquisition, E.P. All authors have read and agreed to the published version of the manuscript.

Funding: Sonder was funded to deliver the HEAL™ program by Country SA PHN. C.A.M. is supported by a Medical Research Future Fund Emerging Leadership Grant (GNT1193862).

Institutional Review Board Statement: The study was conducted according to the guidelines of the Declaration of Helsinki. This analysis of quality assurance data was exempt from ethics approval by the University of South Australia's Human Research Ethics Committee (application no. 204196).

Informed Consent Statement: Patient provided written consent to complete the healthy lifestyle program and for their patient data to be used for quality assurance purposes.

Data Availability Statement: This study is based on patient data. The patients did not provide consent for their individual data to be shared; therefore, the data are not available.

Acknowledgments: We would like to acknowledge the involvement of Sonder staff, including the HEAL™ program team. We would also like to thank participants for supporting the program by attending and providing valuable feedback.

Conflicts of Interest: The authors declare no conflict of interest. The funders had no role in the design of the study; in the collection, analyses, or interpretation of data; in the writing of the manuscript, or in the decision to publish the results.

References

1. Australian Institute of Health and Welfare. *Australia's Health 2014*; Australia's health series no. 14. Cat. no. AUS 178; Australian Institute of Health and Welfare: Canberra, Australia, 2014.
2. Crowley, S.; Antioch, K.; Carter, R.; Waters, A.M.; Conway, L.; Mathers, C. *The Cost of Diet-Related Disease in Australia: A Discussion Paper*; AIHW: Canberra, Australia, 1992.
3. Australian Bureau of Statistics. Daily Intake of Fruit and Vegetables. Australian Health Survey: Updated Results, 2011–2012. 2013. Available online: https://www.abs.gov.au/ausstats/abs@.nsf/Lookup/C549D4433F6B74D7CA257B8200179569?opendocument (accessed on 1 September 2021).
4. Australian Bureau of Statistics. Australian Health Survey: First Results, 2011–12. Available online: https://www.abs.gov.au/ausstats/abs@.nsf/lookup/1DA0C56919DE176BCA257AA30014BFB7?opendocument (accessed on 1 September 2021).
5. Welfare, A. *Australia's Health 2016*; Australia's Health Series No. 15. Cat. No. AUS 199; AIHW: Canberra, Australia, 2016.
6. Ball, K.; Lamb, K.E.; Costa, C.; Cutumisu, N.; Ellaway, A.; Kamphuis, C.B.M.; Mentz, G.; Pearce, J.; Santana, P.; Santos, R.; et al. Neighbourhood Socioeconomic Disadvantage and Fruit and Vegetable Consumption: A Seven Countries Comparison. *Int. J. Behav. Nutr. Phys. Act.* **2015**, *12*, 1–13. [CrossRef]
7. Beenackers, M.A.; Kamphuis, C.B.M.; Giskes, K.; Brug, J.; Kunst, A.E.; Burdorf, A.; Van Lenthe, F.J. Socioeconomic Inequalities in Occupational, Leisure-Time, and Transport Related Physical Activity among European Adults: A systematic review. *Int. J. Behav. Nutr. Phys. Act.* **2012**, *9*, 116. [CrossRef]
8. Andrade-Gómez, E.; García-Esquinas, E.; Ortolá, R.; Martinez-Gomez, D.; Rodríguez-Artalejo, F. Watching TV has a Distinct Sociodemographic and Lifestyle Profile Compared with Other Sedentary Behaviors: A nationwide population-based study. *PLoS ONE* **2017**, *12*, e0188836. [CrossRef]
9. Australian Institute of Health and Welfare. Rural and Remote Health. Available online: https://www.aihw.gov.au/reports/rural-health/rural-remote-health (accessed on 3 October 2019).
10. Australian Institute of Health and Welfare. *Australian Burden of Disease Study: Impact and Causes of Illness and Death in Aboriginal and Torres Strait Islander People 2011*; Cat. no. BOD 7.; AIHW: Canberra, Australia, 2016.
11. Reading, J. *The Crisis of Chronic Disease among Aboriginal Peoples: A Challenge for Public Health, Population Health and Social Policy*; Centre for Aboriginal Health Research: Victoria, BC, Canada, 2009.
12. Hefford, M.; Crampton, P.; Foley, J. Reducing Health Disparities through Primary Care Reform: The New Zealand Experiment. *Health Policy* **2005**, *72*, 9–23. [CrossRef] [PubMed]
13. Cleland, V.; Squibb, K.; Stephens, L.; Dalby, J.; Timperio, A.; Winzenberg, T.; Ball, K.; Dollman, J. Effectiveness of Interventions to Promote Physical Activity and/or Decrease Sedentary Behaviour among Rural Adults: A Systematic Review and Meta-Analysis. *Obes. Rev.* **2017**, *18*, 727–741. [CrossRef]
14. Rhodes, R.E.; Janssen, I.; Bredin, S.; Warburton, D.; Bauman, A. Physical Activity: Health Impact, Prevalence, Correlates and Interventions. *Psychol. Health* **2017**, *32*, 942–975. [CrossRef]

15. Greaves, C.J.; Sheppard, K.E.; Abraham, C.; Hardeman, W.; Roden, M.; Evans, P.H.; Schwarz, P. The IMAGE STUDY Group. Systematic Review of Reviews of Intervention Components Associated with Increased Effectiveness in Dietary and Physical Activity Interventions. *BMC Public Health* **2011**, *11*, 119. [CrossRef]
16. Pignone, M.P.; Ammerman, A.; Fernandez, L.; Orleans, C.; Pender, N.; Woolf, S.; Lohr, K.N.; Sutton, S. Counseling to promote a healthy diet in adults: A summary of the evidence for the U.S. Preventive Services Task Force. *Am. J. Prev. Med.* **2003**, *24*, 75–92. [CrossRef]
17. Conn, V.S.; Hafdahl, A.R.; Brown, S.A.; Brown, L.M. Meta-analysis of patient education interventions to increase physical activity among chronically ill adults. *Patient Educ. Couns.* **2008**, *70*, 157–172. [CrossRef] [PubMed]
18. Shelton, R.C.; Lee, M. Sustaining Evidence-Based Interventions and Policies: Recent Innovations and Future Directions in Implementation Science. *Am. Public Health Assoc.* **2019**, *109*, S132–S134. [CrossRef] [PubMed]
19. Bell, K.J.L.; McCullough, A.; Del Mar, C.; Glasziou, P. What's the uptake? Pragmatic RCTs may be used to estimate uptake, and thereby population impact of interventions, but better reporting of trial recruitment processes is needed. *BMC Med. Res. Methodol.* **2017**, *17*, 174. [CrossRef] [PubMed]
20. Kerner, J.; Rimer, B.; Emmons, K. Introduction to the Special Section on Dissemination: Dissemination Research and Research Dissemination: How Can We Close the Gap? *Health Psychol.* **2005**, *24*, 443–446. [CrossRef] [PubMed]
21. Brownson, R.C.; Jones, E. Bridging the gap: Translating research into policy and practice. *Prev. Med.* **2009**, *49*, 313–315. [CrossRef]
22. Ali, M.K.; Echouffo-Tcheugui, J.B.; Williamson, D.F. How Effective Were Lifestyle Interventions in Real-World Settings That Were Modeled on The Diabetes Prevention Program? *Health Aff.* **2012**, *31*, 67–75. [CrossRef]
23. Hetherington, S.A.; Borodzicz, J.A.; Shing, C.M. Assessing the real world effectiveness of the Healthy Eating Activity and Lifestyle (HEAL™) program. *Health Promot. J. Aust.* **2015**, *26*, 93–98. [CrossRef] [PubMed]
24. Norton, K.; Norton, L. *Pre-Exercise Screening. Guide to the Australian Adult Pre-Exercise Screening System*; Exercise and Sports Science Australia: Adelaide, Australia, 2011.
25. Australian Bureau of Statistics. *Table 3 Correspondence 1270.0.55.005—Australian Statistical Geography Standard (ASGS): Volume 5—Remoteness Structure, July 2016*; Australian Bureau of Statistics: Canberra, Australia, 2018.
26. Australian Bureau of Statistics. *Table 2 Postal Area (POA) Index of Relative Socio-Economic Disadvantage, 2016. 2033.0.55.001—Census of Population and Housing: Socio-Economic Indexes for Areas (SEIFA) Australia, 2016*; Australian Bureau of Statistics: Canberra, Australia, 2018.
27. Australian Institute of Health Welfare. *The Active Australia Survey: A Guide and Manual for Implementation, Analysis and Reporting*; AIHW: Canberra, Australis, 2003.
28. Brown, W.J.; Burton, N.; Marshall, A.; Miller, Y.D. Reliability and Validity of a Modified Self-Administered Version of the Active Australia Physical Activity Survey in a Sample of Mid-Age Women. *Aust. N. Z. J. Public Health* **2008**, *32*, 535–541. [CrossRef]
29. Brown, W.; Bauman, A.; Chey, T.; Trost, S.; Mummery, K. Method: Comparison of Surveys Used to Measure Physical Activity. *Aust. N. Z. J. Public Health* **2004**, *28*, 128–134. [CrossRef]
30. Cora, C.L.; Marshall, A.L.; Sjostrom, M.; Bauman, A.E.; Booth, M.L.; Ainsworth, B.E.; Pratt, M.; Ekelund, U.; Yngve, A.; Sallis, J.F.; et al. International Physical Activity Questionnaire: 12-Country Reliability and Validity. *Med. Sci. Sports Exerc.* **2003**, *35*, 1381–1395. [CrossRef]
31. Wright, J.L.; Scott, J.A. The Fat and Fibre Barometer, a Short Food Behaviour Questionnaire: Reliability, Relative Validity and Utility. *Aust. J. Nutr. Diet.* **2000**, *57*, 33–39.
32. Harada, N.D.; Chiu, V.; Stewart, A.L. Mobility-related function in older adults: Assessment with a 6-minute walk test. *Arch. Phys. Med. Rehabil.* **1999**, *80*, 837–841. [CrossRef]
33. Rikli, R.E.; Jones, C.J. Development and Validation of a Functional Fitness Test for Community-Residing Older Adults. *J. Aging Phys. Act.* **1999**, *7*, 129–161. [CrossRef]
34. Gupta, S.K. Intention-to-Treat Concept: A Review. *Perspect. Clin. Res.* **2011**, *2*, 109–112. [CrossRef] [PubMed]
35. National Health and Medical Research Council. *Australian Dietary Guidelines (Reference N55a)*; National Health and Medical Research Council: Canberra, Australia, 2013.
36. Australian Institute of Health and Welfare. *Towards National Indicators for Food and Nutrition: An AIHW View. Reporting against the Dietary Guidelines for Australian Adults*; Cat. No. PHE 70; AIHW: Canberra, Australia, 2005.
37. Adams, S.A. The Effect of Social Desirability and Social Approval on Self-Reports of Physical Activity. *Am. J. Epidemiol.* **2005**, *161*, 389–398. [CrossRef] [PubMed]
38. Edney, S.M.; Olds, T.; Ryan, J.C.; Vandelanotte, C.; Plotnikoff, R.C.; Curtis, R.; Maher, C.A. A Social Networking and Gamified App to Increase Physical Activity: Cluster RCT. *Am. J. Prev. Med.* **2020**, *58*, e51–e62. [CrossRef]
39. Australian Institute of Health and Welfare. Profile of Indigenous Australians. Available online: https://www.aihw.gov.au/reports/australias-welfare/profile-of-indigenous-australians (accessed on 5 September 2021).
40. Ness, R.B.; Nelson, D.B.; Kumanyika, S.K.; Grisso, J.A. Evaluating Minority Recruitment into Clinical Studies: How Good are the Data? *Ann. Epidemiol.* **1997**, *7*, 472–478. [CrossRef]
41. Moreno-John, G.; Gachie, A.; Fleming, C.M.; Nápoles-Springer, A.; Mutran, E.; Manson, S.M.; Pérez-Stable, E.J. Ethnic Minority Older Adults Participating in Clinical Research. *J. Aging Health* **2004**, *16*, 93S–123S. [CrossRef] [PubMed]

42. Gavarkovs, A.G.; Burke, S.M.; Petrella, R.J. Engaging Men in Chronic Disease Prevention and Management Programs. *Am. J. Men's Health* **2016**, *10*, NP145–NP154. [CrossRef] [PubMed]
43. Brown, C.H.; Curran, G.; Palinkas, L.A.; Aarons, G.A.; Wells, K.B.; Jones, L.; Collins, L.M.; Duan, N.; Mittman, B.S.; Wallace, A.; et al. An Overview of Research and Evaluation Designs for Dissemination and Implementation. *Annu. Rev. Public Health* **2017**, *38*, 1–22. [CrossRef]

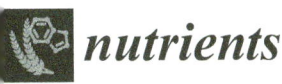

Article

Feasibility Study to Assess the Impact of a Lifestyle Intervention during Colorectal Cancer Screening in France

Inge Huybrechts [1,*], Nathalie Kliemann [1], Olivia Perol [2], Anne Cattey-Javouhey [2], Nicolas Benech [3], Aurelia Maire [2], Tracy Lignini [1], Julien Carretier [2], Jean-Christophe Saurin [3], Beatrice Fervers [2] and Marc J. Gunter [1]

1. International Agency for Research on Cancer, CEDEX 08, 69372 Lyon, France; nathalie.kliemann@gmail.com (N.K.); LigniniT@iarc.fr (T.L.); gunterm@iarc.fr (M.J.G.)
2. Centre Léon Bérard, 69008 Lyon, France; olivia.perol@lyon.unicancer.fr (O.P.); Anne.CATTEY-JAVOUHEY@lyon.unicancer.fr (A.C.-J.); Aurelia.MAIRE@lyon.unicancer.fr (A.M.); julien.carretier@lyon.unicancer.fr (J.C.); beatrice.fervers@lyon.unicancer.fr (B.F.)
3. Service d'Hépato-Gastroentérologie, Hôpital Edouard Herriot, Hospices Civils de Lyon, 69003 Lyon, France; nicolas.benech@chu-lyon.fr (N.B.); jean-christophe.saurin@chu-lyon.fr (J.-C.S.)
* Correspondence: Huybrechtsi@iarc.fr; Tel.: +33-472-738-148

Abstract: Current evidence suggests that 30–50% of cancers are attributable to established lifestyle risk factors. Cancer-screening has been identified as an opportunity for delivering advice on lifestyle behaviour change for cancer prevention. This study aimed to evaluate the feasibility and acceptance of promoting advice on the latest evidence-based lifestyle recommendations for cancer prevention at the time of colorectal cancer screening at two hospitals in Lyon, France. This feasibility study included 49 patients (20 men and 29 women) who were invited for colonoscopy. Patients received a leaflet with lifestyle recommendations for cancer prevention, accompanied with a logbook to plan and monitor their behavioural changes. Feedback from patients, hospital staff, and researchers was received via evaluation questionnaires ($n = 26$) completed after testing the educational material for at least two weeks and via two focus group discussions ($n = 7$ and $n = 9$ respectively) organized at the end of the study. All interviewed patients were interested in lowering their cancer risk, and the majority felt ready to change their lifestyle (88%), although most did not know how to decrease their risk of cancer (61%). All patients found the educational material easy to understand and sufficiently attractive and 50% of the patients reported having achieved at least one of the healthy behaviours recommended within the two weeks following the intervention. All hospital staff and almost all patients (92%) involved found that the screening program and the visits planned for colonoscopy was an appropriate moment to provide them with the educational material. This feasibility study has shown that the content, paper-based format, and time of delivery of the intervention were adequate. Health professionals seem to be willing to provide lifestyle recommendations, and patients appear interested in receiving advice for lowering their cancer risk during screening visits.

Keywords: feasibility; lifestyle intervention; colorectal cancer screening; hospital setting; France

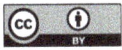

1. Introduction

Colorectal cancer (CRC) is the fourth most commonly diagnosed malignancy and the third leading cause of cancer death in the world, accounting for around 1.9 million new cases and almost 935,000 deaths in 2020 [1]. Given current demographic projections, the global burden of CRC is anticipated to increase by 60% to over 3 million new cases and 1.6 million cancer deaths annually by 2040 [2]. The incidence of CRC varies widely across geographic regions with the highest incidence in higher income countries [3]. In France, for example, CRC is the second most common cancer and the second leading cause of cancer death, accounting for more than 48,061 new cases and 20,953 deaths in 2020 [1].

CRC is a complex disease with a number of recognised risk factors. Advancing age, male sex, family history of CRC, inflammatory bowel disease, smoking, excessive alcohol drinking, overweight and obesity, low levels of physical activity and sedentary lifestyle, diabetes and high consumption of red and processed meat are established risk factors [4–7]. Decades of research have specifically focused on dietary factors: some studies have suggested a protective effect of diets rich in fruit, vegetables, fish, fibre and whole grains, calcium and dairy products against colorectal cancer [5]. Overall, it has been estimated that lifestyle factors could account for up to 40% of CRC cases worldwide [8]. Recent estimates indicate that in France, 56% of CRC cases in men and 74% of CRC cases in women are attributable to modifiable risk factors. Thus, up to 19,000 CRC cases per year could be prevented in France by improving unhealthy lifestyle behaviours [9].

The World Cancer Research Fund's (WCRF) Continuous Update Project (CUP) is the world's largest source of scientific research on cancer prevention and survivorship through diet and physical activity. The CUP analyses global research on how diet and other lifestyle factors are associated with the risk of developing CRC [10], to provide a basis for lifestyle recommendations. More recently, in 2018, the WCRF updated its latest lifestyle recommendations for cancer prevention [10], providing the most up-to-date evidence-based lifestyle recommendations for preventing CRC as well as other cancers. Recent longitudinal studies have demonstrated that adherence to the WCRF recommendations for cancer prevention are associated with 5–17% reductions in CRC incidence and 10–13% reductions in CRC mortality [11–15]. Therefore, developing effective and sustainable interventions promoting lifestyle changes for CRC prevention is of high public health interest. Cancer-screening has been identified as an important milestone that could provide an ideal opportunity for delivering advice on behaviour change for cancer prevention [16]. Berstad and colleagues recently highlighted the importance of including lifestyle counselling as a part of CRC screening since individuals with a positive screening result may be inclined to a less healthy lifestyle compared with those who had a negative screening result [17].

Screening attendance represents a time-window whereby patients may be more receptive to advice on lifestyle change, which has been described as a 'teachable moment' [16]. Screening attendance may influence an individual's perception of their personal risk for CRC, which in turn may prompt motivation to change behaviour. Indeed, a recent study showed that adults eligible for cancer screening and who were not adhering to guidelines were willing to receive lifestyle advice during screening, regardless of its results [18]. While there is little evidence to support the idea that screening prompts spontaneous behaviour change [19], interventions delivered at CRC and mammography screening in the U.K have shown promising results, such as weight loss and increased physical activity [20,21]. However, these interventions were very intensive and there is still a need to test the effect of brief interventions that promote long-term behaviour change as part of screening programs to allow widespread implementation. A recent brief habit-based weight loss intervention promoting a set of everyday healthy eating and physical activity behaviours associated with cancer prevention in patients with obesity from primary care in the UK has shown promising results, such as the maintenance of a significant weight loss over 24 months [22]. Since habit formation advice is simple, easily scalable, and a recommended approach to be used with patients [23], it may be a feasible approach to deliver evidence-based lifestyle recommendations in the cancer screening context.

The CRC screening program in France may be an ideal setting for delivering advice on lifestyle behaviours. This is a population-based nationwide cancer screening program which has been rolling out since 2009. In 2015, the immunochemical test (FIT) replaced the conventional guaiac faecal occult blood test (gFOBT), improving the participation rate [24,25]. The programme targets those aged 50 to 74 years old, who often have other lifestyle related comorbidities, such as obesity, type 2 diabetes mellitus, and cardiovascular disease. Therefore, promoting healthy lifestyle advice to the screened population has the potential to reduce the risk of cancer as well as other related comorbidities and improve prognosis and quality of life. When developing and testing a lifestyle intervention for CRC prevention, it would be the most efficient to first target higher risk population groups before expanding the intervention to the entire screening population. High risk patients include those with positive FIT, a family history of CRC, or patients who score positive (≥ 5) for a validated score consisting of simple clinical factors that successfully estimates the likelihood of detecting advanced colorectal neoplasia in asymptomatic Caucasian patients [26].

Despite this, there is still little evidence on the impact of promoting the evidence-based lifestyle recommendations during CRC screening among individuals at higher risk. There is also a need to extend our efforts to gain understanding of the potential pathways that can explain how lifestyle factors may prevent CRC development [27]. Therefore, the LIFE-SCREEN intervention trial aims to investigate the hypothesis that advice on lifestyle recommendations for cancer prevention at CRC screening among individuals classified as higher risk will promote greater adherence to cancer prevention recommendations, as well as improve the quality of life, biomarkers of cancer risk, physical fitness, and body weight. The current feasibility study presented in this manuscript aimed to evaluate the feasibility and acceptance of the LIFE-SCREEN intervention. Specific objectives were to obtain information on (i) participants' and health professionals' feedback on the educational material; (ii) health professionals' willingness to recruit participants, and (iii) participants' awareness of the risk factors for CRC and willingness to change their lifestyles. In addition, we aimed to conduct focus group meetings with patients, health professionals, and experts in the field in order to explore their feedback on the intervention content, format and delivery in great detail.

2. Materials and Methods

2.1. Study Design and Setting

This study was a single arm, two-center feasibility study of the LIFE-SCREEN intervention that aims to provide advice on evidence-based lifestyle recommendations for cancer prevention at CRC screening among individuals at higher risk of CRC. The feasibility study was carried out in 2019 at two hospitals in Lyon, France, L'hôpital Edouard Herriot (HEH) and Centre Léon Bérard (CLB). The LIFE-SCREEN intervention is registered with clinicaltrials.gov (Ref ClinicalTrials.gov Record PP201907-26) where more details on the feasibility study design and methods can be found. The study was conducted according to the guidelines of the Declaration of Helsinki, and approved by the Institutional Review Board (or Ethics Committee) of International Agency for Re-search on Cancer (IEC Project No. 19-26; reviewed and approved on 3 February 2020).

2.2. Participants

Considering the feasibility study objectives we aimed to recruit at least 30 participants [28]. Eligible patients were adults >18 years without previous cancer diagnosis, who were capable to provide informed consent, and that were attending for colonoscopy as part of CRC screening.

2.3. Lifestyle Intervention

The LIFE-SCREEN intervention aimed to deliver lifestyle advice based upon the most recent recommendations for cancer prevention published by the World Cancer Research Fund (WCRF) [8]. These recommendations entail the following target behaviours: (1) be a healthy weight; (2) move more; (3) enjoy more grains, vegetables, fruits, fish, and dairy products; (4) avoid high-calorie foods rich in fat, salt, and sugar; (5) limit consumption of red and processed meat; (6) limit alcoholic drinks; (7) limit consumption of sugar-sweetened drinks; (8) do not rely on supplements. The behavioural approaches were informed by relevant behaviour change theories and models, such as the Teachable Moments Heuristic model and the Habit formation theory. The concept of Teachable Moments (TMs), that is, naturally occurring life or health events that may prompt risk-reducing health behaviours [16], has been considered a strong foundation for widely-accepted health behaviour models. In addition, the intervention was based on the habit formation theory, in order to promote lasting healthy lifestyle behaviours. Habit-based interventions promote the repetition of target behaviours in a consistent context in order to make them become more automatic and habitual [29–31]. They also promote self-regulatory skills (e.g., goal-setting, planning, self-monitoring, and feedback on performance) in order to translate the intended behaviour into action and override unwanted automated responses [29,32].

The intervention was delivered as a self-coaching leaflet and booklet materials containing the advice on lifestyle recommendations together with strategies on how to achieve and maintain these behaviours. The material also contained instructions on how to set up specific goals (e.g., including what, how, where, and when) to achieve the target behaviours and repeat them at the same time and in the same place in order to improve the patient's likelihood of forming habits and maintaining their behaviour changes. It also provided the participants with instructions on how to track their progress (e.g., using printed booklets to monitor their behaviour), and to amend their plans when these seem inefficient in reaching their target goals.

Health professionals introduced the intervention to eligible patients during pre-colonoscopy (HEH) or post-colonoscopy visit (CLB), depending on the hospital and provided the informed consent letter. During the consultation, health professionals briefly endorsed the importance of the intervention for helping them to achieve and maintain healthy lifestyles and in turn to reduce their colorectal cancer risk. Interested patients, who signed the informed consent for this feasibility study, were provided with the educational material and were instructed to follow the intervention for at least 2 weeks before completing the feasibility evaluation questionnaire.

2.4. Measurements

At baseline, participants were required to answer questions on socio-demographics, reason for the colonoscopy and the type of appointment (pre- or post-colonoscopy), their interest and knowledge on how to reduce colorectal cancer risk, readiness to change their behaviours and interest in following the intervention. At the end of the two-week intervention, participants were invited to complete a feasibility evaluation questionnaire containing closed and open questions to obtain their feedback on the educational material, format, and delivery as well as questions on compliance to the intervention over 15 days. Participants were asked to post their completed evaluation questionnaire back using the pre-paid return envelope or to bring it with them during the focus group meetings. It should be noted that no objective measures were used to control the patient's behaviours in this feasibility study; all measures were self-reported by the patients. Health professionals were also requested to complete an evaluation questionnaire on the intervention delivery and content.

In addition, two focus group discussions were conducted at the end of the feasibility study to discuss in depth the feedback on the intervention content, format, and delivery. One focus group gathered the researchers and (para-)medical staff involved in the feasibility study and the second one invited all the patients who took part in the study. These focus group meetings were logistically organized at one of the hospitals involved in the intervention and moderated by the researcher coordinating the LIFE-SCREEN intervention. Each session began with a PowerPoint presentation that provided an overview of the LIFE-SCREEN study, design, and methods. Next the moderator asked the participants for feedback on the intervention content, format, and delivery. Both focus groups were audio recorded and lasted over one hour each. Participants were offered a free lunch meal to thank them for taking part.

2.5. Data Analysis

Descriptive analysis of the study population was performed. No association analysis was undertaken given the small sample, which was not powered to detect significant differences. Two researchers involved in the study independently assessed the audios and minutes from the focus groups and identified the main suggestions and feedback received.

They met to discuss aspects such as recruitment and delivery acceptability, barriers for lifestyle intervention, content of the educational material and any other issue that should be considered when conducting the full RCT. A consensus list of improvements was then defined and used to optimize the study protocol further.

3. Results

This feasibility study included 49 patients (20 men and 29 women), aged from 23 to 75 years (Table 1). Most of the patients received the invitation and the educational material at their post-colonoscopy visit (84%). All patients who participated in the feasibility study were interested in lowering their CRC risk, although most of them did not know how to decrease their risk (61%). Eighty-eight percent of the respondents felt ready to change their lifestyles with the aim to lower their CRC risk.

Table 1. Baseline information ($n = 49$).

	n (%) or Mean (Min-Max)
Sex	
Men	20 (41%)
Women	29 (59%)
Age	56.6 (23–75) *
Hospital visit at which the intervention was performed	
Pre-colonoscopy	4 (8%)
Post-colonoscopy	41 (84%)
Hospitalization for colonoscopy	4 (8%)
Reason for the colonoscopy	
Family history of Colorectal cancer (CRC)	7 (14%)
CRC symptoms	13 (27%)
CRC screening (positive FIT test)	7 (14%)
Medical follow-up (e.g., Lynch)	22 (45%)
Interested in reducing CRC risk	
Yes	49 (100)
No	0
Knowledge on how to reduce CRC risk	
Yes	19 (39%)
No	30 (61%)
Do healthy lifestyle behaviours help reduce CRC risk?	
Yes	41 (84%)
No	2 (4%)
Don't know	6 (12%)
Ready to change lifestyle behaviours	
Yes	43 (88%)
No	1 (2%)
Don't know	5 (10%)
Interested in taking part in LIFE-SCREEN	
Yes	45 (92%)
No	2 (4%)
Do not know	2 (4%)

* Mean and median age were equal (57 years).

At two-week's follow-up, a total of 26 patients (53%) completed the evaluation questionnaire. Regarding compliance to the intervention, presented in Table 2, half of the patients (50%) reported having achieved at least one target behaviour using the monitoring sheets. Most of them made plans to achieve at least one behaviour (58%) and made amendments to the plans when necessary (58%). Importantly, the majority of patients intended to continue following the intervention after the end of the study (74%).

Table 2. Follow-up information on compliance to the intervention over 15 days ($n = 26$).

Compliance to the Intervention	n (%)
Achieved at least one healthy behaviour using the tick sheets	
Yes	13 (50%)
No	10 (38%)
Missing	3 (12%)
Made plan(s) to achieve at least one healthy behaviour	
Yes	15 (58%)
No	9 (34%)
Missing	2 (8%)
Made adjustment to plan(s) to achieve at least one healthy behaviour	
Yes	14 (58%)
No	9 (34%)
Missing	3 (8%)
Intends to continue following the intervention?	
Yes	19 (74%)
No	7 (26%)
Missing	-

Table 3 shows patients feedback on the intervention delivery and content collected through evaluation questionnaires. All patients said they easily understood the information included in the educational material and most of them found the material sufficiently attractive, complete and in line with their expectations (88%). Although most patients (92%) found the material covered the kind of information they would expect, some reported having suggestions to improve it (27%). Suggestions were made such as providing more plant-based and vegetarian recipes and practical tips on how to achieve their goals (e.g., examples of activities adapted to an ageing population to maintain their fitness, etc.). Interestingly, 54% of the patients preferred to stick to the non-digital (e.g., paper-pencil) tools to monitor their behaviours rather than using digital tools. Most of them found that the CRC screening program and the visits planned for colonoscopy were right/appropriate moments to provide them with the educational material (92%). Similar feedback was obtained in the patients' focus group, composed of three patients (two women and one man) involved in the feasibility study.

Table 3. Follow up information on intervention delivery and content collected via evaluation questionnaires ($n = 26$).

Feedback on the Intervention Delivery and Content	n (%)
Interested in taking part in this intervention if attending cancer screening again in the future	
Not very interested	6 (23%)
Somewhat interested	11 (42%)
Very interested	5 (20%)
Not applicable or missing	4 (15%)
Interested in taking part in this intervention even if randomied to intervention or control condition	
Not very interested	5 (20%)
Somewhat interested	12 (46%)
Very interested	5 (19%)
Not applicable or missing	4 (15%)
Feedback on the Intervention Delivery and Content	**n (%)**
Interested in receiving text-messages and emails reminding about the healthy behaviours	
Not very interested	9 (35%)

Table 3. Cont.

Somewhat interested	9 (35%)
Very interested	6 (23%)
Not applicable or missing	2 (7%)
The educational material was easy to understand	
Yes	26 (100%)
No	0
The educational material covered the kind of information you would expect	
Yes	24 (92%)
No	0
Missing	2 (8%)
The educational materials are attractive and eye-catching	
Yes	23 (88%)
No	1 (4%)
Missing	2 (8%)
Is there any other information or tips that you would like to see in the leaflet or logbook?	
Yes	7 (27%)
No	18 (69%)
Missing	1 (4%)
Was the timing of the delivery adequate?	
Yes	24 (92%)
No	1 (4%)
Missing	1 (4%)
Would it be helpful to have access to a mobile or web-based app to monitor your behaviours?	
Yes	11 (42%)
No	14 (54%)
Missing	1 (4%)

Feedback from experts and health professionals involved in the study was obtained via focus group discussions and evaluation questionnaires. The focus group was conducted with four health professionals and three experts in the field. They suggested to screen participants for their current adherence to the recommendations for cancer prevention at baseline and exclude those with a high score (complying with the recommendations), as they would not have much room to improve their behaviours. However, they emphasized that the study protocol must ensure that the extra work for the surgeons and other health professionals is kept to the minimum (~5 min/patient) to ensure intervention feasibility. They also underlined the importance of testing participants on knowledge about healthy lifestyles and 'knowledge change', as the knowledge of many patients seemed rather low. Regarding the time of the delivery, it was concluded that both pre- and post-colonoscopy are possible. Although it was concluded that both pre- and post-colonoscopy are possible, it was agreed that the most optimal time to deliver the educational material was during the pre-colonoscopy visit, followed by a follow-up intervention (referring to the educational material received at baseline) taking place during the post-colonoscopy visit. Experts and health professionals found that the material could be improved by providing patients with fridge magnets containing messages about the recommendations; recipe books with low-cost vegetarian recipe ideas; and more tips on how to get more active (especially for older patients). They also suggested that the recommendation for quitting smoking should be more prominent.

4. Discussion

The importance of promoting lifestyle changes to prevent cancer has been highlighted in the scientific literature as well as in the lay press [33,34]. Although the time at which an individual undergoes cancer screening could be considered as a teachable moment [20,21], so far evidence regarding the effectiveness of evidence-based lifestyle advice administered during cancer screening is still scarce. Nevertheless, the necessity and importance of including lifestyle counselling as a part of CRC screening has been demonstrated in particular among individuals with a positive screening result, as they may be inclined to a less favourable lifestyle compared with those who tested negative at screening [17]. Therefore, this feasibility study was set up to evaluate the feasibility of an intervention study aimed at delivering evidence-based lifestyle advice during CRC screening among individuals at higher CRC risk, as this may have high public health potential.

In summary, this feasibility study showed that the content, paper-based format, and time of delivery of the intervention (both pre- and post-colonoscopy) were adequate and well accepted by the health professionals and patients.

Previous studies already investigated the impact of lifestyle interventions during cancer screening, though with mixed results [35–40]. Although the colorectal cancer screening has already been evaluated as a potential teachable moment for lifestyle interventions [35], the interventions evaluated so far were rather intensive and personalised lifestyle interventions that require important time investments of (para)-medical staff. Here, our results suggest that a simple, well-documented intervention before or after colonoscopy may be sufficient to impact patient lifestyle. Indeed, following our intervention, half of the patients reported having achieved at least one of the healthy behaviours recommended within the two weeks after the first visit. These results should be confirmed in a larger randomised controlled trial.

Patients and health professionals provided valuable suggestions and feedback for further improvement of the study protocol and educational material, leading us to include a "recipe and practical tips book". The paper-based format of the intervention will be maintained, but patients will also have the option to get access to the electronic (e.g., pdf) version of all documents. Patients will also be allowed to choose whether they wish to receive reminders of the recommendations sent by text-messages and/or emails during the 12-month follow-up. The delivery of the intervention will take place during the pre-colonoscopy visit and a follow-up intervention (referring to the educational material received at baseline) will take place during the post-colonoscopy visit. However, the inclusion in the study will be conditional to the colonoscopy results, as patients who receive CRC diagnosis during the post-colonoscopy visit are not considered eligible for the intervention study that aims at patients at higher risk.

The proposed intervention is expected to promote greater adherence to cancer prevention recommendations and have an effect on quality of life, biomarkers of cancer risk, physical fitness, and body weight among higher CRC risk population groups. The integration of these well-established continuous frameworks, namely the CRC screening program and the WCRF-CUP cancer prevention program that continuously updates the evidence on lifestyle risk factors and cancer risk, ensures the sustainability of this intervention program and the potential for further expansion to other cancer screening programs in France and beyond. If successful, this intervention trial could inspire similar initiatives for other cancer types that have well established cancer screening programs and can be expanded to the full screening population.

The fact that the intervention will be implemented in hospitals, alongside the CRC screening routine procedures, makes the access to blood, faecal, and tissue samples from participants easier and will allow us to explore the effect of the intervention on nutritional, inflammation, metabolic health and microbial biomarkers that could provide important information on the mechanisms of CRC development and prevention targets.

5. Future Perspectives

As stated previously, no standardised protocols or recommendations are available for individuals at higher risk of CRC. If this evidence-based lifestyle intervention confirms the hypothesis that adherence to the latest evidence-based lifestyle guidelines improves following such an intervention, which in turn reduces CRC risk and improves the quality of life, then the intervention can be implemented nationwide and beyond. The recommendations will be developed as a visual representation that is interpretable by non-literate patients to consider and guarantee social equality among the target population. In addition, the lifestyle advice given in this intervention is aimed to limit the burden for the hospital staff involved to a minimum so that it can easily replace routine care when upscaling to a nation-wide intervention.

In the future, this intervention protocol could also be tested in primary care by providing the healthy lifestyle advice to all participants involved in CRC screening, regardless of their FIT test result.

In addition to cancer, rates of other non-communicable diseases (NCDs) continue to rise, affecting the poorest and most vulnerable populations. The intervention targets a higher CRC risk population aged 35 or over, who often have other lifestyle related comorbidities, such as obesity, type 2 diabetes mellitus, and cardiovascular disease. These diseases share common risk factors, as for example, altered lipid levels, inflammation and abnormal glucose metabolism [41,42]. Hence, promoting healthy lifestyle advice to this population has the potential to also reduce the risk of other related NCDs.

Lastly, this intervention will also shed light on changes in biomarkers relevant for cancer prevention, allowing a better understanding of the putative mechanisms involved.

6. Conclusions

This feasibility study has shown that the content, paper-based format, and timing of delivery of the intervention (pre- and/or post-colonoscopy) were adequate and well-accepted by both the health professionals and patients. Health professionals seem to be willing to provide lifestyle recommendations and patients seem interested in receiving advice for lowering their cancer risk during screening visits. Considering the interesting finding that more than half of the patients made plans and adjustments to achieve one of the healthy behaviours recommended in the educational material and that half of the patients reported having achieved at least one of the healthy behaviours recommended within two weeks of receiving the intervention, this LIFE-SCREEN intervention is expected to promote greater adherence to cancer prevention recommendations. Therefore, this LIFE-SCREEN intervention will now be evaluated within the context of a funded randomised-controlled trial.

Author Contributions: Conceptualization, I.H.; M.J.G. and N.K.; methodology, I.H.; N.K.; O.P.; N.B.; A.C.-J.; A.M.; J.C.; J.-C.S.; B.F. and M.J.G.; formal analysis, I.H. and N.K.; Data collection, O.P.; N.B.; A.C.-J. and A.M.; writing—original draft preparation, I.H.; writing—review and editing, I.H.; N.K.; O.P.; N.B.; A.C.-J.; A.M.; J.C.; J.-C.S.; B.F. and M.J.G.; project administration, I.H. and T.L. funding acquisition, I.H.; N.K.; O.P.; N.B.; A.C.-J.; A.M.; J.-C.S.; B.F. and M.J.G. All authors have read and agreed to the published version of the manuscript.

Funding: This research was funded by Institut National du Cancer, grant number INCA RISP20-028.

Institutional Review Board Statement: The study was conducted according to the guidelines of the Declaration of Helsinki, and approved by the Institutional Review Board (or Ethics Committee) of International Agency for Research on Cancer (IEC Project No. 19-26; reviewed and approved on reviewed on 3 February 2020).

Informed Consent Statement: Informed consent was obtained from all subjects involved in the study.

Data Availability Statement: Access to anonymized data and the intervention/educational material can be requested via email through the corresponding author.

Acknowledgments: The authors would like to thank the, L'hôpital Edouard Herriot (HEH), Centre Léon Bérard (CLB) and l'Institut du Cancer for their support in conducting this study. The authors would also like to thank Corrine Casagrande, Genevieve Nicolas, and Karine Racinoux for their support in translations, data entry and analysis.

Conflicts of Interest: The authors declare no conflict of interest.

IARC Disclaimer: Where authors are identified as personnel of the International Agency for Research on Cancer/World Health Organization, the authors alone are responsible for the views expressed in this article and they do not necessarily represent the decisions, policy, or views of the International Agency for Research on Cancer/World Health Organization.

References

1. International Agency for Research on Cancer. Global Cancer Observatory (GCO). Available online: https://gco.iarc.fr/ (accessed on 2 September 2021).
2. Ferlay, J.; Soerjomataram, I.; Ervik, M. *Cancer Incidence and Mortality Worldwide: IARC Cancer Base No. 11*; International Agency for Research on Cancer: Lyon, France, 2013.
3. Arnold, M.; Sierra, M.S.; Laversanne, M.; Soerjomataram, I.; Jemal, A.; Bray, F. Global patterns and trends in colorectal cancer incidence and mortality. *Gut* **2017**, *66*, 683–691. [CrossRef]
4. Johnson, C.M.; Wei, C.; Ensor, J.E.; Smolenski, D.J.; Amos, C.I.; Levin, B.; Berry, D.A. Meta-analyses of colorectal cancer risk factors. *Cancer Causes Control* **2013**, *24*, 1207–1222. [CrossRef]
5. World Cancer Research Fund-American Institute for Cancer Research. Continuous Update Project Expert Report 2018. Diet, Nutrition, Physical ACTIVITY and Colorectal Cancer. Available online: dietandcancerreport.org (accessed on 2 September 2021).
6. Moore, S.C.; Lee, I.M.; Weiderpass, E.; Campbell, P.T.; Sampson, J.N.; Kitahara, C.M.; Keadle, S.K.; Arem, H.; Berrington de Gonzalez, A.; Hartge, P.; et al. Association of Leisure-Time Physical Activity with Risk of 26 Types of Cancer in 1.44 Million Adults. *JAMA Intern. Med.* **2016**, *176*, 816–825. [CrossRef]
7. Morris, J.S.; Bradbury, K.E.; Cross, A.J.; Gunter, M.J.; Murphy, N. Physical activity, sedentary behaviour and colorectal cancer risk in the UK Biobank. *Br. J. Cancer* **2018**, *118*, 920–929. [CrossRef]
8. WCRF/AICR. *Diet, Nutrition, Physical Activity and Cancer: A Global Perspective*; World Cancer Research Fund/American Institute for Cancer Research: Washington, DC, USA, 2018.
9. Marant-Micallef, C.; Shield, K.D.; Vignat, J.; Hill, C.; Menvielle, G.; Dossus, L.; Ormsby, J.N.; Rehm, J.; Rushton, L.; Vineis, P.; et al. Nombre et fractions de cancers attribuables au mode de vie et a l'environnement en France metropolitaine en 2015: Resultats principaux. *Bull. Epidemiol. Hebd.* **2018**, *21*, 442–448.
10. WCRF/AICR. World Cancer Research Fund's (WCRF) Continuous Update Project. Available online: https://www.wcrf.org/diet-and-cancer/continuous-update-project/ (accessed on 2 September 2021).
11. Romaguera, D.; Vergnaud, A.C.; Peeters, P.H.; van Gils, C.H.; Chan, D.S.; Ferrari, P.; Romieu, I.; Jenab, M.; Slimani, N.; Clavel-Chapelon, F.; et al. Is concordance with World Cancer Research Fund/American Institute for Cancer Research guidelines for cancer prevention related to subsequent risk of cancer? Results from the EPIC study. *Am. J. Clin. Nutr.* **2012**, *96*, 150–163. [CrossRef] [PubMed]
12. Romaguera, D.; Ward, H.; Wark, P.A.; Vergnaud, A.C.; Peeters, P.H.; van Gils, C.H.; Ferrari, P.; Fedirko, V.; Jenab, M.; Boutron-Ruault, M.C.; et al. Pre-diagnostic concordance with the WCRF/AICR guidelines and survival in European colorectal cancer patients: A cohort study. *BMC Med.* **2015**, *13*, 107. [CrossRef]
13. Vergnaud, A.C.; Romaguera, D.; Peeters, P.H.; van Gils, C.H.; Chan, D.S.; Romieu, I.; Freisling, H.; Ferrari, P.; Clavel-Chapelon, F.; Fagherazzi, G.; et al. Adherence to the World Cancer Research Fund/American Institute for Cancer Research guidelines and risk of death in Europe: Results from the European Prospective Investigation into Nutrition and Cancer cohort study1,4. *Am. J. Clin. Nutr.* **2013**, *97*, 1107–1120. [CrossRef]
14. Jankovic, N.; Geelen, A.; Winkels, R.M.; Mwungura, B.; Fedirko, V.; Jenab, M.; Illner, A.K.; Brenner, H.; Ordonez-Mena, J.M.; Kiefte de Jong, J.C.; et al. Adherence to the WCRF/AICR Dietary Recommendations for Cancer Prevention and Risk of Cancer in Elderly from Europe and the United States: A Meta-Analysis within the CHANCES Project. *Cancer Epidemiol. Biomark. Prev. A Publ. Am. Assoc. Cancer Res.* **2017**, *26*, 136–144. [CrossRef] [PubMed]
15. Turati, F.; Bravi, F.; Di Maso, M.; Bosetti, C.; Polesel, J.; Serraino, D.; Dalmartello, M.; Giacosa, A.; Montella, M.; Tavani, A.; et al. Adherence to the World Cancer Research Fund/American Institute for Cancer Research recommendations and colorectal cancer risk. *Eur. J. Cancer* **2017**, *85*, 86–94. [CrossRef] [PubMed]
16. Rabin, C. Promoting Lifestyle Change Among Cancer Survivors: When Is the Teachable Moment? *Am. J. Lyfestyle Med.* **2009**, *5*, 142. [CrossRef]
17. Berstad, P.; Loberg, M.; Larsen, I.K.; Kalager, M.; Holme, O.; Botteri, E.; Bretthauer, M.; Hoff, G. Long-term lifestyle changes after colorectal cancer screening: Randomised controlled trial. *Gut* **2015**, *64*, 1268–1276. [CrossRef]
18. Stevens, C.; Vrinten, C.; Smith, S.G.; Waller, J.; Beeken, R.J. Determinants of willingness to receive healthy lifestyle advice in the context of cancer screening. *Br. J. Cancer* **2018**, *119*, 251–257. [CrossRef] [PubMed]
19. Bankhead, C.R.; Brett, J.; Bukach, C.; Webster, R.; Stewart-Brown, S.; Munafo, M.; Austoker, J. Impact of screening on future health-promoting behaviors and health beliefs: A systematic review. *Int. J. Technol. Assess.* **2005**, *21*, 147. [CrossRef]
20. Anderson, A.S.; Craigie, A.M.; Caswell, S.; Treweek, S.; Stead, M.; Macleod, M.; Daly, F.; Belch, J.; Rodger, J.; Kirk, A.; et al. The impact of a bodyweight and physical activity intervention (BeWEL) initiated through a national colorectal cancer screening programme: Randomised controlled trial. *BMJ* **2014**, *348*, g1823. [CrossRef] [PubMed]

21. Anderson, A.S.; Macleod, M.; Mutrie, N.; Sugden, J.; Dobson, H.; Treweek, S.; O'Carroll, R.E.; Thompson, A.; Kirk, A.; Brennan, G.; et al. Breast cancer risk reduction–is it feasible to initiate a randomised controlled trial of a lifestyle intervention programme (ActWell) within a national breast screening programme? *Int. J. Behav. Nutr. Phys. Act.* **2014**, *11*, 156. [CrossRef]
22. Beeken, R.J.; Leurent, B.; Vickerstaff, V.; Wilson, R.; Croker, H.; Morris, S.; Omar, R.Z.; Nazareth, I.; Wardle, J. A brief intervention for weight control based on habit-formation theory delivered through primary care: Results from a randomised controlled trial. *Int. J. Obes.* **2017**, *41*, 246–254. [CrossRef]
23. Gardner, B.; Lally, P.; Wardle, J. Making health habitual: The psychology of 'habit formation' and general practice. *Br. J. Gen. Pract.* **2012**, *62*, 664–666. [CrossRef]
24. Vart, G.; Banzi, R.; Minozzi, S. Comparing participation rates between immunochemical and guaiac faecal occult blood tests: A systematic review and meta-analysis. *Prev. Med.* **2012**, *55*, 87–92. [CrossRef]
25. van Rossum, L.G.; van Rijn, A.F.; Laheij, R.J.; van Oijen, M.G.; Fockens, P.; van Krieken, H.H.; Verbeek, A.L.; Jansen, J.B.; Dekker, E. Random comparison of guaiac and immunochemical fecal occult blood tests for colorectal cancer in a screening population. *Gastroenterology* **2008**, *135*, 82–90. [CrossRef]
26. Kaminski, M.F.; Polkowski, M.; Kraszewska, E.; Rupinski, M.; Butruk, E.; Regula, J. A score to estimate the likelihood of detecting advanced colorectal neoplasia at colonoscopy. *Gut* **2014**, *63*, 1112–1119. [CrossRef]
27. Gunter, M.J.; Alhomoud, S.; Arnold, M.; Brenner, H.; Burn, J.; Casey, J.; Chan, A.T.; Cross, A.J.; Giovannucci, E.; Hoover, R.; et al. International cancer seminars: A focus on colorectal cancer. *Ann. Oncol.* **2018**. Under review.
28. Whitehead, A.L.; Julious, S.A.; Cooper, C.L.; Campbell, M.J. Estimating the sample size for a pilot randomised trial to minimise the overall trial sample size for the external pilot and main trial for a continuous outcome variable. *Stat. Methods Med. Res.* **2016**, *25*, 1057–1073. [CrossRef]
29. Lally, P.; Gardner, B. Promoting habit formation. *Health Psychol. Rev.* **2013**, *7*, S137–S158. [CrossRef]
30. Lally, P.; Van Jaarsveld, C.H.M.; Potts, H.W.W.; Wardle, J. How are habits formed: Modelling habit formation in the real world. *Eur. J. Soc. Psychol.* **2010**, *40*, 998–1009. [CrossRef]
31. Gardner, B.; Sheals, K.; Wardle, J.; McGowan, L. Putting habit into practice, and practice into habit: A process evaluation and exploration of the acceptability of a habit-based dietary behaviour change intervention. *Int. J. Behav. Nutr. Phys. Act.* **2014**, *11*, 135. [CrossRef]
32. Nederkoorn, C.; Houben, K.; Hofmann, W.; Roefs, A.; Jansen, A. Control Yourself or Just Eat What You Like? Weight Gain Over a Year Is Predicted by an Interactive Effect of Response Inhibition and Implicit Preference for Snack Foods. *Health Psychol.* **2010**, *29*, 389–393. [CrossRef]
33. Morin, H. En France, quatre cancers sur dix pourraient être évités. *Le Monde* **2018**, *11*, 142.
34. Elster, N. Modern myths about cancer from 'chemicals' in food to wifi. *Guardian* **2018**, *11*, 452.
35. Robb, K.A.; Power, E.; Kralj-Hans, I.; Atkin, W.S.; Wardle, J. The impact of individually-tailored lifestyle advice in the colorectal cancer screening context: A randomised pilot study in North-West London. *Prev. Med.* **2010**, *51*, 505–508. [CrossRef] [PubMed]
36. LoConte, N.K.; Gershenwald, J.E.; Thomson, C.A.; Crane, T.E.; Harmon, G.E.; Rechis, R. Lifestyle Modifications and Policy Implications for Primary and Secondary Cancer Prevention: Diet, Exercise, Sun Safety, and Alcohol Reduction. *Am. Soc. Clin. Oncol. Educ. Book* **2018**, *93*, 88–100. [CrossRef] [PubMed]
37. Knudsen, M.D.; Hjartåker, A.; Robb, K.A.; de Lange, T.; Hoff, G.; Berstad, P. Improving Cancer Preventive Behaviors: A Randomized Trial of Tailored Lifestyle Feedback in Colorectal Cancer Screening. *Cancer Epidemiol. Biomark. Prev. A Publ. Am. Assoc. Cancer Res.* **2018**, *27*, 1442–1449. [CrossRef]
38. Conway, E.; Wyke, S.; Sugden, J.; Mutrie, N.; Anderson, A.S. Can a lifestyle intervention be offered through NHS breast cancer screening? Challenges and opportunities identified in a qualitative study of women attending screening. *BMC Public Health* **2016**, *16*, 758. [CrossRef] [PubMed]
39. Caswell, S.; Anderson, A.S.; Steele, R.J. Bowel health to better health: A minimal contact lifestyle intervention for people at increased risk of colorectal cancer. *Br. J. Nutr.* **2009**, *102*, 1541–1546. [CrossRef] [PubMed]
40. Stevens, C.; Smith, S.G.; Vrinten, C.; Waller, J.; Beeken, R.J. Lifestyle changes associated with participation in colorectal cancer screening: Prospective data from the English Longitudinal Study of Ageing. *J. Med. Screen.* **2019**, *26*, 84–91. [CrossRef] [PubMed]
41. Klabunde, C.N.; Legler, J.M.; Warren, J.L.; Laura-Mae, B.; Schrag, D. A refined comorbidity measurement algorithm for claims-based studies of breast, prostate, colorectal, and lung cancer patients. *Ann. Epidemiol.* **2007**, *17*, 584–590. [CrossRef]
42. de Bruijn, K.M.J.; Arends, L.R.; Hansen, B.E.; Leeflang, S.; Ruiter, R.; van Eijck, C.H.J. Systematic review and meta-analysis of the association between diabetes mellitus and incidence and mortality in breast and colorectal cancer. *Br. J. Surg.* **2013**, *100*, 1421–1429. [CrossRef] [PubMed]

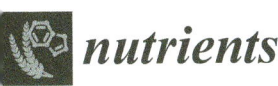

Article

Changes in Dietary Habits and Exercise Pattern of Korean Adolescents from Prior to during the COVID-19 Pandemic

So Young Kim [1], Dae Myoung Yoo [2], Chanyang Min [2,3] and Hyo Geun Choi [2,4,*]

1. Department of Otorhinolaryngology-Head & Neck Surgery, CHA Bundang Medical Center, CHA University, Seongnam 13496, Korea; sossi81@hanmail.net
2. Hallym Data Science Laboratory, Hallym University College of Medicine, Anyang 14068, Korea; ydm1285@naver.com (D.M.Y.); joicemin@naver.com (C.M.)
3. Graduate School of Public Health, Seoul National University, Seoul 08826, Korea
4. Department of Otorhinolaryngology-Head & Neck Surgery, Hallym University College of Medicine, Anyang 14068, Korea
* Correspondence: pupen@naver.com

Abstract: This study aimed to investigate changes in the exercise pattern and dietary habits in adolescents during the COVID-19 pandemic. The 12–18-year-old population in the Korea Youth Risk Behavior Web-Based Survey data of 2019 and 2020 was enrolled. The exercise pattern and dietary habits of 105,600 participants (53,461 in the 2019 group and 52,139 in the 2020 group) were compared. The odds ratios (ORs) for the dietary habits and exercise pattern of the 2020 group compared to the 2019 group were analyzed using multiple logistic regression analysis with complex sampling. The odds of eating fruit, drinking soda, drinking sweet drinks, and consuming fast food were lower in the 2020 group than in the 2019 group (all $p < 0.001$). The odds of eating breakfast were higher in the 2020 group than in the 2019 group (all $p < 0.001$). The 2020 group showed lower odds of frequent vigorous and moderate aerobic exercise and higher odds of frequent anaerobic exercise than the 2019 group (all $p < 0.001$). During the COVID-19 pandemic, adolescents consumed less fruit, soda, and sweet drinks, while they had more breakfast. The frequency of aerobic exercise was lower, while the frequency of anaerobic exercise were higher during the COVID-19 pandemic period.

Keywords: COVID-19; dietary habits; exercise pattern; adolescents; cohort study

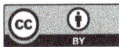

1. Introduction

The outbreak of COVID-19 had various impacts on our daily lives [1]. Due to the high infectivity of SARS-CoV-2, the prevention of contagious infection and the isolation of COVID-19 patients have been among the most important strategies in response to the COVID-19 pandemic. The quarantine maneuvers included social distancing, restriction of social activities, and lockdown. These limitations on social circumferences increased the time spent indoors and eating home-cooked meals, while they decreased outdoor activities and eating out [2]. The lockdown of schools and workplaces changed the schedules of daily life for many people.

A number of researchers have been concerned about the changes in dietary habits and exercise pattern during the COVID-19 pandemic [3–7]. A cross-sectional survey in Poland found that approximately 43% and 52% of adults consumed more food and snacks, respectively, during the COVID-19 lockdown [3]. Approximately 30% of participants gained weight because of the frequent consumption of fast food (3.0 ± 1.6 kg) during the COVID-19 lockdown [3]. Another survey in Italy reported that approximately 33.5% of participants changed their eating habits, and approximately 81% of participants increased frozen food consumption during the COVID-19 lockdown [5]. This survey estimated that home confinement during the COVID-19 crisis was negatively associated with physical activity intensity and positively associated with sedentary time during the COVID-19 lockdown [5].

Importantly, adolescents are in periods of development and are susceptible to acquiring poor lifestyle patterns, including habits related to diet and exercise pattern [5,8,9]. Indeed, an international online survey reported that adolescents consumed more fast food and sweet food during home confinement due to the COVID-19 lockdown (44.6% vs. 64% for fast food; 14% vs. 20.7% for sweet food) [5]. In addition, 70.5% of participants reduced their exercise pattern during the COVID-19 lockdown [5]. An international online survey demonstrated reduced physical activity levels (vigorous, moderate, walking, and overall) during home confinement due to the COVID-19 crisis (5.04 ± 2.51 day/week vs. 3.83 ± 2.82 day/week of physical activities, $p < 0.001$) [6]. However, the information on the respondents was very limited, and the analysis did not consider possible confounders, such as economic status, sleep time, and obesity. As multiple lifestyle factors influence dietary habits and exercise pattern, these factors should be concurrently considered in analyses of the impact of the COVID-19 pandemic on diet and exercise pattern.

As changes in dietary habits and exercise pattern during the COVID-19 pandemic were suggested to increase the risk of metabolic disorders in a previous study [10], we hypothesized that there may have also been changes in the dietary habits and physical activity during the COVID-19 pandemic in Korean adolescents. To test this hypothesis, the dietary habits and exercise pattern were analyzed in adolescents in before and during the COVID-19 pandemic periods. The first patient with COVID-19 was diagnosed on 19 February 2020. Thus, this study compared the 2019 group as a prepandemic population (surveyed from 3 June 2019 to 12 July 2019) with the 2020 group as a COVID-19 pandemic population (surveyed from 3 August 2020 to 13 November 2020 during the social distancing strategies that had been maintained in Korea without complete lockdowns).

2. Materials and Methods

2.1. Study Population and Data Collection

This cross-sectional study used data from the Korea Youth Risk Behavior Web-based Survey (KYRBWS) and covered the nation using statistical methods based on the designed sampling and adjusted weighted values. The KYRBWS obtained data from South Korean adolescents using stratified, two-stage (schools and classes) clustered sampling based on data from the Education Ministry. Sampling was weighted by statisticians, who performed poststratification analyses and considered the nonresponse rates and extreme values. Data from the 2019 and 2020 KYRBWS were analyzed. The details of the sampling methods are described on the KYRBWS website [11]. The KCDC collected the data, and Korean adolescents from 7th through 12th grade voluntarily and anonymously completed the self-administered questionnaire. The validity and reliability of the KYRBWS have been documented by other studies [12,13].

Of the 112,251 total participants (57,303 in 2019; 54,948 in 2020), the following were excluded from this study: participants without information on age ($n = 373$), height or weight ($n = 2596$), and sedentary time ($n = 3682$). Finally, 105,600 participants (53,461 in 2019; 52,139 in 2020), who were 12 through 18 years old, were included in this study (Figure 1).

2.2. Survey

2.2.1. Exposure

In each of the 2019 and 2020 surveys, adolescent participants were selected as stated above to represent the entire adolescent population in Korea. The participants from 2019 were not followed up with. The participants of 2020 were newly selected from the entire Korean adolescent population.

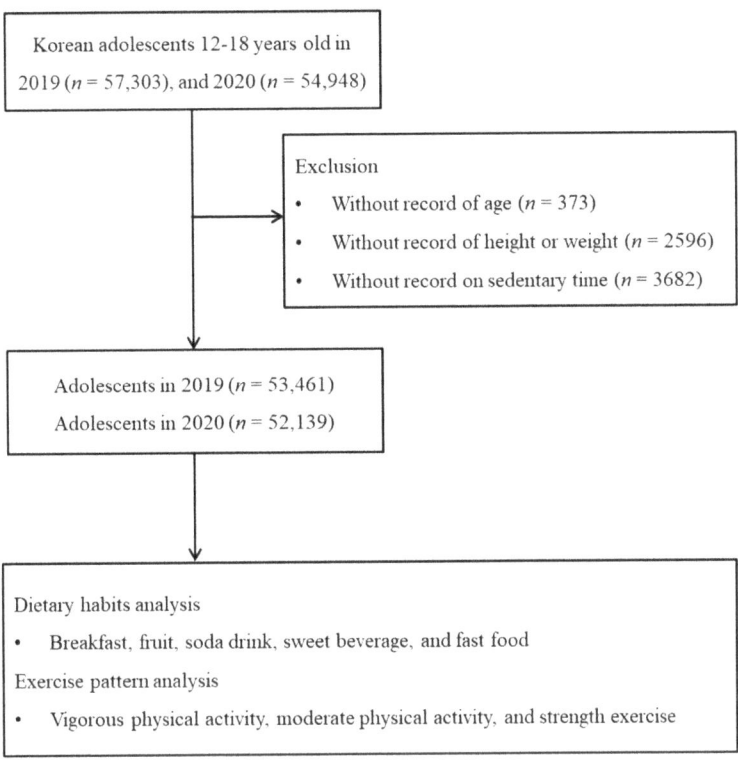

Figure 1. Flowchart of the major steps involved in the conduction of this study.

2.2.2. Outcomes

Dietary habits were surveyed by asking about the frequency of particular dietary habits in the last week. The frequencies of breakfast, fresh fruit, soda beverage (except for pure soda drinks and caffeinated drinks), sweet drinks, and fast food intake were assessed using questionnares. "How many days did you eat breakfast, fresh fruit, soda beverage (except for pure soda drinks and caffeinated drinks), sweet drink, and fast food in the recent 7 days, respectively?".

Regarding exercise pattern, aerobic exercise involving vigorous physical activity was assessed with the following question: "How many days did you exercise with high intense enough to sweat more than 20 min in the recent 7 days?". Aerobic exercise involving moderate physical activity was assessed by asking: "How many days did you exercise until heart rate increase or be short of breath more than 60 min in the recent 7 days?". Anaerobic strength exercises were assessed by asking: "How many days did you exercise to increase muscle power such as sit-up, lift weight, or chin-up bar in the recent 7 days?".

2.2.3. Covariates

Body mass index (BMI, kg/m^2) was calculated using height and weight. Mean sedentary time (h/day) and leisure time were calculated as 5/7 of the time on weekdays plus 2/7 of the time on weekends [14,15]. Sleep times were calculated as 5/7 of the time on weekdays plus 2/7 of the time on weekends [14,15]. The self-reported economic level was categorized into 3 levels: high, middle, and low. Subjective self-reported health status was categorized into 4 levels that ranged from very healthy to unhealthy. Subjective body shape image was categorized into 3 levels, including thin, normal, and obese. Smoking in the last 30 days was assessed and categorized into 3 levels: 0, 1–19, and ≥20 days [16]. Drinking alcohol in the last 30 days was categorized into 3 levels: 0, 1–2, and ≥3 days [16].

2.3. Statistical Analysis

The general characteristics of the data from the 2019 and 2020 surveys were compared using *t*-tests and chi-square tests.

The odds ratios (ORs) for particular dietary habits (breakfast, fresh fruit consumption, soda beverage, sweet drinks, and fast food intake) and exercise pattern (vigorous physical activity, moderate physical activity, and strength exercise) from 2020 compared to 2019 were calculated using multiple logistic regression analysis with complex sampling.

Crude and partially adjusted (age, BMI, sedentary time for study or leisure, sex, economic level, sleep time, subjective health status, subjective body shape image, and smoking and alcohol consumption) and fully adjusted (partial model plus dietary habits and exercise pattern) models were designed. Subgroups determined by sex and school level (middle school vs. high school) were analyzed.

Two-tailed analyses were conducted, and *p*-values lower than 0.05 were considered to indicate significance; 95% confidence intervals (Cis) were also calculated. The weights recommended by the KYRBWS were applied, and thus complex sampling was applied. The data were analyzed using SPSS ver. 25.0 (IBM, Armonk, NY, USA).

2.4. Ethics Approval

The ethics committee of Hallym University approved the use of these data. The study was exempted from the need for written informed consent by the Institutional Review Board (2019-09-005). All Korea Youth Risk Behavior Web-Based Survey (KYRBWS) data analyses were conducted in accordance with the guidelines and regulations provided by the Institutional Review Board of the Centers for Disease Control and Prevention of Korea (KCDC). The understanding, reliability, and validity of each question were investigated by the KCDC to verify the applicability of the surveys [11].

3. Results

The average sedentary time reported in the study was 6.6 (±3.7) hours/day in the 2019 group and 5.9 (±3.4) hours/day in the 2020 group ($p < 0.001$; Table 1). The average sedentary time for leisure was 3.3 (±2.3) hours/day in the 2019 group and 4.3 (±2.8) hours/day in the 2020 group ($p < 0.001$). Reporting subjective body shape image as obese was lower in the 2019 group than in the 2020 group (37.5% vs. 38.5%, $p < 0.001$). The frequencies of smoking and alcohol consumption were higher in the 2019 group than in the 2020 group ($p < 0.001$). The distributions of BMI, sleep time, and subjective health status were different between the 2019 group and the 2020 group (all $p < 0.001$).

In the fully adjusted model, the 2020 group demonstrated lower odds of eating fruit, fast food, drinking soda, and drinking sweet drinks than the 2019 group (all $p < 0.001$; Table 2). On the other hand, the frequency of breakfast was lower in the 2019 group than in the 2020 group ($p < 0.001$). In middle school students, the frequencies of eating fruit, drinking soda, drinking sweet drinks, and eating fast food were lower in the 2020 group than in the 2019 group (all $p < 0.001$; Table S1). In high school students, the frequencies of eating fruit, drinking soda, and drinking sweet drinks were lower in the 2020 group than in the 2019 group (all $p < 0.001$, Table S2). When analyzed by sex, men showed lower frequencies of drinking soda and sweet drinks in the 2020 group than in the 2019 group (all $p < 0.001$; Table S3). In women, the frequencies of eating fruit, drinking sweet drinks, and eating fast food were lower in the 2020 group than in the 2019 group (all $p < 0.05$, Table S4).

Table 1. General Characteristics of Participants.

General Characteristics		2019	2020	p-Value
Total Number, n (%)		53,461 (100.0)	52,139 (100.0)	
Age (years, mean (SD))		15.0 (1.8)	15.1 (1.8)	<0.001 *
BMI (kg/m², mean (SD))		21.3 (3.6)	21.5 (3.7)	<0.001 *
Sedentary time for study (hour/day, mean (SD))		6.6 (3.7)	5.9 (3.4)	<0.001 *
Sedentary time for leisure (hour/day, mean (SD))		3.3 (2.3)	4.3 (2.8)	<0.001 *
Sex, n (%)				0.726
	Male	27,776 (52.0)	27,033 (51.8)	
	Female	25,685 (48.0)	25,106 (48.2)	
Economic level, n (%*)				0.382
	High	20,979 (39.2)	20,367 (39.1)	
	Middle	25,767 (48.2)	25,076 (48.1)	
	Low	6715 (12.6)	6696 (12.8)	
Sleep time, n (%*)				<0.001 †
	Unknown or missing	5018 (9.4)	7923 (15.2)	
	<6 h	12,370 (23.1)	11,911 (22.8)	
	6 h to <7 h	12,155 (22.7)	11,440 (21.9)	
	7 h to <8 h	11,548 (21.6)	10,375 (19.9)	
	≥8 h	12,370 (23.1)	10,490 (20.1)	
Subjective health status, n (%*)				0.007 †
	Very healthy	14,451 (27.0)	14,447 (27.7)	
	Healthy	23,383 (43.7)	22,276 (42.7)	
	Normal	11,848 (22.2)	11,634 (22.3)	
	Unhealthy	3779 (7.1)	3782 (7.3)	
Subjective body shape image, n (%*)				<0.001 †
	Thin	13,768 (25.8)	12,820 (24.6)	
	Normal	19,662 (36.8)	19,220 (36.9)	
	Obese	20,031 (37.5)	20,099 (38.5)	
Smoking in the recent 30 days, n (%*)				<0.001 †
	0 day	50,205 (93.9)	49,886 (95.7)	
	1–19 days	1473 (2.8)	871 (1.7)	
	≥20 days	1783 (3.3)	1382 (2.7)	
Drinking alcohol in the recent 30 days, n (%*)				<0.001 †
	0 day	45,879 (85.8)	46,679 (89.5)	
	1–2 days	4525 (8.5)	3300 (6.3)	
	≥3 days	3057 (5.7)	2160 (4.1)	

* Independent t-test, Significance at $p < 0.05$. † Chi-square test, Significance at $p < 0.05$.

Regarding exercise pattern, the frequencies of vigorous and moderate aerobic exercise were lower in the 2020 group than in the 2019 group (all $p < 0.001$; Table 3). The 2020 group showed lower odds regarding the frequency of vigorous and moderate aerobic exercise than the 2019 group (all $p < 0.001$). In contrast, the frequency of anaerobic exercise was higher in the 2020 group than in the 2019 group ($p < 0.001$). The 2020 group showed higher odds regarding the frequency of anaerobic exercise than the 2019 group ($p < 0.001$). Middle school students showed a lower frequency of vigorous aerobic exercise and a higher frequency of anaerobic exercise in the 2020 group than in the 2019 group (all $p < 0.001$; Table S1). High school students showed lower frequencies of vigorous and moderate aerobic exercise and a higher frequency of anaerobic exercise in the 2020 group than in the 2019 group (all $p < 0.001$; Table S2). When analyzed by sex, both men and women showed a lower frequency of vigorous aerobic exercise and a higher frequency of anaerobic exercise in the 2020 group than in the 2019 group (all $p < 0.001$; Tables S3 and S4).

Table 2. Odd ratios of dietary habits in 2020 compared to 2019 in total participants.

Dietary Habit		Number (%)		OR (95% CI)					
		2019	2020	Crude	p-Value	Partial †	p-Value	Full ‡	p-Value
Breakfast					<0.001 *		0.008 *		<0.001 *
	0–1 time/week	14,455 (27.0)	14,786 (28.4)	1.00 (Ref)		1.00 (Ref)		1.00 (Ref)	
	2–4 times/week	12,471 (23.3)	12,862 (24.7)	1.02 (0.98–1.05)		1.05 (1.01–1.09)		1.07 (1.03–1.11)	
	≥5 times/week	26,535 (49.6)	24,491 (47.0)	0.91 (0.87–0.95)		1.00 (0.96–1.03)		1.01 (0.97–1.05)	
Fruit					<0.001 *		<0.001 *		<0.001 *
	0–2 times/week	22,064 (41.3)	23,334 (44.8)	1.00 (Ref)		1.00 (Ref)		1.00 (Ref)	
	3–4 times/week	14,806 (27.7)	13,922 (26.7)	0.90 (0.87–0.93)		0.93 (0.90–0.97)		0.95 (0.92–0.99)	
	≥5 times/week	16,591 (31.0)	14,883 (28.5)	0.86 (0.82–0.89)		0.91 (0.88–0.95)		0.93 (0.89–0.96)	
Soda drink					<0.001 *		<0.001 *		<0.001 *
	0–2 times/week	33,928 (63.5)	33,667 (64.6)	1.00 (Ref)		1.00 (Ref)		1.00 (Ref)	
	3–4 times/week	12,533 (23.4)	11,482 (22.0)	0.92 (0.88–0.96)		0.87 (0.84–0.90)		0.92 (0.88–0.95)	
	≥5 times/week	7000 (13.1)	6990 (13.4)	0.99 (0.94–1.04)		0.89 (0.85–0.93)		0.94 (0.90–0.99)	
Sweet drinks					<0.001 *		<0.001 *		<0.001 *
	0–2 times/week	26,803 (50.1)	28,229 (54.1)	1.00 (Ref)		1.00 (Ref)		1.00 (Ref)	
	3–4 times/week	15,607 (29.2)	13,350 (25.6)	0.80 (0.77–0.82)		0.79 (0.76–0.81)		0.81 (0.78–0.84)	
	≥5 times/week	11,051 (20.7)	10,560 (20.3)	0.90 (0.86–0.93)		0.85 (0.82–0.89)		0.90 (0.86–0.94)	
Fast food					0.191		<0.001 *		0.001 *
	0–2 times/week	40,236 (75.3)	39,263 (75.3)	1.00 (Ref)		1.00 (Ref)		1.00 (Ref)	
	3–4 times/week	10,487 (19.6)	10,316 (19.8)	1.01 (0.98–1.05)		0.97 (0.93–1.00)		1.02 (0.98–1.05)	
	≥5 times/week	2738 (5.1)	2560 (4.9)	0.96 (0.90–1.02)		0.96 (0.89–0.89)		0.90 (0.85–0.96)	

* Multiple logistic regression analysis with complex sampling, Significance at p < 0.05; † Adjusted for age, BMI, sedentary time for study or leisure, sex, economic level, sleep time, subjective health status, subjective body shape image, smoking, and drinking alcohol histories. ‡ Adjusted for partial model plus dietary habit and exercise pattern.

Table 3. Odd ratios of exercise pattern in 2020 compared to 2019 in total participants.

Physical Activity (PA)		Number (%)		OR (95% CI)					
		2019	2020	Crude	p-Value	Partial †	p-Value	Full ‡	p-Value
Vigorous PA					<0.001 *		<0.001 *		<0.001 *
	0 time/week	16,819 (31.5)	19,859 (38.1)	1.00 (Ref)		1.00 (Ref)		1.00 (Ref)	
	1–2 times/week	19,123 (35.8)	17,411 (33.4)	0.76 (0.73–0.81)		0.78 (0.74–0.81)		0.74 (0.71–0.77)	
	≥3 times/week	17,519 (32.8)	14,869 (28.5)	0.71 (0.67–0.76)		0.71 (0.68–0.75)		0.60 (0.57–0.63)	
Moderate PA					<0.001 *		<0.001 *		0.719
	0 time/week	18,647 (34.9)	20,008 (38.4)	1.00 (Ref)		1.00 (Ref)		1.00 (Ref)	
	1–2 times/week	16,210 (30.3)	15,317 (29.4)	0.88 (0.84–0.92)		0.91 (0.87–0.94)		0.99 (0.95–1.02)	
	≥3 times/week	18,604 (34.8)	16,814 (32.2)	0.84 (0.79–0.89)		0.87 (0.83–0.91)		0.99 (0.96–1.04)	
Strength Exercise					<0.001 *		<0.001 *		<0.001 *
	0 time/week	27,721 (51.9)	26,074 (50.0)	1.00 (Ref)		1.00 (Ref)		1.00 (Ref)	
	1–2 times/week	13,912 (26.0)	13,124 (25.2)	1.00 (0.95–1.05)		1.05 (1.01–1.10)		1.19 (1.14–1.24)	
	≥3 times/week	11,828 (22.1)	12,941 (24.8)	1.15 (1.07–1.23)		1.23 (1.17–1.28)		1.54 (1.46–1.62)	

* Multiple logistic regression analysis with complex sampling, Significance at p < 0.05. † Adjusted for age, BMI, sedentary time for study or leisure, sex, economic level, sleep time, subjective health status, subjective body shape image, smoking, and drinking alcohol histories. ‡ Adjusted for partial model plus dietary habit and physical activities.

4. Discussion

The consumption of fast food, fruit, and drinks such as soda was lower, while the consumption of breakfast was higher during the COVID-19 crisis than in the prepandemic era. The pattern of exercise showed bidirectional changes, with lower aerobic exercise and higher anaerobic exercise during the COVID-19 pandemic when compared with the prepandemic period in this cohort of Korean adolescents. This study improved previous findings on the impact of the COVID-19 pandemic on dietary habits and exercise pattern by concurrently analyzing both the dietary habits and exercise pattern in an adolescent population. In addition, age and sex were subgrouped, and the impact of the COVID-19 pandemic on diet and exercise pattern was analyzed in each subgroup.

The COVID-19 pandemic was associated with decreased intakes of fast food, fruit, soda, and sweet drinks in this cohort of Koreran adolescents. On the other hand, the frequency of breakfast was increased during the COVID-19 pandemic. The decreased consumption of soda, sweet drinks, and fast food could be explained by less frequent eating out due to home confinement. The consumption of fast food and soda intake have mostly been associated with eating out in Korean adolescents [17]. In addition, health-seeking behavior could have decreased the consumption of unhealthy food during the COVID-19 pandemic in this study. The COVID-19 pandemic could have encouraged adolescents to address health-related issues because they were repeatedly exposed to health campaigns and education regarding quarantine maneuvers from school and the mass media. Moreover, the increased time with family and frequency of home cooking could have provided an opportunity for adolescents to discuss healthy behavior with their parents and to alter their unhealthy dietary habits [18,19]. The traditional Korean diet at home includes cooked rice and a number of banchan, such as kimchi. Thus, Koreans could consume sufficient nutrients from vegetables, legumes, and fish, with a low intake of red meat [20]. Frequently cooking dinner was related to a higher Healthy Eating Index-2015 in the US (≥ 7 times/week: +3.57 points, $p < 0.001$) [19]. During the COVID-19 crisis, a cross-sectional survey in Italy demonstrated that approximately 3.3% of respondents quit smoking and 38.3% of respondents increased physical activities, such as bodyweight training [4]. The lockdown and other instances of quarantine could have resulted in difficulties acquiring food, especially fresh food, such as fruit, in some adolescents without caregivers. Indeed, it was reported that over 18% of adults lost weight during the COVID-19 lockdown (-2.9 ± 1.5 kg) [3]. In our cohort, although the BMI was slightly higher in the COVID-19 pandemic group than in the prepandemic group, it was not high enough to have a clinical impact. On the other hand, the increasd time to eat due to the lockdown of schools could have resulted in increasing breakfast consumption, which was observed in this study. Because the restriction of outdoor activities can increase the time available to eat, the increase in breakfast consumption could have been relative to the irregular meal time during school hours.

Anaerobic exercise was higher in the COVID-19 pandemic group than in the prepandemic group in this study. In contrast, vigorous aerobic exercise was lower in the COVID-19 pandemic group than in the prepandemic group. A previous survey estimated 1.3-fold and 1.2-fold higher rates of moderate-to-vigorous physical activity in male and middle-aged populations during the COVID-19 pandemic [21]. The increase in anaerobic exercise could have been a compensation for the decrease in aerobic exercise during the COVID-19 pandemic that was found in the study. A cross-sectional study reported that children spent less time in extracurricular sports (23.5%), and 94.5% of children watched screens for 1.5 (0.5–3.0) hours/day [22]. Quarantine and social distancing maneuvers might have limited outdoor activities [23]. The restrictions on physical activities during the COVID-19 pandemic may have been caused by both individual and community aspects [24,25]. Physical restrictions on outdoor activities may have reduced individuals' aerobic exercise. In addition, the social distancing policy included restrictions on group sports activities, such as football leagues, swimming, and baseball games, all of which are forms of aerobic exercise. On the other hand, the increased time spent at home may have encouraged people to spend time at home training. Moreover, awareness of health-related issues via health promotion campaigns encouraged people to engage in home-based exercises [23,26]. Indeed, a surveillance in Thailand reported a 1.5-fold higher rate of moderate-to-vigorous physical activity in adults who were exposed to fit-from-home campaigns [21]. Furthermore, physical activity was reported to be greatly influenced by personal factors in children, while sedentary behavior was influenced by environmental factors [27]. Thus, physical activity was less influenced by the COVID-19 pandemic, but the geographic area of activity decreased.

The present cohort was composed of a large, nationwide, representative population of Korean adolescents. The validation and regulation of the data were managed by KCDC. Many surveyed items of sedentary time for study, sedentary time for leisure, economic level, sleep time, subjective health status, subjective body shape image, smoking, alcohol consumption, and anthropometric index of BMI were included for analyses. We included these variables as they might have been able to affect diet and exercise pattern. However, because this study was based on the survey, recall bias may have existed. In addition, the amount of food consumption could not be evaluated. The detailed types of physical exercise could not be identified. Furthermore, the study participants could not be longitudinally followed up with; instead, new participants were enrolled in each year. Although numerous factors were surveyed and adjusted for, influential variables may have been unmeasured, such as comorbidities that restrict dietary consumption or exercise pattern. Lastly, because this study included a Korean population, ethnic or regional differences could be present regarding dietary habits or exercise pattern of other ethnic groups [28].

5. Conclusions

There were changes in both the dietary habits and pattern of exercise between the pre- and during COVID-19 pandemic periods in this cohort of Korean adolescents. The consumption of fruit, fast food, soda, and sweet drinks was lower, while the consumption of breakfast was higher during the COVID-19 pandemic than in the prepandemic period. The frequencies of vigorous and moderate aerobic exercise were lower, while the frequency of anaerobic exercise was higher during the COVID-19 pandemic than in the prepandemic period.

Supplementary Materials: The following are available online at https://www.mdpi.com/article/10.3390/nu13103314/s1, Table S1. Odd ratios of dietary habit or exercise pattern in 2020 compared to 2019 in middle school student. Table S2. Odd ratios of dietary habit or exercise pattern in 2020 compared to 2019 in high school student. Table S3. Odd ratios of dietary habit or exercise pattern in 2020 compared to 2019 in men. Table S4. Odd ratios of dietary habit or physical activities in 2020 compared to 2019 in women.

Author Contributions: H.G.C. designed the study; D.M.Y., C.M. and H.G.C. analyzed the data; S.Y.K. and H.G.C. drafted and revised the paper; and H.G.C. drew the figures. All authors have read and agreed to the published version of the manuscript.

Funding: This work was supported in part by research grants (NRF-2018-R1D1A1A02085328 and 2021-R1C1C100498611) from the National Research Foundation (NRF) of Korea. The APC was funded by NRF-2018-R1D1A1A02085328.

Institutional Review Board Statement: The ethics committee of Hallym University (2020-07-022) permitted this study following the guidelines and regulations.

Informed Consent Statement: Written informed consent was waived by the Institutional Review Board.

Data Availability Statement: Releasing of the data by the researcher is not legally permitted. All data are available from the database of the Korea Center for Disease Control and Prevention. The Korea Center for Disease Control and Prevention allows data access, at a particular cost, for any researcher who promises to follow the research ethics. The data of this article can be downloaded from the website after agreeing to follow the research ethics.

Conflicts of Interest: The authors declare no conflict of interest.

References

1. Park, J.H.; Jang, W.; Kim, S.-W.; Lee, J.; Lim, Y.-S.; Cho, C.-G.; Park, S.-W.; Kim, B.H. The Clinical Manifestations and Chest Computed Tomography Findings of Coronavirus Disease 2019 (COVID-19) Patients in China: A Proportion Meta-Analysis. *Clin. Exp. Otorhinolaryngol.* **2020**, *13*, 95–105. [CrossRef] [PubMed]
2. Ferrante, G.; Camussi, E.; Piccinelli, C.; Senore, C.; Armaroli, P.; Ortale, A.; Garena, F.; Giordano, L. Did social isolation during the SARS-CoV-2 epidemic have an impact on the lifestyles of citizens? *Epidemiol. Prev.* **2020**, *44* (Suppl. 2), 353–362. [PubMed]
3. Sidor, A.; Rzymski, P. Dietary Choices and Habits during COVID-19 Lockdown: Experience from Poland. *Nutrients* **2020**, *12*, 1657. [CrossRef] [PubMed]
4. Di Renzo, L.; Gualtieri, P.; Pivari, F.; Soldati, L.; Attinà, A.; Cinelli, G.; Leggeri, C.; Caparello, G.; Barrea, L.; Scerbo, F.; et al. Eating habits and lifestyle changes during COVID-19 lockdown: An Italian survey. *J. Transl. Med.* **2020**, *18*, 229. [CrossRef] [PubMed]
5. Izzo, L.; Santonastaso, A.; Cotticelli, G.; Federico, A.; Pacifico, S.; Castaldo, L.; Colao, A.; Ritieni, A. An Italian Survey on Dietary Habits and Changes during the COVID-19 Lockdown. *Nutrients* **2021**, *13*, 1197. [CrossRef]
6. Ammar, A.; Brach, M.; Trabelsi, K.; Chtourou, H.; Boukhris, O.; Masmoudi, L.; Bouaziz, B.; Bentlage, E.; How, D.; Ahmed, M.; et al. Effects of COVID-19 Home Confinement on Eating Behaviour and Physical Activity: Results of the ECLB-COVID19 International Online Survey. *Nutrients* **2020**, *12*, 1583. [CrossRef]
7. Tulchin-Francis, K.; Stevens, W.; Gu, X.; Zhang, T.; Roberts, H.; Keller, J.; Dempsey, D.; Borchard, J.; Jeans, K.; VanPelt, J. The impact of the coronavirus disease 2019 pandemic on physical activity in U.S. children. *J. Sport Health Sci.* **2021**, *10*, 323–332. [CrossRef] [PubMed]

8. A Moore, S.; Faulkner, G.; Rhodes, R.E.; Brussoni, M.; Chulak-Bozzer, T.; Ferguson, L.J.; Mitra, R.; O'Reilly, N.; Spence, J.C.; Vanderloo, L.M.; et al. Impact of the COVID-19 virus outbreak on movement and play behaviours of Canadian children and youth: A national survey. *Int. J. Behav. Nutr. Phys. Act.* **2020**, *17*, 1–11. [CrossRef] [PubMed]
9. Dunton, G.F.; Do, B.; Wang, S.D. Early effects of the COVID-19 pandemic on physical activity and sedentary behavior in children living in the U.S. *BMC Public Health* **2020**, *20*, 1–13. [CrossRef] [PubMed]
10. Martinez-Ferran, M.; De La Guía-Galipienso, F.; Sanchis-Gomar, F.; Pareja-Galeano, H. Metabolic Impacts of Confinement during the COVID-19 Pandemic Due to Modified Diet and Physical Activity Habits. *Nutrients* **2020**, *12*, 1549. [CrossRef]
11. Kim, Y.; Choi, S.; Chun, C.; Park, S.; Khang, Y.-H.; Oh, K. Data Resource Profile: The Korea Youth Risk Behavior Web-based Survey (KYRBS). *Int. J. Epidemiol.* **2016**, *45*, 1076e. [CrossRef]
12. Bae, J.; Joung, H.; Kim, J.-Y.; Kwon, K.N.; Kim, Y.; Park, S.-W. Validity of Self-Reported Height, Weight, and Body Mass Index of the Korea Youth Risk Behavior Web-Based Survey Questionnaire. *J. Prev. Med. Public Health* **2010**, *43*, 396–402. [CrossRef] [PubMed]
13. Bae, J.; Joung, H.; Kim, J.-Y.; Kwon, K.N.; Kim, Y.T.; Park, S.-W. Test-Retest Reliability of a Questionnaire for the Korea Youth Risk Behavior Web-Based Survey. *J. Prev. Med. Public Health* **2010**, *43*, 403–410. [CrossRef] [PubMed]
14. Min, C.; Kim, H.-J.; Park, I.-S.; Park, B.; Kim, J.-H.; Sim, S.; Choi, H.G. The association between sleep duration, sleep quality, and food consumption in adolescents: A cross-sectional study using the Korea Youth Risk Behavior Web-based Survey. *BMJ Open* **2018**, *8*, e022848. [CrossRef] [PubMed]
15. Kim, S.Y.; Kim, M.-S.; Park, B.; Kim, J.-H.; Choi, H.G. Lack of sleep is associated with internet use for leisure. *PLoS ONE* **2018**, *13*, e0191713. [CrossRef]
16. Kim, S.Y.; Sim, S.; Choi, H.G. Active, passive, and electronic cigarette smoking is associated with asthma in adolescents. *Sci. Rep.* **2017**, *7*, 1–8.
17. Yoon, J.-Y.; Lyu, E.-S.; Lee, K.-A. Korean adolescents' perceptions of nutrition and health towards fast foods in Busan area. *Nutr. Res. Pr.* **2008**, *2*, 171–177. [CrossRef]
18. Fulkerson, J.A.; Friend, S.; Horning, M.; Flattum, C.; Draxten, M.; Neumark-Sztainer, D.; Gurvich, O.; Garwick, A.; Story, M.; Kubik, M.Y. Family Home Food Environment and Nutrition-Related Parent and Child Personal and Behavioral Outcomes of the Healthy Home Offerings via the Mealtime Environment (HOME) Plus Program: A Randomized Controlled Trial. *J. Acad. Nutr. Diet.* **2018**, *118*, 240–251. [CrossRef]
19. A Wolfson, J.; Leung, C.W.; Richardson, C.R. More frequent cooking at home is associated with higher Healthy Eating Index-2015 score. *Public Health Nutr.* **2020**, *23*, 2384–2394. [CrossRef]
20. Soon Hee Kim, M.S.; Lee, M.S.; SoonPark, Y.; Lee, H.J.; Kang, S.; Lee, H.S.; Lee, K.; JeongYang, H.; Kim, M.J.; Lee, Y.; et al. Korean diet: Characteristics and historical background. *J. Ethn. Foods* **2016**, *3*, 26–31.
21. Katewongsa, P.; Widyastari, D.A.; Saonuam, P.; Haemathulin, N.; Wongsingha, N. The effects of the COVID-19 pandemic on the physical activity of the Thai population: Evidence from Thailand's Surveillance on Physical Activity 2020. *J. Sport Health Sci.* **2021**, *10*, 341–348. [CrossRef] [PubMed]
22. Chen, B.; Waters, C.N.; Compier, T.; Uijtdewilligen, L.; A Petrunoff, N.; Lim, Y.W.; van Dam, R.; Müller-Riemenschneider, F. Understanding physical activity and sedentary behaviour among preschool-aged children in Singapore: A mixed-methods approach. *BMJ Open* **2020**, *10*, e030606. [CrossRef] [PubMed]
23. Vancini, R.L.; Andrade, M.S.; Viana, R.B.; Nikolaidis, P.T.; Knechtle, B.; Campanharo, C.R.; de Almeida, A.A.; Gentil, P.; de Lira, C.A. Physical exercise and COVID-19 pandemic in PubMed: Two-months of dynamics and one-year of original scientific production. *Sports Med. Health Sci.* **2021**, *3*, 80–92. [CrossRef] [PubMed]
24. Yeo, T.J. Sport and exercise during and beyond the COVID-19 pandemic. *Eur. J. Prev. Cardiol.* **2020**, *27*, 1239–1241. [CrossRef] [PubMed]
25. Bhatia, R.T.; Marwaha, S.; Malhotra, A.; Iqbal, Z.; Hughes, C.; Börjesson, M.; Niebauer, J.; Pelliccia, A.; Schmied, C.; Serratosa, L.; et al. Exercise in the Severe Acute Respiratory Syndrome Coronavirus-2 (SARS-CoV-2) era: A Question and Answer session with the experts Endorsed by the section of Sports Cardiology & Exercise of the European Association of Preventive Cardiology (EAPC). *Eur. J. Prev. Cardiol.* **2020**, *27*, 1242–1251. [CrossRef]
26. Caputo, E.L.; Reichert, F.F. Studies of Physical Activity and COVID-19 During the Pandemic: A Scoping Review. *J. Phys. Act. Health* **2020**, *17*, 1275–1284. [CrossRef] [PubMed]
27. Schmutz, E.A.; Leeger-Aschmann, C.S.; Radtke, T.; Muff, S.; Kakebeeke, T.H.; Zysset, A.E.; Messerli-Bürgy, N.; Stülb, K.; Arhab, A.; Meyer, A.H.; et al. Correlates of preschool children's objectively measured physical activity and sedentary behavior: A cross-sectional analysis of the SPLASHY study. *Int. J. Behav. Nutr. Phys. Act.* **2017**, *14*, 1–13. [CrossRef] [PubMed]
28. Kim, S.Y.; Kim, D.W. Does the Clinical Spectrum of Coronavirus Disease 2019 (COVID-19) Show Regional Differences? *Clin. Exp. Otorhinolaryngol.* **2020**, *13*, 83–84. [CrossRef] [PubMed]

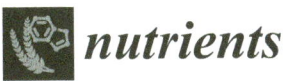

Article

Benefits of Adding an Aquatic Resistance Interval Training to a Nutritional Education on Body Composition, Body Image Perception and Adherence to the Mediterranean Diet in Older Women

Alejandro Martínez-Rodríguez [1,2,*], Bernardo J. Cuestas-Calero [3], María Martínez-Olcina [1] and Pablo Jorge Marcos-Pardo [4,5]

1. Department of Analytical Chemistry, Nutrition and Food Science, Faculty of Sciences, University of Alicante, 03690 Alicante, Spain; maria.martinezolcina@ua.es
2. Alicante Institute for Health and Biomedical Research (ISABIAL Foundation), 03010 Alicante, Spain
3. Faculty of Sport, San Antonio Catholic University of Murcia, 30107 Murcia, Spain; bjcuestas@alu.ucam.edu
4. Department of Education, Faculty of Education Sciences, University of Almería, 04120 Almería, Spain; pjmarcos@ual.es
5. SPORT Research Group (CTS-1024), CERNEP Research Center, University of Almería, 04120 Almería, Spain
* Correspondence: amartinezrodriguez@ua.es

Abstract: The human population is increasing due to lengthening life expectancy, but the quality of life and health of people is moving in the opposite direction. The purpose of this study is to evaluate how aquatic resistance interval training can influence body composition, body image perception and adherence to the Mediterranean diet (MD) in older women participants in a nutrition education program and to study the relation between these variables. Thirty-four participants aged 69 ± 4 years were randomly assigned into two groups: experimental (aquatic resistance interval training plus nutritional intervention) and control (nutritional intervention). The intervention consisted of resistance training in an aquatic environment carried out for 14 weeks (three sessions per week; 60 min each). Body composition, body image perception and adherence to MD diet were evaluated at baseline and 14 weeks. No significant differences were found between groups regarding body image perception and adherence to the MD. There was a significant increase in muscle mass (kg) ($p < 0.001$) and a significant decrease in fat mass (kg) ($p < 0.001$) in the intervention group when compared to the control group. The addition of aquatic resistance interval training to a nutritional intervention was not sufficient to change body image perception and adherence to MD but produced improvement in body composition (through an increase in muscle mass and decrease on fat mass) in older women.

Keywords: geriatric rehabilitation; aging; nutrition education; aquatic resistance training

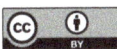

1. Introduction

Aging is characterized by a progressive decline in muscle strength, which potentially impacts mobility and translates into frailty and functional disability, especially in the lower extremities [1].

Around the age of 50 years, women reach menopause. Menopause is characterized by hormonal changes that include a decline in estrogen level, which has an important role in bone remodeling [2], cardiovascular disease and mortality [3] in females. Some researchers explain that the absence of estrogen may be a relevant triggering factor for obesity [4]. Estrogen deficiency enhances metabolic dysfunction, predisposing the human body to diabetes mellitus type 2, metabolic syndrome and cardiovascular disease [4].

The perimenopausal phase—the time in which a woman transitions to menopause— centers around shifts to the hormonal system, which are associated with a weight gain, an increase in fat mass [5] and a reallocation of body fat from the lower body (i.e., hips)

to the upper body (i.e., waist and torso) [6]. Given that these shifts are in direct contrast to Western society's young, thin, beauty standard, menopause could be an especially critical window of vulnerability for the development or exacerbation of disordered eating behaviors and attitudes, highlighting body shape image disorders.

Furthermore, there is a direct relation between loss of bone mass and microarchitectural deterioration of bone tissue, and a decrease in bone strength added to subsequently increased fracture risk, which eventually leads to conditions clinically known as osteopenia and osteoporosis [7], which are major health problems. A mechanical stimulus is then needed in order to maintain bone health.

Many parts of the brain that are related to aging may also be sensitive to shifts in hormone levels: for example, gonadal changes, which usually occur around mid-life, are thought to be associated with changes in cognitive function [8], and mood symptoms are well known to be habitual during the menopause transition period [9,10]. Mood symptoms such as depression and anxiety, along with hot flushes and night sweats, may be affiliated with a negative experience of menopause [8]. The experience of menopause is influenced by the cultural and social context. Women who live with a chronic mental health state can experience additional or increased symptoms throughout menopause [8].

In addition, it is important to consider the eating habits of this population. Some research suggests that postmenopausal women present a greater eating disinhibition and dietary restraint compared to premenopausal women [11]. It has been suggested that higher adherence to a healthy dietary pattern, such as the Mediterranean diet (MD), is contrarily associated with being overweight/obese in perimenopausal and postmenopausal women. High adherence to the Mediterranean dietary pattern and a body mass index (BMI) of 25 kg/m^2 or lower might make a women's quality of life better in the postmenopausal phase [12].

The traditional Mediterranean dietary pattern is distinguished by abundant consumption olive oil (the major source of fat), plant foods (vegetables, fruits, cereals and nuts), fresh fruit as a daily dessert, low to moderate intake of dairy products (cheese and yogurt), low intake of red meat, low to moderate intake of fish and poultry and regular moderate intake of wine, generally consumed during meals.

Regular physical activity (PA) is considered an important element of lifestyle. Numerous epidemiological studies have proved that it has a positive influence on reducing the incidence of many diseases and mortality [13–15]. Regular PA also helps to preserve functional abilities, which play a vital role in motor resourcefulness and self-reliance in everyday life, contributing to a better quality of life and positive self-esteem [16]. In older adults, the best prevention for the accelerated decline in muscle strength and mass is performing resistance training [1], which has been a fundamental part of the American College of Sports Medicine (ACSM) exercise prescription guidelines for older adults since 1998 [17,18]. Safely applied, resistance training has been shown to improve lower and upper body muscle strength in the older adult population, including those suffering from comorbidities such as stroke, postmortem, coronary bypass, hypertension and obesity [1].

Exercise in water, often referred to as water-based exercise, presents a lower risk of traumatic fracture; moreover, the joints are exposed to less stress and impact (reduced loading due to buoyancy) compared to land-based exercise such as running, strength training and resistance training [7]. Furthermore, water-based exercise has been highly recommended for older people, especially those with disability, due to the reduced pain and increased security it can provide, as well as the additional benefits for neuromuscular/functional fitness and cardiometabolic health.

Therefore, menopause marks a period in a woman's life where it is relevant to introduce preventive strategies to reduce the risk of suffering cardiovascular disease, bone health and mortality [2,3].

The main objective of the current study was to evaluate the effect of the addition of aquatic resistance interval training to a nutritional intervention on body composition, body image perception and adherence to MD in older women.

2. Materials and Methods

2.1. Study Design

This study was a randomized clinical trial in which the participants were allocated to an experimental group (aquatic resistance interval training) plus nutritional intervention and a control group (nutritional intervention) in order to determine the effectiveness of aquatic resistance interval training on the variables of body composition, body shape and adherence to the MD. The subjects were assigned electronically in a random way by block design into two arms (control and experimental) using online computer software as stated by published recommendations [19]. This procedure was performed by a researcher who was not involved in the interventions or evaluations of this study.

2.2. Participants

This study included only female older adults. Forty-five women over the age of 65 years from Alicante, Spain, participated. The inclusion criteria were: to be over 65 years old; not to have undergone surgery in the last year; not to present musculoskeletal, neurological or orthopedic diseases that could affect the ability to perform the tests; to be able to walk independently without orthopedic assistance; and not to have previously performed any of the tests included in the study.

Five participants did not meet the inclusion criteria: one declined to participate, and the other four were not able to participate because of musculoskeletal mobility problems, leaving 40 participants who were randomly allocated to an aquatic resistance-training group and a control group. Over the follow-up period, six participants withdrew from the trial, three from each group. Consequently, just 34 women were involved in the analysis. Both groups presented no differences in the demographic variables, and all withdrawals were because of personal reasons (Figure 1).

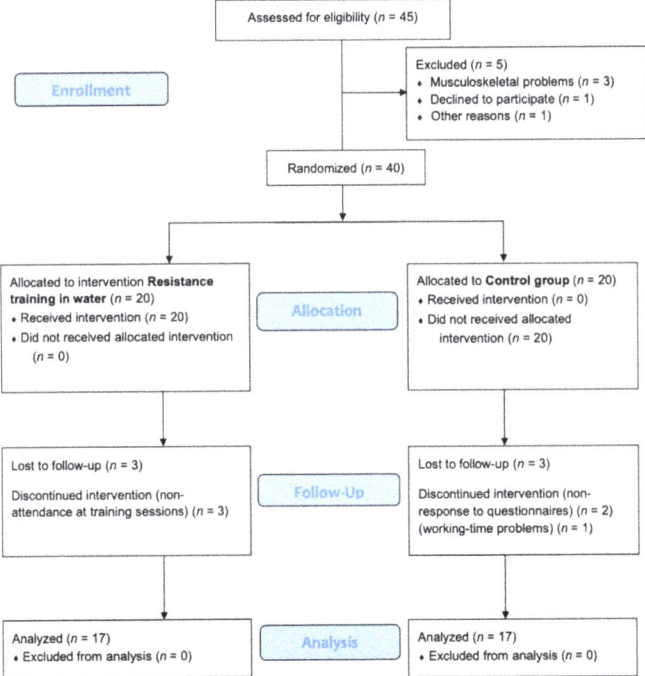

Figure 1. Consort 2010 flow diagram.

2.3. Declarations: Ethical Approval, Consent to Participate and Consent for Publication

The present study was carried out in agreement with the standards of the Helsinki Declaration. The Human Research Ethics Committee of the Catholic University of Murcia (Spain) gave approval to run a randomized trial (CE061920) and prior to the experiment all study participants provided written consent. Furthermore, researchers kept the participants' personal data confidential by codifying all personal information.

2.4. Study Intervention

Evaluation methods regarding body composition, body image perception and adherence to a Mediterranean diet were administered to both groups at baseline and after intervention (14 weeks).

2.4.1. Aquatic Resistance Interval Training

The intervention consisted of a training programme in an aquatic environment. Supervised resistance training was performed for 14 weeks. The sessions were conducted in a heated pool three times a week for 60 min per session. The sessions began with a 15 min warm-up consisting of aerobic and resistance exercises (10 min) and stretching (5 min) of all the muscle groups involved, followed by 30 min of comprehensive interval resistance training involving four 5 min sessions with a 2 min rest between each session.

In each session, the same exercises (pectoral/back, hip flexor/extensor, biceps/triceps, knee flexor/extensor, shoulder and core) were performed for 1 min consecutively, with intervals of 30, 20 and 10 s [20] and at low, moderate and high perceived intensity, respectively [21]. According to the perceived exertion scale, when participants needed to increase the intensity of the upper hemisphere exercises, they put on resistance gloves or resistance dumbbells, whereas for the lower-hemisphere exercises, they put on resistance anklets.

Finally, in the last 10–15 min, stretching (5 min) and relaxation exercises (10 min) were performed. In all the intervention sessions, the perception of effort was controlled using the Borg scale [22].

2.4.2. Nutritional Education

Additionally, all participants received the same nutritional education, based on the MD divided into four theoretical and practical workshops of 60 min for 14 weeks in order to provide updated information about the benefits of following an adequate food pattern. Trained dietitians conducted the sessions. The topics covered in the sessions were: (1) food and nutrition, MD pyramid and a modern lifestyle—daily, weekly and occasional dietary guidelines to achieve a healthy and balanced diet; (2) health and gastronomy—preparation of healthy menus that include components of the MD with an impact on cardiovascular prevention and cognitive deterioration; (3) MD associated with healthy aging, hydration and macro- and micronutrients; and (4) a seminar on sugars and sweeteners—presentation of the effects of sugar consumption on health and the evaluation of different types of sugars and sweeteners and processed products and risk of diseases associated with the consumption of foods not included in the MD. All the participants attended all the sessions, with the aim of standardizing the diet of the sample, to avoid eating habits being a potential confounding factor of the results obtained as an effect of the training.

2.5. Outcome Measurements

2.5.1. Body Composition

Women were profiled by Level 3 International Society for the Advancement of Kinanthropometry (ISAK)-accredited anthropometrists according to ISAK guidelines [23]. The weights and heights of all participants were measured using high-quality electronic calibrated scales and a wall-mounted stadiometer, respectively. Both measurements were determined with participants wearing light clothing and no shoes. With weight in kilograms and height in centimetres, the body mass index (BMI) was calculated as weight/size^2 (kg/m^2). Using the World Health Organization classification, the BMI was interpreted as follows: <18.5, underweight; 18.5–24.99, normal weight; 25–29.9, overweight; and >30, obese).

A mobile anthropometer was used to determine height to the nearest millimetre (Seca 213, SECA Deutschland, Hamburg, Germany), with the participant's head in the Frankfort Horizontal Plane position. Body perimeters were measured in triplicate (with subsequent averaging) with an anthropometric tape. Waist circumference was measured halfway between the last rib and the iliac crest by using an anthropometric tape. The hip circumference was taken horizontally in the maximum extension of the gluteus (larger posterior protrusion). With the result of both measurements, the waist-hip ratio was calculated. All circumferences included in the full ISAK profile were measured [23].

The objective of the measurements is to be able to calculate body composition based on the five-component model (fat mass, residual mass, bone mass, muscle mass and skin) proposed by Kerry Ross [24]. This model is self-evaluated because the sum of all the elements (structured weight) must be equal to the person's actual weight. It is important to note that this model does not calculate percentage fat but percentage adiposity. Put simply, it could be said that fat is the lipid fraction contained within the adipocyte, whereas adiposity would be the lipid fraction plus the adipose cells (i.e., the lipid fraction plus water, minerals, proteins, etc.). Therefore, percentage fat is not interchangeable with percentage adiposity, the latter being 5–10% higher.

The muscle/bone index was calculated as muscle tissue divided by bone tissue in kilograms (muscle/bone). Analysis and distribution of somatotype was done through the method proposed by Heath and Carter [25].

2.5.2. Body Image

The Body Shape Questionnaire, BSQ-34, is a 34-item, self-report measure of body shape and weight preoccupation initially developed to find out body image disturbance among women [26]. The questionnaire asks questions such as 'Have you felt ashamed of your body' and 'Have you been so worried about your shape that you have been feeling you ought to diet'. Each item is scored from 1 to 6 ('Never' = 1 and 'Always' = 6) and the total possible score is 204. Crude cut-off points have proposed that <81 correlates with no body image impairment, 81–110 with mild body image impairment, 111–140 with moderate impairment and >140 with severe impairment; nevertheless, there is no validated level between 'normal' and 'abnormal' [26], and scores were analyzed as both categorical and continuous data.

2.5.3. Mediterranean Diet

To determine the degree of adherence to the MD, a short questionnaire of 14 items was used, validated for the Spanish population and used by the MD Prevention group (Predimed) [27]. For scoring, a value of +1 was assigned to each item with a positive connotation (with regard to mean deviation, MD) and −1 for items with a negative connotation. From the sum of the values obtained for the 14 items, the degree of adherence is set, establishing two different levels: if the total score is ≥9, the diet has a satisfactory level of adherence; and if the total score is <9, the diet has a low level of adherence.

2.6. Statistical Analysis

Statistical analysis of the data was carried out using Jamovi 1.1.3.0. For descriptive statistics (mean ± standard deviation) and inferential analysis, the Shapiro–Wilk test was performed to determine the normality distribution. Afterwards, independent sample t-tests were performed to compare the different values of baseline between groups. Additionally, Levene's test was run for equality of variances, and analysis of covariance (ANCOVA) was applied to analyze the effects of the intervention on outcomes (general linear model; time × group; BMI as covariate). Partial eta-squared (η^2) effect sizes for time × group interaction effects were calculated. For the variables that presented significant main effects, post hoc tests (Bonferroni) were carried out. The level of significance was set at $p \leq 0.05$. The guidelines of Cohen were followed to calculate thee effect size [28].

3. Results

Table 1 shows the baseline descriptive statistics, along with a comparison of baseline values between groups. The general sample is normally homogeneous. However, statistically significant differences are observed between the experimental and control groups regarding height and weight. In all cases, the experimental group presents higher values.

Table 1. Baseline characteristics of study participants.

Variables	Intervention Group (n = 17) Baseline		Control Group (n = 17) Baseline		Baseline Differences		
	Mean	SD	Mean	SD	t	p	ES
Age (Years)	69.6 ±	5.0	67.7 ±	3.6	1.257	0.218	0.431
Height (cm)	162.0 ±	7.9	154.0 ±	5.4	3.347	0.002	1.148
Weight (kg)	75.3 ±	12.8	66.9 ±	10.2	2.122	0.042	0.728
BMI (kg/m^2)	28.8 ±	4.7	28.2 ±	4.2	0.385	0.703	0.132

BSQ = Body Shape Questionnaire; SD = Standard deviation; t = t value; p = p value; ES = Effect size.

Table 2 gives a summary of the ANCOVA statistics. The study's main analysis shows that there was a significant time × group difference in percentage adipose mass ($p \leq 0.001$; $\eta^2 = 0.654$) and muscle mass ($p \leq 0.001$; $\eta^2 = 0.618$). Post hoc analysis showed a decrease in percentage adipose mass between pre- and post-intervention in the experimental group (mean difference (MD): −2.80, $p < 0.001$, effect Size (ES): 0.471) and an increase in the control group (MD: 2.31, $p < 0.001$, ES: 0.471). There were also increases in kilograms of adipose mass (MD: 2.16, $p < 0.001$, ES: 0.357) and percentage muscle mass (MD: −2.541, $p < 0.001$, ES: 0.457) for the experimental group and decreases for the control group (MD: −1.729, $p < 0.001$, ES: 0.357 and MD = 2.035, $p < 0.001$, ES: 0.457, respectively).

Table 2. Comparison of characteristics at baseline and post-intervention (ANCOVA).

Variables	Intervention Group (n = 17) Baseline Mean SD	Intervention Group (n = 17) Post Mean SD	Control Group (n = 17) Baseline Mean SD	Control Group (n = 17) Mean SD	Effect Time F	Effect Time p	Effect Time $\eta^2 p$	Effect Time × Group F	Effect Time × Group p	Effect Time × Group $\eta^2 p$
Body Composition										
Weight (kg)	75.3 ± 12.8	75.3 ± 13.2	66.9 ± 10.2	67.4 ± 10.3	1.065	0.310	0.033	0.329	0.570	0.011
% fat mass	32.3 ± 4.5 *	29.5 ± 3.9 *	34.2 ± 4.1 *	36.5 ± 3.9 *	0.205	0.654	0.007	58.649	<0.001	0.654
% residual mass	11.8 ± 2.5	12.1 ± 2.4	10.6 ± 1.4	10.3 ± 1.2	0.319	0.577	0.010	0.434	0.515	0.014
% muscle mass	40.5 ± 3.4 *	43.0 ± 2.4 *	41.6 ± 2.8 *	39.6 ± 2.7 *	1.160	0.291	0.036	50.09	<0.001	0.618
% bone mass	10.2 ± 1.5	10.2 ± 1.5	8.5 ± 0.9	8.5 ± 0.9	2.164	0.151	0.065	0.194	0.662	0.006
% skin	5.1 ± 0.7 #	5.15 ± 0.8 #	5.0 ± 0.4 #	5.1 ± 0.5 #	4.526	0.041	0.127	3.827	0.060	0.110
kg fat mass	24.5 ± 6.2 *	22.4 ± 5.3 *	22.9 ± 4.3 *	24.7 ± 4.7 *	1.110	0.300	0.035	59.27	<0.001	0.657
kg muscle mass	30.5 ± 5.6 *	32.5 ± 6.1 *	27.8 ± 4.7	26.6 ± 4.5	0.140	0.710	0.005	22.118	<0.001	0.416
kg residual mass	8.9 ± 2.3	9.1 ± 2.1	7.2 ± 1.8	6.9 ± 1.6	1.330	0.258	0.041	2.56	0.120	0.076
kg bone mass	7.6 ± 1.2	7.7 ± 1.2	5.7 ± 0.9	5.7 ± 0.9	3.218	0.083	0.094	0.441	0.511	0.014
kg skin	3.8 ± 0.6	3.8 ± 0.6	3.3 ± 0.3	3.4 ± 0.3	4.120	0.051	0.117	0.202	0.656	0.006
WHR	0.9 ± 0.1	0.9 ± 0.1	0.9 ± 0.1	0.9 ± 0.1	0.297	0.590	0.009	4.377	0.055	0.124
Endomorph	5.79 ± 1.72 *	5.45 ± 1.67 *	6.57 ± 1.22	6.90 ± 1.50	0.000815	0.977	0.000	15.0	<0.001	0.011
Mesomorph	4.87 ± 1.26 *	5.41 ± 1.41 *	5.28 ± 1.56 *	5.03 ± 1.40 *	5.65	0.023	0.003	43.01	<0.001	0.021
Ectomorph	0.59 ± 0.69	0.56 ± 0.60	0.46 ± 0.47	0.45 ± 0.47	0.580	0.451	0.017	0.183	0.672	0.005
Body Image										
BSQ	52.4 ± 17.1	45.9 ± 12.7	57.4 ± 20.4	53.6 ± 20.9	2.050	0.162	0.062	0.482	0.493	0.015
Mediterranean Diet										
Predimed	5.7 ± 2.0	5.9 ± 2.36	6.1 ± 2.1	5.5 ± 2.3	0.198	0.659	0.006	3.128	0.087	0.092

BMI = Body Mass Index; kg = kilograms; WHR: waist-hip ratio; SD = Standard deviation; t = t value; p = p value; ES = Effect size; Mean differences are considered significant when p < 0.05; # differences in time; * differences in time × group.

In terms of kilograms of muscle mass, there were statistically significant differences only in the experimental group; there was an increase (MD: −1.97, $p = 0.001$, ES: 0.473) in muscle mass in terms of weight. However, there were also differences between the control and experimental groups at post-intervention (MD: 5.28, $p = 0.001$, ES: 1.270), with greater kilograms of muscle mass in the experimental group than the control group. About the somatotype variables, an increase in mesomorphism (MD: −0.542, $p < 0.001$, ES: 0.087) and a decrease in endomorphism (MD: 0.339, $p = 0.040$, ES: 0.0812) were observed in the experimental group. In control group, a significant decrease in mesomorphy was observed (MD: −0.254, $p = 0.031$, ES: 0.021). Nevertheless, no significant effects were found for any other variable.

4. Discussion

The objective of this study was to analyze the efficacy of the addition of resistance interval training in an aquatic environment to a nutritional intervention on body composition, body image perception and adherence to the MD in older women. The present study highlights different findings: the addition of resistance training in an aquatic environment to a nutritional intervention was not enough to change the perception of body image or adherence to the MD for older women. However, body composition variables were improved, in terms of loss of fat mass and gain of muscle mass.

In recent years, fat mass has been one of the most studied parameters in terms of body composition, due to its close relationship with health status. In this sense, it has been found that a greater fat mass is related to an increase in the probability of suffering cardiovascular diseases, overweight and obesity, arterial hypertension, diabetes and metabolic syndrome [29].

Although there are no data on body composition in women doing resistance training, there are data on body composition in women doing pilates training [29]. Comparing the results shows that, overall the women in the study of Raquel et al., 2015 [29], had lower values both before and after the intervention, whereas the level of improvement in fat percentage seems to be higher after resistance training (2.1 ± 5.75 kg), than pilates (1.04 ± 3.6 kg). No improvement occurred in the case of women in the control group, as an increase in this compartment is observed.

For bone mass and residual mass, an increase of 0.03 ± 1.04 kg was observed in women doing pilates and 0.1 ± 1.2 kg in women doing resistance training. It appears that resistance training increases bone mineral content. This was expected, as it has been previously seen [30,31] that resistance training improves bone strength indices and functional performance in postmenopausal women. The control group in the present study was unchanged.

Muscle mass is another parameter closely related to the state of health, especially at aging and menopause stages of life, when the process of sarcopenia and other age-related muscle dysfunctions start appearing [32]. After 14 weeks of resistance training, an increase of 2 ± 5.85 kg of muscle mass was observed, while in the control group, there was a decrease of −1.2 ± 4.6 kg. If we compare with the results of Raquel et al. [29] the increase is slightly lower; 0.94 ± 4.48 kg.

In addition, coinciding with other research [33,34], it has been observed that the 14 weeks of 10–20–30 s training reduced the percentage fat mass along with an increase in percentage muscle mass. These arguments confirm the current evidence on interval training [35,36], which consists of repeated sets of high-intensity exercise interspersed with passive/active recovery because it has been shown to induce metabolic adaptations and improve body composition. In general, studies that have used exercise protocols with an intervention period of 8–24 weeks, a frequency of 2–5 times per week and a low to moderate level of exercise intensity have reported significant improvements in body composition, as indicated by significant decreases in fat mass and increases in lean mass [37]. The subjects in the present study not only lost fat mass but also increased muscle mass, which is favorable because age-related muscle mass is an important determinant of strength and physical function in older adults [38].

Another method proposed to estimate body composition and shape is the somatotype [39]. However, there are no studies conducted in older women that analyze this variable; there is just one that evaluated the effectiveness of the pilates method [29]. In the present study, both women in the intervention (5.79–4.87–0.59) and control (6.57–5.28–0.46) groups presented an endomorph–mesomorph somatotype in the pretest. After 14 weeks of intervention, in the intervention group, the "endomorph" component decreased and the "mesomorph" increased significantly ($p < 0.001$); (5.45–4.41–0.56). In the control group, no significant changes were observed (6.90–5.03–0.45).

As well is kown, the gold standard for measuring body composition is the Dual-energy X-ray absorptiometry (DXA), although the data are not comparable; note that the % of fat in women aged 69 ± 4 years measured by anthropometry is around 33.27 ± 4.19%, while in DXA, overweight women aged 63 ± 6 years have a % of fat mass of 38.1 ± 4.9 and women with normal weight of 31.1 ± 4.2% [40].

The concept of self-image (i.e., how we see ourselves) undergoes changes throughout the entire life cycle. Body image suffers modifications over the years that require adaptation and psychological accommodation [41]. The physical changes that aging entails, in a more or less gradual way, suppose a modification of the subject's own self-image, and on many occasions, there is an abyss between the desired and the real image [41]. Studies show that approximately 50% of young women show great dissatisfaction with their physical appearance, and this is also evident in older women [42,43].

The relation between diet-related behaviours and body self-perception is a current theme for healthcare professionals. In a systematic review by Cristina Bouzas [44], it was noted that, generally, bodyweight satisfaction was related to having less intent to lose weight or change lifestyles. In contrast, body weight dissatisfaction was associated with a greater intent to change lifestyle or weight, a higher BMI and, specifically in women, dietary restraint. In addition, it has been reported that the body image of women can be improved only by increasing exercise, regardless of any weight change [45].

If the sample is classified according to score, as has been done previously in other research [46], only one participant in the intervention group was slightly preoccupied (97 pre- and 86 post-scores). In the control group, although again only one participant was slightly preoccupied, the scores were slightly higher (121 pre- and 118 post-scores). This information suggests, as previously noted [46], that the prevalence of older people suffering from body image concern is between 2.5% and 6% [46,47]. Although the differences were not significant, it has been observed that there are greater differences in the intervention group between the pre- and post-scores (52.4 ± 17.1 and 45.9 ± 12.7, respectively) than in the control group (57.4 ± 20.4 and 53.6 ± 20.9), which suggests that doing physical exercise helps to improve body image perception.

Resistance training is widely used among older adults because physical function is closely related to strength and muscle mass, thus improving psychological well-being and health-related quality of life as well as decreasing anxiety and depression levels [48]. However, this was not observed in the present study because the perception of body image did not improve after the intervention. One of the reasons could be a lack of motivation, as it has been seen that team aerobic training or team sports training is more intrinsically motivating than resistance training, mainly due to the higher degree of social connectedness [48].

No significant differences were observed in terms of body image dissatisfaction variables, either in adherence to the MD between groups or between pre- and post-intervention. As with the Predimed score, no significant differences were observed between groups or between pre- and post-intervention. Overall, adherence to the MD was moderate in both the intervention group (5.65 ± 2.03 and 5.94 ± 2.36 pre- and post-intervention, respectively) and the control group (6.06 ± 2.14 and 5.53 ± 2.35 pre- and post-intervention, respectively).

Compared to other studies, the recent scores obtained by Luigi Barrea et al. [49] and Naomi Cano-Ibáñez et al. [50] were higher.

These data suggest that because the participants did not receive an individualized nutritional program, the nutritional education they received was not sufficient to change the total Predimed score. For this type of population, individualized and specialized dietary–nutritional treatment would be recommended, with the aim of achieving greater adherence to treatment and therefore better results, as it has been noted that greater adherence to the MD is related to lower percentages of fat mass and higher BMI values in this population [51].

The present study has some limitations. Firstly, the study included only female patients. Because of the gender-specific response, our results may not be generalizable to all elderly populations. The levels of daily PA were not assessed using self-reported questionnaires such as the International Physical Activity Questionnaire or using measurement devices such as accelerometers or smart watches. In addition, the method of measuring body composition must be considered, since anthropometry was used and not DXA, which is considered the gold standard for body composition assessments. Finally, diet control or nutritional supplementation during the intervention was not analyzed; there could also be an association with body composition. Food quality was assessed, but it was not feasible to evaluate the quantity.

Future research should consider the limitations presented above. Researchers in the field are asked to evaluate more specific information on the amount of food and supplements ingested by the participants. In addition to assessing total daily PA, the activity bracelets should consider the training sessions they performed in the intervention.

5. Conclusions

The addition of resistance training in an aquatic environment to a nutritional intervention was not sufficient to change the perception of body image and adherence to the MD in older women. However, it does produce an improvement in body composition, through the increase of muscle mass and decrease of fat mass. To improve eating habits and body image perception, specific intervention and individualized treatment is necessary for this population.

Author Contributions: Conceptualization, A.M.-R. and P.J.M.-P.; methodology, A.M.-R. and P.J.M.-P.; software, M.M.-O. and A.M.-R.; validation, A.M.-R., B.J.C.-C. and P.J.M.-P.; formal analysis, M.M.-O. and A.M.-R.; investigation, A.M.-R., P.J.M.-P. and B.J.C.-C.; resources, B.J.C.-C. and P.J.M.-P.; data curation, A.M.-R., B.J.C.-C. and M.M.-O.; writing—original draft preparation, A.M.-R. and B.J.C.-C.; writing—review and editing, P.J.M.-P.; visualization, A.M.-R., B.J.C.-C. and M.M.-O.; supervision, P.J.M.-P. All authors have read and agreed to the published version of the manuscript.

Funding: This research received no external funding.

Institutional Review Board Statement: The study was conducted according to the guidelines of the Declaration of Helsinki and approved by the University Human Research Ethics Committee of the Catholic University of San Antonio (Murcia), code: CE061920 and data: 07/06/2019.

Informed Consent Statement: Informed consent was obtained from all subjects involved in the study.

Data Availability Statement: The data presented in this study are available on request from the corresponding author. The data are not publicly available due to the fact that they consist in personal health information.

Acknowledgments: The authors are grateful to all the subjects for their participation in this study.

Conflicts of Interest: The authors declare no conflict of interest.

References

1. Buch, A.; Kis, O.; Carmeli, E.; Keinan-Boker, L.; Berner, Y.; Barer, Y.; Shefer, G.; Marcus, Y.; Stern, N. Circuit resistance training is an effective means to enhance muscle strength in older and middle aged adults: A systematic review and meta-analysis. *Ageing Res. Rev.* **2017**, *37*, 16–27. [CrossRef] [PubMed]
2. Marín-Cascales, E.; Alcaraz, P.E.; Ramos-Campo, D.J.; Rubio-Arias, J.A. Effects of multicomponent training on lean and bone mass in postmenopausal and older women: A systematic review. *Menopause* **2018**, *25*, 346–356. [CrossRef] [PubMed]
3. Colpani, V.; Baena, C.P.; Jaspers, L.; van Dijk, G.M.; Farajzadegan, Z.; Dhana, K.; Tielemans, M.J.; Voortman, T.; Freak-Poli, R.; Veloso, G.G.V.; et al. Lifestyle factors, cardiovascular disease and all-cause mortality in middle-aged and elderly women: A systematic review and meta-analysis. *Eur. J. Epidemiol.* **2018**, *33*, 831–845. [CrossRef]
4. Lizcano, F.; Guzmán, G. Estrogen deficiency and the origin of obesity during menopause. *BioMed Res. Int.* **2014**, *2014*, 757461. [CrossRef] [PubMed]
5. Ho, S.C.; Wu, S.; Chan, S.G.; Sham, A. Menopausal transition and changes of body composition: A prospective study in Chinese perimenopausal women. *Int. J. Obes.* **2010**, *34*, 1265–1274. [CrossRef]
6. Thompson, K.A.; Bardone-Cone, A.M. Menopausal status and disordered eating and body image concerns among middle-aged women. *Int. J. Eat. Disord.* **2019**, *52*, 314–318. [CrossRef]
7. Simas, V.; Hing, W.; Pope, R.; Climstein, M. Effects of water-based exercise on bone health of middle-aged and older adults: A systematic review and meta-analysis. *Open Access J. Sport. Med.* **2017**, *8*, 39–60. [CrossRef]
8. Perich, T.; Ussher, J.; Meade, T. Menopause and illness course in bipolar disorder: A systematic review. *Bipolar Disord.* **2017**, *19*, 434–443. [CrossRef]
9. Bromberger, J.T.; Epperson, C.N. Depression during and after the perimenopause: Impact of hormones, genetics, and environmental determinants of disease. *Obstet. Gynecol. Clin. N. Am.* **2018**, *45*, 663–678. [CrossRef]
10. Gibbs, Z.; Lee, S.; Kulkarni, J. What factors determine whether a woman becomes depressed during the perimenopause? *Arch. Women's Ment. Health* **2012**, *15*, 323–332. [CrossRef]
11. Drobnjak, S.; Atsiz, S.; Ditzen, B.; Tuschen-Caffier, B.; Ehlert, U. Restrained eating and self-esteem in premenopausal and postmenopausal women. *J. Eat. Disord.* **2014**, *2*, 23. [CrossRef]
12. Sayón-Orea, C.; Santiago, S.; Cuervo, M.; Martínez-González, M.A.; Garcia, A.; Martínez, J.A. Adherence to Mediterranean dietary pattern and menopausal symptoms in relation to overweight/obesity in Spanish perimenopausal and postmenopausal women. *Menopause* **2015**, *22*, 750–757. [CrossRef]
13. Cicero, A.F.G.; D'Addato, S.; Santi, F.; Ferroni, A.; Borghi, C. Leisure-time physical activity and cardiovascular disease mortality: The brisighella heart study. *J. Cardiovasc. Med.* **2012**, *13*, 559–564. [CrossRef] [PubMed]
14. Chen, L.J.; Stevinson, C.; Ku, P.W.; Chang, Y.K.; Chu, D.C. Relationships of leisure-time and non-leisure-time physical activity with depressive symptoms: A population-based study of Taiwanese older adults. *Int. J. Behav. Nutr. Phys. Act.* **2012**, *9*, 28. [CrossRef]
15. Petersen, C.B.; Severin, M.; Hansen, A.W.; Curtis, T.; Grønbæk, M.; Tolstrup, J.S. A population-based randomized controlled trial of the effect of combining a pedometer with an intervention toolkit on physical activity among individuals with low levels of physical activity or fitness. *Prev. Med.* **2012**, *54*, 125–130. [CrossRef] [PubMed]
16. Nawrocka, A.; Mynarski, W.; Cholewa, J. Adherence to physical activity guidelines and functional fitness of elderly women, using objective measurement. *Ann. Agric. Environ. Med.* **2017**, *24*, 632–635. [CrossRef]
17. Chodzko-Zajko, W.J.; Proctor, D.N.; Fiatarone Singh, M.A.; Minson, C.T.; Nigg, C.R.; Salem, G.J.; Skinner, J.S. American college of sports medicine position stand. exercise and physical activity for older adults. *Med. Sci. Sports Exerc.* **1998**, *41*, 992–1008.
18. Pollock, M.L.; Wenger, N.K. Physical activity and exercise training in the elderly: A position paper from the society of geriatric cardiology. *Am. J. Geriatr. Cardiol.* **1998**, *7*, 45–46. [PubMed]
19. Saghaei, M. An overview of randomization and minimization programs for randomized clinical trials. *J. Med. Signals Sens.* **2011**, *1*, 55–61. [CrossRef]
20. Gunnarsson, T.P.; Bangsbo, J. The 10-20-30 training concept improves performance and health profile in moderately trained runners. *J. Appl. Physiol.* **2012**, *113*, 16–24. [CrossRef]
21. Andrade, L.S.; Kanitz, A.C.; Häfele, M.S.; Schaun, G.Z.; Pinto, S.S.; Alberton, C.L. Relationship between oxygen uptake, heart rate, and perceived effort in an aquatic incremental test in older women. *Int. J. Environ. Res. Public Health* **2020**, *17*, 8324. [CrossRef]
22. Borg, G. Psychophysical scaling with applications in physical work and the perception of exertion. *Scand. J. Work. Environ. Health* **1990**, *16*, 55–58. [CrossRef]
23. Norton, K.I. Standards for Anthropometry Assessment. In *Kinanthropometry and Exercise Physiology*; Routledge: London, UK, 2019; pp. 68–137.
24. Ross, W.D.; Kerr, D.A. Fraccionamiento de la Masa Corporal: Un Nuevo Método para Utilizar en Nutrición, Clínica y Medicina Deportiva. *Revista de Actualización en Ciencias del Deporte*. **1993**, *3*, 1.
25. Carter, J.E.L. *The Heath-Carter Anthropometric Somatotype-Instruction Manual-Somatotype Instruction Manual 2 Part 1: The Heath-Carter Anthropometric Somatotype-Instruction Manual*; TeP and ROSSCRAFT: Surrey, BC, Canada, 2002.
26. Cooper, P.J.; Taylor, M.J.; Cooper, Z.; Christopher, G.; Fairbum, M.D. The development and validation of the body shape questionnaire. *Int. J. Eat. Disord.* **1987**, *6*, 485–494. [CrossRef]

27. Martínez-González, M.A.; García-Arellano, A.; Toledo, E.; Salas-Salvadó, J.; Buil-Cosiales, P.; Corella, D.; Covas, M.I.; Schröder, H.; Arós, F.; Gómez-Gracia, E.; et al. A 14-item mediterranean diet assessment tool and obesity indexes among high-risk subjects: The predimed trial. *PLoS ONE* **2012**, *7*, e43134. [CrossRef]
28. Gignac, G.E.; Szodorai, E.T. Effect size guidelines for individual differences researchers. *Pers. Individ. Differ.* **2016**, *102*, 74–78. [CrossRef]
29. Vaquero-Cristóbal, R.; Alacid, F.; Esparza-Ros, F.; López-Plaza, D.; Muyor, J.M.; López-Miñarro, P.A. The effects of a reformer Pilates program on body composition and morphological characteristics in active women after a detraining period. *Women Health* **2016**, *56*, 784–806. [CrossRef] [PubMed]
30. Watson, S.L.; Weeks, B.K.; Weis, L.J.; Harding, A.T.; Horan, S.A.; Beck, B.R. High-intensity resistance and impact training improves bone mineral density and physical function in postmenopausal women with osteopenia and osteoporosis: The liftmor randomized controlled trial. *J. Bone Miner. Res.* **2018**, *33*, 211–220. [CrossRef] [PubMed]
31. Villareal, D.T.; Aguirre, L.; Gurney, A.B. Aerobic or resistance exercise, or both, in dieting obese older adults. *N. Engl. J. Med.* **2017**, *376*, 1943–1955. [CrossRef]
32. Correa-de-Araujo, R.; Hadley, E. Skeletal muscle function deficit: A new terminology to embrace the evolving concepts of sarcopenia and age-related muscle dysfunction. *J. Gerontol. A. Biol. Sci. Med. Sci.* **2014**, *69*, 591–594. [CrossRef]
33. Baasch-Skytte, T.; Lemgart, C.T.; Oehlenschläger, M.H.; Petersen, P.E.; Hostrup, M.; Bangsbo, J.; Gunnarsson, T.P. Efficacy of 10-20-30 training versus moderate-intensity continuous training on HbA1c, body composition and maximum oxygen uptake in male patients with type 2 diabetes: A randomized controlled trial. *Diabetes Obes. Metab.* **2020**, *22*, 767–778. [CrossRef] [PubMed]
34. Boukabous, I.; Marcotte-Chénard, A.; Amamou, T.; Boulay, P.; Brochu, M.; Tessier, D.; Dionne, I.; Riesco, E. Low-volume high-intensity interval training versus moderate-intensity continuous training on body composition, cardiometabolic profile, and physical capacity in older women. *J. Aging Phys. Act.* **2019**, *27*, 879–889. [CrossRef] [PubMed]
35. Zhang, H.; Tong, T.K.; Qiu, W.; Zhang, X.; Zhou, S.; Liu, Y.; He, Y. Comparable effects of high-intensity interval training and prolonged continuous exercise training on abdominal visceral fat reduction in obese young women. *J. Diabetes Res.* **2017**, *2017*, 1–9. [CrossRef]
36. Keating, S.E.; Johnson, N.A.; Mielke, G.I.; Coombes, J.S. A systematic review and meta-analysis of interval training versus moderate-intensity continuous training on body adiposity. *Obes. Rev.* **2017**, *18*, 943–964. [CrossRef] [PubMed]
37. Lee, J.S.; Kim, C.G.; Seo, T.B.; Kim, H.G.; Yoon, S.J. Effects of 8-week combined training on body composition, isokinetic strength, and cardiovascular disease risk factors in older women. *Aging Clin. Exp. Res.* **2015**, *27*, 179–186. [CrossRef]
38. Perry, C.A.; Van Guilder, G.P.; Kauffman, A.; Hossain, M. A calorie-restricted DASH diet reduces body fat and maintains muscle strength in obese older adults. *Nutrients* **2020**, *12*, 102. [CrossRef]
39. Boldsen, J.L.; Carter, J.E.L.; Honeyman, B. Lindsay carter, barbara honeyman heath. In *Somatotyping: Development and Applications*; Cambridge University Press: Cambridge, UK, 2005.
40. Li, S.; Xue, J.; Hong, P. Relationships between serum omentin-1 concentration, body composition and physical activity levels in older women. *Medicine* **2021**, *100*, e25020. [CrossRef] [PubMed]
41. Cobo, C.M.S. Body image in older. Descriptive studie. *Gerokomos* **2012**, *23*, 15–18.
42. Allaz, A.F.; Bernstein, M.; Rouget, P.; Archinard, M.; Morabia, A. Body weight preoccupation in middle-age and ageing women: A general population survey. *Int. J. Eat. Disord.* **1998**, *23*, 287–294. [CrossRef]
43. Webster, J.; Tiggemann, M. The relationship between women's body satisfaction and self-image across the life span: The role of cognitive control. *J. Genet. Psychol.* **2003**, *164*, 241–252. [CrossRef]
44. Bouzas, C.; Bibiloni, M.D.M.; Tur, J.A. Relationship between body image and body weight control in overweight ≥55-year-old adults: A systematic review. *Int. J. Environ. Res. Public Health* **2019**, *16*, 1622. [CrossRef]
45. Fougner, M.; Bergland, A.; Lund, A.; Debesay, J. Aging and exercise: Perceptions of the active lived-body. *Physiother. Theory Pract.* **2019**, *35*, 651–662. [CrossRef]
46. Dean, E.; Haywood, C.; Hunter, P.; Austin, N.; Prendergast, L. Body image in older, inpatient women and the relationship to BMI, anxiety, depression, and other sociodemographic factors. *Int. J. Geriatr. Psychiatry* **2020**, *35*, 182–187. [CrossRef]
47. Latorre Román, P.A.; García-Pinillos, F.; Huertas Herrador, J.A.; Cózar Barba, M.; Muñoz Jiménez, M. Relacion entre sexo, Composicion corporal, Velocidad de la marcha y satisfaccion corporal en ancianos. *Nutr. Hosp.* **2014**, *30*, 851–857.
48. Pedersen, M.T.; Vorup, J.; Nistrup, A.; Wikman, J.M.; Alstrøm, J.M.; Melcher, P.S.; Pfister, G.U.; Bangsbo, J. Effect of team sports and resistance training on physical function, quality of life, and motivation in older adults. *Scand. J. Med. Sci. Sport.* **2017**, *27*, 852–864. [CrossRef] [PubMed]
49. Barrea, L.; Muscogiuri, G.; Di Somma, C.; Tramontano, G.; De Luca, V.; Illario, M.; Colao, A.; Savastano, S. Association between Mediterranean diet and hand grip strength in older adult women. *Clin. Nutr.* **2019**, *38*, 721–729. [CrossRef] [PubMed]
50. Cano-Ibáñez, N.; Gea, A.; Martínez-González, M.A.; Salas-Salvadó, J.; Corella, D.; Zomeño, M.D.; Romaguera, D.; Vioque, J.; Aros, F.; Wärnberg, J.; et al. Dietary diversity and nutritional adequacy among an older Spanish population with metabolic syndrome in the predimed-plus study: A cross-sectional analysis. *Nutrients* **2019**, *11*, 958. [CrossRef] [PubMed]
51. Martí, A.Z.; Martínez, M.J.C.; Sánchez, J.A.H.; Pérez, A.L. Adherencia a la dieta mediterránea y su relación con el estado nutricional en personas mayores. *Nutr. Hosp.* **2015**, *31*, 1667–1674.

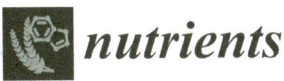

Article

Utilizing Participatory Research to Engage Underserved Populations to Improve Health-Related Outcomes in Delaware

Shannon M. Robson [1,*], Samantha M. Rex [1,2], Katie Greenawalt [1,3], P. Michael Peterson [1] and Elizabeth Orsega-Smith [1]

1. Department of Behavioral Health and Nutrition, University of Delaware, 26 N College Avenue, Newark, DE 19713, USA; srex2@jhmi.edu (S.M.R.); keg5293@psu.edu (K.G.); pmpeter@udel.edu (P.M.P.); eosmith@udel.edu (E.O.-S.)
2. Department of International Health, Bloomberg School of Public Health, Johns Hopkins University, 615 N Wolfe Street, Baltimore, MD 21205, USA
3. PennState Extension, College of Agricultural Sciences, The Pennsylvania State University, 323 Agricultural Administration Building, University Park, PA 16802, USA
* Correspondence: robson@udel.edu; Tel.: +1-302-831-6674

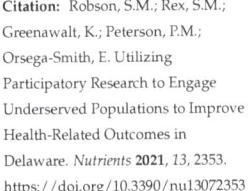

Citation: Robson, S.M.; Rex, S.M.; Greenawalt, K.; Peterson, P.M.; Orsega-Smith, E. Utilizing Participatory Research to Engage Underserved Populations to Improve Health-Related Outcomes in Delaware. *Nutrients* 2021, *13*, 2353. https://doi.org/10.3390/nu13072353

Academic Editor: Carlos Vasconcelos

Received: 15 May 2021
Accepted: 6 July 2021
Published: 9 July 2021

Publisher's Note: MDPI stays neutral with regard to jurisdictional claims in published maps and institutional affiliations.

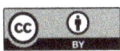

Copyright: © 2021 by the authors. Licensee MDPI, Basel, Switzerland. This article is an open access article distributed under the terms and conditions of the Creative Commons Attribution (CC BY) license (https://creativecommons.org/licenses/by/4.0/).

Abstract: Cooperative Extension is a community outreach program. Despite its large reach, there is a need for the evaluation of changes in health-related outcomes for individuals engaged with Cooperative Extension. A team-based challenge was developed using community-engaged participatory research integrated with Cooperative Extension to encourage healthy eating and physical activity behaviors through Cooperative Extension programming. Thus, the primary purpose of this secondary analysis was to (1) evaluate changes in anthropometric outcomes and (2) evaluate changes in health behavior outcomes. Associations of anthropometric changes and health behavior changes with engagement in the three-month team-based challenge were explored. Anthropometrics were measured using standard procedures, and intake of fruits and vegetables and physical activity were self-reported. Of the 145 participants in the community-engaged participatory research portion of the study, 52.4% ($n = 76$) had complete anthropometrics before and after the team-based challenge and were included in this study. At 3 months, there was a significant reduction in body mass index (-0.3 kg/m^2, $p = 0.024$) and no significant change in waist circumference ($p = 0.781$). Fruit and vegetable intake significantly increased (+0.44 servings/day, $p = 0.018$). Physical activity did not significantly change based on (1) the number of days 30 or more minutes of physical activity was conducted ($p = 0.765$) and (2) Godin Leisure-Time Exercise Questionnaire scores ($p = 0.612$). Changes in anthropometrics and health behaviors were not associated with engagement in the team-based challenge. Using community-engaged participatory research with community outreach programs, such as Cooperative Extension, can improve health-related outcomes in underserved populations. However, despite a participatory approach, changes in anthropometrics and health behaviors were not associated with engagement in the developed team-based challenge.

Keywords: community-based; participatory research; anthropometrics; fruit and vegetable intake; physical activity; Cooperative Extension

1. Introduction

Poor dietary habits and low levels of physical activity are often associated with poor health outcomes, including overweight and obesity [1–3]. In the USA, approximately 70% of the adult population is classified as being overweight or obese [4]. Racial/ethnic and socioeconomic disparities exist in obesity with Hispanic and Black populations often experiencing a higher prevalence than White and Asian populations, and lower income populations having higher rates of overweight and obesity than higher income populations [5]. While several social, biological and environmental determinants influence overweight and obesity, nutrition and physical activity are considered to be key factors [6].

In particular, a diet of higher quality has been associated with lower risk of overweight and obesity in adults [7–9] and consumption of fruits and vegetables contributes to better diet quality [10]. In addition, regular physical activity is important for maintaining and achieving a healthy weight [11].

In 1914, Cooperative Extension was established with the purpose of providing educational outreach services through land-grant institutions dedicated to delivering science-based programs to people, businesses and communities, with a particular focus on programming promoting health [12]. Cooperative Extension has a wide reach across the USA with extension agents in approximately 3000 counties. Cooperative Extension is a trusted source of information within communities and can often provide known and respected connections to local networks and community leaders. Despite its reach, there has been a continuous call for greater engagement across the Extension system [13,14]. Within Cooperative Extension, participatory research has been suggested as one method of increasing community engagement that may lead to more impactful outcomes [15]. Community-engaged participatory research is a technique that can be used to plan community acceptable programs (interventions) as the community engages as an equal partner in the research.

Improvements in health behaviors (including diet and physical activity) associated with participatory research have been well documented [16–21]; however, the integration of community-engaged participatory research with Cooperative Extension has been limited. Thus, among a sample of adults engaged with Cooperative Extension in Delaware (USA), the purpose of this secondary analysis was to (1) examine changes in anthropometric outcomes (body mass index and waist circumference) and (2) examine changes in the health behaviors (fruit and vegetable intake and physical activity) of participants with complete anthropometric measures before and after the team-based challenge. Associations between changes in anthropometrics and changes in health behaviors and engagement in the team-based challenge developed through a community-engaged participatory research process were explored.

2. Methods

2.1. Participants' Eligibility and Recruitment

Participants were recruited through personal contact among the Cooperative Extension agents, local churches and community groups. Adults (≥18 years-old) living in Kent or New Castle County, Delaware (USA), were eligible to participate in a community-based participatory research study to develop a program for increased engagement in healthy lifestyle behaviors. Of the 145 adults that were involved in the participatory research portion of the study that created the team-based challenge, 76 had complete anthropometric measures at baseline and end of the team-based challenge (three months) and were included in this secondary analysis with the primary purpose of examining changes in anthropometrics. The study was approved by the Institutional Review Board at the University of Delaware. All participants signed informed consent forms.

2.2. Study Procedures

Using community-engaged participatory research, input from community members was collected through key informant interviews, focus groups and community advisory boards. The information collected was used to inform the development of a 3-month team-based challenge. The team-based challenge was created with the purpose of engaging the community in healthy lifestyle behaviors. In teams, anyone from the community could enroll and accrue points each month. Points were awarded based upon participation in a variety of individual and team-based activities. Points were assigned to various health behaviors and activities, such as steps walked per day, parking the car further away, preparing a new recipe, or getting a health screening. Points were allocated based on complexity or effort required to complete an activity; for example, parking the car further away would equate to five points, while walking 10,000 steps a day would equate to 20 points. Participants could also earn points by attending the Cooperative Extension educational programming. Points allocated for participation in these Cooperative Extension programs were based on the number of sessions. For example, participation in Cooperative Extension education sessions, such as "Dining with Diabetes", would equate to 100 points for multiple class sessions (or partial points if individual classes were attended). Single education session programs, such as "Get Your Snack on Track", would be worth 50 points. Participants tracked their total points on a log each day, and at the end of the month, team members turned in their logs to the Cooperative Extension health educator, who totaled and averaged the points by number of team members. Participants received incentives, such as gift cards and prizes, as goals were achieved to promote engagement.

2.3. Measures

Anthropometrics were measured and a comprehensive questionnaire, which was available in English and Spanish, that included questions regarding demographics and health conditions, servings of fruit and vegetables and physical activity, was completed by participants at baseline and after the three-month time period of the team-based challenge.

Anthropometrics. The weight and height of each participant were measured by research personnel using standard procedures [22]. Weight and height were used to calculate body mass index (BMI) by dividing weight in kilograms by the square of height in meters. BMI was used to classify weight status (normal weight: <25 kg/m^2; overweight: 25–29.9 kg/m^2; obesity: ≥ 30 kg/m^2). The mean of three consecutive waist measurements was taken at the smallest point of the waist [23] in inches and recorded when the tape measure was snug around the waist, but not constricting. Mean waist measurements were converted to centimeter for reporting.

Demographics and Health Conditions. Basic demographic information related to age, education level, marital status and income was collected. Participants self-report (yes or no) of having diabetes, hypertension and/or high cholesterol was collected at baseline.

Servings of Fruits and Vegetables. Fruit and vegetable intake, defined as fresh, frozen, canned, dried, and 100% juice, were assessed based on servings (with one serving equal to a half cup equivalent) with the question "How many fruits and vegetables do you usually eat each day?" Response options ranged from none to five or more servings per day.

Physical Activity. Physical activity was assessed based on the response of 0–7 days to the question "How many days was 30 or more minutes of purposeful physical activity accumulated in a typical week?" and the Godin Leisure-Time Exercise Questionnaire [24]. The Godin Leisure-Time Exercise Questionnaire asks participants "During a typical 7-day period, how many times on average do you do the following kinds of exercise for more than 15 min during your free time?" with response options of "strenuous exercise" (e.g., running, jogging, hockey, football and soccer), "moderate exercise" (e.g., fast walking, basketball, tennis, easy bicycling and volleyball), or "mild exercise" (e.g., yoga, archery, fishing, bowling and golfing). The number of times per option was multiplied by 9, 5 and 3, respectively, then summed to generate a Godin Leisure-Time Exercise score. Scores were categorized into three levels of physical activity: active (≥ 24 or more), moderately active (14–23), or insufficiently active/sedentary (<14) [25].

Engagement. Engagement was measured through the total number of points accumulated by teams each month in this team-based challenge. Participants earning one or more points over the course of the three-month team-based challenge were considered engaged, but if an individual did not participate or earned zero points, they were considered to have not engaged.

2.4. Statistical Analysis

Analyses were conducted using SPSS (IBM, Chicago, IL, USA, version 26). Means and frequencies were used to analyze continuous and categorical data, respectively, for demographics, engagement, anthropometrics, fruit and vegetable intake and physical activity. Paired t-tests examined changes from baseline to three months for anthropometrics, fruit and vegetable intake and physical activity, as measured by the number of days participants accumulated at least 30 min of physical activity and the Godin Leisure-Time Exercise score. The marginal homogeneity test was used to examine the change in the proportion of individuals in each Godin Leisure-Time physical activity category (active, moderately active and insufficiently active/sedentary) from baseline to three months. Chi-square tests were conducted to determine the association between change in anthropometrics, change in servings of fruit and vegetable and change in the level of physical activity outcomes based on the Godin Leisure-Time Exercise score and engagement (yes vs. no). An *alpha* < 0.05 was considered significant *a priori*.

3. Results

Of the 145 individuals who participated in the participatory research portion of the study, 52.4% ($n = 76$) participated in the team-based challenge and had complete anthropometrics measures at baseline and three months. Participants were on average 51.3 ± 17.4 years old, 77.0% female, with 59.2% identifying as non-Hispanic, African American, and 34.2% identifying as Hispanic, White. Of those who reported household income, 45.4% reported an annual household income < USD 20,000 per year. The median reported income in the USA in 2017 (when the study was conducted) was USD 61,372 [26]. Among participants, 23.6% reported having diabetes, 39.2% reported having hypertension and 41.3% reported having high cholesterol (Table 1).

Table 1. Baseline demographics and health condition characteristics of adults participating in the Cooperative Extension team-based challenge with complete anthropometrics.

Characteristics	$N = 76$ [1]
	M ± SD or n (%)
Age, years	51.3 ± 17.4
Sex [$n = 74$]	
Male	17 (23.0%)
Female	57 (77.0%)
Race/Ethnicity	
Non-Hispanic, Black or African American	45 (59.2%)
Hispanic, White	26 (34.2%)
Other	5 (6.6%)
Education [$n = 73$]	
No high school degree	13 (17.8%)
High School or GED degree	22 (30.1%)
Some college	15 (20.5%)
College degree	17 (23.3%)
Postgraduate/professional degree	6 (8.2%)
Marital Status	
Married	37 (48.7%)
Widowed	4 (5.3%)
Divorced	10 (13.2%)
Separated	4 (5.3%)
Never married	21 (27.6%)
Household Income [$n = 66$]	
<USD 20,000	30 (45.5%)
USD 20,000 to <USD 50,000	27 (40.9%)
>USD 50,000	9 (13.6%)
Diabetes [$n = 72$]	
Yes	17 (23.6%)
No	55 (76.4%)

Table 1. Cont.

	N = 76 [1]
Characteristics	M ± SD or n (%)
Hypertension [n = 74]	
Yes	29 (39.2%)
No	45 (60.8%)
High Cholesterol [n = 75]	
Yes	31 (41.3%)
No	44 (58.7%)

[1] Sample sizes vary due to missing data for the following variables: sex (n = 74), education (n = 73), household income (n = 66), diabetes (n = 72), hypertension (n = 74), and high cholesterol (n = 75).

As shown in Table 2, on average, participant weight significantly decreased over the three-month time period (t (75) = −2.405; $p = 0.019$). BMI also significantly decreased over the three-month program (t (75) = −2.298; $p = 0.024$). Waist circumference measurements of participants did not significantly change with participation in a three-month program. Participant (n = 74) consumption of daily servings of fruits and vegetables significantly increased over time (t (73) = 2.414, $p = 0.018$). There was no statistically significant change reported by participants for the number of days participants accumulated at least 30 min of physical activity or the Godin Leisure-Time Exercise score over the three months. The proportion of individuals within each level of physical activity based on the Godin Leisure-Time Exercise score did not significantly change over time. Changes in weight, BMI, waist circumference, daily servings of fruit and vegetable intake, and Godin Leisure-Time Exercise score for physical activity were not significantly different between individuals who actively engaged versus those who did not.

Table 2. Participant (n = 76) [1] anthropometrics, fruit and vegetable intake and physical activity measures at baseline and after the 3-month team-based challenge.

	Baseline	3-Months	p-Value
	M ± SD or n (%)	M ± SD or n (%)	
Height [2], m	1.6 ± 0.1	N/A	-
Weight, kg	82.9 ± 19.1	82.0 ± 18.3	0.019 *
Waist Circumference, cm	98.6 ± 16.1	98.5 ± 15.8	0.781
Body Mass Index, kg/m^2	30.7 ± 7.4	30.4 ± 7.1	0.024 *
Fruit and Vegetable Intake, servings/day	2.7 ± 1.4	3.2 ± 1.4	0.018 *
Physical Activity, days/week of 30+ minute	3.0 ± 2.1	3.0 ± 2.1	0.765
Godin Leisure-Time Exercise Score	28.8 ± 30.8	30.9 ± 28.4	0.612
Godin Leisure-Time Exercise Categories			
Insufficiently active/Inactive	20 (34.5%)	18 (31.0%)	0.376
Moderately active	11 (19.0%)	9 (15.5%)	
Active	27 (46.6%)	31 (53.4%)	

[1] Sample sizes vary due to missing data for the following variables: fruit and vegetable intake (n = 74), Godin Leisure-Time Exercise Score and exercise categories (n = 58). [2] Given an adult population, height was only measured at the pre-assessment. * $p < 0.05$.

4. Discussion

Impacts of community-based participatory research on health-related outcomes are less established in the literature [27]. This secondary analysis is one of few reporting on anthropometrics and health behaviors [17,19]. The utilization of community-based participatory research to develop a team-based challenge integrated with Cooperative Extension programming found an improvement in anthropometric outcomes based upon BMI and an increase in fruit and vegetable intake (a health behavior). Despite the decrease in BMI being statistically significant, it may have limited the clinical impact on health outcomes. Recommendations suggest 5–10% weight loss for an improvement in health outcomes; however, these recommendations are heavily based upon intensive lifestyle interventions delivered in clinical or research settings [28]. It is known that the dissemination of lifestyle interventions through community-based programs produce smaller weight losses [29] since the goals of community-level interventions are more often focused on increasing reach or increasing access to interventions [30]. Similarly, while there was a significant increase in fruit and vegetable intake over the three-month program, the change was small, equivalent to about a half serving or a one-quarter cup equivalent. Despite the increase, these data demonstrate that the participants still consumed less than the amounts recommended by the US Dietary Guidelines for Americans [31]. Waist circumference did not significantly change, and longer-term evaluation data are needed to better understand a possible maintenance effect. The physical activity level did not significantly change. The majority of participants were engaging in some type of physical activity upon starting the team-based challenge. While non-significant, there was an increase in the number of participants classified as "active" according to the Godin Leisure-Time Exercise categories. While findings suggest that the team-based challenge, developed through community-based participatory research and integrated with Cooperative Extension programming, can have a positive impact on health-related outcomes, changes in health-related outcomes were not associated with engagement.

It was unexpected that engagement in the team-based challenge was not correlated with outcomes; however, few studies report on engagement in the literature [32], particularly in community-based programs, limiting the ability to understand this finding in a broader context. Furthermore, the concept or definition of community engagement is inconsistent [33] and has more often focused on engaging the community during the development of interventions and programs, such as the community-engaged research paradigm used to develop the team-based challenge as opposed to engagement in the intervention or program developed [34]. Despite variable definitions, interventions that use community engagement, particularly for vulnerable populations, have been shown to be effective in improving health behaviors [35]. Relying on input to develop programs and interventions from individuals already engaged with established community-based outreach programs, such as Cooperative Extension, may further promote engagement in nutrition and physical activity interventions due to the community's familiarity with the established program. Zoellner and colleagues [20] found that the process of developing and implementing a walking program through community engaged participatory research and partnership with the Mississippi State Cooperative Extension was successful.

Due to the high prevalence of overweight and obesity in the USA, many community-based programs, such as Cooperative Extension, aim to encourage healthy behaviors related to eating and physical activity to promote a healthier weight. Fruits and vegetables are a large focus due to under-consumption, particularly among lower socioeconomic groups [6,36] who are served by Cooperative Extension outreach programs. There was a significant increase in fruit and vegetable intake over the three-month program, but the change was small, equivalent to about a half serving or a one-quarter cup equivalent. This small change may diminish any potential clinically meaningful impact on health. Although the increase was similar to many other findings investigating fruit and vegetable intake, these data demonstrate that participants consumed less than that recommended by the Dietary Guidelines for Americans [37].

This study is the result of a team-based challenge developed through community-based participatory research and implemented in the community utilizing an existing community resource, Cooperative Extension. Reporting health outcomes as a result of community-based participatory research is a strength of this study that is often cited as a limitation of this type of work. Study personnel measured height, weight and waist circumference of participants, providing a more accurate measurement than self-reporting. Additional study limitations include the cross-sectional nature of the data not allowing for comparison to a control condition and the use of self-reporting for fruit and vegetable intake and physical activity. These measures of fruit and vegetable intake and physical activity may not accurately reflect actual consumption or engagement in activity. Missing data are an additional limitation of this secondary analysis as of the 76 participants with anthropometric data at both time points, two were missing fruit and vegetable data, and 18 were missing the Godin Leisure-Time Exercise Score. The generalizability of the findings is limited given the results are representative of lower-income adults in the state of Delaware (USA) engaging with Cooperative Extension.

5. Conclusions

The integration of programming developed through community-engaged participatory research with established community outreach programs, such as Cooperative Extension, may be a novel way to create programs to improve health outcomes in underserved populations. While changes were small, improvements in weight, BMI and fruit and vegetable intake did occur, indicating the potential beneficial impact of programs developed by the community for the community on healthy lifestyle behaviors. However, despite the use of a community-engaged participatory research process, changes to health-related outcomes were not associated with engagement in the team-based challenge.

Author Contributions: Conceptualization, P.M.P. and E.O.-S.; Methodology, S.M.R. (Shannon M. Robson), S.M.R. (Samantha M. Rex), K.G. and E.O.-S.; Data Curation, S.M.R. (Shannon M. Robson), K.G. and E.O.-S.; Formal Analysis, S.M.R. (Shannon M. Robson) and S.M.R. (Samantha M. Rex); Writing—Original Draft Preparation, S.M.R. (Shannon M. Robson) and S.M.R. (Samantha M. Rex); Writing—Review and Editing, S.M.R. (Shannon M. Robson), S.M.R. (Samantha M. Rex), K.G., P.M.P. and E.O.-S.; Funding Acquisition, P.M.P. and E.O.-S. All authors have read and agreed to the published version of the manuscript.

Funding: This research was funded by the Delaware Department of Health and Human Services, Division of Public Health. The APC was funded by authors Shannon M. Robson, P.M.P. and E.O.-S.

Institutional Review Board Statement: The study was conducted according to the guidelines of the Declaration of Helsinki, and approved by the Institutional Review Board of the University of Delaware (protocol code 81196-3 and date of approval: 22 September 2015).

Informed Consent Statement: Informed consent was obtained from all subjects involved in the study.

Data Availability Statement: The data presented in this study are not publicly available, but available on request from the corresponding author.

Conflicts of Interest: The authors declare no conflict of interest. The funders had no role in the design of the study; in the collection, analyses, or interpretation of data; in the writing of the manuscript, or in the decision to publish the results.

References

1. Hill, J.O.; Wyatt, H.R.; Peters, J.C. Energy balance and obesity. *Circulation* **2012**, *126*, 126–132. [CrossRef] [PubMed]
2. Sparling, P.B.; Franklin, B.A.; Hill, J.O. Energy balance: The key to a unified message on diet and physical activity. *J. Cardiopulm. Rehabil. Prev.* **2013**, *33*, 12–15. [CrossRef] [PubMed]
3. Hills, A.P.; Byrne, N.M.; Lindstrom, R.; Hill, J.O. 'Small changes' to diet and physical activity behaviors for weight management. *Obes. Facts* **2013**, *6*, 228–238. [CrossRef]
4. Hales, C.M.; Carroll, M.D.; Fryar, C.D.; Ogden, C.L. *Prevalence of Obesity and Severe Obesity Among Adults: United States, 2017–2018*; Brief, N.D., Ed.; National Center for Health Statistics: Hyattsville, MD, USA, 2020.
5. Krueger, P.M.; Reither, E.N. Mind the gap: Race/ethnic and socioeconomic disparities in obesity. *Curr. Diab. Rep.* **2015**, *15*, 95. [CrossRef] [PubMed]
6. James, W.P.; Nelson, M.; Ralph, A.; Leather, S. Socioeconomic determinants of health. The contribution of nutrition to inequalities in health. *BMJ* **1997**, *314*, 1545–1549. [CrossRef]
7. Asghari, G.; Mirmiran, P.; Yuzbashian, E.; Azizi, F. A systematic review of diet quality indices in relation to obesity. *Br. J. Nutr.* **2017**, *117*, 1055–1065. [CrossRef] [PubMed]
8. Hiza, H.A.; Casavale, K.; Guenther, P.; Davis, C.A. Diet quality of Americans differs by age, sex, race/ethnicity, income, and education level. *J. Acad Nutr. Diet.* **2013**, *113*, 297–306. [CrossRef]
9. Livingstone, K.M.; McNaughton, S.A. Diet quality is associated with obesity and hypertension in Australian adults: A cross sectional study. *BMC Public Health* **2016**, *16*, 1037. [CrossRef] [PubMed]

10. Krebs-Smith, S.M.; Pannucci, T.E.; Subar, A.F.; Kirkpatrick, S.I.; Lerman, J.L.; Tooze, J.A.; Wilson, M.M.; Reedy, J. Update of the Healthy Eating Index: HEI-2015. *J. Acad. Nutr. Diet.* **2018**, *118*, 1591–1602. [CrossRef]
11. Chin, S.H.; Kahathuduwa, C.N.; Binks, M. Physical activity and obesity: What we know and what we need to know. *Obes. Rev.* **2016**, *17*, 1226–1244. [CrossRef]
12. Sternberg, R.J. *The Modern Land-Grant University*; Purdue University Press: West Lafayette, IL, USA, 2014.
13. Franz, N.K. Measuring and articulating the value of community engagement: Lessons learned from 100 years of Cooperative Extension work. *J. High. Educ. Outreach Engagem.* **2014**, *18*, 5.
14. Vines, K.A. Exploration of engaged practice in Cooperative Extension and implications for higher education. *J. Ext.* **2018**, *56*, 24.
15. Franz, N.K.; Piercy, F.; Donaldson, J.; Richard, R.; Westbrook, J. How farmers learn: Implications for agricultural educators. *J. Rural. Soc. Sci.* **2010**, *25*, 37–59.
16. Fleischhacker, S.; Roberts, E.; Camplain, R.; Evenson, K.R.; Gittelsohn, J. Promoting physical activity among native American youth: A systematic review of the methodology and current evidence of physical activity interventions and community-wide initiatives. *J. Racial. Ethn. Health Disparities* **2016**, *3*, 608–624. [CrossRef] [PubMed]
17. Wieland, M.L.; Weis, J.A.; Palmer, T.; Goodson, M.; Loth, S.; Omer, F.; Abbenyi, A.; Krucker, K.; Edens, K.; Sia, I.G. Physical activity and nutrition among immigrant and refugee women: A community-based participatory research approach. *Womens Health Issues* **2012**, *22*, e225–e232. [CrossRef]
18. Coughlin, S.S.; Smith, S.A. Community-based participatory research to promote healthy diet and nutrition and prevent and control obesity among African-Americans: A literature review. *J. Racial. Ethn. Health Disparities* **2017**, *4*, 259–268. [CrossRef]
19. Pazoki, R.; Nabipour, I.; Seyednezami, N.; Imami, S.R. Effects of a community-based healthy heart program on increasing healthy women's physical activity: A randomized controlled trial guided by Community-based Participatory Research (CBPR). *BMC Public Health* **2007**, *7*, 216. [CrossRef]
20. Zoellner, J.; Connell, C.L.; Santell, R.; Fungwe, T.; Strickland, E.; Avis-Williams, A.; Yadrick, K.; Lofton, K.; Rowser, M.; Powers, A.; et al. Fit for life steps: Results of a community walking intervention in the rural Mississippi delta. *Prog. Community Health Partn.* **2007**, *1*, 49–60. [CrossRef]
21. de la Torre, A.; Sadeghi, B.; Green, R.D.; Kaiser, L.L.; Flores, Y.G.; Jackson, C.F.; Shaikh, U.; Whent, L.; Schaefer, S.E. Ninos sanos, familia sana: Mexican immigrant study protocol for a multifaceted CBPR intervention to combat childhood obesity in two rural California towns. *BMC Public Health* **2013**, *13*, 1033. [CrossRef]
22. Lohman, T.; Roche, A.; Martorell, K. *Anthropometric Standarization Reference Manual*; Human Kinetics Books: Champaign, IL, USA, 1988.
23. Ross, R.; Berentzen, T.; Bradshaw, A.J.; Janssen, I.; Kahn, H.S.; Katzmarzyk, P.T.; Kuk, J.L.; Seidell, J.C.; Snijder, M.B.; Sorensen, T.I.; et al. Does the relationship between waist circumference, morbidity and mortality depend on measurement protocol for waist circumference? *Obes. Rev.* **2008**, *9*, 312–325. [CrossRef]
24. Godin, G.; Shephard, R. Godin leisure-time exercise questionnaire. *Med. Sci. Sports Exerc.* **1997**, *29*, 36–38.
25. Godin, G. The godin-shephard leisure-time physical activity questionnaire. *Health Fit. J. Can.* **2011**, *4*, 18–22.
26. Fontenot, K.; Semega, J.; Kollar, M.; Bureau, U.S.C. *Income and Poverty in the United States: 2017*; Government Printing Office: Washington, DC, USA, 2018.
27. Luger, T.M.; Hamilton, A.B.; True, G. Measuring community-engaged research contexts, processes, and outcomes: A mapping review. *Milbank Q.* **2020**, *98*, 493–553. [CrossRef]
28. Jensen, M.D.; Ryan, D.H.; Apovian, C.M.; Ard, J.D.; Comuzzie, A.G.; Donato, K.A.; Hu, F.B.; Hubbard, V.S.; Jakicic, J.M.; Kushner, R.F.; et al. 2013 AHA/ACC/TOS guideline for the management of overweight and obesity in adults: A report of the American College of Cardiology/American heart association task force on practice guidelines and the obesity society. *Circulation* **2014**, *129* (Suppl. S2), S102–S138. [CrossRef]
29. Webb, V.L.; Wadden, T.A. Intensive lifestyle intervention for obesity: Principles, practices, and results. *Gastroenterology* **2017**, *152*, 1752–1764. [CrossRef] [PubMed]
30. Raynor, H.A.; Champagne, C.M. Position of the academy of nutrition and dietetics: Interventions for the treatment of overweight and obesity in adults. *J. Acad Nutr. Diet.* **2016**, *116*, 129–147. [CrossRef]
31. U.S. Department of Health and Human Service; U.S. Department of Agriculture. 2015–2020 Dietary Guidelines for Americans, 8th ed. 2015. Available online: https://health.gov/our-work/food-nutrition/previous-dietary-guidelines/2015 (accessed on 7 July 2021).
32. Concannon, T.W.; Fuster, M.; Saunders, T.; Patel, K.; Wong, J.B.; Leslie, L.K.; Lau, J. A systematic review of stakeholder engagement in comparative effectiveness and patient-centered outcomes research. *J. Gen. Intern. Med.* **2014**, *29*, 1692–1701. [CrossRef] [PubMed]
33. Brunton, G.; Thomas, J.; O'Mara-Eves, A.; Jamal, F.; Oliver, S.; Kavanagh, J. Narratives of community engagement: A systematic review-derived conceptual framework for public health interventions. *BMC Public Health* **2017**, *17*, 944. [CrossRef] [PubMed]
34. Wallerstein, N.; Duran, B. Community-based participatory research contributions to intervention research: The intersection of science and practice to improve health equity. *Am. J. Public Health* **2010**, *100* (Suppl. S1), S40–S46. [CrossRef]

35. O'Mara-Eves, A.; Brunton, G.; Oliver, S.; Kavanagh, J.; Jamal, F.; Thomas, J. The effectiveness of community engagement in public health interventions for disadvantaged groups: A meta-analysis. *BMC Public Health* **2015**, *15*, 129. [CrossRef] [PubMed]
36. Kamphuis, C.B.; Giskes, K.; de Bruijn, G.J.; Wendel-Vos, W.; Brug, J.; van Lenthe, F.J. Environmental determinants of fruit and vegetable consumption among adults: A systematic review. *Br. J. Nutr.* **2006**, *96*, 620–635. [PubMed]
37. U.S. Department of Agriculture; U.S. Department of Health and Human Services. Dietary Guidelines for Americans, 2020–2025. 9th Edition. December 2020. Available online: DietaryGuidelines.gov (accessed on 7 July 2021).

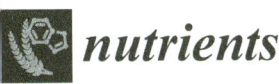

Article

Targeting Diet Quality at the Workplace: Influence on Cardiometabolic Risk

Samira Amil [1,2], Isabelle Lemieux [1], Paul Poirier [1,3], Benoît Lamarche [2,4], Jean-Pierre Després [1,5,6] and Natalie Alméras [1,5,*]

1. Centre de recherche de l'Institut universitaire de cardiologie et de pneumologie de Québec—Université Laval, Québec, QC G1V 4G5, Canada; samira.amil@criucpq.ulaval.ca (S.A.); isabelle.lemieux@criucpq.ulaval.ca (I.L.); paul.poirier@criucpq.ulaval.ca (P.P.); Jean-Pierre.Despres@criucpq.ulaval.ca (J.-P.D.)
2. École de nutrition, Faculté des sciences de l'agriculture et de l'alimentation, Université Laval, Québec, QC G1V 0A6, Canada; Benoit.Lamarche@fsaa.ulaval.ca
3. Faculty of Pharmacy, Université Laval, Québec, QC G1V 0A6, Canada
4. Centre Nutrition, santé et société (NUTRISS), Institut sur la nutrition et les aliments fonctionnels (INAF), Université Laval, Québec, QC G1V 0A6, Canada
5. Department of Kinesiology, Faculty of Medicine, Université Laval, Québec, QC G1V 0A6, Canada
6. VITAM—Centre de recherche en santé durable, CIUSSS de la Capitale-Nationale, Québec, QC G1J 0A4, Canada
* Correspondence: natalie.almeras@criucpq.ulaval.ca; Tel.: +1-418-656-8711 (ext. 3600)

Abstract: The American Heart Association criteria for cardiovascular health include overall diet quality (DQ). The present study evaluated the effect of a workplace health promotion program targeting DQ and physical activity on features of cardiometabolic risk (CMR). Before and after the 3-month intervention, 2260 employees (1462 men and 798 women) completed a health and fitness evaluation including assessment of DQ using a validated food-based questionnaire. After the 3-month lifestyle modification program, DQ increased significantly in both sexes ($p < 0.0001$) as well as physical activity level ($p < 0.0001$). A reduction in waist circumference ($p < 0.0001$) and improved lipid levels were also observed. Significant associations were found between changes in DQ index and changes in CMR variables in both men (standardized regression coefficients ranged from -0.19 (95% confidence interval: -0.26 to -0.12) to -0.29 (95% confidence interval: -0.34 to -0.25)) and women (standardized regression coefficients ranged from -0.18 (95% confidence interval: -0.25 to -0.11) to -0.27 (95% confidence interval: -0.41 to -0.13)). Multiple linear regression analyses showed a significant contribution of changes in the DQ index to the variation in some CMR variables, independent from changes in physical activity level and cardiorespiratory fitness. This study provides evidence that targeting DQ at the workplace is relevant to improve cardiometabolic health.

Keywords: abdominal obesity; cardiorespiratory fitness; hypertriglyceridemic waist phenotype; lifestyle intervention; diet quality index

1. Introduction

According to the World Health Organization, 41 million deaths annually are attributed to noncommunicable diseases, representing 71% of worldwide mortality [1]. Cardiovascular diseases (CVD) are the first cause of deaths accounting for 31% of global deaths [2]. This proportion increases to 37% in people under the age of 70. Thus, the prevalence of chronic diseases remains high despite advances in medical treatments and procedures as well as in efforts invested in primary prevention. As a consequence, the societal and economic burden linked to these diseases represents a major public health issue which may be not sustainable by health systems in the future. Such a situation emphasizes the relevance of developing upstream prevention strategies to slow the CVD tide and its associated socioeconomic consequences.

In order to address this issue, the American Heart Association (AHA) proposed in 2010 to move the focus from fighting CVD to promoting cardiovascular health and introduced the concept of ideal cardiovascular health as an approach to reduce the burden of CVD [3]. The AHA recommended to target seven heart-healthy metrics (Life's Simple 7), four of which are lifestyle-based (not smoking, increasing physical activity, having a normal body mass index (BMI), eating a healthy diet), while the three others are based on achieving ideal clinical and laboratory measures (having normal blood cholesterol and glucose levels and normal blood pressure). Maintaining these metrics as close as possible to ideal levels has been shown to be associated with markedly low CVD incidence and mortality as well as with a low incidence of cancer [4–6]. Among the seven metrics of cardiovascular health, studies have reported that the least prevalent healthy behavior was a high diet quality (DQ), a criterion which was found to be met by less than 1% of individuals, making DQ the most deteriorated parameter among ideal cardiovascular health metrics [7,8].

Therefore, considering that only a very small proportion of the population adopts a high DQ, modifying this factor could have a major beneficial impact on cardiovascular health [9]. Although there is no consensus definition on how to assess DQ, several indices have been developed for assessing a population's adherence to dietary patterns associated with cardiovascular health [10]. In this regard, DQ indices based on food items or food groups consumed rather than nutrients have been shown to provide good discrimination of CMR [11,12].

Among opportunities available, the workplace has been proposed as a relevant setting for implementing health promotion strategies [13,14]. According to 2019 statistics, the labor force participation rate in Canada was 65.8% [15], workers spending 6 to 9 h a day on average at their workplace. Thus, the environment provided by public/private employers has the potential to play a key role in the adoption of behaviors compatible with either maintenance of health or development of chronic diseases. In 2014, the World Health Organization proposed the workplace as a priority setting for health promotion [16]. To our knowledge, there is a paucity of published intervention studies conducted at the workplace that have targeted the adoption of healthy lifestyle habits including food-based overall DQ. The present study was therefore conducted to evaluate the relevance of assessing and targeting food-based overall DQ in the context of a workplace health promotion program and its effects on various indices of cardiometabolic health.

2. Materials and Methods

2.1. Participants

Our cohort is a convenience sample of employees involved in the "Grand Défi Entreprise" (GDE) project, a workplace health and wellness program which provided comprehensive cardiometabolic and cardiorespiratory health evaluations using a mobile risk assessment unit. Once the baseline evaluation is completed, the GDE also involves a 3-month lifestyle intervention where participating employees are asked to increase their physical activity level (PAL), improve their eating habits (DQ), and stop smoking [17,18].

All participants were volunteers. The intervention program took place between 2011 and 2019 and involved 28 participating organizations of the Province of Québec. No inclusion or exclusion criteria were used. This paper compares the CMR data at baseline and after the 3-month lifestyle intervention program obtained on a sample of 2260 workers (1462 men and 798 women) derived from an initial cohort of 5122 workers. Therefore, participants who did not participate to the intervention were excluded as well as participants with missing DQ data either at baseline or at the 3-month evaluation (see Figure 1 for Flowchart).

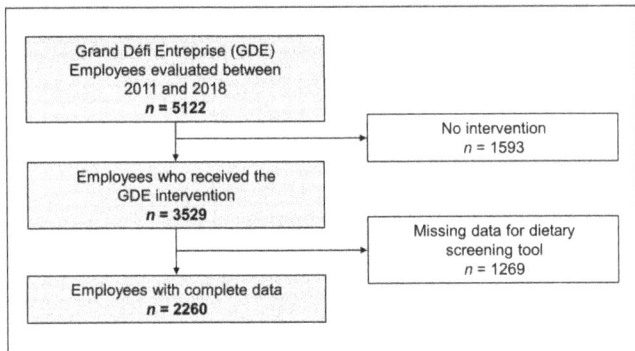

Figure 1. Flowchart of participants and reasons for exclusion for the present analyses.

All measurements were performed in a single visit at baseline and at 3 months by trained healthcare professionals. All participants completed standardized questionnaires on medical history, current medication, and lifestyle behaviors (DQ, PAL, and smoking status). Data included anthropometric variables, body composition, waist circumference, lipid profile, and cardiorespiratory fitness (CRF). The local Institutional Review Board approved the study (20636), and participants provided their informed consent.

2.2. Assessment of Overall Diet Quality

The dietary screening tool (DST) [19] was selected to assess DQ. This questionnaire has been found helpful to provide personalized food-based nutritional recommendations to workers. Further details on this tool have already been published [20]. Compared to other DQ indices, this tool does not evaluate adherence to nutrition guidelines or dietary patterns [21,22]. The DST is based on the frequency of consumption of several food items or food groups (vegetables and fruits, grain products, dairy products, meat, and substitutes) as well as on the assessment of certain dietary habits such as the addition of sugar and fat, the consumption of alcohol, or the use of nutritional supplements. This questionnaire consists of 25 food- and behavior-specific questions associated with dietary habits and generates a DQ score, which varies from 0 (low DQ) to 100 (high DQ) [19]. The DST is therefore useful to identify, in 10 min, individuals at high nutritional risk which is one of its strengths.

2.3. Physical Activity Level

Reported PAL was measured at baseline using a self-administered, validated questionnaire that assesses leisure-time aerobic physical activity (cycling, walking, running, swimming, etc.) for each season during the year preceding the intervention [23]. During the 3-month intervention, using an electronic journal, workers compiled each aerobic period of 15 min of physical activity in their leisure time for the assessment of the cumulative physical activity time during a week. An average number of total minutes per week was subsequently calculated.

2.4. Anthropometric Measurements and Body Composition

Height and weight were obtained both at baseline and post-intervention according to standardized procedures, and BMI was calculated [24]. Waist circumference was assessed using standardized procedures [25]. Body composition (fat mass and body fat) was estimated with the Tanita body composition analyzer TBF-300A (Tanita Corporation, Arlington Heights, IL, USA) for the employees from organizations evaluated between 2011 and 2017. From 2018, the InBody 570 body composition analyzer was used (InBody Co., Seoul, Korea).

2.5. Lipid Profile

Nonfasting blood samples obtained from the forearm vein were collected into lithium heparin tubes and analyzed with an Abaxis Piccolo Xpress Chemistry Analyzer (Union City, CA, USA) to assess cholesterol fractions and triglyceride (TG) concentrations.

2.6. Cardiorespiratory Fitness

As already published, a submaximal treadmill exercise test was performed to assess CRF [17,26]. Maximal oxygen consumption (VO$_2$max) was estimated by linear extrapolation [27] to age estimated maximal heart rate (220-age) [28] using ACSM's Metabolic Equations and the least square method [29]. Two parameters were used as CRF endpoints: the heart rate at the standardized submaximal exercise workload (3.5 mph, 2% slope) and the estimated VO$_2$max.

2.7. Hypertriglyceridemic Waist Phenotype

The hypertriglyceridemic waist (hyperTG waist) phenotype was used to identify individuals with visceral obesity and at risk for cardiometabolic abnormalities [30,31]. Criteria used were waist circumference ≥ 90.0 cm and TG ≥ 2.0 mmol/L for men or waist circumference ≥ 85.0 cm and TG ≥ 1.5 mmol/L for women [30,31].

2.8. Lifestyle Intervention

Details on the intervention have been published elsewhere [17]. After the baseline evaluation, workers were invited to form teams of five individuals to participate in an in-house competition. Throughout the 3-month intervention, physical activity and nutritional objectives were compiled on a web platform. Such ongoing collection of participants' key behaviors made it possible to establish the team's ranking in real time. The platform served as a lifestyle journal as well as a means to share and communicate progress within the team and at the workplace. Workers also received tips and recommendations. This friendly competition favored peer support helping individual changes in lifestyle habits. At the end of the intervention, prize incentives were offered by the management of participating organizations.

2.9. Statistical Analyses

Sex differences in baseline characteristics were tested by an unpaired t-test. A repeated measures analysis of variance was used to examine changes in variables between baseline and the 3-month follow-up. The normality assumption was verified with the Shapiro–Wilk test on residuals from the statistical model. The Brown and Forsythe's variation of Levene's test statistic was used to verify the homogeneity of variances. For most of the variables, these assumptions were not fulfilled. A repeated measures analysis of variance on ranks was therefore performed using the approach proposed by Brunner et al. [32]. As a significant sex*time interaction term was found for many cardiometabolic variables, analyses have been performed by sex. The McNemar's test for paired data was performed to analyze changes in the proportion of hyperTG waist carriers. Pearson's correlations were computed to measure the association between changes in the DQ index or PAL and changes in CMR variables. To investigate the relationship between changes in DQ or changes in PAL with changes in CMR risk variables, multiple linear regression models were performed. All statistical regression models were adjusted for medication use for lipids, hypertension, and diabetes as well as menopausal status in women. A second model including waist circumference was also performed, and the effect of potential confounding variables such as medication use for lipids, hypertension, and diabetes as well as menopausal status (in women) was further examined. Lastly, the potential contribution of interaction terms among studied variables was also assessed in regression analyses. Models with the lowest Akaike information criterion (AIC) were chosen. Finally, a one-way analysis of variance adjusted for baseline DQ index was performed to compare changes in CMR variables between quartiles of changes in the DQ index with Tukey–Kramer's post hoc corrections for multiple comparisons. A p value ≤ 0.05

was considered as statistically significant. All statistical analyses were performed using SAS statistical package version 9.4 (SAS Institute, Cary, NC, USA).

3. Results

The mean age of the 2260 participants was 44.3 ± 10.1 years in men and 42.4 ± 10.6 years in women (range: 19 to 76 years of age), and 64.7% of participants were men. Almost half of participants were blue-collar workers (46.8%). Additional sociodemographic characteristics are presented in Table 1. At baseline, 40.5% of employees were overweight and 25.6% met the criteria for obesity (BMI $\geq$ 30 kg/m^2). The prevalence of pre-existing treated diabetes and hypertension was 2.7% and 11.1%, respectively, and 10.2% of participants self-reported a history of dyslipidemia. Moreover, 13.7% of workers were active smokers or former smokers <12 months, and 56.9% of participants had never smoked.

Table 1. Employees' sociodemographic characteristics.

Variables	%
Sex	
Male	64.7
Female	35.3
Ethnicity	
Caucasian	94.3
Afro-Canadian	1.3
Latino-Canadian	0.9
Asian	0.4
First Nations	0.3
Others	2.9
Marital status	
Married/cohabiting	74.8
Unmarried	18.1
Separated/divorced	6.6
Widow/widower	0.5
Employee categories	
White collar	39.7
Blue collar	46.8
Unknown	13.5
Household income	
Low (<CAN 50,000)	26.6
Medium (CAN 50,000–80,000)	14.1
High (>CAN 80,000)	54.2
Unknown	5.2
Education	
<High school	3.9
High school	36.9
College	29.3
University	19.9
Post-graduate	10.0

Table 2 presents anthropometric, body composition, and lifestyle variables as well as CRF before and after the 3-month lifestyle modification program. A significant improvement of 7 units in the DQ index was observed in both sexes ($p < 0.0001$). At the end of the intervention, participants became significantly more active as revealed by the increase in PAL ($p < 0.0001$). Accordingly, the estimated VO$_2$max also improved significantly in men ($p < 0.0001$), whereas the increase was of borderline significance in women ($p = 0.055$). As an additional CRF indicator, heart rate at a standardized exercise workload decreased significantly in both sexes ($p < 0.0001$ and $p < 0.05$ in men and women, respectively). These changes were accompanied by significant reductions in BMI, waist circumference, fat mass, and percent body fat in both sexes ($p < 0.0001$).

Table 2. Employees' characteristics as well as markers of lifestyle habits before and after the 3-month lifestyle modification program.

	Baseline	3 Months	Δ
Men			
Anthropometric measurements and body composition (n)	1430–1462	1459–1462	1429–1462
Body mass index (kg/m^2)	27.4 (24.9, 30.4)	26.8 (24.3, 29.4)	−0.5 (−1.1, 0.0) *
Waist circumference (cm)	97.0 (89.3, 104.9)	92.9 (85.9, 100.6)	−3.4 (−5.8, −1.2) *
Fat mass (kg)	20.4 (15.3, 26.8)	18.6 (14.1, 24.5)	−1.3 (−3.1, −0.1) *
Body fat (%)	24.4 (20.1, 28.7)	22.8 (18.9, 26.8)	−1.2 (−2.8, 0.0) *
Lifestyle habits (n)	1462	1452–1462	1452–1462
Diet quality index	61 (52, 70)	69 (60, 76)	7 (1, 14) *
Physical activity level (min/week)	210 (84, 378)	222 (131, 339)	18 (−108, 121) *
Cardiorespiratory profile (n)	1384–1441	684–708	669–702
Exercise heart rate (bpm)	112 (103, 121)	108 (100, 115)	−4 (−10, 2) *
Estimated VO$_2$max (mL/min/kg)	41.5 (35.5, 48.3)	43.2 (36.7, 51.5)	1.9 (−3.0, 7.2) *
Women			
Anthropometric measurements and body composition (n)	793–798	798	793–798
Body mass index (kg/m^2)	25.0 (22.1, 28.9)	24.5 (21.7, 28.4)	−0.4 (−0.9, 0.1) *
Waist circumference (cm)	85.3 (77.1, 96.8)	82.8 (75.2, 93.4)	−2.5 (−5.1, −0.1) *
Fat mass (kg)	21.7 (15.9, 30.0)	20.8 (14.6, 28.3)	−1.1 (−2.5, 0.1) *
Body fat (%)	33.0 (27.2, 39.5)	31.7 (25.7, 38.1)	−1.2 (−2.5, 0.1) *
Lifestyle habits (n)	798	798	798
Diet quality index	65 (57, 72)	72 (65, 79)	7 (1, 13) *
Physical activity level (min/week)	168 (84, 294)	211 (132, 314)	37 (−61, 126) *
Cardiorespiratory profile (n)	725–776	170–176	164–173
Exercise heart rate (bpm)	125 (114, 135)	120 (109, 131)	−3 (−9, 5) ‡
Estimated VO$_2$max (mL/min/kg)	33.0 (27.7, 39.8)	34.1 (28.9, 40.5)	1.0 (−2.7, 5.1) §

Data represent median and interquartile range (25th and 75th percentile). n: range of participants. ‡ $p < 0.05$; * $p < 0.0001$; § $p = 0.055$.

The plasma lipid profile also improved significantly after the 3-month lifestyle modification program (Table 3). For instance, total cholesterol, TG, and non-high-density lipoprotein (non-HDL) cholesterol concentrations declined significantly in both men ($p < 0.0001$) and women ($p < 0.05$). Significant decreases in low-density lipoprotein (LDL) cholesterol levels and the cholesterol/HDL cholesterol ratio were also observed in men ($p < 0.0001$). HDL cholesterol increased in men ($p < 0.0001$), whereas it decreased in women ($p < 0.001$) (Table 3).

Table 3. Plasma lipid profile before and after the 3-month lifestyle modification program.

	Baseline	3 Months	Δ
Men			
Lipid variables (n)	1418–1462	721–728	712–728
Total cholesterol (mmol/L)	4.70 (4.10, 5.30)	4.40 (3.90, 5.00)	−0.20 (−0.50, 0.10) *
LDL cholesterol (mmol/L)	2.50 (2.00, 3.00)	2.40 (2.00, 2.80)	−0.10 (−0.40, 0.20) *
HDL cholesterol (mmol/L)	1.25 (1.07, 1.47)	1.25 (1.07, 1.45)	0.03 (−0.07, 0.13) *
Non-HDL cholesterol (mmol/L)	3.40 (2.85, 3.95)	3.16 (2.64, 3.65)	−0.20 (−0.50, 0.09) *
Cholesterol/HDL cholesterol	3.70 (3.10, 4.30)	3.50 (3.00, 4.20)	−0.20 (−0.56, 0.10) *
Triglycerides (mmol/L)	1.81 (1.23, 2.72)	1.44 (1.00, 2.26)	−0.26 (−0.85, 0.22) *
Women			
Lipid variables (n)	780–794	180–182	179–182
Total cholesterol (mmol/L)	4.60 (4.10, 5.10)	4.40 (4.00, 5.10)	−0.10 (−0.40, 0.20) †
LDL cholesterol (mmol/L)	2.40 (2.00, 2.80)	2.40 (2.00, 2.80)	0.00 (−0.30, 0.20) ‡
HDL cholesterol (mmol/L)	1.60 (1.34, 1.80)	1.44 (1.28, 1.68)	−0.02 (−0.15, 0.10) †
Non-HDL cholesterol (mmol/L)	2.97 (2.48, 3.51)	2.94 (2.48, 3.41)	−0.12 (−0.34, 0.13) ‡
Cholesterol/HDL cholesterol	2.90 (2.50, 3.40)	3.10 (2.60, 3.50)	−0.10 (−0.30, 0.10)
Triglycerides (mmol/L)	1.18 (0.87, 1.69)	1.05 (0.79, 1.55)	−0.10 (−0.40, 0.14) *

Data represent median and interquartile range (25th and 75th percentile). HDL: high-density lipoprotein; LDL: low-density lipoprotein; n: range of participants. ‡ $p < 0.05$; † $p < 0.001$; * $p < 0.0001$.

Figure 2 presents changes in the proportion of hyperTG waist [30,31] in response to the workplace intervention program. Although the proportion of the hyperTG waist phenotype decreased in both sexes, the reduction only reached significance in men ($p < 0.0001$). In addition, relative changes in TG levels were significantly correlated with relative changes in waist circumference (r = 0.29, $p < 0.0001$, for both men and women).

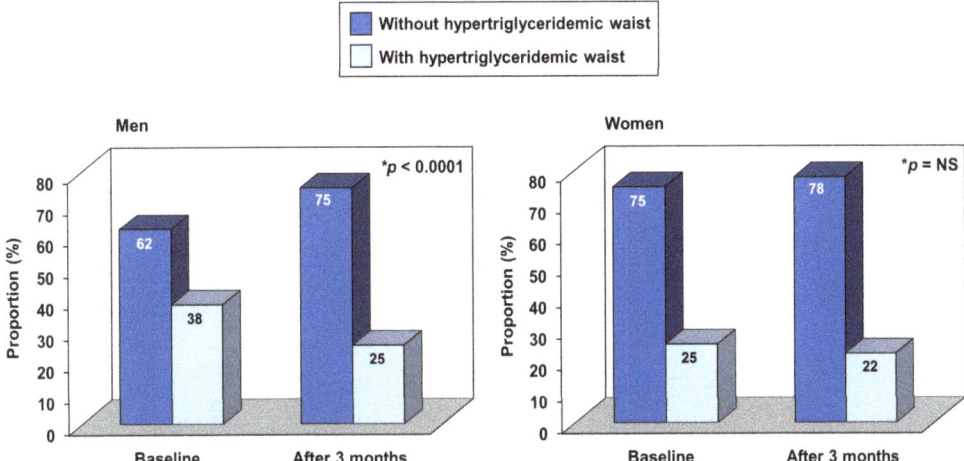

Figure 2. Changes in carriers of the hypertriglyceridemic waist phenotype in response to the 3-month lifestyle modification program. * The statistical difference has been quantified according to the McNemar's test.

Several significant negative relationships were observed between changes in the DQ index or PAL and changes in CMR markers (Figure 3). For instance, increases in the DQ index and PAL were associated with decreases in BMI, waist circumference, total cholesterol, non-HDL cholesterol, and TG. To examine the relationship between changes in the DQ index and changes in the CMR profile further, quartiles of changes in the DQ index were compared (Figure 4). This analysis revealed that men in the top quartile of change in the DQ index were also those who showed the most substantial reduction in waist circumference ($p < 0.0001$). They were also characterized by greater reductions in TG and non-HDL cholesterol levels compared to men in the first two quartiles ($p < 0.05$). In women, only changes in TG were significantly different across quartiles of changes in the DQ index ($p < 0.05$).

To quantify the independent associations of changes in the DQ index, PAL, and submaximal exercise heart rate to the 3-month variation in CMR markers, multiple linear regression analyses were performed (Table 4). In men, changes in anthropometric measures and body composition variables were mainly associated with the change in the DQ index ($p < 0.0001$) with smaller but significant associations of changes in PAL and exercise heart rate. On the other hand, in women, changes in PAL significantly contributed to explain changes in body composition indices, while changes in waist circumference and BMI were more associated with changes in the DQ index. Moreover, in men, changes in the lipid profile were explained by changes in the DQ index, PAL, and exercise heart rate. However, in women, changes in PAL contributed the most to overall changes in blood lipids ($p < 0.05$) except for changes in TG levels which were only associated with changes in the DQ index ($p < 0.001$). Finally, in order to examine to what extent the beneficial effect of DQ and PAL on CMR factors could be confounded by concurrent changes in waist circumference, this variable was added to the linear regression analysis (Table 5). In men, adjusting for waist circumference largely attenuated the association between changes in DQ and lipid variables. In women, changes in DQ and in PAL remained significantly associated with changes in several lipid variables even after adjustment for concurrent changes in waist circumference.

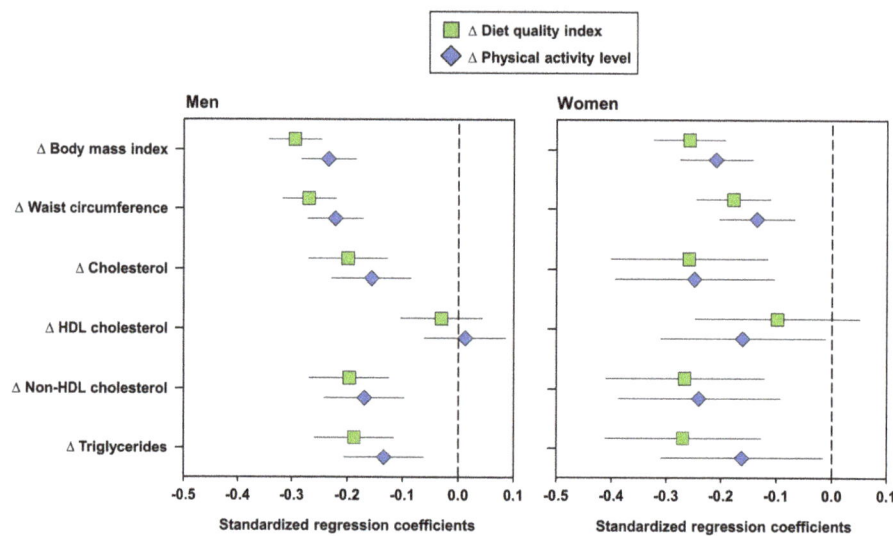

Figure 3. Standardized regression coefficients (with 95% confidence intervals) for the association between changes in diet quality index or physical activity level and changes in cardiometabolic risk markers in men and women. Models are adjusted for medication use (lipids, hypertension, and diabetes) and menopausal status in women. HDL: high-density lipoprotein.

Table 4. Multiple linear regression models showing the independent associations of changes in diet quality index, physical activity level, and exercise heart rate on changes in cardiometabolic markers.

	Total $R^2 \times 100$	Partial $R^2 \times 100$ Δ DQ Index	Partial $R^2 \times 100$ Δ PAL	Partial $R^2 \times 100$ Δ Exercise HR
Men				
Anthropometric measurements and body composition (n = 669–697)				
Δ Body mass index	15.7	10.5 *	1.5 †	3.6 *
Δ Waist circumference	13.8	10.7 *	1.8 †	1.3 ‡
Δ Fat mass	13.7	11.0 *	1.2 ‡	1.5 †
Δ Body fat	9.6	8.3 *	0.9 ‡	0.5
Lipid profile (n = 678–694)				
Δ Total cholesterol	5.8	4.1 *	1.7 †	–
Δ LDL cholesterol	0.4	0.4	–	–
Δ HDL cholesterol	1.8	0.4	–	1.5 ‡
Δ Non-HDL cholesterol	5.8	3.8 *	2.0 †	–
Δ Cholesterol/HDL cholesterol	4.4	0.9 ‡	2.4 *	1.1 ‡
Δ Triglycerides	5.9	3.2 *	1.3 ‡	1.5 ‡
Women				
Anthropometric measurements and body composition (n = 168–173)				
Δ Body mass index	9.7	6.4 †	3.3 ‡	–
Δ Waist circumference	9.5	5.9 ‡	3.5 ‡	–
Δ Fat mass	14.5	3.0 ‡	11.5 *	–
Δ Body fat	11.5	–	11.5 *	–
Lipid profile (n = 170–173)				
Δ Total cholesterol	14.0	4.6 ‡	9.4 *	–
Δ LDL cholesterol	2.4	–	2.4 ‡	–
Δ HDL cholesterol	4.3	–	4.3 ‡	–
Δ Non-HDL cholesterol	12.9	4.6 ‡	8.3 †	–
Δ Cholesterol/HDL cholesterol	–	–	–	–
Δ Triglycerides	9.2	7.9 †	1.3	–

DQ: diet quality; HDL: high-density lipoprotein; HR: heart rate; LDL: low-density lipoprotein; PAL: physical activity level; n: range of participants; – not included in the model due to lack of significance; ‡ p < 0.05; † p < 0.001; * p < 0.0001.

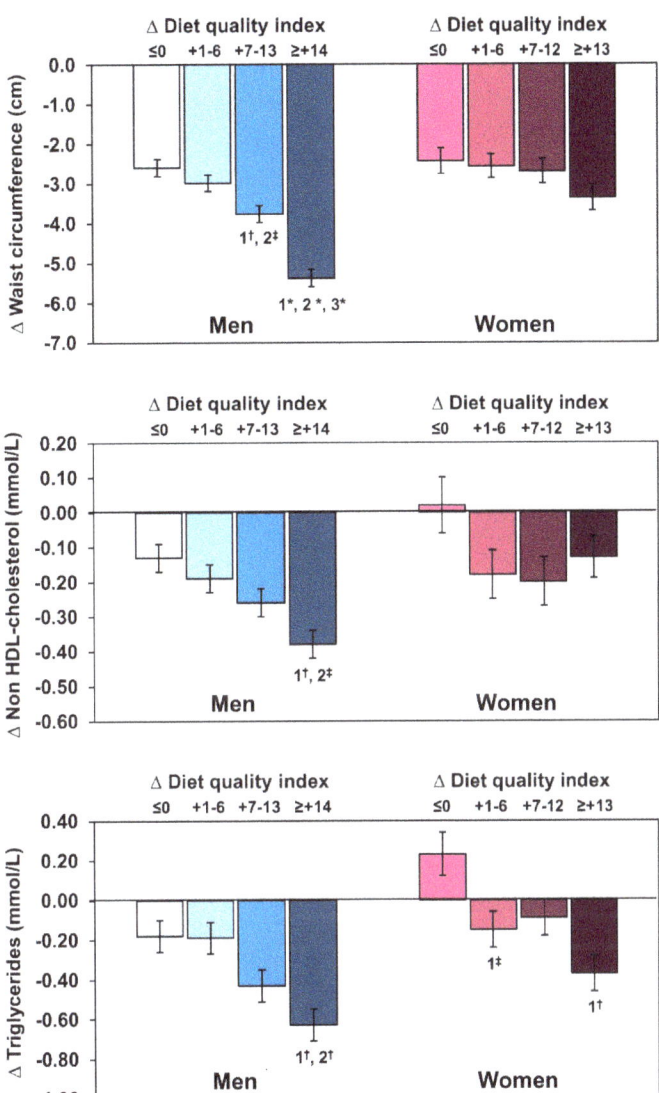

Figure 4. Changes in waist circumference, non-HDL cholesterol, and triglycerides according to quartiles of changes in diet quality index in response to the 3-month lifestyle modification program. Data represent least-squares means ± standard error to the mean adjusted for the baseline diet quality index. ‡ $p < 0.05$; † $p < 0.001$; * $p < 0.0001$.

Table 5. Multiple linear regression models showing the independent associations of changes in diet quality index, physical activity level, exercise heart rate, and waist circumference on changes in lipid variables.

	Total $R^2 \times 100$	Partial $R^2 \times 100$ Δ DQ Index	Partial $R^2 \times 100$ Δ PAL	Partial $R^2 \times 100$ Δ Exercise HR	Partial $R^2 \times 100$ Δ Waist
Men					
Lipid profile (n = 678–694)					
Δ Total cholesterol	9.8	1.4 ‡	1.0 ‡	–	7.3 *
Δ LDL cholesterol	0.8	–	–	0.3	0.5
Δ HDL cholesterol	1.8	0.4	–	1.5 ‡	–
Δ Non-HDL cholesterol	12.4	0.6 ‡	1.3 ‡	–	10.5 *
Δ Cholesterol/HDL cholesterol	9.9	–	1.0 ‡	0.5	8.4 *
Δ Triglycerides	11.4	0.5	0.8 ‡	0.8 ‡	9.4 *
Women					
Lipid profile (n = 170–173)					
Δ Total cholesterol	17.1	3.1 ‡	9.4 *	–	4.6 ‡
Δ LDL cholesterol	2.4	–	2.4 ‡	–	–
Δ HDL cholesterol	4.3	–	4.3 ‡	–	–
Δ Non-HDL cholesterol	16.1	3.0 ‡	8.3 †	–	4.8 ‡
Δ Cholesterol/HDL cholesterol	–	–	–	–	–
Δ Triglycerides	13.4	4.6 ‡	–	–	8.9 *

DQ: diet quality; HDL: high-density lipoprotein; HR: heart rate; LDL: low-density lipoprotein; PAL: physical activity level; n: range of participants; – not included in the model due to lack of significance; ‡ $p < 0.05$; † $p < 0.001$; * $p < 0.0001$.

Additional statistical analyses were performed in order to control for menopausal status and medication use (lipids, hypertension, diabetes). After taking into account these potential confounding variables, similar findings were observed (Supplementary Table S1). Lastly, the potential contribution of interaction terms among studied variables was assessed. In women, results did not change following the addition of interaction terms into multiple linear regression analyses. In men, interaction terms only significantly contributed to changes in the cholesterol/HDL cholesterol ratio and changes in TG levels. The interaction between changes in PAL and changes in waist circumference (R^2: 1.7%, $p < 0.001$) as well as changes in waist circumference (R^2: 8.4%, $p < 0.0001$) and changes in exercise heart rate (R^2: 0.5%, $p \leq 0.05$) contributed to explain changes in the cholesterol/HDL cholesterol ratio. In addition, the interaction between changes in exercise heart rate and changes in waist circumference (R^2: 1.2%, $p < 0.05$) contributed to explain changes in TG levels along with changes in waist circumference (R^2: 9.4%, $p < 0.0001$), changes in PAL (R^2: 0.8%, $p < 0.05$), and changes in DQ (R^2: 0.5%, $p \leq 0.05$).

4. Discussion

In the present study, our objectives were to evaluate whether: 1—DQ could be improved by our workplace lifestyle modification program; and 2—changes in DQ would have a favorable influence on features of cardiometabolic health. Results of the present study provide evidence that food markers of overall DQ can be assessed and targeted at the workplace in order to improve cardiometabolic health substantially. For instance, a large proportion of participants (76%) improved their DQ index (by at least 1 unit) after the 3-month intervention program. Among these participants, the median increase in DQ index was 10 (interquartile range: 5, 16) in men and was 9 (interquartile range: 5, 16) units in women. In a previous cross-sectional analysis conducted on our cohort of male and female workers that used the same DQ assessment tool, we had previously reported marked differences in features of CMR when employees were classified on the basis of their DQ index [20].

Results of this intervention show that DQ can be assessed and targeted at the workplace. Indeed, in our study, changes in a simple food-based index were accompanied by significant reductions in waist circumference and by improved lipid levels. To our knowledge, there are only a few published intervention studies targeting lifestyle changes at the workplace that included a large number of employees which assessed a comprehensive

CMR profile (e.g., body fat distribution, lipid levels, submaximal treadmill exercise test). In a workplace-based lifestyle intervention program conducted in a sample of employees at high risk of CVD and involving a team of health professionals (nurse practitioner, registered dietician, exercise physiologist, certified diabetic educator, and registered nurse), Rouseff et al. [33] reported significant improvements in several CMR markers such as percent body fat, blood pressure, lipid parameters, as well as CRF. One novel aspect of our study is our finding that it appears possible to target overall DQ with a food-based approach instead of using traditional nutritional interventions focused on dietary fat reduction and/or caloric restriction in order to have beneficial impacts on cardiometabolic health. Such an approach is in line with recent recommendations of nutrition experts [9,11,34,35]. As previously reported [20], we found significant differences in DQ, men having a poorer DQ index than women at baseline (mean ± SD: 60.5 ± 12.3 and 64.2 ± 11.6, for men and women, respectively, $p < 0.0001$). However, both sexes significantly improved their DQ in response to the program (by 7 units). Additionally, men of the present study were characterized by a more deteriorated baseline CMR profile than women (data not shown), although significant changes were observed in both sexes. In this regard, greater improvements in CMR markers are expected in men since lifestyle interventions have a greater effect on CVD risk factors in higher-risk populations [17,33,36–38]. In addition, in both men and women, changes in DQ were found to be associated with changes in adiposity and lipid levels (Figure 3). These findings show that the food-based index of DQ could discriminate CMR. In addition, our findings indicate that being successful in implementing meaningful changes in DQ as measured by this index predicted significant changes in CMR variables. Targeting DQ with a brief and food-based strategy has been effectively shown to improve DQ and reported to be as effective as other lifestyle interventions in improving CMR markers [39–44].

One unique feature of this workplace intervention aiming at improving DQ is that we also simultaneously considered PAL and CRF as important potential confounders of cardiometabolic health in our statistical analyses. Of course, one cannot exclude the possibility that employees who showed the most substantial improvements in their DQ were also those who became the most physically active. In this regard, it has been reported that the most active individuals are also those characterized by a better DQ [45]. In line with this possibility, we found a weak but significant association between changes in the DQ index and changes in PAL ($r = 0.22$, $p < 0.0001$ and $r = 0.27$, $p < 0.0001$ in men and women, respectively). In the present study, we found that whereas CRF assessed by estimated VO_2max was significantly increased in men, the change in VO_2max was only of borderline significance in women. However, submaximal HR was decreased in both men and women, a finding clearly showing that the change in PAL induced an improvement in submaximal working capacity in both sexes, while not being enough to improve maximal oxygen consumption in women. These results suggest that women may have responded to the lifestyle intervention by improving further their DQ and by doing more physical activity of moderate intensity, whereas men may have performed more vigorous physical activity. Although we did not assess physical activity intensity in the present study, it has been reported that VO_2max is more likely to be improved with higher-intensity endurance exercise [46,47], while low-intensity exercise may not always be sufficient to improve CRF [48,49]. This sex difference in how workers adopted different strategies to improve their lifestyle habits will require further investigation.

Therefore, changes in PAL observed at the end of the 3-month intervention program may have also contributed to explain the beneficial changes found in CMR markers. This notion is supported by findings showing that across quartiles of DQ index changes, a reduction in waist circumference was observed (Figure 4). Moreover, in both sexes, changes in PAL were also associated with changes in features of cardiometabolic health (Figure 3). Thus, one novel aspect of our workplace intervention was to quantify the respective contributions of changes in the DQ index vs. changes in PAL to the improvement of cardiometabolic health. To examine this issue, we performed multiple linear regression analyses which revealed that in men, changes in the DQ index were related to changes in most features of CMR, with a modest but significant additional contribution of changes in PAL and CRF (Table 4). In women, whereas changes in the DQ index were independently associated with changes in CMR variables, changes in PAL had a major influence on the variation in adiposity variables, with no independent influence of CRF. While we propose that such potential sex differences should deserve further attention, we put forward the hypothesis that since women had a better DQ and were less physically active than men at baseline, their increase in physical activity, despite not being performed at the intensity required to improve maximal oxygen consumption (estimated by the VO_2max), it could have nevertheless played a role in inducing weight loss and loss of abdominal fat (waist circumference). In men, we propose that since their DQ was lower than women at baseline, improving their DQ and performing more vigorous physical activity which translated into improved CRF could be key contributing factors to explain the beneficial effects of the program on their cardiometabolic health.

Finally, as both men and women reduced their waist circumference in response to the program, a key remaining question was to test whether improving DQ had an influence on CMR after controlling for concomitant changes in waist circumference. Our findings are concordant with the notion that changes in waist circumference in men largely explained the influence of changes in DQ on lipid variables, whereas in women changes in DQ and PAL remained associated with changes in several lipid variables after controlling for changes in waist circumference (Table 5). These results suggest that while targeting food-based DQ is relevant to improve cardiometabolic health, the concomitant effect of such an intervention (diet and physical activity) on waist circumference is an important contributor to the association between DQ and cardiometabolic health. As already highlighted in a consensus paper [50], the reduction in waist circumference through lifestyle changes is likely to generate a decrease in morbidity and mortality risk by improving intermediate CMR markers. One of the reasons explaining this beneficial association would be the mobilization of the high-risk visceral fat generated by the lifestyle modification program [51]. Although not measured, we can speculate that employees of the present study for whom a reduction in waist circumference was observed were also characterized by a reduction in visceral fat as suggested by the decrease in carriers of the hyperTG waist phenotype, a clinical marker of visceral obesity [30,31].

A strength of our workplace lifestyle intervention program is the collection of a comprehensive CMR profile including the evaluation of CRF by a submaximal exercise treadmill test. In addition, our study sample was heterogeneous in terms of education level, socio-economic status, health profile, and job characteristics and demands. In order to make sure that we could evaluate the effects of our program on a population as heterogeneous as possible in terms of baseline characteristics, we had no criteria for employees' inclusion or exclusion. Furthermore, this study is a unique "real world intervention", as it took place in different and uncontrolled work environments. The DST allows us to assess overall DQ without any intermediate method (24 h recall, quantitative food frequency questionnaire, etc.).

However, our study has some limitations. Firstly, despite the fact that we did not have inclusion/exclusion criteria, it is obvious that our sample of workers is not representative of the entire workforce as all participants were volunteers, an obvious selection bias. These participants are most likely to be more health-conscious and consequently may had responded to the program to a greater extent compared to the general population. Moreover, although we used a validated questionnaire, PAL is notoriously over-reported when compared to direct measurements [52] at baseline. Thereby, the change in PAL may be underestimated by an overestimation of baseline PAL. Thus, its independent contribution to variations in the CMR profile may have been underestimated in the regression model. Secondly, as our intervention is short term (3 months), there is clearly a need to document the long-term impact of that type of program. As a consequence, we cannot speculate about the long-term effect and adherence to our intervention.

5. Conclusions

In summary, this pragmatic 3-month lifestyle intervention provides evidence that a key behavior influencing cardiometabolic health such as DQ can be assessed and targeted at the workplace using a simple food-based questionnaire. Furthermore, the contribution of changes in DQ to the improvement in CMR remained significant after controlling for changes in PAL. Improving DQ through lifestyle interventions in the workplace may have direct effects on CMR, particularly in women, as well as indirect effects on both men and women through effects on abdominal adiposity. Finally, findings of the present study support the proposal from a recent consensus group that waist circumference is a simple and useful marker of the influence of healthy/unhealthy behaviors [50].

Supplementary Materials: The following are available online at https://www.mdpi.com/article/10.3390/nu13072283/s1, Table S1: Multiple linear regression models showing the independent associations of changes in diet quality index, physical activity level, exercise heart rate, waist circumference, medication use (lipids, hypertension, diabetes) and menopausal status on changes in lipid variables.

Author Contributions: P.P., J.-P.D., N.A. designed the study (project conception, development of overall research plan, and study oversight) and managed the research (hands-on conduct of the experiments and data collection); J.-P.D., N.A. provided the database; S.A., I.L., J.-P.D., N.A. examined data or performed statistical analyses; S.A. drafted the manuscript; S.A. and I.L. prepared figures; and I.L., P.P., B.L., J.-P.D., N.A. edited and revised the manuscript; S.A., I.L., J.-P.D., N.A. reviewed and approved the final version of the manuscript. All authors have read and agreed to the published version of the manuscript.

Funding: This study was partly supported by an unrestricted grant from Pfizer, by the Foundation of the Institut universitaire de cardiologie et de pneumologie de Québec, as well as by a Foundation grant from the Canadian Institutes of Health Research (FDN-167278). The project is the result of a consortium between the Grand Défi Entreprise Inc. and the Institut universitaire de cardiologie et de pneumologie de Québec—Université Laval. Jean-Pierre Després is the Scientific Director of the International Chair on Cardiometabolic Risk, which is based at Université Laval.

Institutional Review Board Statement: The present study was conducted according to the guidelines laid down in the Declaration of Helsinki, and all procedures involving human subjects were approved by the local Institutional Review Board (20636).

Informed Consent Statement: Informed consent was obtained from all subjects involved in the study. Participants provided written informed consent prior to enrollment into the study.

Data Availability Statement: The data presented are available on request from the corresponding author.

Acknowledgments: The authors would like to express their gratitude to all companies and participating employees for their commitment to the Grand Défi Entreprise workplace health program.

Conflicts of Interest: The authors declare no conflict of interest. The Grand Défi Entreprise Inc. was not involved in the analysis and interpretation of the data, nor in the writing of this paper.

References

1. World Health Organization. Noncommunicable Diseases: Key Facts. 2018. Available online: https://www.who.int/news-room/fact-sheets/detail/noncommunicable-diseases (accessed on 20 February 2021).
2. World Health Organization. Cardiovascular Diseases (CVDs): Key Facts. 2017. Available online: https://www.who.int/news-room/fact-sheets/detail/cardiovascular-diseases-(cvds) (accessed on 21 February 2021).
3. Lloyd-Jones, D.M.; Hong, Y.; Labarthe, D.; Mozaffarian, D.; Appel, L.J.; Van Horn, L.; Greenlund, K.; Daniels, S.; Nichol, G.; Tomaselli, G.F.; et al. Defining and setting national goals for cardiovascular health promotion and disease reduction: The American Heart Association's strategic Impact Goal through 2020 and beyond. *Circulation* **2010**, *121*, 586–613. [CrossRef]
4. Dong, C.; Rundek, T.; Wright, C.B.; Anwar, Z.; Elkind, M.S.; Sacco, R.L. Ideal Cardiovascular Health Predicts Lower Risks of Myocardial Infarction, Stroke, and Vascular Death Across Whites, Blacks, and Hispanics: The northern Manhattan study. *Circulation* **2012**, *125*, 2975–2984. [CrossRef]
5. Rasmussen-Torvik, L.J.; Shay, C.M.; Abramson, J.G.; Friedrich, C.A.; Nettleton, J.A.; Prizment, A.E.; Folsom, A.R. Ideal cardiovascular health is inversely associated with incident cancer: The Atherosclerosis Risk in Communities study. *Circulation* **2013**, *127*, 1270–1275. [CrossRef] [PubMed]

6. Younus, A.; Aneni, E.C.; Spatz, E.S.; Osondu, C.U.; Roberson, L.; Ogunmoroti, O.; Malik, R.; Ali, S.S.; Aziz, M.; Feldman, T.; et al. A Systematic Review of the Prevalence and Outcomes of Ideal Cardiovascular Health in US and Non-US Populations. *Mayo Clin. Proc.* **2016**, *91*, 649–670. [CrossRef]
7. Virani, S.S.; Alonso, A.; Aparicio, H.J.; Benjamin, E.J.; Bittencourt, M.S.; Callaway, C.W.; Carson, A.P.; Chamberlain, A.M.; Cheng, S.; Delling, F.N.; et al. Heart disease and stroke statistics—2021 update: A report From the American Heart Association. *Circulation* **2021**, *143*, e254–e743. [CrossRef]
8. Harrison, S.; Couillard, C.; Robitaille, J.; Vohl, M.C.; Bélanger, M.; Desroches, S.; Provencher, V.; Rabasa-Lhoret, R.; Bouchard, L.; Langlois, M.F.; et al. Assessment of the American Heart Association's "Life's simple 7" score in French-speaking adults from Quebec. *Nutr. Metab. Cardiovasc. Dis.* **2019**, *29*, 684–691. [CrossRef]
9. Mozaffarian, D. Dietary and Policy Priorities for Cardiovascular Disease, Diabetes, and Obesity: A Comprehensive Review. *Circulation* **2016**, *133*, 187–225. [CrossRef]
10. Waijers, P.M.C.M.; Feskens, E.; Ocké, M.C. A critical review of predefined diet quality scores. *Br. J. Nutr.* **2007**, *97*, 219–231. [CrossRef] [PubMed]
11. Liu, A.G.; Ford, N.A.; Hu, F.B.; Zelman, K.M.; Mozaffarian, D.; Kris-Etherton, P.M. A healthy approach to dietary fats: Understanding the science and taking action to reduce consumer confusion. *Nutr. J.* **2017**, *16*, 1–15. [CrossRef]
12. Mozaffarian, D.; Appel, L.J.; Van Horn, L. Components of a cardioprotective diet: New insights. *Circulation* **2011**, *123*, 2870–2891. [CrossRef] [PubMed]
13. Dishman, R.K.; Oldenburg, B.; O'Neal, H.; Shephard, R.J. Worksite physical activity interventions. *Am. J. Prev. Med.* **1998**, *15*, 344–361. [CrossRef]
14. Plotnikoff, R.C.; McCargar, L.J.; Wilson, P.M.; Loucaides, C.A. Efficacy of an E-Mail Intervention for the Promotion of Physical Activity and Nutrition Behavior in the Workplace Context. *Am. J. Health Promot.* **2005**, *19*, 422–429. [CrossRef] [PubMed]
15. Statistics Canada. Labour Force Survey. April 2019. Available online: https://www150.statcan.gc.ca/n1/daily-quotidien/190510/dq190510a-eng.htm (accessed on 22 February 2021).
16. World Health Organization. Occupational Health. Available online: https://www.Who.Int/occupational_health/topics/workplace/en/ (accessed on 4 October 2020).
17. Lévesque, V.; Vallières, M.; Poirier, P.; Després, J.-P.; Alméras, N. Targeting Abdominal Adiposity and Cardiorespiratory Fitness in the Workplace. *Med. Sci. Sports Exerc.* **2015**, *47*, 1342–1350. [CrossRef]
18. Lévesque, V.; Poirier, P.; Després, J.-P.; Alméras, N. Relation Between a Simple Lifestyle Risk Score and Established Biological Risk Factors for Cardiovascular Disease. *Am. J. Cardiol.* **2017**, *120*, 1939–1946. [CrossRef] [PubMed]
19. Bailey, R.L.; Miller, P.E.; Mitchell, D.C.; Hartman, T.J.; Lawrence, F.R.; Sempos, C.T.; Smiciklas-Wright, H. Dietary screening tool identifies nutritional risk in older adults. *Am. J. Clin. Nutr.* **2009**, *90*, 177–183. [CrossRef] [PubMed]
20. Buteau-Poulin, D.; Poirier, P.; Després, J.-P.; Alméras, N. Assessing nutritional quality as a 'vital sign' of cardiometabolic health. *Br. J. Nutr.* **2019**, *122*, 195–205. [CrossRef]
21. Günther, A.L.; Liese, A.D.; Bell, R.A.; Dabelea, D.; Lawrence, J.M.; Rodriguez, B.L.; Standiford, D.A.; Mayer-Davis, E.J. Association Between the Dietary Approaches to Hypertension Diet and Hypertension in Youth with Diabetes Mellitus. *Hypertension* **2009**, *53*, 6–12. [CrossRef]
22. Rumawas, M.E.; Dwyer, J.T.; McKeown, N.M.; Meigs, J.B.; Rogers, G.; Jacques, P.F. The Development of the Mediterranean-Style Dietary Pattern Score and Its Application to the American Diet in the Framingham Offspring Cohort. *J. Nutr.* **2009**, *139*, 1150–1156. [CrossRef]
23. Khaw, K.-T.; Jakes, R.; Bingham, S.; Welch, A.; Luben, R.; Day, N.; Wareham, N. Work and leisure time physical activity assessed using a simple, pragmatic, validated questionnaire and incident cardiovascular disease and all-cause mortality in men and women: The European Prospective Investigation into Cancer in Norfolk prospective population study. *Int. J. Epidemiol.* **2006**, *35*, 1034–1043. [CrossRef]
24. Gordon, C.C.; Chumlea, W.C.; Roche, A.F. Stature, Recumbent Length, and Weight. In *Anthropometric Standardization Reference Manual*; Lohman, T.G., Roche, A.F., Martorell, R., Eds.; Human Kinetics Books: Champaign, IL, USA, 1988; pp. 3–8.
25. National Institutes of Health. Clinical guidelines on the identification, evaluation, and treatment of overweight and obesity in adults-the evidence report. *Obes. Res.* **1998**, *6*, 51S–209S.
26. Côté, C.-E.; Rhéaume, C.; Poirier, P.; Després, J.-P.; Alméras, N. Deteriorated Cardiometabolic Risk Profile in Individuals with Excessive Blood Pressure Response to Submaximal Exercise. *Am. J. Hypertens.* **2019**, *32*, 945–952. [CrossRef] [PubMed]
27. Wyndham, C.H. Submaximal tests for estimating maximum oxygen intake. *Can. Med. Assoc. J.* **1967**, *96*, 736–745. [PubMed]
28. Astrand, P.O.; Ryhming, I. A nomogram for calculation of aerobic capacity (physical fitness) from pulse rate during sub-maximal work. *J. Appl. Physiol.* **1954**, *7*, 218–221. [CrossRef]
29. American College of Sports Medicine. *ACSM's Guidelines for Exercise Testing and Prescription*, 10th ed.; Riebe, D., Ehrman, J.K., Liguori, G., Magal, M., Eds.; Wolters Kluwer Health: Philadelphia, PA, USA, 2018.
30. Arsenault, B.J.; Lemieux, I.; Després, J.-P.; Wareham, N.J.; Kastelein, J.J.P.; Khaw, K.-T.; Boekholdt, S.M. The hypertriglyceridemic-waist phenotype and the risk of coronary artery disease: Results from the EPIC-Norfolk Prospective Population Study. *Can. Med. Assoc. J.* **2010**, *182*, 1427–1432. [CrossRef] [PubMed]

31. Lemieux, I.; Pascot, A.; Couillard, C.; Lamarche, B.; Tchernof, A.; Alméras, N.; Bergeron, J.; Gaudet, D.; Tremblay, G.; Prud'homme, D.; et al. Hypertriglyceridemic waist. A marker of the atherogenic metabolic triad (hyperinsulinemia, hyperapolipoprotein B, small, dense LDL) in men? *Circulation* **2000**, *102*, 179–184. [CrossRef]
32. Brunner, E.; Domhof, S.; Langer, F. *Nonparametric Analysis of Longitudinal Data in Factorial Experiments*; John Wiley & Sons: New York, NY, USA, 2002.
33. Rouseff, M.; Aneni, E.C.; Guzman, H.; Das, S.; Brown, D.; Osondu, C.U.; Spatz, E.; Shaffer, B.; Santiago-Charles, J.; Ochoa, T.; et al. One-year outcomes of an intense workplace cardio-metabolic risk reduction program among high-risk employees: The My Unlimited Potential. *Obesity* **2015**, *24*, 71–78. [CrossRef] [PubMed]
34. Jacobs, D.R., Jr.; Tapsell, L.C. Food, not nutrients, is the fundamental unit in nutrition. *Nutr. Rev.* **2007**, *65*, 439–450. [CrossRef]
35. Mozaffarian, D.; Ludwig, D.S. Dietary Guidelines in the 21st Century—A Time for Food. *JAMA* **2010**, *304*, 681–682. [CrossRef] [PubMed]
36. Barnard, R.; Inkeles, S.B. Effects of an intensive diet and exercise program on lipids in postmenopausal women. *Women Health Issues* **1999**, *9*, 155–161. [CrossRef]
37. Groeneveld, I.F.; Proper, K.I.; Van Der Beek, A.J.; Hildebrandt, V.H.; Van Mechelen, W. Lifestyle-focused interventions at the workplace to reduce the risk of cardiovascular disease—A systematic review. *Scand. J. Work. Environ. Health* **2010**, *36*, 202–215. [CrossRef] [PubMed]
38. Couillard, C.; Després, J.-P.; Lamarche, B.; Bergeron, J.; Gagnon, J.; Leon, A.S.; Rao, D.C.; Skinner, J.S.; Wilmore, J.H.; Bouchard, C. Effects of endurance exercise training on plasma HDL cholesterol levels depend on levels of triglycerides: Evidence from men of the Health, Risk Factors, Exercise Training and Genetics (HERITAGE) Family Study. *Arterioscler. Thromb. Vasc. Biol.* **2001**, *21*, 1226–1232. [CrossRef]
39. Petrogianni, M.; Kanellakis, S.; Kallianioti, K.; Argyropoulou, D.; Pitsavos, C.; Manios, Y. A multicomponent lifestyle intervention produces favourable changes in diet quality and cardiometabolic risk indices in hypercholesterolaemic adults. *J. Hum. Nutr. Diet.* **2013**, *26*, 596–605. [CrossRef]
40. Remy, C.; Shubrook, J.H.; Nakazawa, M.; Drozek, D. Employer-Funded Complete Health Improvement Program: Preliminary Results of Biomarker Changes. *J. Am. Osteopat. Assoc.* **2017**, *117*, 293–300. [CrossRef]
41. Després, J.-P.; Alméras, N.; Gauvin, L. Worksite Health and Wellness Programs: Canadian Achievements & Prospects. *Prog. Cardiovasc. Dis.* **2014**, *56*, 484–492. [CrossRef] [PubMed]
42. Mastrangelo, G.; Marangi, G.; Bontadi, D.; Fadda, E.; Cegolon, L.; Bortolotto, M.; Fedeli, U.; Marchiori, L. A worksite intervention to reduce the cardiovascular risk: Proposal of a study design easy to integrate within Italian organization of occupational health surveillance. *BMC Public Health* **2015**, *15*, 12. [CrossRef]
43. Reed, J.L.; Prince, S.A.; Elliott, C.G.; Mullen, K.A.; Tulloch, H.E.; Hiremath, S.; Cotie, L.M.; Pipe, A.L.; Reid, R.D. Impact of workplace physical activity interventions on physical activity and cardiometabolic health among working-age women: A systematic review and meta-analysis. *Circ. Cardiovasc. Qual. Outcomes* **2017**, *10*, e003516. [CrossRef] [PubMed]
44. Mulchandani, R.; Chandrasekaran, A.M.; Shivashankar, R.; Kondal, D.; Agrawal, A.; Panniyammakal, J.; Tandon, N.; Prabhakaran, D.; Sharma, M.; Goenka, S. Effect of workplace physical activity interventions on the cardio-metabolic health of working adults: Systematic review and meta-analysis. *Int. J. Behav. Nutr. Phys. Act.* **2019**, *16*, 1–16. [CrossRef]
45. Monfort-Pires, M.; Folchetti, L.D.; Previdelli, A.N.; Siqueira-Catania, A.; De Barros, C.R.; Ferreira, S.R.G. Healthy Eating Index is associated with certain markers of inflammation and insulin resistance but not with lipid profile in individuals at cardiometabolic risk. *Appl. Physiol. Nutr. Metab.* **2014**, *39*, 497–502. [CrossRef]
46. Gormley, S.E.; Swain, D.P.; High, R.; Spina, R.J.; Dowling, E.A.; Kotipalli, U.S.; Gandrakota, R. Effect of Intensity of Aerobic Training on VO2max. *Med. Sci. Sports Exerc.* **2008**, *40*, 1336–1343. [CrossRef]
47. Helgerud, J.; Høydal, K.; Wang, E.; Karlsen, T.; Berg, P.; Bjerkaas, M.; Simonsen, T.; Helgesen, C.; Hjorth, N.; Bach, R.; et al. Aerobic High-Intensity Intervals Improve VO2max More Than Moderate Training. *Med. Sci. Sports Exerc.* **2007**, *39*, 665–671. [CrossRef] [PubMed]
48. Swain, D.P.; Franklin, B.A. VO(2) reserve and the minimal intensity for improving cardiorespiratory fitness. *Med. Sci. Sports Exerc.* **2002**, *34*, 152–157. [CrossRef] [PubMed]
49. Ross, R.; de Lannoy, L.; Stotz, P.J. Separate Effects of Intensity and Amount of Exercise on Interindividual Cardiorespiratory Fitness Response. *Mayo Clin. Proc.* **2015**, *90*, 1506–1514. [CrossRef] [PubMed]
50. Ross, R.; Neeland, I.J.; Yamashita, S.; Shai, I.; Seidell, J.; Magni, P.; Santos, R.D.; Arsenault, B.; Cuevas, A.; Hu, F.B.; et al. Waist circumference as a vital sign in clinical practice: A Consensus Statement from the IAS and ICCR Working Group on Visceral Obesity. *Nat. Rev. Endocrinol.* **2020**, *16*, 177–189. [CrossRef] [PubMed]
51. Neeland, I.J.; Ross, R.; Després, J.-P.; Matsuzawa, Y.; Yamashita, S.; Shai, I.; Seidell, J.; Magni, P.; Santos, R.D.; Arsenault, B.; et al. Visceral and ectopic fat, atherosclerosis, and cardiometabolic disease: A position statement. *Lancet Diabetes Endocrinol.* **2019**, *7*, 715–725. [CrossRef]
52. Prince, S.A.; Adamo, K.B.; Hamel, E.M.; Hardt, J.; Gorber, S.C.; Tremblay, M. A comparison of direct versus self-report measures for assessing physical activity in adults: A systematic review. *Int. J. Behav. Nutr. Phys. Act.* **2008**, *5*, 56–64. [CrossRef]

Article

Hunger and Health: Taking a Formative Approach to Build a Health Intervention Focused on Nutrition and Physical Activity Needs as Perceived by Stakeholders

Kelsey Fortin *[ID] and Susan Harvey

Department of Health, Sport and Exercise Sciences, School of Education and Human Sciences, Lawrence Campus, University of Kansas, Lawrence, KS 66045, USA; Suharvey@ku.edu
* Correspondence: Kelseyf123@ku.edu

Abstract: The intersections between hunger and health are beginning to gain traction. New interventions emphasize collaboration between the health and social service sectors. This study aimed to understand the nutrition and physical activity (PA) needs as perceived by food pantry stakeholders to inform a health intervention approach. The study used formative research incorporating mixed methods through surveying and semi-structured interviews with three food pantry stakeholder groups: Clients ($n = 30$), staff ($n = 7$), and volunteers ($n = 10$). Pantry client participants reported; high rates of both individual (60%, $n = 18$) and household (43%, $n = 13$) disease diagnosis; low consumption (0–1 servings) of fruits (67%, $n = 20$) and vegetables (47%, $n = 14$) per day; and low levels (0–120 min) of PA (67%, $n = 20$) per week. Interviews identified five final convergent major themes across all three stakeholder groups including food and PA barriers, nutrition and PA literacy, health status and lifestyle, current pantry operations and adjustments, and suggestions for health intervention programming. High rates of chronic disease combined with low health literacy among pantry clients demonstrate the need to address health behaviors. Further research piloting the design and implementation of a comprehensive health behavior intervention program in the food pantry setting is needed.

Keywords: food insecurity; hunger and health; nutrition; physical activity; health intervention; formative research

1. Introduction

Food pantries offer important resources in the federal aid system. Food insecurity is defined by the USDA as "limited or uncertain availability of nutritionally adequate and safe foods," and 14 million U.S. households were food insecure in 2018 [1]. Despite the availability of federal nutrition assistance programs (e.g., SNAP, WIC, TANF), there is a gap in services, leaving organizations like Feeding America, a network of 60,000 food pantries and meal programs, still serving roughly 4.3 million meals to hungry people [2]. These emergency food services are reaching the most vulnerable populations needing both food and health services. The number of chronic diseases for adults in households with low food security, is on average, 18 percent higher than those with high food-security [2], and one out of three chronically ill food insecure adults are unable to afford medicine, food, or both [3].

Significant financial constraints leave food insecure individuals frequently limited to food pantry availability and low-cost food items. This translates into coping strategies promoting low nutrient diets high in processed foods [4]. In general, poor dietary intake (e.g., excess saturated or trans-fat intake, a diet low in fruits and vegetables) has been linked to a number of chronic diseases, including cardiovascular disease, Type 2 diabetes, some types of cancer and osteoporosis [5,6]. Overall, those living in food insecure households often have disrupted eating patterns and diets that are inadequate in nutrient-dense foods, contributing to malnourishment and an increased risk for poor health and chronic disease [7]. Beyond the quality of food, the existence of medical conditions associated with a poor diet can interfere with medication adherence [8]. Clients accessing a mobile food pantry reported that food insecurity impacts medication adherence due to the requirement that some medication be taken with food [9]. Therefore, gaps in the pantry schedule, lack of transportation or conflicting commitments may prevent individuals from accessing the food they need to meet medication recommendations.

Pantry clients have reported similar barriers, such as lack of transportation, inadequate kitchen equipment, lack of nutrition knowledge and skills, and few social support networks impacting their ability to eat healthy [10]. Other than adherence to medication for existing conditions, pantry clients are lacking in access, knowledge, and the to eat healthy diets to prevent disease onset. Begley et al. (2019) postulates that poor food and nutrition literacy behaviors contribute to food insecurity. Behaviors related to food planning and management, shopping, preparation, and cooking all show an association between food literacy behaviors and food security status [11]. In other words, the higher level of food literacy, the more food and nutritional behaviors individuals engage in that are associated with greater food security (e.g., food storage and preparation). Health literacy and self-efficacy have also been found to be predictors of food label use, which positively predict individuals diet quality [12]. As health professionals work to address hunger and health among food insecure populations, issues of food and health literacy are important interventional considerations.

The Department of Health and Human services (DHSS) recommends that American adults engage in a minimum of 150-minutes of moderately intense physical activity (PA) per week to experience health benefits [13]. PA rates among adults are low across the U.S. with nearly 80% of adults not meeting PA-recommended guidelines [13]. Common barriers associated with PA include a lack of confidence performing exercises, lack of time, lack of financial resources, and having diseases that create exercise limitations [13–15]. Food insecurity has demonstrated a significant association with adherence to PA guidelines among both adults and children [16]. Outside of the traditional barriers that prevent adults from engaging in PA, food insecure adults experience higher levels of stress and have poorer health, with a greater number of chronic diseases, creating larger obstacles to engaging in PA [16]. Additionally, food insecurity is associated perceptions, and readiness to engage in PA [17,18]. Within the context of disease, food insecure individuals report physical limitations that may prevent them from activities of daily life, including PA [19]. Connections between food insecurity and PA, particularly among adults, are the areas of hunger and health literature, which merit further research development.

According to the World Health Organization, non-communicable diseases (e.g., diabetes and cardiovascular disease) account for two-thirds of premature deaths worldwide [20]. Food insecure individuals are reporting broader disease prevalence and comorbidities, such as obesity, disability and mental health disorders that warrant the need for a broader approach and multi-sector collaboration among medical providers, public health practitioners, social workers and food banks [21]. Within the space of chronic disease management, health coaching interventions have shown promise in the medical setting [22,23]. Health coaching often makes use of motivational interviewing techniques that promote collaboration, client evocation and autonomy, leading to successful behavior change across a variety of contexts, populations and health behaviors [24]. Health coaching uses a relationship building strategy in health behavior change through activities, such as health education sessions and individual practical support [25]. Health coaching shows positive results when targeting a range of diseases and populations, including diabetes, heart disease, hyperlipidemia and low-income patients [26]. If food pantries can implement a broader intervention design (e.g., health coaching), incorporating more holistic behavioral components (e.g., both nutrition and PA), can be developed that captures a broader range of food insecure individuals with comorbidities, and address lifestyle health behaviors leading to those disease.

The Academy of Nutrition and Dietetics released a position paper stressing the importance for nutrition practitioners to build partnerships with food pantries [27]. Health professionals are beginning to recognize the importance of targeted interventions among food insecure populations [28]. Recent intervention research relating to diabetes, nutrition education, and dietary and food purchasing behaviors within the food pantry setting resulted in positive health outcomes for food insecure pantry clients [29–31]. Among the literature, a recent systematic review of food pantry interventions revealed nutrition literacy and diabetic management interventions have been dominant in the field [32]. The cited studies indicate innovation and promise, yet present gaps in assisting individuals outside of the diabetic and nutrition scope. Only one study in the review of the literature utilized a more holistic health coaching approach within the food pantry setting [23]. Although, the study yielded positive pantry client health outcomes, it was still focused predominantly on nutritional behaviors, disregarding PA as an important disease prevention and management strategy.

As scientists and practitioners develop and implement interventions aimed at food pantry clients, little is known about the design and implementation of health intervention that combine both nutrition and PA health behaviors within a holistic health intervention model. This study uses formative research to understand nutrition and PA needs as perceived by food pantry stakeholders (pantry clients, volunteers, and staff) to inform a health intervention approach at a county-wide Midwest food pantry. This formative approach makes use of a community participatory model [33] to gain buy-in and consultation from the community of interest. The study aims to fill a gap in the literature by; (1) understanding more about PA behaviors and needs among food insecure adult pantry users; and (2) explore the program components of a comprehensive health intervention that incorporates both PA and nutrition as perceived by pantry stakeholders. This study will act as phase one to a multiphase intervention design research project.

2. Materials and Methods

The Institutional Review Board at a large Midwest research institution approved this study. Formative research using mixed methods incorporated surveys, individual interviews, and one focus group with three stakeholder groups (food pantry staff, volunteers, and clients). All data were collected on site at a local county-wide Midwest food pantry.

2.1. Pantry Context

The food pantry in the current study is the largest food pantry within the county it's located serving roughly 13,000 residents in 2017 [34]. The county has a food insecurity rate of nearly 17% and overall poverty rate of 19% [34]. The pantry saw a 15% increase in overall client visits between 2017 and 2018 [35], with 51% of clients surveyed reporting having to skip meals between one and three times, on average, per week [31]. Demographically, over half of their clients (65%) identify as white and fall between the 18–64 age group (62%) [35]. Due to chronic disease concerns, with 62% of pantry clients surveyed reporting a household member with type 2 diabetes, the pantry has begun to offer health screenings on-site [35]. Additionally, the pantry offers a variety of nutrition programs including cooking and gardening classes, and an intensive culinary training program to encourage self-sufficiency among pantry clients [35]. The pantry utilizes seven full-time staff members and a fleet of volunteers.

2.2. Sample

Convenience sampling occurred focusing on three stakeholder groups ($n = 47$) (1) pantry staff ($n = 7$); (2) pantry volunteers ($n = 10$); and (3) pantry clients ($n = 30$). All staff currently employed by the pantry were included in the study, volunteers and pantry client participants were recruited until data saturation occurred. All participants were recruited in-person via direct communication with study staff during regularly scheduled pantry hours (M-F, 9 a.m.–5 p.m.). Inclusion criteria included individuals starting at age 18 to capture those of adult status and ending at age 75. This age range is representative of the majority age range of clients served (18–65) plus an extended age range (65–75) to capture the retired volunteer population. Additionally, stakeholder group classification (pantry staff, volunteer, or client), and ability to speak, read and write English were inclusion requirements. Participants incentives consisted of a "healthy eating goodie bag" containing a reusable grocery tote, cooking oil, one cooking utensil (wooden spoon, fork, or spatula), recipe cards, and informational brochures on various healthy eating topics. Only pantry clients were encouraged and received a "healthy eating goodie bag" upon completion of the study.

Demographic Characteristics

Table 1 displays pantry client ($n = 30$) demographics, and individual and household health status information. Majority of clients were Caucasian (80%, $n = 24$) and female (73%, $n = 22$). Disease prevalence was high with 60% ($n = 18$) reporting at least one chronic disease and 37% ($n = 11$) reporting more than one. Additional health status and demographic information is displayed in Tabe 1 below. Staff ($n = 7$) participant age ranged from 23 to 39, with majority of the participants (71%, $n = 5$) identifying as Caucasian/white, and two identified as mixed race. All staff work full-time, with years of experience ranging between one to six years. Lastly, Volunteer ($n = 10$) participants included individuals ages 18 to 79, primarily identifying as Caucasian (90%, $n = 9$), with one identifying as African American. Volunteer employment status ranged from full-time to retired.

Table 1. Pantry client demographic Characteristics and health status.

Demographic Category	Food Pantry Client Characteristics ($n = 30$)	n	%
Gender	Male	8	26.7
	Female	22	73.3
Age, years	20–30	4	13.3
	31–40	2	6.7
	41–50	9	30.0
	51–60	9	30.0
	61–73	6	20.0
Race	Caucasian/White	24	80.0
	African American/Black	5	16.7
	Hispanic/Latino	1	3.3
Annual Household Income	<$10,000	13	43.3
	$10,000–$24,999	15	50.0
	$25,000–$49,999	2	6.7
Occupational Status	Working full-time	5	16.7
	Working part-time	4	13.3
	Unemployed, currently seeking	8	26.7
	Unemployed, not currently seeking	7	23.3
	Retired	6	20.0
Education Level	Some high school	1	3.3
	High school graduate or GED	5	16.7
	Some college	14	46.7
	Associate degree	6	20.0
	Bachelor's degree	3	10.0
	Master's degree	1	3.3
Number of health conditions (individual)	Zero chronic disease listed	1	3.3
	One chronic disease listed	18	60.0
	More than one chronic disease listed	11	36.7

Table 1. Cont.

Demographic Category	Food Pantry Client Characteristics (n = 30)	n	%
Specification of health condition (individual)	Diabetes	4	13.3
	High Blood Pressure	11	36.7
	High Cholesterol	7	23.3
	Heart Disease	3	10.0
	Metabolic Syndrome	5	16.7
Overall Health	Excellent	1	3.3
	Very Good	9	30.0
	Good	11	36.7
	Fair	9	30.0
Last Doctor Visit	1–3 months	21	70.0
	4–6 months	5	16.7
	>1 yr.	4	13.3
Health Insurance Status	Insured	22	73.3
	Uninsured	8	26.7
Number of health conditions (household)	Zero chronic disease listed	12	40.0
	One chronic disease listed	13	43.3
	More than one chronic disease listed	5	16.7
Specification of health condition (household)	Diabetes	5	16.7
	High Blood Pressure	7	23.3
	High Cholesterol	5	16.7
	Heart Disease	4	13.3
	Metabolic Syndrome	4	13.3

2.3. Measures

Primary data collection involved three investigator-designed surveys and corresponding interview guides using a combination of newly developed questions based on the current study's aims, and questions modified based on validated measures previously found in the literature. All survey measures were collected via hard copy, in-person, direct participant response. A researcher was present to answer participant questions.

2.3.1. Client Survey Measures

The client survey included validated measures through questions on self-reported health [36] and the Behavioral Risk Factor Surveillance Survey nutrition and PA module measures [37]. Investigator-designed measures included categorical questions (yes or no) on individual and household chronic disease diagnosis (e.g., diabetes), and barriers to healthy eating (e.g., healthy foods are too expensive) and PA (e.g., I don't know enough about physical activity). Last, the survey asked participants to report individual demographic characteristics (race/ethnicity, gender, annual household income, employment status, and level of education). The survey consisted of 28 questions and the full details can be reviewed under Supplementary File S1.

2.3.2. Client Semi-Structured Interviews

An investigator-designed moderator's guide, which corresponded with survey questions, guided semi-structured interviews. Sample questions included, "What are some of the challenges and barriers to choosing and cooking healthy options?" and "What current health issues are you and/or members of your household facing? Last, questions pertaining to intervention components included "What do you think are some critical characteristics of this program? (Probe: How often meetings are, time of day, days of the week, how long, educator characteristics, location, electronic vs. in-person)?" The moderator's guide consisted of 14 questions and the full details can be reviewed under Supplementary File S2.

2.3.3. Volunteer/Staff Survey Measures

Volunteer and staff measures included an investigator-designed survey informed by the study aims and topics represented in the client survey. Example questions include categorical questions (often, sometimes, never) related to client engagement within the topics of health, nutrition and PA (e.g., "How often do you engage with clients about the cost of food?). Last, the survey asked participants to report individual demographic characteristics (race/ethnicity, gender, annual household income, employment status, level of education and number of years of service at the current food pantry). The survey consisted of 16 questions and the full details can be reviewed under Supplementary File S3.

2.3.4. Volunteer/Staff Semi-Structured Interviews

Interviews consisted of an investigator-designed moderator's guide corresponding to the survey. Sample questions included, "What questions do clients most commonly ask about (a) Food/food products, (b) Nutrition, (c) Physical Activity, (d) Health (e) Programs/resources offered by the pantry" and "What important topics within nutrition, physical activity, and health should be covered in an intervention program?" The moderator's guide consisted of 8 questions and the full details can be reviewed under Supplementary File S4.

2.4. Data Collection

Participants completed a written informed consent prior to data collection. Collection occurred through in-person hard copy surveys completed by participants, individual semi-structured interviews with pantry clients and volunteers, and one focus group with pantry staff.

2.4.1. Participant Surveys

Survey responses were collected from all three-stakeholder groups (staff, volunteers, and clients) immediately before conducting interview questions. Surveys were administered in hard copy using paper and pencil, and were completed independently by study participants. Study staff were available for participant support.

2.4.2. Participant Interviews and Focus Group

Volunteer and client groups participated in follow-up individual semi-structured interviews, while staff participated in a single focus group during a routine staff meeting. All interviews and focus groups were semi-structured, immediately followed survey completion, and were located in a secure private room on-site at the food pantry. All correspondence was audio recorded with sessions lasting between roughly 30 to 60 min in length. A single investigator (the PI) with training and experience in qualitative methods and the interview protocol conducted interviews and took field notes. Member checks and debriefings occurred during interviews to ensure accuracy of participant statements and to increase trustworthiness [38].

2.5. Data Analysis

All data were reviewed and analyzed separately, then brought back together to find convergent themes across all sources and stakeholder groups. All survey responses were input into IBM SPSS Statistics 26 software for descriptive data analysis.

Interview/Focus group Analysis

All interviews were audio recorded and transcribed verbatim by the PI of the study. Once transcribed, a priori categories, based on categories within the semi-structured interview guide, directed the initial coding process and were combined with exploratory findings to generate final themes [39]. Last, data triangulation occured between the existing literature, stakeholder surveys and stakeholder interviews/focus group to informed research findings [39,40]. This process included two co-investigators of the research team.

3. Results

This section will provide a detailed description of each stakeholder group's results separately, followed by a joining of the data generating final convergent themes. Final convergent major themes include food and PA barriers, nutrition and PA literacy, health status and lifestyle, current pantry operations and adjustments and suggestions for health intervention programming.

3.1. Client Results

Client survey responses revealed low consumption of fruits and vegetables with over half (67%, $n = 20$) reporting zero to one servings of fruits per day, and 47% ($n = 14$) reporting zero to one servings of vegetables per day. Commonly reported healthy eating barriers include: healthy food being too expensive (40%, $n = 12$), not knowing enough about healthy cooking (37%, $n = 11$), not knowing enough about general nutrition to make healthy meals (30%, $n = 9$), and not knowing how to choose and store fresh produce (27%, $n = 8$). A high rate of participants (67%, $n = 20$) reported low PA between zero to 120 min per week. Common barriers preventing participants from engaging in regular PA, included having health conditions that restrict activity (30, $n = 9$), lack of enjoyment for PA (27%, $n = 8$), lack of access to a facility to engage in PA (23%, $n = 7$), and having a job that is physically demanding (20%, $n = 6$).

During client interviews, four themes emerged, including Food and PA barriers, Nutrition and PA literacy, Health Status and Lifestyle, and Suggestions for Health Intervention Programming. In the first major theme, participants reported things such as cost, and food preparation restrictions as leading roadblocks to improving nutrition. One participant reported, "Right now, I live in a camper out in the park, and I don't have electricity in it, so mostly it's the food banks, or going to get something that's cooked in the store. Unless I can get a fire going, so that limits me and what I can do." Barriers to PA, included mental and physical limitations and occupational restrictions. Occupational restrictions include sedentary jobs and lack of time due to multiple jobs.

The second major theme, Nutrition and PA Literacy is associated with general nutrition and PA education. Within nutrition, categories, such as cooking, specialty diets, and produce storage and preparation were noted. Within PA most feedback was focused on general strength exercises, and exercises for physical limitations. Participants also mentioned a desire for weight management education with statements like, "Losing weight. What I would need to do to really lose some weight. And not just do strange starving eating type of things. The healthy way to do it."

Third, the Health Status and Lifestyle theme corresponded with the depth of physical and mental illness across participants with one participant sharing "I have anxiety, depression, migraines, frontal lobe seizures, turrets, treated for blood clots, get treated for low vitamin B, Arthritis." Additionally, there were reports on impacts to lifestyle due to disease. These related to both positive impacts, such as disease translating to improvements in health behaviors, and negative impacts with connections to disease affecting quality of life in examples like "She took me off work for two months to see if we could get it under control [high blood pressure], so hopefully."

In the fourth major theme, Suggestions for Health Intervention Programming, pertained to programmatic and structural recommendations from pantry clients. Structurally, participants were interested in both electronic services and face-to-face services, as well as group and individual formats. They reflected on the idea of social support from both the health educator or coach, and other pantry client intervention participants in a group setting. Recommendations for intervention content included statements such as "It should be the holistic approach. Teaching people to eat better sooner, instead of waiting until the point of diabetes or the health issues." Last, participants demonstrated support and excitement for a health intervention program by stating comments, such as "I think this is a fabulous idea I think it is doable with a lot of your hard work and I look forward to you moving forward and changes ahead."

3.2. Staff Results

Staff survey responses demonstrated that within the category of health, staff reported often engaging with clients about health insurance (29%, $n = 2$) and local health services (29%, $n = 2$). Within nutrition, staff reported often engaging with clients about cost of food (86%, $n = 6$), quick meal options (57%, $n = 4$), and food restrictions (57%, $n = 4$). Within PA, staff indicated often engaging with clients about physical limitations (57%, $n = 4$).

Staff participated in a follow-up focus group instead of interviews to capture collaborative staff ideas as a part of a monthly staff meeting. Three themes emerged. Themes included Specialty Diet Questions, Pantry Operations, and Client Education. Specialty Diet questions included clients coming in with specific recommendations from medical providers with one staff member reporting, "I am finding more hyper specificity. [clients reporting] This is my diet, I have talked to my doctor, and they say I need to be eating these specific items, do you have any of those?"

Within the theme of Pantry Operations, staff proposed a variety of pantry operational changes that may assist clients with questions and food choice. This theme included creating general handouts, nutritional nudges, and increased meal kit options. Last, the Client Education theme, informed by direct client experience and observations, led to recommending general nutrition and PA education. For example, one staff member said the following: "Helping people understand how to be more realistic [portion size], my immediate thought goes to My Healthy Plate campaign."

3.3. Volunteer Results

Volunteer survey responses demonstrated that within the category of health, volunteers reported often communicating with clients about high blood pressure (30%, $n = 3$) and local health services (30%, $n = 3$). Volunteers reported sometimes engaging about unusual food items (50%, $n = 5$), building healthy meals ($n = 4$), and food storage ($n = 4$). Volunteers indicated never engaging with clients about PA in nearly all categories.

During semi-structured interviews, four themes emerged including Pantry Questions, Pantry Shopping Adjustments, Client Education, and Volunteer Training. Within the theme of Pantry Questions, volunteers highlighted frequent client questions related to either food products or preparation. One volunteer indicated: "Sometimes people will ask about what would be a good way to prepare this vegetable or meat," or pantry logistics "not too many questions other than how many points is this [food item]".

Volunteers offered recommendations for Pantry Shopping Adjustments addressing the topics of food products/preparation and pantry logistics. Recommendations included adding information for use and preparation of unusual produce and including simple recipes directly with these items. Major topics highlighted within the Client Education theme included general nutrition and PA guidelines with comments like, "Most people don't have a general understanding of nutrition," and shopping strategies, "Educating on how to effectively use their points. Some people only have 10 points and they get 4 sandwiches and that is going to last you a max of 2 days."

The Volunteer Training theme emphasized conflicting opinions. Regarding volunteer training, some volunteers indicated interest in receiving training related to "Food stamp options. How or where; opportunities to talk about options for food," with other volunteers indicated a lack of interest in further training with rationales like, "A lot of us are retired and not wanting to fill that role [health specific volunteer role]."

3.4. Final Convergent Major Themes

There were five identified final convergent major themes including Food and PA Barriers, Nutrition and PA Literacy, Health Status and lifestyle, Current Pantry Operations and Adjustments, and Suggestions for Health Intervention Programming.

Food and PA Barriers, include identification of life circumstance that make healthy eating and PA difficult among pantry clients. Barriers that were reported included cost of food, produce storage and self-life, physical limitations to exercise, and the perception that PA is a privilege based on social status.

Nutrition and PA Literacy, the second theme, pertains to gaps in knowledge about healthy eating, selection and preparation of foods, PA recommendations based on limitations both identified by the clients through personal experience, and volunteers and staff based on client interactions and questions.

Similarly, clients' personal reports, and volunteer and staff interactions with clients demonstrate how food insecurity and limitations due to disease influence clients lives under the Health Status and Lifestyle major theme. This included reporting on how much disease clients were experiencing daily and coping strategies such as seeking out dietary recommendations from staff at the pantry.

The fourth major theme, Current Pantry Operations and Adjustments, relates to volunteer and staff experience with the current climate within the pantry associated with nutrition and PA among clients, and ideas for adjustments to create a more informed and positive experience. This included ideas for inclusion of nutrient information in meal kits and throughout the pantry, as well as guidance on how to use their pantry points and potential training opportunities for volunteers.

Suggestions for Health Intervention Programming highlights the perspectives from all three stakeholder groups related to intervention program components consisting of nonjudgmental, supportive, coaching, with the inclusion of PA and nutrition education, and support for hosting such a health intervention program in the pantry setting. A summary of these final convergent themes and corresponding client, volunteer, and staff quotes can be found in Table 2.

Table 2. Final convergent Major Themes and Quotes.

Major Theme	Participant Quotes
Nutrition and physical activity barriers	"Mostly the prices [referring to barriers]. The cheaper it is, the less healthy it is. I have walked through a few organic isles, but it is just off the charts, even for food stamps." (C.1) "I am a single person and I can't buy a whole chicken, I just want one or two pieces, if I buy a roast, I want to buy a small one. I don't want to have a whole bunch of spoiled stuff." (C.9) "The short life of the produce, some of the stuff from the farmers market here will last a week, but some of the stuff from the supermarkets is old." (C.21) "The hip, back pain or issues [barrier to PA]. I found out I have first stage emphysema so breathing issues." (C.14) "Honestly, when my depression gets bad I have issues with that [motivation for physical activity] (C.15) "I don't think people quite understand the importance of nutrition and physical activity because they are just trying to survive." (V.8) "Sometimes I see the specific recipes and I think there is no way they are going to have those ingredients." (V.5) "There is a high proportion of individuals who also have physical limitations or physical barriers to physical activity" (S.5) "I have experience direct interactions with clients that view physical activity as perhaps a luxury that they can't afford yet." (S.3) "I would say in my experience I get very little interaction with clients who are on a preventative track [related to disease, diet, exercise]." (S.3)
Nutrition and Physical Activity Literacy	Sometimes the knowledge of what to do with certain food. Not knowing how to cook it or what to do with it. Knowing how to use different ingredients or spices." (C. 26) "A lot of health issues, when you have diabetes or that other stuff, how to incorporate that into your daily life or eating. Foods that you're able to make to help you with your health challenges like diabetes and other things." (C.10) "I think I would be interested in learning what type of activities I could do, due to the fact of arthritis in the knees." (C.20) "It would always be nice to know types of exercises you could do. I was in wrestling in high school, and all we did was like weights and stretch. So that is all I know." (C.1) "Even stuff like the plate [referencing MyPlate]. It is basic, but it is useful for people to know" (V.5) "Maybe explaining you can walk and it's still exercise. The little things that are PA and the benefits so like losing weight and the actual health benefits to your heart" (V.3) "I get a lot of recipe questions, or what does this go with, or does this go together, what can I do with these three things." (S.2) "I think partially, it is a lack of knowledge about preparation, but also there is an assumption that I can't prepare something a certain way because I don't have the specialized machinery for it." (S.3)

Table 2. Cont.

Major Theme	Participant Quotes
Health Status and Lifestyle	"I have PTSD and Depression, high blood pressure, the knee injury, the hand injury, my boyfriend he has high cholesterol. He also has PTSD from Afghanistan and Iraq." (C.6) "Hip problems and osteoporosis in the hip, stage one emphysema, I have problems that I feel are manageable as far as, yeah, I have been diagnosed with depression and I have been for years." (C.14) "I have a 13-year-old now that has prediabetes and I am scared to death. We all have ADHD, we control it with medication. I also have schizoaffective disorder. I am living in recovery from drugs and alcohol. My sons are high anxiety. I just began taking antianxiety meds. Because of the stress I was being put under, I am a survivor of child sex abuse, so I am still very affected. It's more like coming back to the surface. It took just 10 pounds more to make me just start getting really sensitive again." (C.19) I have had gastric sleeve surgery, so pretty much 80% of everything I eat needs to be protein. Since the surgery, my stomach is real finicky so even stuff I am supposed to eat I can't. I am limited by what surgery did to me." (C.2) "I have a thyroid condition that I am supposed to be working on. And I supposed to be on a diet for it. But it's hard to get the meal planning to get it situated." (C.4) "People asking about health related things. I am finding more and more hyper specificity for [clients requesting] this is my diet, I have talked to my doctor and they say I need to be eating these specific items, can you help me find those, or do you have any of those?" (S.3) "I keep going back to mental and emotional health. So we know that majority of our clients live in really high stress situations for a number of reasons, so I think food can be, I have seen clients in the past that had food addiction, and this place can be incredibly triggering." (S.1)
Current Pantry operations and adjustments	"Identification of vegetables that are a bit different. We have had them here before, but they are incredibly passive, so that is people to sign up for SNAP." (V.9) "Maybe you could be [pantry name] certified to help with that kind of thing [specialty diet recommendations]. Then if somebody has that issue then put it on their profile and you know what volunteers are certified to help with that. So specific volunteers can be certified in certain things and not everything." (V.3) "If you train more in blood pressure and things like that, it would be nice, but I don't know if I have time for something like that." (V.9) "From a programmatic standpoint, I am asked about every type of chronic disease and nutrition for those specific diseases." (S.5) "It would be kind of cool to have point guides [referencing how to get the most out of your allowable pantry points]." (S.6) "Nutrition facts placed around the place. Like what is the average suggested caloric intake for a day, and sodium intake." (S.1) "I would love to know more nutritional information [reference to additional training]. Honestly, I don't know much of any. Maybe, I know my ways of stretching meals, but that doesn't mean it will work for everybody, like how can I help support." (S.1)
Health Intervention Program logistics	"I don't do technology, so I would want face-to-face. I think maybe a lot of people don't have the money, if they are coming here, they maybe can't afford internet" (C.3) "You might get more people there if you reward them somehow. Like food or gift certificates to some place. Preferably some place healthy." (C.3) "Individual [intervention delivery] because everyone has individual difference. Because you have your physical limits, but you also have your health. Some are disabilities. everybody is different." (C.8) "If you can make it available online face-to-face like through zoom, wouldn't that be great. Just the touching base." (C.19) "If you go at them, I guess too forcefully or judgmental, you push them away. Approaching something with a positive outline." (C.12) "Accountability, you need to be able to hold people accountable. If you don't do that you aren't going to get a good result." (C. 27) "Ideally how to eat healthier. Healthy eating. Do that, but not do it in a patronizing way. It is too often it's blamed on the individual." (V.9) "I think that is one of the biggest one. Educating on how to effectively use their points. Some people only have 10 points and they get 4 sandwiches and that is going to last you max of 2 days." (V.2) "Like the meal kits stuff they come up with [referencing premade meal kits available to clients]. Like super simple stuff that doesn't require a lot of time or something I can maybe order a lot that [food items] we could use every week." (S.4) "Budget stuff, I think talking to them about process of food acquisition, do you come here first or do you go to the grocery store first, you should come here first see what you can get with your points, and then build recipes off what you can make with what you get kind of thing." (S.6) "We have had a lot of people recently asking specifically for items. So they want to do it, but sometimes they can't. So maybe it would help to get together with the coach and say hey this week we are going to have this, or I can order this, then we can really encourage people to go down this route." (S.4)

Note: C = Client quote, S = Staff quote, V = Volunteer quote.

4. Discussion

Consistent with previous research, pantry clients reported high levels of individual and household chronic diseases [40,41], which are compounded by client reported gaps in doctors' visits and health insurance coverage [41]. As more research connects the dots between food insecurity and insufficient medical care, organizations work to provide solutions in both pantry and clinical settings. Within clinical settings, screenings, referrals, and connecting patients with emergency food services is becoming a more common practice [19]. Additionally, interventions in the form of food pharmacy programs are connecting patients with food and nutrition resources within medical facilities [42,43]. Medical interventions are surfacing and have shown promise in food pantry settings [44]. Within the pantry setting, disease specific interventions (e.g., diabetes management interventions) have shown success among pantry clients [22,45]. However, disease specific interventions leave an unmet gap in serving pantry clinics with co-morbidities outside of the scope of that intervention. Additionally, little is known about targeting nutrition and PA behaviors in a holistic health intervention framework to address chronic disease among food pantry users. Health coaching frameworks with the use of motivational interviewing techniques have demonstrated effectiveness in chronic illness management [46]. Only one study was found with the employment of health coaching as a component of a more comprehensive intervention model within the food pantry [28]. By providing interventions around a health coaching framework, using a combination of health education and motivational interviewing, health coaches can address a broader range of clients providing clients with both nutrition and physical activity education, and social support, thereby increasing self-efficacy [47].

All three-stakeholder groups identified poor nutrition and PA literacy as a contributor to poor health outcomes. Research has shown low food and nutrition literacy may contribute to food insecurity in developing countries [15], while health literacy and self-efficacy have been found to predict food label use, which is positively related with diet quality [16]. As health education contributes to relationship building between health coaches and patients [30], further education through health intervention programming using these program components within the pantry setting could lead to improvements in food security status and diet quality [15,16]. The lack of skills in preparing fresh produce and irregularity of food supply have been noted in the literature as pantry client barriers to utilizing fresh produce [48]. The current study found consistencies with all three-stakeholder groups reporting barriers in using and preparing unusual produce. Interventions targeting weekly cooking classes within a six-week format have been shown to improve diet quality and decrease food cost within the pantry setting [21] by teaching food preparation skills. Little is known about using a similar program structure targeting PA, and further a holistic program targeting both, PA and nutrition as a comprehensive chronic disease health intervention program.

Staff report more "hyper specificity" in the types of foods clients are requesting due to doctor recommendations through food prescriptions, yet neither staff nor volunteers have the expertise to address these client needs. Thus, trained health educators and/or health coaches could help fill this void [49]. Health professionals could provide services such as pantry shopping assistance, food item identification, recipes, and food skills training that match specific client needs [50]. Due to this gap in expertise among current volunteers and staff, health intervention programming within the food pantry setting would require, either a hired staff member, additional recruitment and training of volunteers, and/or a partnership with local health organizations.

Nutrition and PA knowledge gaps across a diverse range of categories were recognized between all three stakeholder groups. This ranged from healthy cooking on a budget to exercising with limitations, giving direction to health content as an educational component to health intervention programming. Clients advocated for a positive, non-judgmental climate, entailing goal setting and accountability components. This is consistent with elements used within health coaching models that are linked to improvements in health lifestyle behaviors [49]. Health coaching can combine traditional health education strategies with motivational interviewing techniques to increase knowledge, skills, individual motivation, autonomy, and self-efficacy, promoting changes in health behaviors [29]. Last, support for health intervention programing was generated by all three stakeholder groups, particularly among the priority population. By using a formative community participatory approach [33] to gain support and develop intervention components, there will be a greater chance for intervention success and adoption by pantry clients during implementation.

Study Limitations

The current study only included one county-wide Midwest food pantry with a small sample of the key stakeholders creating generalization limitations. Additionally, the tools included in the study were designed by an investigator and were not first tested for reliability or validity.

5. Conclusions

High rates of chronic disease combined with low nutrition and PA literacy among pantry clients demonstrates the need to address health behaviors. In this study, each stakeholder group provided program component recommendations and indicated support for a health intervention program within the food pantry setting. Further research piloting the design and implementation of such a program in the pantry setting is needed. More specifically, design and implementation of a more holistic approach incorporating both nutrition and PA aimed at individual needs and disease prevention. The results will be used to prepare phase two, design and implement a health intervention program within a county-wide Midwest food pantry. Furthermore, key highlights from this research work that could be transferable into the field include:

- High rates of disease combined with low nutrition and PA literacy highlight the importance of holistic health intervention programming targeting health behaviors and chronic disease among food pantry clients. This includes considering intervention designs that go beyond addressing a single disease (e.g., diabetes) and work within a broader framework to address disease prevention and management (e.g., health coaching).
- A lack of expertise among volunteers and staff suggests program implementation will require hired staff members, specialized volunteers, and/or partnerships with local health organizations. This warrants the need to build community partnerships and create opportunities for additional training within pantry staff and volunteers to include an ecological approach to intervention design and implementation.
- Key characteristics of health intervention programming included accountability, incentives and individual attention. Mixed results regarding the program delivery platform lend to hybrid format options (in-person, virtual, group, and individual). Health coaching incorporates elements such as individual attention, social support, motivational interviewing, and accountability that match these intervention characteristics. This approach has been minimally tested in the food pantry setting.
- All three stakeholder groups recognized individual-level client needs and gaps in programming, aimed at prevention, prior to disease onset. Intervention programming that is focused on individual level need, such as health coaching, can lend to an intervention, which meets both disease management and disease prevention needs of food insecure pantry clients.

Supplementary Materials: The following are available online at https://www.mdpi.com/article/10.3390/nu13051584/s1, File S1: Shaping a Food Pantry Health Intervention-Client Survey, File S2: Shaping a Food Pantry Health Intervention-Client Interview Questions, File S3: Shaping a Food Pantry Health Intervention-Staff/volunteer Survey, File S4: Shaping a Food Pantry Health Intervention-Staff/volunteer Interview Questions.

Author Contributions: K.F., primary investigator (PI), co-designed instruments, collected and analyzed data, and co-wrote manuscript; S.H. advisor to the project, co-PI, co-designed instruments, and co-wrote manuscript. Both authors have read and agreed to the published version of the manuscript.

Funding: This research work was supported by the University of Kansas office of Graduate Studies Summer Research Scholarship. The article processing charges related to the publication of this article were supported by The University of Kansas (KU) One University Open Access Author Fund sponsored jointly by the KU Provost, KU Vice Chancellor for Research & Graduate Studies, and KUMC Vice Chancellor for Research and managed jointly by the Libraries at the Medical Center and KU-Lawrence.

Institutional Review Board Statement: The study was conducted according to the guidelines of the Declaration of Helsinki and approved by the Institutional Review Board of The University of Kansas (STUDY00144140, approved 11 June 2019).

Informed Consent Statement: Informed consent was obtained from all subjects involved in the study.

Data Availability Statement: The data presented in this study are available on request from the corresponding author.

Acknowledgments: The authors would like to thank all of the individuals that were willing to participate and tell their stories. Additionally, we would like to thank Elizabeth Keever and the staff at the Just Food food bank for providing secondary data and hosting the project work.

Conflicts of Interest: The authors declare no conflict of interest.

References

1. Coleman-Jensen, A.; Rabbitt, M.P.; Gregory, C.A.; Singh, A. Household Food Security in the United States in 2018. 2019. Available online: https://www.ers.usda.gov/webdocs/publications/94849/err270_summary.pdf?v=963.1 (accessed on 13 October 2020).
2. Gregory, C.A.; Coleman-Jensen, A. Food insecurity, chronic disease, and health among working-age adults. In *Economic Research Report Number 235*; USDA: Washington, DC, USA, 2017.
3. Berkowitz, S.A.; Basu, S.; Gundersen, C.; Seligman, H.K. State-Level and county-level estimates of health care costs associated with food insecurity. *Prev. Chronic Dis.* **2019**, *16*, E90. [CrossRef]
4. Hoisington, A.; Shultz, J.A.; Butkus, S. Coping strategies and nutrition education needs among food pantry users. *J. Nutr. Educ. Behav.* **2002**, *34*, 326–333. [CrossRef]
5. Ziliak, J.P.; Gundersen, C. The health consequences of senior hunger in the united states: Evidence from the 1999–2010 NHANES. In *Prepared for the National Foundation to End Senior Hunger*; Feeding America: Chicago, IL, USA, 2014; Available online: https://www.feedingamerica.org/research/senior-hunger-research/senior (accessed on 13 October 2020).
6. Dietary Guidelines Advisory Committee. *Scientific Report of the 2015 Dietary Guidelines Advisory Committee. Washington, DC: U.S. Department of Agriculture & U.S. Department of Health and Human Services, 2015*; Dietary Guidelines Advisory Committee: Washington, DC, USA, 2016.
7. Holben, D.H.; Marshall, M.B. Position of the academy of nutrition and dietetics: Food insecurity in the united states. *J. Acad. Nutr. Diet.* **2017**, *117*, 1991–2002. [CrossRef]
8. McGuire, S.; Nord, M.; Coleman-Jensen, A.; Andrews, M.; Carlson, S. Household food security in the united states, 2009. EER-108, U.S. Dept. of Agriculture, Econ. Res. Serv. November 2010. *Adv. Nutr.* **2009**, *2*, 153–154. [CrossRef]
9. Bradley, S.; Vitous, C.A.; Walsh-Felz, A.; Himmelgreen, D. Food insecurity and healthcare decision making among mobile food pantry clients in Tampa Bay. *Ecol. Food Nutr.* **2018**, *57*, 206–222. [CrossRef]
10. Dave, J.M.; Thompson, D.I.; Svendsen-Sanchez, A.; Cullen, K.W. Perspectives on barriers to eating healthy among food pantry clients. *Health Equity* **2017**, *1*, 28–34. [CrossRef]
11. Begley, A.; Paynter, E.; Butcher, L.M.; Dhaliwal, S.S. Examining the association between food literacy and food insecurity. *Nutrients* **2019**, *11*, 445. [CrossRef]
12. Cha, E.; Kim, K.H.; Lerner, H.M.; Dawkins, C.R.; Bello, M.K.; Umpierrez, G.; Dunbar, S.B. Health literacy, self-efficacy, food label use, and diet in young adults. *Am. J. Health Behav.* **2014**, *38*, 331–339. [CrossRef]
13. U.S. Department of Health and Human Services. *Physical Activity Guidelines for Americans*, 2nd ed.; Department of Health and Human Services: Washington, DC, USA, 2018.
14. To, Q.G.; Frongillo, E.A.; Gallegos, D.; Moore, J.B. Household food insecurity is associated with less physical activity among children and adults in the U.S. population. *J. Nutr.* **2014**, *144*, 1797–1802. [CrossRef] [PubMed]
15. Abe, T.; Mitsukawa, N.; Loenneke, J.P. Walking past barriers to physical activity. *J. Trainol.* **2020**, *9*, 9–10. [CrossRef]
16. Rech, C.; Camargo, E.; Almeida, M.; Bronoski, R.; Okuno, N.; Reis, R. Barriers for physical activity in overweight adults. *Rev. Bras. Ativ. Física Saúde* **2016**, *21*, 272–279. [CrossRef]
17. Bruening, M.; van Woerden, I.; Todd, M.; Laska, M.N. Hungry to learn: The prevalence and effects of food insecurity on health behaviors and outcomes over time among a diverse sample of university freshmen. *Int. J. Behav. Nutr. Phys. Act.* **2018**, *15*, 9. [CrossRef]
18. Gunter, K.B.; Jackson, J.; Tomayko, E.J.; John, D.H. Food insecurity and physical activity insecurity among rural Oregon families. *Prev. Med. Rep.* **2017**, *8*, 38–41. [CrossRef] [PubMed]
19. Gundersen, C.; Ziliak, J.P. Food insecurity and health outcomes. *Health Aff.* **2015**, *34*, 1830–1839. [CrossRef]
20. WHO. World Health Statistics 2018: Monitoring Health for the SDGs, Sustainable Development Goals. 2018. [Cited 14 September 2020]. Available online: https://apps.who.int/iris/bitstream/handle/10665/272596/9789241565585-eng.pdf?ua=1 (accessed on 13 October 2020).
21. Chiu, C.-Y.; Brooks, J.; An, R. Beyond food insecurity. *Br. Food J.* **2016**, *118*, 2614–2631. [CrossRef]
22. Thom, D.H.; Hessler, D.; Willard-Grace, R.; Bodenheimer, T.; Najmabadi, A.; Araujo, C.; Chen, E.H. Does health coaching change patients' trust in their primary care provider? *Patient Educ. Couns.* **2014**, *96*, 135–138. [CrossRef]

23. Williams, A.; Gattuso, J.; Adams, A.; Stockslager, S.; Boston, J. Food pantry to food farmacy: Design of a multi-faceted quality improvement program for low-income diabetes patients. *J. Nutr. Educ. Behav.* **2018**, *50*, S62. [CrossRef]
24. Hecht, J.; Borrelli, B.; Breger, R.K.; DeFrancesco, C.; Ernst, D.; Resnicow, K. Motivational interviewing in community-based research: Experiences from the field. *Ann. Behav. Med. A Publ. Soc. Behav. Med.* **2005**, *29*, 29–34. [CrossRef]
25. Thom, D.H.; Wolf, J.; Gardner, H.; DeVore, D.; Lin, M.; Ma, A.; Ibarra-Castro, A.; Saba, G. A qualitative study of how health coaches support patients in making health-related decisions and behavioral changes. *Ann. Fam. Med.* **2016**, *14*, 509–516. [CrossRef] [PubMed]
26. Willard-Grace, R.; DeVore, D.; Chen, E.H.; Hessler, D.; Bodenheimer, T.; Thom, D.H. The effectiveness of medical assistant health coaching for low-income patients with uncontrolled diabetes, hypertension, and hyperlipidemia: Protocol for a randomized controlled trial and baseline characteristics of the study population. *BMC Fam. Pract.* **2013**, *14*, 1–10. [CrossRef] [PubMed]
27. Byker Shanks, C. Promoting food pantry environments that encourage nutritious eating behaviors. *J. Acad. Nutr. Diet.* **2017**, *117*, 523–525. [CrossRef]
28. Holben, D.H. Position of the american dietetic association: Food insecurity and hunger in the united states. *J. Am. Diet. Assoc.* **2006**, *106*, 446–458. [CrossRef]
29. Flynn, M.M.; Schiff, A.R. A six week cooking program using a plant-based, olive oil diet improves the diet quality and the food purchased by food pantry clients. *J. Am. Diet. Assoc.* **2010**, *110*, A12. [CrossRef]
30. Seligman, H.K.; Lyles, C.; Marshall, M.B.; Prendergast, K.; Smith, M.C.; Headings, A.; Bradshaw, G.; Rosenmoss, S.; Waxman, E. A pilot food bank intervention featuring diabetes-appropriate food improved glycemic control among clients in three states. *Health Aff.* **2015**, *34*, 1956–1963. [CrossRef]
31. Martin, K.S.; Wu, R.; Wolff, M.; Colantonio, A.G.; Grady, J. A novel food pantry program: Food security, self-sufficiency, and diet-quality outcomes: Food security, self-sufficiency, and diet-quality outcomes. *Am. J. Prev. Med.* **2013**, *45*, 569–575. [CrossRef] [PubMed]
32. An, R.; Wang, J.; Liu, J.; Shen, J.; Loehmer, E.; McCaffrey, J. A systematic review of food pantry-based interventions in the USA. *Public Health Nutr.* **2019**, *22*, 1704–1716. [CrossRef]
33. Rabinowitz, P. Section 2. Participatory Approaches to Planning Community Interventions. n.d. [Cited 27 October 2020]. Available online: https://ctb.ku.edu/en/table-of-contents/analyze/where-to-start/participatory-approaches/main (accessed on 27 January 2021).
34. Just Food. Just Food Assessment and 5-Year. Strategic Plan 2018–2023. 2018. Available online: https://0198a7cc-03cc-4169-a240-5b50c131d308.filesusr.com/ugd/ec97f8_55cf1f39f92e49b18f75dbd4c5f43370.pdf (accessed on 13 October 2020).
35. Just Food. Annual Report 2018-2019. *Belf. North. Irel. Soc. Care Counc.* **2018**. Available online: https://0198a7cc-03cc-4169-a240-5b50c131d308.filesusr.com/ugd/ec97f8_59c555574ec14c1f9dc82d5e8d55f097.pdf (accessed on 13 October 2020).
36. Prinja, S.; Jeet, G.; Kumar, R. Validity of self-reported morbidity. *Indian J. Med. Res.* **2012**, *136*, 722–724.
37. Center for Disease Control and Prevention. BRFSS Questionnaires. 2019. Available online: https://www.cdc.gov/brfss/questionnaires/index.htm (accessed on 24 January 2021).
38. Lincoln, Y.; Guba, E. *Naturalistic Inquiry*; Sage Publications: London, UK, 1985.
39. Merriam, S.B.A. *Qualitative Research: A Guide to Design and Implementation*, 4th ed.; Tisdell, E.J.A., Ed.; Jossey-Bass, a Wiley Brand: San Francisco, CA, USA, 2016.
40. American Hospital Association. Improvement, EXECUTIVE BRIEFING 3: Hospitals and Food Insecurity. *Trustee* **2017**, *70*. Available online: https://trustees.aha.org/articles/1299-hospitals-and-food-insecurity (accessed on 24 November 2020).
41. FRAC Hunger & Health. *The Impact of Poverty, Food Insecurity, and Poor Nutrition on Health and Well-Being*; FRAC Hunger & Health: Washington, DC, USA, 2017; pp. 1–6.
42. Wetherill, M.S. Design and implementation of a clinic-based food pharmacy for food insecure, uninsured patients to support chronic disease self-management. *J. Nutr. Educ. Behav.* **2018**, *50*, 947–949. [CrossRef]
43. AAFP. Food is Health Pilot Improves Patients' Diabetes Markers. 2019. Available online: https://www.aafp.org/news/education-professional-development/20190410foodishealth.html (accessed on 24 November 2020).
44. Long, C.R.; Rowland, B.; Steelman, S.C.; McElfish, P.A. Outcomes of disease prevention and management interventions in food pantries and food banks: A scoping review. *BMJ Open* **2019**, *9*, e029236. [CrossRef] [PubMed]
45. Cheyne, K. Food bank-based diabetes prevention intervention to address food security, dietary intake, and physical activity in a food-insecure cohort at high risk for diabetes. *Prev. Chronic Dis.* **2020**, *17*, E04. [CrossRef] [PubMed]
46. Linden, A.; Butterworth, S.W.; Prochaska, J.O. Motivational interviewing-based health coaching as a chronic care intervention. *J. Eval. Clin. Pract.* **2010**, *16*, 166–174. [CrossRef] [PubMed]
47. Cinar, A.B.; Schou, L. The role of self-efficacy in health coaching and health education for patients with type 2 diabetes. *Int. Dent. J.* **2014**, *64*, 155–163. [CrossRef] [PubMed]
48. Kihlstrom, L.; Long, A.; Himmelgreen, D. Barriers and facilitators to the consumption of fresh produce among food pantry clients. *J. Hunger Environ. Nutr.* **2019**, *14*, 168–182. [CrossRef]
49. Feeding America. Why Should We Think about Food Insecurity and Health? n.d. Available online: https://hungerandhealth.feedingamerica.org/explore-our-work/community-health-care-partnerships/ (accessed on 26 April 2021).
50. USDA. Healthy Pantry Initiative. 2016. Available online: https://snaped.fns.usda.gov/success-stories/healthy-food-pantry-initiative (accessed on 26 April 2021).

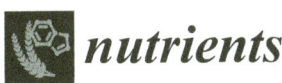

Article

The Combined Effects of Milk Intake and Physical Activity on Bone Mineral Density in Korean Adolescents

Jae Hyun Lee [1,†], Ae Wha Ha [2,†], Woo Kyoung Kim [2] and Sun Hyo Kim [3,*]

1. Department of Sport Science, College of Natural Sciences, Chungnam National University, Daejeon City 34134, Korea; leejh1215@cnu.ac.kr
2. Department of Food Science and Nutrition, College of Natural Science, Dankook University, Chungcheongnam-do, Cheonan City 31116, Korea; aewhaha@dankook.ac.kr (A.W.H.); wkkim@dankook.ac.kr (W.K.K.)
3. Department of Technology and Home Economics Education, Kongju National University, Chungcheongnam-do, Gongju City 32588, Korea
* Correspondence: shkim@kongju.ac.kr
† These authors contributed equally to this work.

Abstract: The purpose of this study was to examine the combined effects of milk intake and physical activity on bone mineral density in adolescents. This study was conducted using data from the 2009–2011 Korea National Health and Nutrition Examination Survey (KNHANES), which provided measurements of bone mineral density (BMD) in addition to basic health-related data. This study included 1061 adolescents aged 13 to 18 years (557 males and 504 females) whose data on milk intake and participation time in moderate to vigorous physical activity were available. BMD was measured by dual-energy X-ray absorptiometry (DXA). Milk intake was assessed using the 24-h recall method, and the levels of physical activity were examined using a questionnaire. The physical activity questions of 2009–2011 KNHANES were based on the Korean version of the International Physical Activity Questionnaire (IPAQ) short form. The subjects were classified into four groups according to milk intake and physical activity level: no milk intake + low-level physical activity group ($M_{no}P_{low}$), no milk intake + high-level physical activity group ($M_{no}P_{high}$), milk intake + low-level physical activity group ($M_{yes}P_{low}$), and milk intake + high-level physical activity group ($M_{yes}P_{high}$). The results of partial correlation controlling for age, body mass index (BMI), and energy intake showed that the BMD variables were associated significantly with physical activity in both males and females. Among males, the $M_{no}P_{low}$ group had the lowest BMD in all BMD variables, showing a significant difference from the high-level physical activity groups ($M_{no}P_{high}$, $M_{yes}P_{high}$) by multiple logistic regression analysis. Among females, the $M_{yes}P_{high}$ group showed a significantly higher lumbar BMD value than the other groups. The $M_{no}P_{low}$ group had approximately 0.3 to 0.5 times lower odds ratio for median or higher BMD values, compared to $M_{yes}P_{high}$ group. These results show that milk intake and physical activity have a combined effect on BMD, and suggest that to achieve healthy bone growth, it is important to encourage both moderate to vigorous physical activity and milk intake during adolescence.

Keywords: bone mineral density; milk intake; physical activity; adolescence

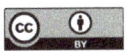

1. Introduction

Bones are major organs that determine the body's physique and perform various functions, such as protection of internal organs, mineral storage, and blood cell formation. Bone ossification begins in the prenatal period and almost reaches the total peak bone mass by the end of teenage growth [1,2]. During puberty, the bone mineral accrual rate reaches a peak, and approximately one quarter of the total bone minerals of adults are accumulated within two years at this time [3]. In Koreans, the peak bone mass of the femoral neck and total hip is achieved around the age of 20, and the greatest increase in lumbar bone mineral density (BMD) occurs between 11–13 years of age in females and 12–14 years of age in males [4,5]. Hence, adolescence is a very important period of life for the formation of healthy bones. People who fail to achieve optimal peak bone mass and strength during childhood and adolescence have been reported to be more likely to develop osteoporosis later in life [6,7], and low BMD is associated with a higher risk of fractures even in healthy children and adolescents, just as it is a risk factor for fracture in adults with osteoporosis [8,9]. Therefore, to obtain the benefits of healthy bones for life, appropriate interventions are required to help children and adolescents build healthy and strong bones during the growth period.

Peak bone mass, which means the maximum accumulation of bone mineral content, is determined by genetic and environmental factors. Environmental factors include physical activity, sedentary lifestyle, and dietary factors such as milk intake [10–14]. The consumption of milk and dairy products helps maximize the bone mineral content during puberty, which is the second period of the growth spurt [15,16]. Milk has a high calcium content, and calcium in milk has high digestibility and bioavailability [17]. This is because milk contains lactose, vitamin D, and peptides promoting calcium absorption, which help the body to absorb calcium, and contains calcium and phosphorus in an appropriate ratio that increases the rate of calcium absorption [18]. The consumption of milk and dairy products during the growth period can be a good source of calcium as well as energy, macronutrients, and micronutrients important for the growth and development of children and adolescents [13,14,17–20]. A four-year follow-up study of 19,991 children in eight European countries reported that the consumption of milk and dairy products (yogurt and cheese) as snacks was associated with better diet quality [21]. Therefore, the daily consumption of milk and dairy products for children and adolescents can be a good strategy for maintaining a balanced diet during the growth period.

Mechanical stimulation is an important determinant of bone growth and formation. Exercises that provide physical and physiological stimulation improve muscular strength, cartilage preservation, and bone remodeling [22,23], and they have a positive effect on increasing BMD [24,25]. Most studies on the effects of weight-bearing exercises on the accumulation of bone mineral content during childhood and adolescence reported that such exercises have positive effects, and this phenomenon is particularly pronounced in early puberty [26]. The performance of the activities of high intensity or impact and participation in sports activities have also found to have a positive effect on the BMD or cortical bone size [25,27,28].

As described above, various studies have been conducted on the effects of milk intake or physical activity alone on BMD during the growth period. Limited studies suggested an important interaction between physical activity and the intake of dietary calcium, not milk intake, to increase bone mass. When physical activity and calcium intake were combined, bone density formation was greater than either physical activity or calcium intake alone [29–31]. In addition, those studies have been conducted in preschool or school children. Therefore, this study aims to evaluate the combined effects of milk intake and physical activity on BMD during adolescence. We hypothesized that adolescents who had a high level of physical activity and consumed milk would have higher BMD than those who had a low level of physical activity and did not consume milk.

2. Methods

2.1. Data Collection

This study examined the relationship of BMD with milk intake and physical activity using 2009 to 2011 data from the fourth (2007–2009) and fifth (2010–2012) Korea National Health and Nutrition Examination Survey (KNHANES). The KNHANES survey began in 1998 and has been conducted annually, with BMD measurements conducted from July 2008 to May 2011. Data of 1731 people aged 13–18 (1198 males and 812 females) who underwent BMD measurements using dual energy X-ray absorptiometry (DXA) were collected. Subjects with missing data regarding milk intake or physical activity and those whose data showing extreme outliers were excluded. Ultimately, the data of 1061 people (557 males and 504 females) were included in the final analysis.

This study used the data from the KNHANES approved by the Institutional Review Board of the Korea Centers for Disease Control and Prevention (2009-01CON-03-2C, 2010-02CON-21-C, 2011-02CON-06-C), which was conducted after receiving an exempt determination from the Institutional Review Board of Kongju National University (KNU_IRB_2020-65).

2.2. Milk Intake

The analysis of milk intake was conducted using data from a dietary intake survey by the 24-h recall method among the raw data sets of the KNHANES. According to the food-group classification standard codes presented in the guidelines on the use of the KNHANES data, the food name of 'milk' among the secondary food names was first classified. The type of milk consumed was then examined using the primary food names, and the participant was classified as a person consuming milk when the type of milk consumed was white milk.

2.3. Physical Activity

The level of physical activity was calculated by the time of moderate or vigorous physical activity performed per week (number of days per week (days/week) × activity time (minutes/day)). The questions on moderate and vigorous physical activity in KNHANES were as follows:

- Questions on moderate physical activity:
  - On how many days in the past week did you perform moderate physical activity that made you feel slightly more tired than usual, or during which you felt a little short of breath for at least 10 min?
  - On the days when you performed moderate physical activities, how many minutes per day did you usually perform them?

Examples of moderate physical activities: vocational and physical activities, such as slow swimming, doubles tennis, volleyball, badminton, table tennis, moving, or carrying light items.

- Questions on vigorous physical activity:
  - On how many days in the past week did you perform vigorous physical activity that made you feel much more exhausted than usual, or during which you felt very short of breath?
  - On the days when you performed vigorous physical activities, how many minutes per day did you usually perform them?

Examples of vigorous activities: vocational and physical activities, such as jogging or running, mountain climbing, fast cycling, fast swimming, soccer, basketball, jumping rope, squash, singles tennis, moving or carrying heavy objects.

In this study, based on the guidelines on physical activity presented by the Ministry of Health and Welfare for calculating weekly physical activity time, it was assumed that one minute of vigorous physical activity is equal to two minutes of moderate physical activity [32]. Using this guideline, the total physical activity time was calculated by converting vigorous physical activity time to moderate physical activity time. The physical activity questions of the 2009–2011 KNHANES were based on the Korean version of the International Physical Activity Questionnaire (IPAQ) short form.

2.4. Subject Grouping

The subjects were divided into the milk intake group (M_{yes} group: milk intake >0 g/day) and the no milk intake group (M_{no} group: milk intake = 0 g/day). For physical activity grouping, the median of the weekly participation time of moderate-to-vigorous physical activity was calculated by converting vigorous physical activity times to moderate physical activity time. Subjects with a value below the median were classified as the low-level physical activity (P_{low}) group. Those with a value equivalent or higher than median were classified as the high-level physical activity (P_{high}) group. Groups can also be classified according to the satisfaction of the physical activity guidelines of 60 min of moderate-to-vigorous activities every day. However, only 5.1% of men and 1.9% of women actually meet these criteria (420 min per week), making it impossible to compare the groups using statistical analysis. Therefore, in this study, groups were classified using the median of converted physical activity time per week. The physical activity questions of the 2009–2011 KNHANES were based on the Korean version of the International Physical Activity Questionnaire (IPAQ) short form.

By combining these two classifications, the subjects were finally classified into four groups according to milk intake and physical activity level: no milk intake + low-level physical activity group ($M_{no}P_{low}$), no milk intake + high-level physical activity group ($M_{no}P_{high}$), milk intake + low-level physical activity group ($M_{yes}P_{low}$), and milk intake + high-level physical activity group ($M_{yes}P_{high}$).

2.5. Bone Mineral Density

BMD was measured using dual-energy X-ray absorptiometry (DXA; DISCOVERY-W fan-beam densitometer Hologic Inc., Bedford, MA, USA) and each subject's whole body, lumbar spine, and femur were scanned. When measuring the lumbar spine, a lumbar positioner was used to reduce spinal lordosis, and the lumbar spine was positioned straight so as to be in line with the vertical central axis of the image. The image included the midsection of T12 and L5, and to determine whether the lumbar spine was correctly positioned, it was checked whether the 12th rib and iliac crest were visible in the image, and whether the intervertebral disc of L4–L5 passed in line with the iliac crest. When measuring the femur, the angle of the leg was adjusted so that the femoral shaft was positioned straight in line with the vertical central axis of the image. When measuring DXA, it was checked if there were any artifacts such as coins or keys, buttons, wires, jewelry, or metal objects in the pocket. Among the various DXA measurement indices, total body, femur, femur neck, and lumbar spine (L1–4) BMD were analyzed statistically, and total body BMD was calculated using the BMD values of the whole body except for head BMD.

2.6. Statistical Analysis

The data of the KNHANES were collected not by simple random sampling but by stratified multistage probability sampling. Hence, the weight, strata (KSTRATA), and cluster (primary sampling unit, PSU) were included in the analysis. The sociodemographic characteristics of the subjects were expressed as frequency and percentage, and differences in distribution between the groups were compared using PROC SURVEYFREQ (chi-squared test). For the continuous variables, descriptive statistical analysis was performed to calculate the mean and standard error. Partial correlation analysis was performed to identify the relationship of BMD with physical activity and milk intake while controlling for age, body mass index (BMI), and energy intake. The differences in explanatory variables between the four groups ($M_{no}P_{low}$, $M_{no}P_{high}$, $M_{yes}P_{low}$, and $M_{yes}P_{high}$ groups) were analyzed by PROC SURVEYREG analysis after adjusting for age, BMI, and energy intake. For a post-hoc test of the differences among the groups, the *p*-values were assessed using a Bonferroni test considering the design effect of complex sampling design. The PROC SURVEYLOGISTIC analysis was performed (after adjusting for age, BMI, and energy intake) to calculate the risk ratio of each BMD index of the three groups compared to the reference group (the $M_{yes}P_{high}$ group). The analysis results were expressed as an odds ratio (OR) and 95% confidence interval (CI).

All statistical analyses were conducted using SAS version 9.4 (Statistical Analysis System, SAS Institute, Cary, NC, USA), and *p* values <0.05 were considered significant.

3. Results

Table 1 lists the sociodemographic characteristics of the subjects. Significant differences in school year and gender were observed among the four groups. Of the 1061 subjects, high-school students (57.0%) comprised a larger proportion than middle-school students (43.0%), and the difference in the percentage between middle school and high school was the largest in the $M_{no}P_{low}$ group. The subjects consisted of 557 males (52.5%) and 504 females (47.5%), and the difference in the percentage between males and females was the largest in the $M_{yes}P_{high}$ group (68.0% in males vs. 32.0% in females). Therefore, the analysis was conducted separately for males and females, and data analysis was conducted by controlling for age. There were no significant differences in the distribution of income levels or residential areas.

Table 1. Sociodemographic characteristics of the subjects.

	Variables	$M_{no}P_{low}$ [1]	$M_{no}P_{high}$	$M_{yes}P_{low}$	$M_{yes}P_{high}$	Total	p-Value [2]
School year	Middle school (7th–9th year)	146(34.6) [3]	100(49.5)	108(41.2)	102(58.3)	456(43.0)	<0.001
	High school (10th–12th year)	276(65.4)	102(50.5)	154(58.8)	73(41.7)	605(57.0)	
Gender	Male	203(48.1)	105(52.0)	130(49.6)	119(68.0)	557(52.5)	0.044
	Female	219(51.9)	97(48.0)	132(50.4)	56(32.0)	504(47.5)	
Income	Low	125(30.0)	49(24.7)	65(25.0)	35(20.2)	274(26.1)	0.086
	Middle–low	108(25.9)	47(23.7)	60(23.1)	43(24.9)	258(24.6)	
	Middle–high	96(23.0)	51(25.8)	61(23.4)	42(24.3)	250(23.9)	
	High	88(21.1)	51(25.8)	74(28.5)	53(30.6)	266(25.4)	
Region (Living area)	Large city	172(40.8)	76(37.6)	105(40.1)	80(45.7)	433(40.8)	0.719
	Medium or small city	183(43.3)	98(48.5)	113(43.1)	77(44.0)	471(44.4)	
	Rural area	67(15.9)	28(13.9)	44(16.8)	18(10.3)	157(14.8)	

[1] $M_{no}P_{low}$: no milk intake + low physical activity; $M_{no}P_{high}$: no milk intake + high physical activity; $M_{yes}P_{low}$: milk intake + low physical activity; $M_{yes}P_{high}$: milk intake + high physical activity (P_{low}: physical activity less than 50th percentile; P_{high}: physical activity of 50th percentile or more); [2] p-value by chi-square test. [3] n (%).

Regarding the distribution of daily milk intake among subjects, the milk intake ranged from 0 to 1484 mL/day among males and from 0 to 848 mL/day among females. Approximately 55.4% of males and 62.6% of females did not consume milk, and in both males and females, the proportion of people drinking 200–400 mL/day was highest, accounting for 24.2 and 20.9%, respectively. According to the dietary reference intakes for Koreans (KDRIs), it is recommended that adolescents drink two glasses (400 mL) of milk a day [33], and the percentage of adolescents consuming the recommended amount or more of milk was 14.7% in males and 8.1% in females; females tended to drink less milk than males (Figure 1).

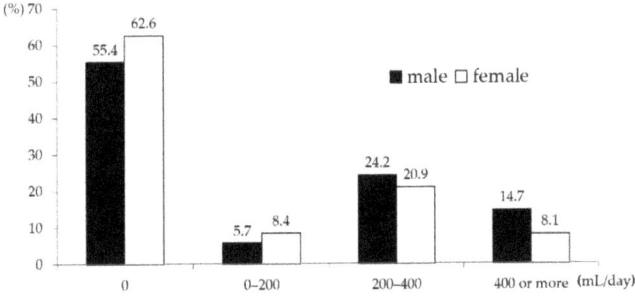

Figure 1. Distribution of daily milk intake.

The converted time of physical activity ranged from 0 to 780 min/week among males and 0 to 600 min/week among females. The weekly participation time of moderate to vigorous physical activity except for walking was 0 min in 31.2% of males and 49.7% of females. For both males and females, the proportion of adolescents showing a converted physical activity time of 60–120 min per week was highest, accounting for 14.6% and 16.3%, respectively. The proportion of those participating in physical activity for 300 min or more per week was 12.9% in males and 4.9% in females. Hence, the level of participation in physical activity was significantly lower among females than among males (Figure 2).

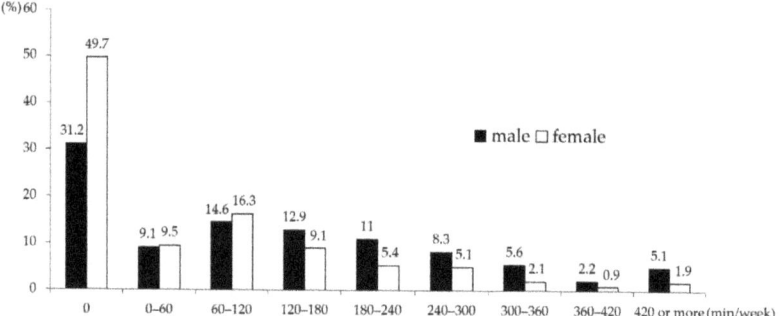

Figure 2. Distribution of physical activity.

Table 2 lists the milk intake and physical activity time of each group. Because the subjects were classified according to whether they consumed milk or not, the daily milk intake of the no milk intake groups ($M_{no}P_{low}$, $M_{no}P_{high}$) was 0 mL. In the milk intake groups, the milk intake levels for males in the $M_{yes}P_{low}$ and $M_{yes}P_{high}$ groups were 360.1 mL and 349.0 mL, respectively. For females, the milk intake levels in the $M_{yes}P_{low}$ and $M_{yes}P_{high}$ were 280.8 mL and 278.8 mL, respectively. There was a large difference in the physical activity time between the high-level physical activity groups ($M_{no}P_{high}$, $M_{yes}P_{high}$) and low-level physical activity groups ($M_{no}P_{low}$, $M_{yes}P_{low}$). For groups with high physical activity, weekly physical activity time among males was 227.3 min for $M_{no}P_{high}$ and 230 min for $M_{yes}P_{low}$. Among females, the physical activity time in the $M_{no}P_{high}$ and $M_{yes}P_{high}$ groups was 130.7 min and 175.9 min per week, respectively. The weekly physical activity time among males was 11.8 ± 1.9 min for $M_{no}P_{low}$ and 26.3 ± 3.7 min for $M_{yes}P_{low}$.

Table 2. Milk intake and physical activity according to the group.

Gender	Variables	$M_{no}P_{low}$ [1]	$M_{no}P_{high}$	$M_{yes}P_{low}$	$M_{yes}P_{high}$	p-Value [2]	Total
Male	N	203	105	130	119		557
	Milk intake (mL/day)	0.0 ± 0.0 [3][a][4]	0.0 ± 0.0 [a]	360.1 ± 30.3 [b]	349.0 ± 28.1 [b]	<0.001	146.2 ± 12.2
	Physical activity (min/week)	11.8 ± 1.9 [a]	227.3 ± 12.2 [b]	26.3 ± 3.7 [c]	230.0 ± 14.3 [b]	<0.001	120.7 ± 7.9
Female	N	219	97	132	56		504
	Milk intake (mL/day)	0.0 ± 0.0 [a]	0.0 ± 0.0 [a]	280.8 ± 19.6 [b]	278.8 ± 18.6 [b]	<0.001	100.1 ± 9.1
	Physical activity (min/week)	0.0 ± 0.0 [a]	130.7 ± 11.1 [b]	0.0 ± 0.0 [a]	175.9 ± 22.7 [c]	<0.001	70.4 ± 7.9

[1] $M_{no}P_{low}$: no milk intake + low physical activity; $M_{no}P_{high}$: no milk intake + high physical activity; $M_{yes}P_{low}$: milk intake + low physical activity; $M_{yes}P_{high}$: milk intake + high physical activity (P_{low}: physical activity less than 50th percentile; P_{high}: physical activity of 50th percentile or more); [2] p-value by PROC SURVEYREG adjusted for age, body mass index, and energy intake; [3] Mean ± SE; [4][abc]: values with different alphabets in the same row are significantly different at $p = 0.05$ by a Bonferroni test.

Table 3 lists the general characteristics of each of the four groups classified according to milk intake and the level of physical activity. In both males and females, the mean age was highest in the $M_{no}P_{low}$ group and lowest in the $M_{yes}P_{high}$. For BMI, there was a significant difference only in females, showing that the $M_{no}P_{low}$ and $M_{yes}P_{low}$ groups with low levels of physical activity had a significantly lower mean BMI than the groups with high levels of physical activity. However, the mean BMI of these four groups were not largely different from 20.9 kg/m^2, the median BMI (50th percentile) of 15.4-year-old boys in the 2017 Korean National Growth Charts for Children and Adolescents published by the Ministry of Health and Welfare [34]. For reference, the BMI corresponding to overweight (from the 85th percentile to less than the 95th percentile) for a 15.4-year-old Korean girl is 23.7~25.5 kg/m^2, and the BMI corresponding to obesity (95th percentile or more) is 25.5 kg/m^2 or more [34].

Table 3. Physical characteristics of subjects.

Gender	Variables	$M_{no}P_{low}$ [1]	$M_{no}P_{high}$	$M_{yes}P_{low}$	$M_{yes}P_{high}$	p-Value [2]	Total
Male	Age (year)	15.9 ± 0.2 [3a4]	15.6 ± 0.2 [ab]	15.3 ± 0.2 [b]	15.1 ± 0.2 [b]	0.005	15.5 ± 0.1
	Height (cm)	171.0 ± 0.9	172.0 ± 0.8	169.9 ± 0.9	170.4 ± 0.7 [NS 5]	0.416	171.2 ± 0.4
	Weight (kg)	61.3 ± 1.2	64.1 ± 1.3	62.5 ± 1.7	62.3 ± 1.4 [NS]	0.745	62.5 ± 0.6
	BMI (kg/m^2) [6]	20.9 ± 0.4	21.8 ± 0.4	21.1 ± 0.5	21.4 ± 0.4 [NS]	0.307	21.2 ± 0.2
	%Fat (%)	20.2 ± 0.7	21.3 ± 0.7	20.0 ± 0.8	22.2 ± 0.9 [NS]	0.425	20.8 ± 0.4
Female	Age (year)	15.9 ± 0.2 [a]	15.3 ± 0.2 [bc]	15.3 ± 0.2 [bc]	14.8 ± 0.2 [b]	<0.001	15.4 ± 0.1
	Height (cm)	159.7 ± 0.6	160.4 ± 0.5	160.4 ± 0.7	160.0 ± 0.6 [NS]	0.551	160.2 ± 0.3
	Weight (kg)	53.0 ± 0.8	56.2 ± 1.1	52.5 ± 1.1	55.3 ± 1.7 [NS]	0.890	54.1 ± 0.6
	BMI (kg/m^2)	20.8 ± 0.3 [a]	21.8 ± 0.3 [b]	20.3 ± 0.3 [a]	21.6 ± 0.6 [b]	0.036	21.0 ± 0.2
	%Fat (%)	31.9 ± 0.5	33.6 ± 0.6	31.8 ± 0.6	33.0 ± 1.0 [NS]	0.195	32.7 ± 0.4

[1] $M_{no}P_{low}$: no milk intake + low physical activity; $M_{no}P_{high}$: no milk intake + high physical activity; $M_{yes}P_{low}$: milk intake + low physical activity; $M_{yes}P_{high}$: milk intake + high physical activity (P_{low}: physical activity less than 50th percentile; P_{high}: physical activity of 50th percentile or more); [2] p-value by PROC SURVEYREG adjusted for age, body mass index (BMI) and energy intake; [3] Mean ± SE; [4 abc]: values with different alphabets in the same row are significantly different at p = 0.05 by Bonferroni test; [5 NS]: not significant; [6] BMI = weight(kg)/height(m^2).

There was no difference in body fat (%) between groups in both male and females. Regarding the percentage of body fat in each group, the lowest and highest mean values were 20.0% and 22.2% among males and 31.8% and 33.6% among females. For reference, the mean body fat percentages of the male groups correspond to the 50–75th percentile of the percent body fat of Korean male adolescents, and the mean body fat percentages of female groups correspond to the 25–75th percentile of Korean female adolescents [35].

In order to identify the association of physical activity and milk intake with BMD, a partial correlation analysis for each gender group was conducted while controlling for age, BMI, and energy intake (Table 4). The results of this analysis showed that milk intake had no significant correlation with BMD. On the other hand, physical activity was found to have a weak but significant correlation with total body, femur, femur neck, and lumbar BMD.

Table 5 lists the results of comparative analysis of BMD among the four groups. Among males, there was a significant difference among the groups in all BMD variables, and the $M_{no}P_{low}$ group, the group of adolescents who did not consume milk and had a low level of physical activity, had a significantly lower BMD than the $M_{no}P_{high}$ and $M_{yes}P_{high}$ groups, which had a high level of physical activity. The BMD values of the $M_{no}P_{low}$ group were lower than the median BMD value among 15-year-old Korean boys and higher than the 10th percentile [4]. In the case of females, there was a significant difference among the groups only in lumbar BMD. The $M_{yes}P_{high}$ group, the group of females who consumed milk and had a high level of physical activity, showed a significantly higher lumbar BMD value of 0.931 (g/cm^2) than the other groups ($M_{no}P_{low}$: 0.902, $M_{no}P_{high}$: 0.900, $M_{yes}P_{low}$: 0.898). For reference, the median lumbar BMD value among 15-year-old Korean girls was 0.875 g/cm^2 [4].

Table 4. Relationships of bone mineral density with milk intake and physical activity.

Milk Intake and Physical Activity	Variables of BMD [1]	Male (n = 557)		Female (n = 504)	
		r	p-Value [2]	r	p-Value
Milk intake	Total BMD (g/cm^2)	0.025	0.574	0.038	0.426
	Femur BMD (g/cm^2)	0.017	0.707	0.017	0.718
	Femur neck BMD (g/cm^2)	−0.001	0.991	0.029	0.545
	Lumbar BMD (g/cm^2)	0.049	0.274	0.075	0.112
Physical activity time	Total BMD (g/cm^2)	0.212	<0.001	0.120	0.019
	Femur BMD (g/cm^2)	0.257	<0.001	0.142	0.005
	Femur neck BMD (g/cm^2)	0.250	<0.001	0.135	0.008
	Lumbar BMD (g/cm^2)	0.120	0.020	0.180	<0.001

[1] BMD: bone mineral density; [2] p-value by partial correlation controlled by age, body mass index, and energy intake.

Table 5. Bone mineral density among the groups of the combination of milk intake and physical activity.

Gender	Variables	$M_{no}P_{low}$ [2]	$M_{no}P_{high}$	$M_{yes}P_{low}$	$M_{yes}P_{high}$	p-Value [3]	Total
Male	Total BMD [1] (g/cm^2)	0.916 ± 0.012 [4][a][5]	0.952 ± 0.010 [b]	0.917 ± 0.014 [ac]	0.947 ± 0.012 [bc]	0.003	0.939 ± 0.005
	Femur BMD (g/cm^2)	0.896 ± 0.015 [a]	0.952 ± 0.016 [b]	0.917 ± 0.017 [ab]	0.952 ± 0.013 [b]	0.003	0.934 ± 0.006
	Femur neck BMD (g/cm^2)	0.813 ± 0.014 [a]	0.866 ± 0.014 [b]	0.817 ± 0.018 [ac]	0.863 ± 0.014 [c]	0.002	0.847 ± 0.006
	Lumbar BMD (g/cm^2)	0.839 ± 0.015 [a]	0.881 ± 0.016 [b]	0.850 ± 0.020 [ab]	0.866 ± 0.015 [b]	0.019	0.865 ± 0.007
Female	Total BMD (g/cm^2)	0.868 ± 0.010	0.866 ± 0.009	0.860 ± 0.010	0.866 ± 0.011 [NS][6]	0.094	0.866 ± 0.005
	Femur BMD (g/cm^2)	0.868 ± 0.014	0.876 ± 0.012	0.859 ± 0.015	0.885 ± 0.011 [NS]	0.416	0.873 ± 0.006
	Femur neck BMD (g/cm^2)	0.760 ± 0.013	0.769 ± 0.014	0.755 ± 0.015	0.770 ± 0.011 [NS]	0.700	0.765 ± 0.006
	Lumbar BMD (g/cm^2)	0.902 ± 0.011 [a]	0.900 ± 0.013 [a]	0.898 ± 0.014 [a]	0.931 ± 0.015 [b]	0.030	0.904 ± 0.007

[1] BMD: bone mineral density; [2] $M_{no}P_{low}$: no milk intake + low physical activity; $M_{no}P_{high}$: no milk intake + high physical activity; $M_{yes}P_{low}$: milk intake + low physical activity; $M_{yes}P_{high}$: milk intake + high physical activity (P_{low}: physical activity less than 50th percentile, P_{high}: physical activity of 50th percentile or more); [3] p-value by PROC SURVEYREG adjusted for age, body mass index, and energy intake; [4] Mean ± SE; [5] abc: Values with different alphabets in the same row are significantly different at p = 0.05 by Bonferroni test; [6] NS: not significant.

Table 6 lists the odds ratio and confidence interval (CI) for the 50th or higher percentile of the BMD value in each BMD variable for each group compared to the $M_{yes}P_{high}$ group. Among males, the $M_{no}P_{low}$ group had significantly lower odds ratio for the 50th percentile or higher of the BMD value than the $M_{yes}P_{high}$ group in all BMD variables. More specifically, the $M_{no}P_{low}$ group was 0.317 times less likely to have the 50th or higher percentile of total body BMD value than the $M_{yes}P_{high}$ group. For femur, femur neck, and lumbar BMD, the $M_{no}P_{low}$ group had 0.289, 0.512, and 0.493 times lower odds ratio for the 50th or higher percentile of the BMD compared to the $M_{yes}P_{high}$ group. In other words, the ratio of individuals with a median or higher BMD was significantly lower among the males who did not drink milk and had a low level of physical activity than the males who consumed milk and had a high level of physical activity. Among the females, the $M_{no}P_{low}$ group and $M_{yes}P_{low}$ group were 0.433 and 0.434 times less likely, respectively, to have the 50th or higher percentile of lumbar BMD than the $M_{yes}P_{high}$ group.

Table 6. Odds ratios on the bone mineral density according to the combination of milk intake and physical activity.

Variables	Group	Male		Female	
		Odds Ratio	CI [1]	Odds Ratio	CI
Total BMD [2] ≥50th percentile, 0.896 (Reference)	$M_{no}P_{low}$ [3] vs. $M_{yes}P_{high}$	0.317	(0.151, 0.663) * [4]	0.635	(0.301, 1.342)
	$M_{no}P_{high}$ vs. $M_{yes}P_{high}$	1.539	(0.729, 3.249)	0.654	(0.332, 1.289)
	$M_{yes}P_{low}$ vs. $M_{yes}P_{high}$	0.582	(0.248, 1.363)	0.652	(0.307, 1.384)
Femur BMD ≥50th percentile, 0.897 (Reference)	$M_{no}P_{low}$ vs. $M_{yes}P_{high}$	0.289	(0.154, 0.539) *	0.684	(0.339, 1.380)
	$M_{no}P_{high}$ vs. $M_{yes}P_{high}$	0.773	(0.394, 1.517)	0.752	(0.388, 1.461)
	$M_{yes}P_{low}$ vs. $M_{yes}P_{high}$	0.485	(0.234, 1.007)	0.545	(0.261, 1.141)
Femur neck BMD ≥50th percentile, 0.801 (Reference)	$M_{no}P_{low}$ vs. $M_{yes}P_{high}$	0.512	(0.274, 0.958) *	0.843	(0.405, 1.754)
	$M_{no}P_{high}$ vs. $M_{yes}P_{high}$	1.551	(0.798, 3.012)	0.918	(0.454, 1.857)
	$M_{yes}P_{low}$ vs. $M_{yes}P_{high}$	0.636	(0.30, 1.35)	0.894	(0.409, 1.951)
Lumbar BMD ≥50th percentile, 0.875 (Reference)	$M_{no}P_{low}$ vs. $M_{yes}P_{high}$	0.493	(0.245, 0.992) *	0.433	(0.21, 0.895) *
	$M_{no}P_{high}$ vs. $M_{yes}P_{high}$	1.140	(0.58, 2.24)	0.485	(0.233, 1.009)
	$M_{yes}P_{low}$ vs. $M_{yes}P_{high}$	1.149	(0.568, 2.322)	0.434	(0.203, 0.928) *
	$M_{yes}P_{high}$	1.000	(ref)	1.000	(ref)

[1] CI: confidence interval; [2] BMD: bone mineral density; [3] $M_{no}P_{low}$: no milk intake + low physical activity; $M_{no}P_{high}$: no milk intake + high physical activity; $M_{yes}P_{low}$: milk intake + low physical activity; $M_{yes}P_{high}$: milk intake + high physical activity (P_{low}: physical activity less than the 50th percentile; P_{high}: physical activity of the 50th percentile or more); [4] *: $p<0.05$ by PROC SURVEYLOGISTIC.

4. Discussion

Adolescence is a very important period for lifelong bone health. Several studies have reported that the factors that positively affect the increase in bone mineral content and density have greater effects during this period than in adulthood, and that the effects of such factors continue into adulthood [2,3,15,16,36,37].

The two methods for building strong bones or improving bone strength are ingesting sufficient nutrients related to the bone matrix or bone metabolism and applying appropriate mechanical stimulation to the bones. Typically, when the former method is used, people consume milk, which has a high calcium content and high digestibility and bioavailability of calcium. Weight-bearing physical activities are performed when the latter method is used. Consequently, the study was designed to examine the combined effects of milk intake and physical activity on BMD.

In a partial correlation analysis controlling for age, BMI, and energy intake, physical activity had a significant positive correlation with total, femur, femur neck, and lumbar BMD in both males and females. Physical activity has beneficial effects on bone health in all age groups, including adolescents. In particular, bone mineral content is higher among children and adolescents participating in activities involving the exertion of high impact force than among those who participate in non-weight bearing exercises, such as swimming, or in low-impact activities, such as walking [38,39]. Therefore, activities involving high ground-reaction forces, such as jumping, skipping, and running, are recommended as exercises for strengthening the bones during the growth period [40,41]. A cross-sectional analysis of the relationship between physical activity and hip BMD in 724 adolescents found that high impact (>4.2 g) activities, such as jumping and running (speeds>10 km/h), were associated with hip BMD, but moderate impact activity, such as jogging, had little effect [25]. However, the physical activity variable analyzed in this study was the time of participation in moderate to vigorous physical activities. The physical activities with moderate intensity examined in this study included sports, such as slow swimming, doubles tennis, badminton, and table tennis. Walking was excluded from the analysis because it was examined separately with a different format. Given these facts, it seems that the low correlation between physical activity and BMD might be related to the type and intensity of physical activity analyzed in this study. Nevertheless, physical activity was consistently related to the BMD variable in both males and females.

On the other hand, milk intake and BMD had no significant correlation, which is inconsistent with previous studies reporting a quantitative relationship between the intake of milk and dairy products and bone mineralization. Several studies on the relationship between the intake of calcium, vitamin D, and dairy products and bone frailty during growth have reported conflicting or inconsistent results [42]. In this study, calcium and vitamin D intakes were not included as control variables. The reason is that it was confirmed that the calcium intake of Korean adolescents was very low, and milk was the major source of calcium. Besides, when the bone mineral density variable was analyzed using calcium as a parameter, the same result was obtained as from using milk intake. Also, vitamin D intake was excluded from the control variable as there was no significant difference between groups. There might be a threshold in the expression of the effect of calcium intake. Eating above a certain level of calcium does not affect the bone mass significantly but eating less than this can lead to an inadequate balance [1]. In addition, the effect of nutritional intake may vary depending on the nutritional status of the subjects. In cases where the intake of minerals or high-quality protein may be insufficient, the subjects may show a distinct increase in bone growth after the supply of dairy products [1,43]. On the other hand, Ren et al. reported that children with a good nutritional status did not show a clear positive correlation between major bone nutrients and bone outcomes compared to children with nutritional deficiencies [44]. In considering the results of this study that concern the relationship between milk intake and BMD, it is also necessary to consider that the overall milk intake level of the subjects was low, with an average daily milk intake of less than one glass (200 mL), and that 58.8% of subjects did not drink any milk. Therefore, additional studies will be needed to investigate the relationship between milk intake and BMD considering the distribution of milk intake and the basic nutritional status of subjects.

No linear relationship was observed between milk intake and BMD, but physical activity and milk intake had a statistically significant combined effect on BMD. Among males, the $M_{no}P_{low}$ group had the lowest BMD in all BMD variables, showing the statistical difference from the groups with a high level of physical activity, the $M_{no}P_{high}$ group and the $M_{yes}P_{high}$ group. Among females, the $M_{yes}P_{high}$ group had a significantly higher lumbar BMD than the other groups.

In particular, an analysis of the odds ratios of male subjects showed that those who did not consume milk and had a low level of physical activity ($M_{no}P_{low}$) were significantly less likely to have a high BMD than those who consumed milk and had a high level of physical activity ($M_{yes}P_{high}$). Specifically, the $M_{no}P_{low}$ group was approximately 0.5 times less likely to have a high femur neck BMD and lumbar BMD and was approximately 0.3 times less likely to have high BMD for the total body and the femur than the $M_{yes}P_{high}$ group.

These results suggest that milk intake and physical activity have combined effects in strengthening bones. Branca et al. (2001) reported that bone anabolism could be increased by weight-bearing exercise during adolescence, and adequate calcium intake is necessary for exercises to have a bone stimulating effect [36]. In a review study on the interactions between physical activity and nutrients in children and adolescents, Julián-Almárcegui (2015) reported that the combined effects of exercise and calcium intake were greater than the effects of exercise or calcium intake alone, and physical activity required calcium intake to have a positive effect on bones [45]. According to a clinical report of the American Academy of Pediatrics, routine calcium supplementation is not required for healthy children and adolescents for bone health, and it is necessary to increase the supply of calcium through dietary intake to meet daily recommended levels [46]. Therefore, drinking milk, a major source of calcium, combined with moderate to vigorous physical activity that provides mechanical stimulation to the bones during growth, is considered an effective strategy to maximize bone growth potential.

In females, the effect of milk intake and physical activity was found only in lumbar BMD. The positive effect of physical activity or physical activity combined with nutrients on BMD was relatively insignificant in females, because the overall physical activity of females was low. The converted weekly moderate physical activity time was only 70.4 ± 47.9 min for females, compared to 120.7 ± 7.9 min for males. Probably due to the fact that a mechanical load has an impact on the bones in a region-specific and tissue-specific manner [44,47,48], there was no difference in the BMD of the femur and femur neck among groups, which are the areas where the mechanical impact is applied more directly during physical activity. In addition, the increase in the total body BMD and leg BMD slows down in females after the age of 13 years, whereas the lumbar BMD shows a relatively continuous increase during adolescence [4]. Therefore, the lumbar BMD of females seemed to reflect the effects of lifestyle more sensitively during adolescence.

The results of this study showed that a combination of moderate to vigorous physical activity with milk intake during adolescence, which is a very important period for laying the foundation for lifelong bone health, is an effective strategy for maximizing the growth potential of BMD. Nevertheless, there is a need to consider the following limitations when interpreting and applying the findings of this study. First, this study was a cross-sectional survey study. A longitudinal study will be needed to elucidate and verify the causal relationships among physical activity, milk intake, and BMD with respect to the combined effects of the two factors on BMD. Second, the level of physical activity was assessed based on the participation time of moderate to vigorous physical activity, but the time spent walking was not included. The intensity of walking can vary from low to moderate. Although there was a separate questionnaire item on walking, it was excluded from the analysis because it did not quantify the intensity of walking. Third, the KNHANES used in this study does not investigate type of physical activity. Therefore, non-weight bearing physical activity participation time, such as slow swimming, included as an example of moderate intensity activity, could not be considered separately to be analyzed, possibly reducing the correlation between physical activity and BMD. Fourth, in this study, the level of physical activity was examined through a questionnaire survey. Hence, this study has inherent limitations regarding the objectivity and reliability of the self-report measures of physical activity, compared to objective, direct measures of physical activity. Fifth, when carrying out subject grouping, in terms of physical activity, the subjects were divided into high- and low-level physical activity groups. In the case of milk intake, however, because a considerable proportion of people did not consume milk, the subjects were classified into two milk groups: those who did not drink milk at all or those who did. In interpreting the results, it will be necessary to consider these differences in the criteria for evaluating impact of milk intake and physical activity. Sixth, due to dietary variation within the individual, there is a limit to grasp accurately the usual intake status with a single-day survey through the 24-h recall method.

In conclusion, adolescents who did not drink milk and had a low level of physical activity were less likely to have a high BMD than those who drank milk and had a high level of physical activity. These results show that there is a synergistic effect of physical activity and milk intake on BMD, suggesting that practicing both moderate to vigorous physical activity and milk consumption in adolescence is an effective way to build healthy bones. The findings of the present study are expected to be useful as empirical data for establishing strategies for promoting healthy bone growth during adolescence.

Author Contributions: Conceptualization by J.H.L., A.W.H., S.H.K. and W.K.K., Formal analysis by A.W.H. and J.H.L., Funding acquisition by S.H.K. Investigation by J.H.L. and A.W.H., Methodology by A.W.H. and J.H.L., Project administration by S.H.K. and W.K.K., Resources by S.H.K. and W.K.K., Supervision by S.H.K. and W.K.K., Writing original draft by J.H.L., Writing, review & editing by S.H.K., W.K.K. and A.W.H. All authors have read and agreed to the published version of the manuscript.

Funding: This research was funded by a 2017 grant from the Korea Dairy & Beef Farmers Association and the Korea Milk Marketing Board (2017-0243-01).

Institutional Review Board Statement: The study was conducted according to the guidelines of the Declaration of Helsinki, and approved by the Institutional Review Board of Kongju National University (protocol code: KNU_IRB_2020-65, date of approval: 21 August 2020).

Informed Consent Statement: Informed consent was obtained from all subjects involved in the study.

Data Availability Statement: Data were obtained from the Korean National Health and Nutrition Examination Survey (KNHANES) and are available from the KNHANES website (at http://knhanes.cdc.go.kr (accessed on 26 June 2017)).

Conflicts of Interest: The authors declare no conflict of interest.

References

1. De Lamas, C.; De Castro, M.J.; Gil-Campos, M.; Gil, Á.; Couce, M.L.; Leis, R. Effects of dairy product consumption on height and bone mineral content in children: A systematic review of controlled trials. *Adv. Nutr.* **2019**, *10*, S88–S96. [CrossRef] [PubMed]
2. Baxter-Jones, A.D.G.; Kontulainen, S.A.; Faulkner, R.A.; Bailey, D.A. A Longitudinal study of the relationship of physical activity to bone mineral accrual from adolescence to young adulthood. *Bone* **2008**, *43*, 1101–1107. [CrossRef]
3. Kohrt, W.M.; Bloomfield, S.A.; Little, K.D.; Nelson, M.E.; Yingling, V.R. Physical activity and bone health. *Med. Sci. Sports Exerc.* **2004**, *36*, 1985–1996. [CrossRef]
4. Yi, K.H.; Hwang, J.S.; Kim, E.Y.; Lee, J.A.; Kim, D.H.; Lim, J.S. Reference values for bone mineral density according to age with body size adjustment in Korean children and adolescents. *J. Bone Miner. Metab.* **2014**, *32*, 281–289. [CrossRef]
5. Lee, E.Y.; Kim, D.; Kim, K.M.; Kim, K.J.; Choi, H.S.; Rhee, Y.; Lim, S.K. Age-related bone mineral density patterns in Koreans (KNHANES IV). *J. Clin. Endocrinol. Metab.* **2012**, *97*, 3310–3318. [CrossRef]
6. Cooper, C.; Westlake, S.; Harvey, N.; Javaid, K.; Dennison, E.; Hanson, M. Review: Developmental origins of osteoporotic fracture. *Osteoporos. Int.* **2006**, *17*, 337–347. [CrossRef] [PubMed]
7. Baim, S.; Leonard, M.B.; Bianchi, M.L.; Hans, D.B.; Kalkwarf, H.J.; Langman, C.B.; Rauch, F. Official positions of the international society for clinical densitometry and executive summary of the 2007 ISCD Pediatric Position Development Conference. *J. Clin. Densitom.* **2008**, *11*, 6–21. [CrossRef] [PubMed]
8. Ferrari, S.L.; Chevalley, T.; Bonjour, J.P.; Rizzoli, R. Childhood fractures are associated with decreased bone mass gain during puberty: An early marker of persistent bone fragility? *J. Bone Miner. Res.* **2006**, *21*, 501–507. [CrossRef]
9. Clark, E.M.; Ness, A.R.; Bishop, N.J.; Tobias, J.H. Association between bone mass and fractures in children: A prospective cohort study. *J. Bone Miner. Res.* **2006**, *21*, 1489–1495. [CrossRef]
10. Nikander, R.; Sievänen, H.; Heinonen, A.; Daly, R.M.; Uusi-Rasi, K.; Kannus, P. Targeted exercise against osteoporosis: A systematic review and meta-analysis for optimising bone strength throughout life. *BMC Med.* **2010**, *8*, 1–16. [CrossRef]
11. Tan, V.P.S.; Macdonald, H.M.; Kim, S.J.; Nettlefold, L.; Gabel, L.; Ashe, M.C.; McKay, H.A. Influence of physical activity on bone strength in children and adolescents: A systematic review and narrative Synthesis. *J. Bone Miner. Res.* **2014**, *29*, 2161–2181. [CrossRef] [PubMed]
12. Iuliano-Burns, S.; Stone, J.; Hopper, J.L.; Seeman, E. Diet and exercise during growth have site-specific skeletal effects: A co-twin control study. *Osteoporos. Int.* **2005**, *16*, 1225–1232. [CrossRef]
13. Alexy, U.; Remer, T.; Manz, F.; Neu, C.M.; Schoenau, E. Long-term protein intake and dietary potential renal acid load are associated with bone modeling and remodeling at the proximal radius in healthy children. *Am. J. Clin. Nutr.* **2005**, *82*, 1107–1114. [CrossRef] [PubMed]
14. Moyer-Mileur, L.J.; Xie, B.; Ball, S.D.; Pratt, T. Bone mass and density response to a 12-month trial of calcium and vitamin D supplement in preadolescent girls. *J. Musculoskelet. Neuronal Interact.* **2003**, *3*, 63–70. [PubMed]
15. Lanou, A.J.; Berkow, S.E.; Barnard, N.D. Calcium, dairy products, and bone health in children and young adults: A reevaluation of the evidence. *Pediatrics* **2005**, *115*, 736–743. [CrossRef]
16. Lee, B.K.; Lee, Y.K.; Lee, H.L.; Park, S.M. Maternal and lifestyle effect on bone mineral density in Korean children and adolescents aged 8-19. *Korean J. Nutr.* **2013**, *46*, 147–155. [CrossRef]
17. Pereira, P.C. Milk nutritional composition and its role in human health. *Nutrition* **2014**, *30*, 619–627. [CrossRef]
18. Séverin, S.; Wenshui, X. Milk biologically active components as nutraceuticals: Review. *Crit. Rev. Food Sci. Nutr.* **2005**, *45*, 645–656. [CrossRef]
19. Lee, J.H.; Kim, W.K.; Kim, S.H. Participation in the school milk program contributes intake by middle school students in South Korea. *Nutrients* **2019**, *11*, 2386. [CrossRef]
20. Rangan, A.M.; Flood, V.M.; Denyer, G.; Webb, K.; Marks, G.B.; Gill, T. Dairy consumption and diet quality in a sample of Australian children. *J. Am. Coll. Nutr.* **2012**, *31*, 185–193. [CrossRef]
21. Iglesia, I.; Intemann, T.; De Miguel-Etayo, P.; Pala, V.; Hebestreit, A.; Wolters, M.; Russo, P.; Veidebaum, T.; Papoutsou, S.; Nagy, P.; et al. Dairy consumption at snack meal occasions and the overall quality of diet during childhood. Prospective and cross-sectional analyses from the IDEFICS/I.family cohort. *Nutrients* **2020**, *12*, 642. [CrossRef]
22. Musumeci, G. The use of vibration as physical exercise and therapy. *J. Funct. Morphol. Kinesiol.* **2017**, *2*, 17. [CrossRef]
23. Castrogiovanni, P.; Trovato, F.M.; Szychlinska, M.A.; Nsir, H.; Imbesi, R.; Musumeci, G. The importance of physical activity in osteoporosis. From the molecular pathways to the clinical evidence. *Histol. Histopathol.* **2016**, *31*, 1183–1194. [CrossRef]
24. Fujita, Y.; Iki, M.; Ikeda, Y.; Morita, A.; Matsukura, T.; Nishino, H.; Yamagami, T.; Kagamimori, S.; Kagawa, Y.; Yoneshima, H. Tracking of appendicular bone mineral density for 6 years including the pubertal growth spurt: Japanese population-based osteoporosis kids cohort study. *J. Bone Miner. Metab.* **2011**, *29*, 208–216. [CrossRef] [PubMed]

25. Deere, K.; Sayers, A.; Rittweger, J.; Tobias, J.H. Habitual levels of high, but not moderate or low, impact activity are positively related to hip BMD and geometry: Results from a population-based study of adolescents. *J. Bone Miner. Res.* **2012**, *27*, 1887–1895. [CrossRef] [PubMed]
26. Hind, K.; Burrows, M. Weight-bearing exercise and bone mineral accrual in children and adolescents: A review of controlled trials. *Bone* **2007**, *40*, 14–27. [CrossRef]
27. Lorentzon, M.; Mellström, D.; Ohlsson, C. Association of amount of physical activity with cortical bone size and trabecular volumetric BMD in young adult men: The GOOD study. *J. Bone Miner. Res.* **2005**, *20*, 1936–1943. [CrossRef]
28. Sayers, A.; Mattocks, C.; Deere, K.; Ness, A.; Riddoch, C.; Tobias, J.H. Habitual levels of vigorous, but not moderate or light, physical activity is positively related to cortical bone mass in adolescents. *J. Clin. Endocrinol. Metab.* **2011**, *96*, 793–802. [CrossRef]
29. Courteix, D.; Jaffré, C.; Lespessailles, E.; Benhamou, L. Cumulative effects of calcium supplementation and physical activity on bone accretion in premenarchal children: A double-blind randomised placebo-controlled trial. *Int. J. Sports Med.* **2005**, *26*, 332–338. [CrossRef]
30. Specker, B.; Binkley, T. Randomized trial of physical activity and calcium supplementation on bone mineral content in 3 to 5-year-old children. *J. Bone Miner Res.* **2003**, *18*, 885–892. [CrossRef] [PubMed]
31. Bass, S.L.; Naughton, G.; Saxon, L.; Iuliano-Burns, S.; Daly, R.; Briganti, E.M.; Hume, C.; Nowson, C. Exercise and calcium combined results in a greater osteogenic effect than either factor alone: A blinded randomized placebo-controlled trial in boys. *J. Bone Miner. Res.* **2007**, *22*, 458–464. [CrossRef]
32. Ministry of Health and Welfare. *The Physical Activity Guide for Koreans*; Company, H.C., Ed.; Ministry of Health and Welfare: Seoul, Korea, 2013.
33. Korean Ministry of Health and Welfare, The Korean Nutrition Society. *2020 Dietary Reference Intakes for Koreans: Energy and Macronutrients*; The Korean Nutrition Society: Seoul, Korea, 2020.
34. Korea Centers for Disease Control and Prevention; Division of Chronic Diseases Surveillance; Committee for the Development of Growth Standard for Korean Children and Adolescents; Korean Pediatric Society; Committee for School Health and Public Health Statistics. *2017 Korean Children and Adolescents Growth Standard*; Korea Centers for Disease Control and Prevention: Cheongju, Korea, 2017.
35. Park, H.W.; Chung, S. Body composition and obesity in Korean adolescents and its impact on diabetes mellitus. *Korean J. Obes.* **2013**, *22*, 137–144. [CrossRef]
36. Branca, F.; Valtuena, S. Calcium, physical activity and bone health – Building bones for a stronger future. *Public Health Nutr.* **2001**, *4*, 117–123. [CrossRef]
37. Kalkwarf, H.J.; Khoury, J.C.; Lanphear, B.P. Milk intake during childhood and adolescence, adult bone density, and osteoporotic fractures in US women. *Am. J. Clin. Nutr.* **2003**, *77*, 257–265. [CrossRef] [PubMed]
38. Elhakeem, A.; Heron, J.; Tobias, J.H.; Lawlor, D.A. Physical activity throughout adolescence and peak hip strength in young adults. *JAMA Netw.* **2020**, *3*, e2013463. [CrossRef]
39. Gomez-Bruton, A.; Montero-Marín, J.; González-Agüero, A.; García-Campayo, J.; Moreno, L.; Casajús, J.A.; Vicente-Rodríguez, G. The effect of swimming during childhood and adolescence on bone mineral density: A systematic review and meta-analysis. *Sport. Med.* **2016**, *46*, 365–379. [CrossRef] [PubMed]
40. Weaver, C.M.; Gordon, C.M.; Janz, K.F.; Kalkwarf, H.J.; Lappe, J.M.; Lewis, R.; O'Karma, M.; Wallace, T.C.; Zemel, B.S. The national osteoporosis foundation's position statement on peak bone mass development and lifestyle factors: A systematic review and implementation recommendations. *Osteoporos. Int.* **2016**, *27*, 1281–1386. [CrossRef] [PubMed]
41. American College of Sports Medicine. *ACSM's Guidelines for Exercise Testing and Prescription*, 10th ed.; Lippincott: Philadelphia, PA, USA, 2017.
42. Händel, M.N.; Heitmann, B.L.; Abrahamsen, B. Nutrient and food intakes in early life and risk of childhood fractures: A systematic review and meta-analysis. *Am. J. Clin. Nutr.* **2015**, *102*, 1182–1195. [CrossRef] [PubMed]
43. Huncharek, M.; Muscat, J.; Kupelnick, B. Impact of dairy products and dietary calcium on bone-mineral content in children: Results of a meta-analysis. *Bone* **2008**, *43*, 312–321. [CrossRef]
44. Ren, J.; Brann, L.S.; Bruening, K.S.; Scerpella, T.A.; Dowthwaite, J.N. Relationships among diet, physical activity, and dual plane dual-energy X-ray absorptiometry bone outcomes in pre-pubertal girls. *Arch. Osteoporos.* **2017**, *12*, 19. [CrossRef]
45. Julián-Almárcegui, C.; Gómez-Cabello, A.; Huybrechts, I.; González-Agüero, A.; Kaufman, J.M.; Casajús, J.A.; Vicente-Rodríguez, G. Combined effects of interaction between physical activity and nutrition on bone health in children and adolescents: A systematic review. *Nutr. Rev.* **2015**, *73*, 127–139. [CrossRef] [PubMed]
46. Golden, N.H.; Abrams, S.A. Optimizing Bone Health in Children and Adolescents. *Pediatrics* **2014**, *134*, e1229-43. [CrossRef] [PubMed]
47. Dowthwaite, J.N.; Scerpella, T.A. Skeletal geometry and indices of bone strength in artistic gymnasts. *J. Musculoskelet. Neuronal Interact.* **2009**, *9*, 198–214.
48. Dowthwaite, J.N.; Rosenbaum, P.F.; Scerpella, T.A. Site-specific advantages in skeletal geometry and strength at the proximal femur and forearm in young female gymnasts. *Bone* **2012**, *50*, 1173–1183. [CrossRef] [PubMed]

MDPI
St. Alban-Anlage 66
4052 Basel
Switzerland
Tel. +41 61 683 77 34
Fax +41 61 302 89 18
www.mdpi.com

Nutrients Editorial Office
E-mail: nutrients@mdpi.com
www.mdpi.com/journal/nutrients

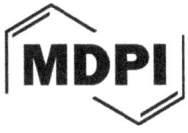

www.ingramcontent.com/pod-product-compliance
Lightning Source LLC
LaVergne TN
LVHW070206100526
838202LV00015B/2005